St. Anthony Publishing/Medicode

DRG
Desk Reference

The ultimate resource for improving DRG assignment practices

2004

Notice

DRG Desk Reference has been prepared based upon subjective medical judgment and upon the information available as of the date of publication. This publication is designed to provide accurate and authoritative information in regard to the subject covered, and every reasonable effort has been made to ensure the accuracy of the information contained within these pages. *DRG Desk Reference* serves only as a guide. Ingenix, Inc., its employees, agents, and staff make no representation or guarantee that the use of this manual will prevent differences of opinion or disputes with Medicare or other payers as to the amounts that will be paid to providers of services. Ingenix, Inc., its employees, agents, and staff make no representation or guarantee that this manual is free of errors and will bear no responsibility or liability for the results or consequences of its use.

Acknowledgments

Anita C. Hart, RHIA, CCS, CCS-P, *Product Manager/Technical Editor*
Elizabeth Boudrie, *Vice President, Publisher*
Karen Schmidt, BSN, *Technical Editor*
Lynn Speirs, *Senior Director, Publishing Services*
Stacy Perry, *Desktop Publishing Manager*
Tracy Betzler, *Desktop Publishing Specialist*
Irene Day, *Desktop Publishing Specialist*
Nora Fitzpatrick, *Desktop Publishing Specialist*
Regina Heppes, *Copy Editor*

Copyright

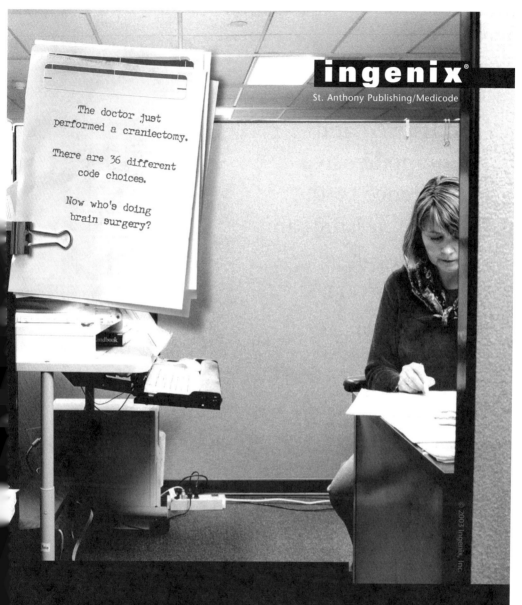

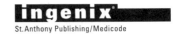

St.Anthony Publishing/Medicode

A Trusted and Comprehensive Reference to the DRG Classification System for Twenty Years.

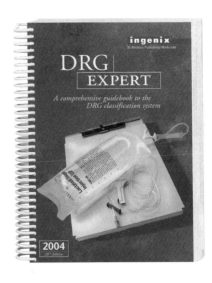

2004 DRG Expert

Item No. 5579 **$99.95**

Available September 2003   ISBN: 1-56337-483-8

Formerly called the DRG Guidebook, this has been a trusted reference to the DRG classification system for twenty years. The convenient and innovative book that is organized by Major Diagnostic Category (MDC) follows the logical DRG decision process and is designed specifically for those who need a comprehensive resource to accurately assign DRGs concurrently and retrospectively or verify DRG information.

- **Medicare CMS Rate Structure.** Updated to provide current relative weight, geometric length of stay, and average length of stay for each DRG under both the IPPS and LTCH PPS system.

- **Exclusive — Color Coding.** Visual alerts for surgical/medical partitioning, CCs and age restrictions, and principal or secondary diagnosis qualifications.

- **Exclusive —Transfer DRG Symbol.** Indicates a DRG selected as a qualified discharge that may be paid at the per diem rate.

- **Exclusive —Target DRG symbol.** Know when specific documentation and coding guidelines must be followed when assigning these DRGs targeted by OIG for audit.

- **Exclusive — Main Term Code Search.**

- **Exclusive — Average National Payment Table.**

- **Exclusive — Optimizing Potential Indicator.**

- **Surgical Hierarchy Table.** Quickly find the DRG hierarchy for multiple procedure cases to help you assign the code that reflects the greatest resource utilization.

- **Invalid DRG Conversion Table.** Easily track the reassignment of codes to the new DRG.

SAVE 5% when you order at www.ingenixonline.com (reference source code FOBW4)

or call toll-free 1.800.INGENIX (464.3649), option 1.

Also available from your medical bookstore or distributor.

2004 Publications

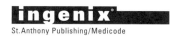

2004 ICD-9-CM Code Books for Hospitals

ICD-9-CM Professional for Hospitals, Vols. 1, 2, & 3

Softbound
Item No. 5586 **$84.95**
Available: September 2003
ISBN: 1-56337-478-1

Compact
Item No. 5588 **$79.95**
Available: September 2003
ISBN: 1-56337-479-X

ICD-9-CM Expert for Hospitals, Vols. 1, 2, & 3

Spiral
Item No. 5580 **$94.95**
Available: September 2003
ISBN: 1-56337-480-3

Binder
Item No. 3539 **$154.95**

These code books offer accurate and official code information integrated with all Medicare code edits crucial to appropriate reimbursement.

Professional and Expert editions feature:

- New and Revised Code Symbols.
- Fourth or Fifth-digit Alerts.
- Complete Official Coding Guidelines
- Age and Sex Edits.
- AHA's *Coding Clinic* references.
- Illustrations and Definitions.
- Manifestation Code Alert
- Complex Diagnosis and Major Complication Alerts
- HIV Major Related Diagnosis Alert
- CC Principal Diagnosis Exclusion
- CC Diagnosis Symbol
- Crucial Medicare Procedure Code Edits

Expert editions also include these enhancements:

- Special Reports Via E-mail
- PDX/MDC/DRG List
- Pharmacological List
- Valid Three-Digit Category List
- CC Code List

Expert Updateable Binder Subscriptions feature:

- Three Updates a Year. (Sept, Feb, and July)
  –Full text update with new code set in September.
  –February update with new illustrations, definitions, code edits, and AHA's *Coding Clinic* references.
  –July update newsletter with a preview of the new codes.
- Summary of topics covered in the the latest AHA's *Coding Clinic*

100% Money Back Guarantee:

If our merchandise* ever fails to meet your expectations, please contact our Customer Service Department toll-free at 1.800.INGENIX (464.3649), option 1, for an immediate response.

Software: Credit will be granted for unopened packages only.

SAVE 5% when you order at www.ingenixonline.com (reference source code FOBW4)

or call toll-free 1.800.INGENIX (464.3649), option 1.

Also available from your medical bookstore or distributor.

FOBA 4

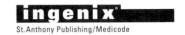

2004 Publications

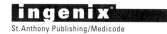

The Best Physicians' Current Procedural Terminology (CPT®) Reference in the Industry!

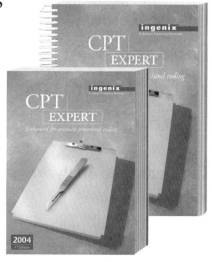

2004 CPT® Expert

Spiral bound **$89.95** Item No. 4531
Available: December 2003   ISBN: 1-56337-444-7

Compact **$79.95** Item No. 4532
Available December 2003   ISBN: 1-56337-445-5

Publisher's Note: CPT® Expert is not a replacement for the American Medical Association's CPT® 2003 Standard and Professional code books.

The CPT® Expert offers physicians' offices codes and icons denoting new, changed, and deleted language from the latest release (CPT® 2004), plus information that will help the coder find and use CPT® codes more easily. An extensive index, terms to know, and other additions help clarify the codes and speed assigning accurate codes. The product also provides valuable information about CPT® coding for Medicare Part B.

Inside you'll find:

- **New!** Crosswalk from CPT® to equivalent HCPCS codes helps Medicare billing

- **Exclusive** — Color Keys and Icons. Color keys reveal comprehensive NCCI edits, and icons denote Medicare, CLIA, and other common coding rules.

- **Exclusive** — Code-specific Definitions, Rules, and Tips pulled from the Medicare Carriers Manual and Coverage Issues Manual, among others.

- Complete—All 2004 CPT® codes and official, full descriptions

- 2004 Deleted codes with full descriptions and strike-outs to help you finish outstanding claims.

- ASC icon denoting ASC group.

- Color keys help you identify easily miscoded codes, unlisted codes, and codes not covered by Medicare

- Common icons from the AMA CPT® code book help you match information with the official book

- Simple, short introductions to each chapter describe how best to assure accuracy and speed claims

- Terms found in the nomenclature, defined, in glossary.

- Extensive, improved Index makes navigating easy.

- **Easy To Use.** Quick color references throughout, identifying unique nomenclature and rules, along with commonly misreported procedures that could impact your coding decisions.

- **Illustrated.** Detailed illustrations orient you to the procedures.

100% Money Back Guarantee:

If our merchandise* ever fails to meet your expectations, please contact our Customer Service Department toll-free at 1.800.INGENIX (464.3649), option 1, for an immediate response.

*Software: Credit will be granted for unopened packages only.

CPT is a registered trademark of the American Medical Association.

SAVE 5% when you order at www.ingenixonline.com (reference source code FOBW4)

or call toll-free 1.800.INGENIX (464.3649), option 1.

Also available from your medical bookstore or distributor.

2004 Publications

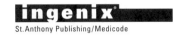

Easily Review, Edit, and Maintain Your Chargemaster Electronically!

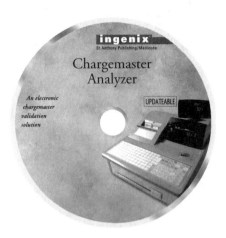

Chargemaster Analyzer

$2495.95   Item No. 2101

Available: Now

Introducing the first, affordable e-solution for maintaining an accurate and complete chargemaster for Medicare billing purposes.

- **NEW – Import Wizard.** Save time and avoid data manipulation with our new and improved process for importing your chargemaster. Now allows you to import a hospital identifier and utilization statistics.

- **NEW – Charge Data Comparison.** Identify potential revenue opportunities and analyze competitive pricing with charge data for hospital outpatient services for your Metropolitan Statistical Area (MSA).

- **NEW – CCI Edits.** Understand comprehensive and component code relationships for faster, more efficient coding.

- **NEW – Best Practices.** Identifies additional revenue potential by analyzing your CDM file for CPT™ codes and HCPCS Level II codes that may be missing.

- **NEW – Payment Lookup.** Locate hospital-specific APC payments and fee schedule payment amounts with ease by using this simple code lookup tool.

- **NEW – Enhanced Sort Capabilities.** Analyze and compare your CDM data more effectively with multiple sort scenarios.

- **Chargemaster Validation.** Reduce the risk of inaccuracies caused by outdated information. Chargemaster data is substantiated against comprehensive data definitions, tables, and relationships to improve reimbursement for your facility.

- **Browse Code Function.** Easily look up, compare, and search for codes, code descriptions, and relationships, and use the data to populate your CDM file.

- **Audit Trail and Reporting.** Diminish concerns about revised records. Modify chargemaster file entries and produce revised files with complete audit trails, customizable with Sticky Notes to track and report changes on a line-by-line basis.

- **Reviews Charges and Code Descriptions.** Improve consistency of CDM data with our automated review that verifies descriptions to accurately reflect the services performed.

CPT is a trademark of the American Medical Association.

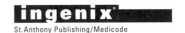

St.Anthony Publishing/Medicode

Keep Up with Medicare's National Coverage Guidelines!

Complete Guide to Medicare Coverage Issues

$279.95

Available: Now

Item No. 3036

ISBN: 1-56337-493-5

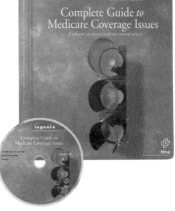

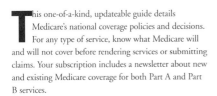

This one-of-a-kind, updateable guide details Medicare's national coverage policies and decisions. For any type of service, know what Medicare will and will not cover before rendering services or submitting claims. Your subscription includes a newsletter about new and existing Medicare coverage for both Part A and Part B services.

- **New—Now Includes Pending National Decisions.** Provides all draft and pending national decisions in one resource to help you and your staff manage all national coverage issues affecting Part A and Part B services.

- **Exclusive—Color-coded Coverage Prompts.** Know at a glance whether an item or procedure has restricted coverage, enabling you to make accurate coverage decisions promptly and submit bills correctly the first time.

- **Contains over 300 National Policies.** Helps prevent costly denials and claim resubmissions. Provides guidance regarding proper documentation for medical necessity, and helps you know when to issue an advance beneficiary notice for noncovered services. Also helps health plans understand Medicare coverage policies.

- **Fully Indexed.** Permits you to easily locate a specific item or service.

- **Updates and Coverage Alert Newsletter.** Keeps you up to date on all new national Medicare coverage policies and revisions to existing policies.

- **Full Text of Manual—in PDF Format.** Provides an electronic solution for researching national coverage decisions and medical necessity issues. Allows you to find key coverage issues and/or specific items and services with the click of a mouse. Other easy-to-use features include hypertext links and electronic bookmarks to take you quickly to the sections of the manual that you use the most.

- **HFMA Co-labeled Product.** Validates the relevance of the product content.

100% Money Back Guarantee:

If our merchandise* ever fails to meet your expectations, please contact our Customer Service Department toll-free at 1.800.INGENIX (464.3649), option 1, for an immediate response.

*Software: Credit will be granted for unopened packages only.

CPT is a registered trademark of the American Medical Association.

SAVE 5% when you order at www.ingenixonline.com (reference source code FOBW4)

or call toll-free 1.800.INGENIX (464.3649), option 1.

Also available from your medical bookstore or distributor.

PUBLICATION ORDER AND FAX FORM

FOBA4

Customer No._____

Contact No._____

Purchase Order No._____
(Attach copy of Purchase Order)

Source Code_____

Contact Name _____

Title_____

Company_____

Specialty_____

Address _____
(no P.O. Boxes, please)

City_____ State_____ Zip_____

Phone (_____)_____
(in case we have questions about your order)

Fax (_____)_____

IMPORTANT: E-MAIL REQUIRED FOR ORDER CONFIRMATION AND SELECT PRODUCT DELIVERY.

E-mail _____

Ingenix respects your right to privacy. We will not sell or rent your e-mail address or fax number to anyone outside Ingenix and its business partners. If you would like to remove your name from Ingenix promotions, please call 1.800.INGENIX (464.3649), option 1.

Order Toll-Free
1.800.INGENIX
(464.3649), Option 1

Item #	Qty	Item Description	Price	Total
4025	1	(SAMPLE) DRG Guidebook	$89.95	$89.95

Shipping and Handling	
No. of Items	Fee
1	$10.95
2-4	$12.95
5-7	$14.95
8-10	$19.95
11+	Call

Sub Total _____

TX, UT, OH, and VA residents please add applicable sales tax _____

Shipping & handling (see chart) _____
(11 plus items, foreign, Canadian, AK, and HI orders, please call for shipping costs)

Total enclosed _____

Payment Options

☐ Check enclosed. (Make payable to Ingenix, Inc.)

☐ Charge my: ☐ MasterCard ☐ VISA ☐ AMEX ☐ Discover

Card # | | | | | | | | | | | | | | | | | | Exp. Date: | | | | |
                                                                    MM   YR

☐ Bill Me P.O.#_____

Signature _____

EASY WAYS TO ORDER!

1 **MAIL** this order form with payment and/or purchase order to: **Ingenix, PO Box 27116, Salt Lake City, UT 84127-0116.**

2 **CALL** toll-free **1.800.INGENIX (464.3649), option 1** and mention the Source Code: FOBA4.

3 **FAX** this order form with credit card information and/or purchase order to **(801) 982-4033.**

4 **SHOP** on line at www.ingenixonline.com. Reference Source Code FOBW4 and save 5%.

100% Money Back Guarantee:

If our merchandise* ever fails to meet your expectations, please contact our Customer Service Department toll-free at 1.800.INGENIX (464.3649), option 1, for an immediate response.

*Software: Credit will be granted for unopened packages only.

©2003 Ingenix, Inc. All prices subject to change without notice.

FOBA4

Contents

Introduction

The *DRG Desk Reference* is the most comprehensive diagnosis-related group (DRG) resource library offering a simplified solution to DRG assignment practices. This all-in-one portable desk reference is ideal for the coder, DRG/utilization review coordinators and compliance auditors to efficiently and effectively manage hospital financial success through easy access to critical coding information. This resource primarily provides

- a basic history and understanding of the DRG system
- a step-by-step approach to coder DRG assignment, tips for the encoder user, key abstracting fields for reimbursement, and how to establish a DRG audit process that will survive regulatory scrutiny
- supplemental information to assess whether the DRG assigned is the most appropriate DRG (This is clinical documentation that justifies moving a case to a higher paying DRG [formerly *DRG Companion*].)
- compilation of clinical information that identifies complications and comorbidities that may affect DRG assignment (formerly *Clinical Coder*)
- coding and documentation requirements for the 22 DRGs targeted by the Office of Inspector General (OIG) for potential fraud (this information is necessary to self audit claims and prepare for quality improvement organization [QIO, formerly known as PRO] audit of targeted DRGs [formerly *DRG Compliance Auditor*].)

There are three basic steps of accurate DRG assignment. Step 1: assign the working DRG accurately using a DRG guide. Step 2: assess the working DRG assignment using all the information in the completed medical record to identify any conditions that cause higher facility resource use and, therefore, may qualify for higher reimbursement. Step 3: determine whether all the required documentation is present to support assignment of the DRG. The *DRG Desk Reference* will primarily provide all the necessary information to complete steps 2 and 3 of the DRG assignment process.

DRG History

The Medicare program began in 1965 to pay a portion of the cost of health care for its beneficiaries. Until 1982, the method of payment for eligible Medicare beneficiaries was based on costs reported by the hospitals to the government. In 1982, a section of the Tax Equity and Fiscal Responsibility Act mandated limits on Medicare payments to hospitals. Medicare began using the inpatient prospective payment system (IPPS) in late 1983.

Centers for Medicare and Medicaid Services (CMS), the agency responsible for the administration of Medicare, funded studies seeking ways to decrease the cost of health care. One of the studies was based on DRGs, originally developed by Yale University researchers for utilization review purposes in the late 1960s. It was this revised study of DRGs, updated and changed to an ICD-9-CM version by Yale, that became the Medicare prospective payment (PPS). Today, correct assignment of DRGs is still dependent on ICD-9-CM diagnosis and procedure codes. CMS remains the lead agency for the maintenance and modification of DRGs; revisions to the system have been contracted to 3M Health Information Systems (HIS).

Researchers at Yale University developed the early application of the ICD-9-CM version of DRGs based on the concept of patient case mix complexity. The researchers identified patient attributes that contributed most to resource demands. Key among them were the following:

- severity of illness
- prognosis
- treatment difficulty

- need for intervention
- resource intensity

Researchers next sought to classify patients based on information routinely collected in hospital medical records. The goal was to identify a manageable number of patient groups that shared demographic, diagnostic, and therapeutic attributes. The classifications that resulted were of clinically similar patients that consume hospital resources in a similar fashion.

DRGs provide the basis for payment to hospitals for care of Medicare, Medicaid, and an increasing number of commercially insured patients. Approximately 60 percent of hospital reimbursement comes from the IPPS based upon the DRG system. Through the DRG-based PPS, hospitals are reimbursed a flat rate based on a patient's diagnosis and treatment. On the assumption that patients with similar illnesses undergoing similar procedures will require similar care, each category of illness/treatment is assigned a DRG that is the main factor in determining reimbursement.

Because DRG payments are standardized by illness and treatment, DRGs allow payers and providers to predict reimbursement prospectively—before the care is provided. This type of reimbursement is called a PPS.

The scope of DRGs has expanded far beyond Medicare and private payer costs and claims. Personnel in health information management departments now influence the financial health of hospitals, as DRGs are based on patient records that list principal and secondary diagnoses, age, complications, discharge status, and comorbidities. Documentation is crucial. Hospital executives closely evaluate case mix—the clientele that the hospital serves—since the nature and severity of overall patient illnesses play heavily in budget projections. DRGs affect literally everyone within a hospital—from nurses to department heads, social workers to utilization review coordinators, physicians to patients—because some standardization of treatments is necessary to keep costs in line with flat-rate reimbursements.

Although DRGs may appear intimidating to the lay person or professional exposed to them for the first time, DRGs are easy to understand if first you learn about their origins.

Basic Characteristics of DRG Classification

A DRG is one of 518 currently valid groups that classify patients into clinically cohesive groups that demonstrate similar consumption of hospital resources and length-of-stay patterns.

The DRG system organizes ICD-9-CM diagnosis and procedure codes into a complex, comprehensive system based on a few simple principles.

Understanding how the DRG system works enables providers to recover the appropriate payment for services rendered, which is consistent with the intent of the federal government when it devised the DRG system. The *DRG Desk Reference* assists providers in understanding DRGs, thus ensuring appropriate payment.

In addition to calculation of reimbursement, DRGs have the following two major functions:

- The first is to evaluate the quality of care. Critical pathways are designed around DRGs. Benchmarking and outcomes analysis can be launched using the DRG clinical frame work, and quality reviews can be performed to assess coding practices and physician documentation. Ongoing education of physicians, coders, nurses, and utilization review personnel can be guided by the results of DRG analysis.
- Secondly, DRGs assist in evaluating the utilization of services. Each DRG represents the average resources needed to treat patients grouped to that DRG relative to the national average of resources used to treat all Medicare patients. The DRG assigned to each hospital in a patient stay also relates to the hospital case mix (i.e., the types of patient the hospital treats). The hospital case mix index (CMI) is determined by dividing the sum

of all DRG relative weights (RWs) for every DRG used by Medicare patients (counting each patient populating the DRG separately) by the total number of Medicare inpatient cases for the hospital.

Medicare computes the case mix adjustment for each fiscal year for all hospitals based upon the case mix data received. This CMI is then used to adjust the hospital base rate, which is a factor in computing the total hospital payment under the PPS. The formula for computing the hospital payment for each DRG is as follows:

DRG RW x Hospital base rate = Hospital payment

The hospital case mix complexity includes the following patient attributes:

- severity of illness—the level of loss of function or mortality associated with disease
- prognosis—defined as probable outcome of illness
- treatment difficulty—patient management problems
- need for intervention—severity of illness that would result due to lack of immediate or continuing care
- resource intensity—volume and types of services required for patient management

The purpose for which the DRG system was developed is to relate case mix to resource utilization. Reimbursement is adjusted to reflect the resource utilization and does not take into consideration severity of illness, prognosis, treatment difficulty, or need for intervention.

Case mix and complexity can be analyzed and monitored in relation to cost and utilization of services. In addition, high-volume conditions and services can be identified and monitored, and DRG trend analysis can aid in forecasting future staff and facility requirements. One important operating parameter is the CMI, which measures the cost of a hospital's Medicare patient mix in relation to the cost of all Medicare patients. A low case mix may indicate unnecessary revenue loss.

MDC and DRG Hierarchies

DRGs divide all possible principal diagnoses into 25 mutually exclusive categories, referred to as major diagnostic categories (MDCs). The MDCs were further subdivided into DRGs:

- First—Principal diagnosis linked to anatomical system (MDC)
- Second—Patient's surgical status
  - principal diagnosis (nonsurgical DRG),
  - extent of surgical procedure (surgical DRG)
- Third—Comorbidities, complications, age, sex, discharge status, and birth weight of neonates

MDC Categories

The diagnoses that define each MDC fall under the umbrella of a single organ system or etiology and are usually grouped by medical specialty, as in MDC 19, Mental Diseases and Disorders or MDC 14, Pregnancy, Childbirth and the Puerperium. Two other MDCs were added to the original list to cover multiple trauma and human immunodeficiency virus (HIV) infections.

MDC Categories

MDC 1   Diseases and Disorders of the Nervous System (DRGs 1–35, 524, 528–534)

MDC 2   Diseases and Disorders of the Eye (DRGs 36–48)

MDC 3   Diseases and Disorders of the Ear, Nose, Mouth and Throat
(DRGs 49–74, 168–169, 185–187)

MDC 4   Diseases and Disorders of the Respiratory System (DRGs 75–102, 475)

MDC 5   Diseases and Disorders of the Circulatory System
          (DRGs 104–145, 478–479, 514–518, 525–527, 535–536)

MDC 6   Diseases and Disorders of the Digestive System
          (DRGs 146–167, 170–184, 188–190)

MDC 7   Diseases and Disorders of the Hepatobiliary System and Pancreas
          (DRGs 191–208, 493–494)

MDC 8   Diseases and Disorders of the Musculoskeletal System and Connective Tissue
          (DRGs 209–213, 216–220, 223–256, 471, 491, 496–503, 519–520, 537–538)

MDC 9   Diseases and Disorders of the Skin, Subcutaneous Tissue and Breast
          (DRGs 257–284)

MDC 10   Endocrine, Nutritional and Metabolic Diseases and Disorders (DRGs 285–301)

MDC 11   Diseases and Disorders of the Kidney and Urinary Tract (DRGs 302–333)

MDC 12   Diseases and Disorders of the Male Reproductive System (DRGs 334–352)

MDC 13   Diseases and Disorders of the Female Reproductive System (DRGs 353–369)

MDC 14   Pregnancy, Childbirth and the Puerperium (DRGs 370–384, 469)

MDC 15   Newborns and Other Neonates with Conditions Originating in the Perinatal
          Period (DRGs 385–391, 469–470)

MDC 16   Diseases and Disorders of the Blood and Blood Forming Organs and
          Immunological Disorders (DRGs 392–399)

MDC 17   Myeloproliferative Diseases and Disorders, and Poorly Differentiated Neoplasms
          (DRGs 400–414, 473, 492, 539–540)

MDC 18   Infectious and Parasitic Diseases (Systemic or Unspecified Sites) (DRGs 415–423)

MDC 19   Mental Diseases and Disorders (DRGs 424–432)

MDC 20   Alcohol/Drug Use and Alcohol/Drug Induced Organic Mental Disorders
          (DRG 433, 521–523)

MDC 21   Injuries, Poisonings and Toxic Effects of Drugs (DRGs 439–455)

MDC 22   Burns (DRGs 504–511)

MDC 23   Factors Influencing Health Status and Other Contacts with Health Services
          (DRGs 461–467)

MDC 24   Multiple Significant Trauma (DRGs 484–487)

MDC 25   Human Immunodeficiency Virus Infections (DRGs 488–490)

Pre-MDC   Heart Transplant (DRG 103)
          Liver Transplant (DRG 480)
          Bone Marrow Transplant (DRG 481)
          Tracheostomy (DRGs 482–483)
          Lung Transplant (DRG 495)
          Simultaneous Pancreas/Kidney Transplant (DRG 512)
          Pancreas Transplant (DRG 513)

Since the MDCs represent clinically coherent groups based upon diagnosis, cases are defined by the principal diagnosis, the condition established after study to be chiefly responsible for occasioning the admission of the patient to the hospital.   Once a patient is assigned to an MDC, the next step is to determine whether the case should be designated as surgical or medical.

Surgical Cases

Cases are considered surgical if there is a valid operating room procedure performed or other non-operating room procedure that affects DRG assignment. The performance of OR procedures brings into play a host of inpatient resources, including anesthesia, nursing care, recovery room, and the operating suite. As a result, DRGs are separated into categories of surgical or medical (nonsurgical) cases.

For one group of DRGs, the Pre-DRGs, the initial step in DRG assignment is based upon the procedure performed, not the principal diagnosis.

Surgical DRGs are chosen based on the ICD-9-CM Volume 3 procedural code assigned. Keep in mind that a case is first grouped to the MDC according to the principal diagnosis assigned. As an example, in order to be assigned to DRG 191 Pancreas, Liver and Shunt Procedures with CC, the case must first be assigned a principal diagnosis assigned to MDC 7, Diseases and Disorders of the Hepatobiliary System and Pancreas. In addition the OR procedure performed must be one that is listed under DRG 191. And there must be a condition that is considered a complication or comorbidity. Other factors that contribute to the DRG assignment process for a case include: complications, comorbidities, age, sex, discharge status, and birth weight of neonates. For patients undergoing multiple procedures, the most complex, applicable DRG in the hierarchy of major surgery, minor surgery, other surgery, and surgery unrelated to principal diagnosis that applies is chosen as driving DRG assignment.

Medical Cases

If no procedures were perfomed, a medical DRG is assigned. Medical diagnoses are divided into categories in the medical DRGs. These categories include neoplasms and symptoms and conditions related to a single anatomical system. The level of service required for medical DRGs is generally less resource-intense than that for patients who undergo surgery.

Other Factors

A patient's age can occasionally be a defining factor in DRG assignment. Patients younger than 17 or older than 17 years of age are often assigned age-sensitive DRGs. For instance, DRG 342 is assigned to a patient older than 17 undergoing a circumcision. A male age 17 or younger would be assigned DRG 343 instead.

The patient's status upon discharge from the hospital is also considered a variable in the definition of a DRG. For example, DRG 122, Circulatory disorders with acute myocardial infarction without major complications, discharged alive. Separate DRGs were designed for patients who leave the hospital against medical advice.

Complications and Comorbidities (CCs)

Both medical and surgical classes are sometimes further defined by the presence of complications or comorbidities (CCs) which affect the consumption of hospital resources. For example, patients admitted for pleural effusion may exhibit numerous CCs, such as atrial fibrillation or hypovolemia, and their length of stay in the hospital and use of other services could be higher than other patients with pleural effusion who don't exhibit an arrhythmia or hypovolemia.

Examples of the most commonly missed CCs are listed below:
- alcoholism, acute/chronic
- anemia due to blood loss, acute/chronic
- angina pectoris
- atrial fibrillation/flutter
- atelectasis
- cachexia
- cardiogenic shock
- cardiomyopathy
- cellulitis

- CHF
- chronic obstructive pulmonary disease (COPD)
- decubitus ulcer
- dehydration
- diabetes mellitus, insulin dependent (IDDM)
- furuncles
- hematuria
- hematemesis
- hypertensive heart disease with CHF
- hyponatremia
- malnutrition
- melena
- pleural effusion
- pneumothorax
- renal failure, acute/chronic
- respiratory failure
- urinary retention
- urinary tract infection

The validity of CCs is dependent on the principal diagnosis. There are some diagnoses that may not function as a CC condition under certain circumstances because they are too closely related to the principal diagnosis. For example, atrial fibrillation is a CC for a patient admitted for syncope and collapse but not for a patient admitted for circulatory disease. The following parameters are used to determine those secondary diagnoses that are excluded from the CC list:

- Chronic and acute manifestations of the same condition should not be considered CCs for one another.
- Specific and nonspecific diagnosis codes for a condition should not be considered CCs for one another.
- Conditions that may not coexist such as partial/total, unilateral/bilateral, obstructed/ unobstructed, and benign/malignant should not be considered CCs for one another.
- The same condition in anatomically proximal sites should not be considered CCs for one another.
- Closely related conditions should not be considered CCs for one another.

ICD-9-CM Coding Accuracy

Correct ICD-9-CM coding is essential for correct DRG assignment. Coding references, whether hard copy or electronic, will probably feature some level of support material to steer the user toward the most specific code selection. The hospital edition of volume 1 features Medicare code edit (MCE) indicators for codes that affect DRG assignments, including unacceptable principal diagnoses, CCs, questionable admissions, and nonspecific diagnoses. Volume 3 tabular references also usually feature an indicator for codes that affect DRG assignments, including OR or non-OR procedures, noncovered procedures, or nonspecific OR procedures.

Principal Diagnosis

To assign a DRG, first determine and code the principal diagnosis, then all secondary diagnoses, and CCs. With the principal and secondary diagnoses in mind, consult volume 3 to assign any procedure code(s) that might apply to the patient's case.

Principal Procedure

The principal procedure is usually the procedure that is necessary in treating a complication, or is performed for definitive treatment, not for diagnostic or exploratory purposes. It is the procedure most closely related to the principal diagnosis. If two procedures seem to meet the principal procedure definition, the one most closely related to the principal diagnosis should be designated as the principal procedure.

DRG Assignment Process

In total, there are now 25 MDCs and eight pre-MDCs subdivided into 518 DRGs. Both the medical and surgical classes within an MDC are organized by principles of anatomy, surgical approach, diagnostic approach, pathology, etiology, and the treatment process.

DRGs are assigned using the principal diagnosis, up to eight additional diagnoses, the principal procedure and up to five additional procedure codes, and age, sex, and discharge status. One DRG is as signed to each inpatient stay.

Diagnoses and procedures are designated by ICD-9-CM codes. The following describes the typical decision process used to assign a DRG to a case. A case is assigned to one of the 25 MDCs based on its principal diagnosis. DRG assignment is based upon the following considerations:

- principal and secondary diagnosis and procedure codes
- sex
- age
- discharge status
- presence or absence of CCs
- birthweight for neonates

There were two DRGs created especially to report cases assigned invalid principal diagnoses (DRG 469) or ungroupable principal diagnoses (DRG 470).

Each year, effective October 1 through September 30, DRG assignments are adjusted based on relative weight, arithmetic mean length of stay, and geometric mean of stay. Annually, new ICD-9-CM codes are also incorporated into the existing DRGs and new DRGs may be added for that fiscal year.

Government Scrutiny

In the "Message from Inspector General" that precedes the Semiannual Report to Congress for the time period of October 1, 2002 through March 31, 2003, it states the OIG will continue to be vigilant in examining payments made to providers to ensure they are accurate. The OIG in conjunction with CMS plans to continue its effort to decrease the fee-for-service error rate. As noted in our previous edition, a Medicare report for fiscal year 2001 Medicare fee-for-service payments (A-17-01-02002), involved the review of 6,594 Medicare claims and the associated medical records. The records were reviewed to determine whether the services were provided to eligible beneficiaries, paid correctly by Medicare contractors, and whether they were medically necessary, properly coded, and sufficiently documented in the medical record. Results of the audit revealed an estimated $12.1 billion in improper payments and that 6.3 percent of all audited claims were incorrect. Insufficient or no documentation was the most prevalent error, accounting for $5.1 billion of the improper payments. Lack of medical necessity, the second most common error, accounted for $5.2 billion, and incorrect coding, which constituted 17 percent of the total, accounted for another $2 billion in improper payments.

In addition to the above audit, one of the focus areas addressed in the OIG's 2003 work plan is the "Update on Diagnosis-Related Group Coding Project." This initiative focuses on DRGs that have a history of aberrant coding to determine whether some acute hospitals are exhibiting aberrant coding patterns. The OIG plans to determine coding payment error rates and incorporate the results of a recent review by quality improvement organizations.

In the OIG report, "Monitoring the Accuracy of Hospital Coding" (OEI-01-98-00420), the inspector general recommended that CMS, require all QIOs (formerly known as PROs) to engage in DRG validation under the Sixth Scope of Work (SOW), which was effective on August 1, 1999. Abusive as well as fraudulent coding and billing practices are being targeted. In 1996, the False Claims Act was amended to include claims made to the government in deliberate ignorance or reckless disregard of the truth or falsity of the information. It's not necessary that there be any specific intent to defraud under that provision of the law. A mere pattern or practice of overbilling is sufficient, and that can spell fines of not less than $5,000 and as much as $10,000 per claim, plus treble damages. What's more, government enforcers are using that clause to the maximum effect; numerous settlements have been in the tens and hundreds of millions of dollars.

Federal regulatory agency initiatives to validate documentation and coding as well as proper DRG assignment comes as a result of

- the shift in responsibility for accuracy of diagnosis and procedure codes from physicians to hospitals
- the internal pressures to increase case mix from one fiscal year to the next
- the fact that "optimizing DRGs" has been ingrained into coders since the 1983 inception of the Medicare PPS

Keys to a Financially Successful DRG Program

Each DRG is assigned a relative weight by CMS based upon charge data for all Medicare inpatient hospital discharges. Each hospital has a customized base rate designed to adjust payment commensurate with the hospital's cost of providing services. The type of hospital and the wage index for the geographic area determines the hospital base rate. DRG relative weights and hospital base rates are adjusted yearly (effective October 1 through September 30) to reflect changes in health care resource consumption as well as economic factors. Payment is determined by multiplying the DRG relative weight by the hospital base rate. The DRG with the highest relative weight is the highest-paying DRG. Regardless of actual costs incurred, the hospital receives only the calculated payment.

The DRG payment system is based on averages. Payment is determined by the resource needs of the average Medicare patient for a given set of diseases or disorders. These resources include the length of stay and the number and intensity of services provided. Therefore, the more efficiently a provider delivers care, the greater its operating margin will be.

The keys to a financially successful DRG program are

- decreased length of stay
- decreased resource utilization (tests/procedures)
- increased intensity of case management services resulting in optimal length of stay for the patient and facility
- increased preadmission testing
- improved medical record documentation

The Future

Refinements that would further divide DRGs by degrees of severity are being considered by CMS. While plans are made to launch a new system of expanded DRGs, other changes in current coding systems could require a complete overhaul of the DRG system within a few years. CMS intends to replace ICD-9-CM with ICD-10-CM/PCS, a new alphanumeric coding system for diseases and procedures, by middecade. The National Center for Health Statistics (NCHS) recently published an updated draft of ICD-10-CM. AHIMA will be using the June 2003 release in its ICD-10-CM testing project. The procedural section of ICD-10-PCS, administered by CMS, is currently being tested at sites across the United States.

Since DRGs are all based on ICD-9-CM codes, the change to ICD-10-CM/PCS would greatly affect DRG decision trees and assignments. The same issues of mapping will be at work when ICD-10 is adopted. Once CMS formally presents the proposed DRG and ICD-10-CM/PCS changes, the hospital industry can begin to analyze the effects these changes will have upon their businesses.

Under Medicare PPS, any revision of the DRG system must redistribute reimbursement among hospitals according to the case mix, but may not increase or decrease aggregate Medicare payments to hospitals. Individual hospitals, however, could see significant changes in reimbursement under the new DRGs depending on their case mix as generated by the new DRGs.

DRG Desk Reference Organization

Key Fields for Coder Abstracting—Several key fields on the abstracting form significantly impact the reimbursement process for inpatient stays. Key fields such as discharge status and UB-92 billing data and their impact on reimbursement are discussed in-depth.

DRG Assignment Tutorial—Step-by-step guide to improving DRG assignment practices. With complete information in the medical record, coders will be able to properly analyze, code, and report the required information. This ensures that proper payment is received. For example, if the physician documents that a patient with a skull fracture was in a coma for less than one hour, DRG 28 is assigned. If the physician documents that the coma lasted for more than one hour, DRG 27 is assigned, with a resulting payment difference.

DRG Decision Trees—A visual representation of the decision making process of determining the DRG assignment.

DRG Listing with Potential DRG for Optimizing Payment—Each DRG listed with potential DRG along with the diagnosis and/or procedure codes that are required in order to be assigned to that DRG.

- **Tips for the Encoder User**—Encoder programs are built using the Boolean logic process demanding a yes/no answer. There are many crucial decision points that will significantly impact reimbursement. Tips to avoid making the wrong decision are identified.

Complications and Comorbidities (CCs)

- **Complete List of CCs**
- **Documentation Linked to Most Commonly Missed CC Conditions**—The most common signs and symptoms indicating CC conditions that affect DRG assignment are listed for quick review. According to coding guidelines these CCs must affect patient care in terms of requiring clinical evaluation; therapeutic treatment; further evaluation by diagnostic studies, procedures, or consultation; extended length of stay; or increased nursing care and/or monitoring for reporting purposes.

- **CC Principal Diagnosis Exclusion List**—Listing of all complications and comorbidity condition codes and the excluded principal diagnoses for which the CC does not affect DRG assignment. In this section, column 1 is the CC code with the excluded principal diagnoses in the second column to the right.

Diagnostic Implications of Abnormal Electrocardiogram (EKG)—Link commonly overlooked CCs that affect DRG assignment with EKG reports. Drugs that may be used to treat each problem, signs and symptoms that may be present, and possible conditions associated with the abnormality are listed.

Diagnostic Implications of Abnormal Laboratory—Link commonly overlooked CCs that affect DRG assignment with laboratory results. A reference range of normal values is provided for each laboratory test.

Diagnostic Implications of Drug Usage—Link commonly overlooked or undocumented CCs that affect DRG assignment by reviewing drug usage. Quick review of a patient's medication record may indicate a list of prescribed drugs for which a diagnosis is not clearly documented. This section will help the coder locate the drug and determine the drug action and the indications for the drug.

Listing of Organisms—Link commonly overlooked CCs that affect DRG assignment with lab results noting pathogens in specimens. This information is listed, for each body site, under the heading "Normal Condition of Flora." The source and site of each specimen are identified for further clarification.

DRG Assignment Implications for Major Cardiovascular Diagnoses—Link commonly overlooked cardiovascular complications that affect DRG 121, Circulatory Disorders with Acute Myocardial Infarction and Cardiovascular Complication, Discharged Alive. Signs and symptoms and ancillary report findings that indicate complications are also listed.

DRG Assignment Implications for Complex Cardiovascular Diagnoses—Link commonly overlooked complex diagnoses that affect DRG 124, Circulatory Disorders except Myocardial Infarction with Cardiac Catheterization and Complex Diagnosis. The list contains complex diagnoses, their signs and symptoms and the ancillary report findings that indicate the presence of certain conditions.

Diagnostic Implications of Noninvasive Diagnostic Test—Link commonly overlooked CCs that affect DRG assignment associated with specific diagnostic tests. Diagnostic tests do not in and of themselves affect DRG assignment but may link to a diagnosis that does. The tests are arranged alphabetically and are grouped by each specialty section for quick reference.

Diagnostic Implications of Durable Medical Equipment (DME) and Supplies—Link commonly overlooked CCs that affect DRG assignment associated with the use of DME such as oxygen, catheters, or specialized mattresses. The listed terms are arranged alphabetically and include alternative names, information about the purpose of the DME/supply, indications for its use, and commonly associated procedures.

Developing an Audit Process—Format for establishing a plan to audit DRG assignments in a proactive and retrospective manner to avoid regulatory scrutiny and provide an education feedback loop to coders and physicians.

Targeted DRG Listing—Complete list of DRGs targeted for potential abuse. ICD-9-CM official coding guidelines and advice for the most commonly assigned principal diagnosis codes that group to the targeted DRGs.

New Services and Technology Under IPPS—This section provides a summary of the changes for fiscal year 2004 and which service/new technology passed the test for additional add-on payment.

DRG List—Provides the most current list of DRGs and their descriptors, along with their respective relative weights.

Glossary of Terms—This section contains definitions of terms associated with the DRG classification system.

Instructions for Using Your *DRG Desk Reference*

Basic Protocols for DRG Assignment

A basic functional understanding of the DRG assignment process is a prerequisite to using this manual. However, several sections provide building blocks to help validate DRG assignment practices. The following are the basic steps for validating DRGs:

Step 1: Identify assigned DRG. Reviewing the complete DRG title is necessary to understand the nature of the cases it comprises.

Step 2: Identify similar DRGs.

Step 3: Compare assigned DRG with similar DRGs. Many diagnoses and procedure codes will group to more than one DRG. Be sure to check every DRG referenced.

The following are key chapters that provide supporting references in applying DRG assignments:

- Key Fields for Coder Abstracting
- DRG Assignment Tutorial
- Developing an Effective DRG Audit Process
- New Medical Services and Technologies Under IPPS
- DRG List
- Glossary of Terms

The key application chapters, which will assist in every day DRG challenges, are described below.

DRG Decision Trees

Introduction to Decision Trees

The general structure of a typical MDC is shown by the tree diagram found in this section. This is followed by MDC specific decision trees for each of the current 25 MDCs.

The tree diagrams describing the DRG structure for each MDC uses several symbols to describe the different types of decisions made in the process of assigning a DRG. Within each decision tree symbol will be text that indicates the precise decision being made.

A diamond indicates that a decision is being made on a single variable as opposed to several variables. This symbol is used when the variable is principal diagnosis, discharge status, or age.

A circle indicates a decision is being made that involves several variables. A circle is also used when the decision in the DRG structure involves the presence of an operating room procedure or the presence of a particular diagnosis as either the principal diagnosis or a secondary diagnosis.

A square indicates that a DRG has been assigned.

A pointer indicates that the tree diagram is continued on another page.

DRG Listing with Potential DRG for Optimizing Payment

Once the appropriate DRG is assigned, this section helps provide a careful, methodical walk-through of proven steps that can improve DRG assignment practices for Medicare reimbursement.

Each page provides potential DRGs that create a more accurate DRG assignment when appropriate. Some DRGs have no known potential optimization; therefore, no alternative DRGs are provided.

The DRGs are grouped by the MDC into which they fall. Some DRGs, such as pre-DRGs and DRGs associated with all MDCs, are not associated with a particular MDC; these appear in the "Other DRGs" section.

Using DRG 080 as an example, the instructions walk you through the steps to accurately assign the most appropriate DRG.

Once you have completed the exercise in the instructions, simply find the DRG to which a case is grouped and follow the same steps.

The symbol ◆ indicates an encoder tip that provides key terms or other critical decisive hints in guiding the coder to select the appropriate encoder logic and ultimately accurate DRG assignment.

The symbol ■ indicates a coding tip that could function as a compliance alert or a coding guideline to support the assignment of a code for validation of accurate DRG assignment.

The symbol ● indicates documentation tips to provide you with terms you might find in the medical record indicating an additional or alternative code choice. Note that there are code citations for the diagnoses and procedures mentioned.

Step 1: To use this section, first turn to the page of the DRG to which your case is grouped. Use the DRG index at the back of the book to find the page. The DRG system contains many DRGs that are nearly identical in terms of the diagnoses and/or procedures they include.

Step 2: Although the potential DRGs listed appear to be similar, they contain elements that give them different reimbursement levels. To determine which DRG is most accurate for your case and has the highest reimbursement, you must analyze the detailed components of each of the DRGs.

Note: A code citation with an asterisk (*) indicates an inclusive code range. For example, *806 is a reference for all subcategories and subclassification codes that begin with 806.

First, identify the differences in the potential DRGs that are available. DRGs may be similar in terms of diagnoses and/or procedures. The differences have been placed in boldface type for quick and easy identification.

Once you have identified the differences, finding the DRG with the highest level of reimbursement is easy. The DRG with the highest RW is the highest-paying DRG.

Do not assume that a DRG listed as nonoptimized can never be optimized. It is entirely possible that a very unusual combination of diagnoses or procedures could legitimately offer optimization potential. This book has not endeavored to identify any extraordinary optimization potentials. In the circulatory MDC, all major complicating diagnoses are consolidated one time under DRG 122. DRGs that are identified as potential regulatory targets for audit are identified by the yield symbol (▼).

Step 3: To determine whether a more accurate assignment would be made by grouping the case to a different DRG, look at the listings in the table below the potential DRG descriptions. The column titled "Principal Diagnosis/Procedure" provides you with a list of the key elements for grouping to each DRG. No attempt has been made to compile a complete, or even representative listing of potential diagnoses/procedures. See *The DRG Expert 2003* for the complete array of complete codes. Each suggestion is merely a guide. To ensure accurate DRG assignment, it is important to review the entire medical record to compile a complete diagnosis/procedure list and to check for any additional diagnoses that are CCs.

If the column directs you to the list of the most commonly missed CCs, check the complete list of CC conditions in the CC section of the *DRG Desk Reference*.

Step 4: Finally, you will need to find documentation within the medical record to support the assignment to the appropriate DRG. The DRG can change because of additions or changes to the principal diagnosis, secondary diagnoses, surgical and nonsurgical procedures, age, and discharge status. To support this DRG change, the secondary diagnosis must be compatible with the uniform hospital discharge data set (UHDDS) definition of "other diagnosis" (see the *AHA's Coding Clinic for ICD-9-CM*, second quarter 1990, for additional information on secondary diagnoses).

As with any DRG change, documentation supporting the DRG change is necessary to meet DRG validation requirements and to ensure accurate and complete data quality.

For example, upon review of the laboratory values, you note that the patient had a urine culture that showed over 100,000 colony growth of an organism called *Escherichia coli (E. coli)*. This abnormal finding should alert you to a possible urinary tract infection, which is listed as a commonly missed CC.

First look to see whether there was any indication that the condition had an effect on the patient's hospital care in terms of requiring one or more of the following:

- clinical evaluation
- therapeutic treatment
- diagnostic studies or procedures
- increased length of stay
- increased nursing care and/or monitoring

Investigating the medical record reveals that the patient received therapy in the form of Septra, an antibiotic commonly used to treat urinary tract infection.

Next, ask the physician to verify and document the omitted condition based on the clinical findings and treatment listed in the record. Then add the appropriate codes as documented, such as 599.0 for urinary tract infection NOS, or 595.0 for acute cystitis, and the additional code 041.4 for the *E. coli*.

Step 5: After inserting the additional diagnosis code, regroup the codes to the most appropriate DRG.

Clinical Reference Sections

General Instructions

The *DRG Desk Reference* is used by a variety of health care professionals—utilization review and quality assurance coordinators, QIO (formerly known as PRO) reviewers, DRG coordinators, compliance auditors, third-party payer reviewers, and medical record coders. It also serves as a quick reference in hospital, physician, or freestanding laboratories.

The *DRG Desk Reference* assists health care professionals in determining whether potentially overlooked conditions can be coded. Accurate code assignment depends on the record reviewer identifying physician documentation in the medical record for reportable conditions that may require

- clinical evaluation
- therapeutic treatment
- further evaluation by diagnostic studies, procedures, or consultation
- extended length of hospital stay
- increased nursing care and/or other monitoring

Example:

A patient's principal diagnosis is pneumonia. The medical record documentation lacks physician identification of the organism causing the pneumonia and the coder may suspect a causative organism based on the laboratory reports. The numerous ICD-9-CM diagnoses codes for pneumonia and the impact that this coding has on hospital reimbursement under the DRG system challenges the coder to communicate with the physician for accurate reporting.

Turn in the *DRG Desk Reference* to the organisms section, arranged by site of specimen. Note from the laboratory findings in the medical record that a sputum culture grew *Staphylococcus aureus (S. aureus)*. Look under "Sputum," the specimen source, in the organisms section. Notice that *S. aureus* is pathogenic in this instance. After verification with the physician that *S. aureus* is the causative organism of the patient's pneumonia, the physician modifies the principal diagnosis to read "pneumonia due to *S. aureus*."

The *DRG Desk Reference* can also be a valuable resource to determine whether there are any secondary diagnoses, requiring additional resources used to treat the patient. Although the physician documentation may not clarify the addition of a secondary diagnosis, a review of the medical record, especially ancillary reports, may suggest additional diagnoses or conditions.

In this example, the *DRG Desk Reference* can be used to compare the patient's laboratory test results with the results listed in the abnormal laboratory values section. This section lists various abnormal test results, a general test reference range, a blank line where a hospital-specific reference range for the test may be listed, the possible conditions indicated by the abnormal test result, and the signs, symptoms, and treatment of those conditions. If the test results fall outside of the general reference range, and the hospital's reference range for the test, which is indicated in the upper left hand corner of each page in the section, the patient could have one of the conditions listed beneath the test.

Remember that the medical record must include physician documentation confirming the presence of the condition. Clinical evidence must support principal and subsequent diagnoses before they can be reported.

In this instance, investigating the laboratory values reveals that the patient had a urine culture that showed an *E. coli* colony growth of greater than 100,000. According to the abnormal laboratory values section, under "Urine Culture—Presence of Pathogens," this abnormal finding indicates the possible presence of a urinary tract infection.

To determine whether a 100,000 colony count of *E. coli* is significant in this instance, look under "Urine" in the organisms section. The information under "Possible Pathogens" lists any organism with a count greater than 100,000 as infectious.

Next, check the medication record for evidence that the patient was treated for a urinary tract infection. For this example, the physician prescribed Cipro. Look up "Cipro" in the drug usage section of the *DRG Desk Reference*. Note that the medication frequently is used to treat urinary tract infections.

This example shows that the coder can detect evidence of a urinary tract infection by reviewing the patient's medical record, along with referencing the appropriate sections in the *DRG Desk Reference*. The evidence includes the abnormal results of the patient's urine culture and the medication record, which indicates that Cipro was prescribed during the patient's hospital stay.

The next step is to query the physician and ask, when appropriate, an addendum to the medical record documentation be written, based on the clinical findings and treatment documented in the record. For correct coding and appropriate reimbursement, it is important to include the additional diagnosis code to complete the patient's profile.

Target DRG Listing

The DRGs included in this section were chosen based on the "Medicare Provider Analysis and Review" (MedPAR) file, which contains records for 100 percent of Medicare beneficiaries using hospital inpatient services in the United States. Using 2001 MedPAR data, the 22 DRGs selected are those that have a potential for "upcoding" or "DRG creep." According to the OIG's *Compliance Program Guidance for Hospitals,* "upcoding" is using a billing code that has a higher payment rate than the appropriate code, and "DRG creep" is the practice of billing using a DRG code that provides a higher payment rate than the DRG code that accurately reflects the service furnished to the patient.

Once the 22 most error-prone DRGs were identified, a corresponding DRG was selected. This similar or "paired" DRG is the one that the case would most likely group to when the documentation and code assignment does not support the assignment to the higher paying DRG.

DRG "pairs" are arranged numerically. Below each DRG pair, the ICD-9-CM codes commonly assigned to them are listed numerically, as well. For the chosen DRGs, the ICD-9-CM codes included under each DRG are those that were most likely to be assigned by coding staff, based on a 5 percent threshold of all codes listed for a particular DRG in the 2001 MedPAR file. This means that 95 percent of all cases assigned to the particular DRG were assigned one of the listed diagnosis codes as a principal diagnosis.

The guidelines for the ICD-9-CM codes contained in this book are based on the ICD-9-CM code book, the American Hospital Association's (AHA's)*Coding Clinic for ICD-9-CM* and CMS's UHDDS definitions and reporting requirements. *Coding Clinic for ICD-9-CM* provides specific diagnostic information and guidelines that should be followed to determine proper diagnosis coding and is the only publication endorsed by CMS (*Federal Register,* vol. 54, no. 139, 1989). In addition, all guidelines published in *Coding Clinic for ICD-9-CM* are approved by the cooperating parties: AHA, the American Health Information Management Association, the CMS, and the National Center for Health Statistics. Whenever possible, the date that the coding advice is effective is included. This is an important element in determining whether you are in compliance with the rules applicable to the case based on the discharge date under review. Any internal guidelines developed by the facility must be consistent with *Coding Clinic for ICD-9-CM* advice.

The UHDDS is a minimum data set that hospitals are required to complete and report for individual hospital discharges in the Medicare and Medicaid programs. The principal diagnosis, other diagnoses, the principal procedure and other procedures are selected by hospital coders based on UHDDS definitions. Proper DRG assignment is dependent on the correct reporting of diagnoses and procedures according to UHDDS rules.

Step 1: Locating a DRG

To locate a DRG and its documentation and coding guidelines for the selected ICD-9-CM codes, review the table of contents for the DRG and/or ICD-9-CM code you wish to review. Then, turn to the referenced page to quickly get the answers you need.

Step 2: DRG Groups

The DRGs are grouped in similar groups. The first DRG listed is the "target" DRG, and the second or third DRG is the DRG to which the case would most likely be assigned if the documentation does not support assignment for the "target" DRG.

For example, to validate that your medical record documentation will support the assignment of DRG 079, Respiratory Infections and Inflammations, and to review the coding guidelines, turn to the table of contents and determine the page where DRG 079 is located. Turn to that page, where the following DRG would be found.

DRG 079   Respiratory Infections and Inflammations, Age Greater than 17 with CC

DRG 089   Simple Pneumonia and Pleurisy, Age Greater than 17 with CC

Step 3: The Issue

For each grouped pair an explanation of the issue concerning the accurate assignment of the appropriate DRG is provided.

Issues

The coding of pneumonia is one of the most frequent problems encountered by hospital inpatient coders today. It is problematic because of the lack of physician documentation on the organism causing the pneumonia when the causative organism is known or suspected and the complexity of the ICD-9-CM diagnosis codes and coding guidelines for pneumonia. The following represent the major issues affecting the DRG pairs 079 and 089:

- failure of the physician documentation in clearly confirming the type (bacterial versus viral) and organism causing pneumonia (gram-negative versus gram-positive) after study
- presence of coexisting conditions such as septicemia on admission, and lack of support of physician documentation to determine sequencing of principal versus secondary diagnoses, which may or may not be equally treated
- symptoms of pneumonia overlap with other chronic forms of respiratory disease such as acute bronchitis and chronic obstructive pulmonary disease

Step 4: Most Common Principal Diagnoses List

For the DRGs in the pair, a list of diagnoses that were most likely to be assigned by coding staff is provided, based on a 5 percent threshold of all codes listed for a particular DRG in the MedPAR file. Using the above pair as an example, the following information is provided for DRG 079 and DRG 089.

Using a 5 percent threshold of 2001 MedPAR data, the most commonly assigned ICD-9-CM codes assigned as the principal diagnosis that group to DRG 079 are *Pseudomonas* (482.1), *S. aureus* (482.41), gram-negative organisms (482), and pneumonia due to aspiration of food or vomitus (507.0). The principal diagnosis code that most commonly grouped to DRG 089 was due to pneumonias not otherwise specified (486).

If one of the above codes is chosen as the principal diagnosis, review the record against the following review standards to validate the documentation and code assignment to ensure coding compliance and accurate DRG assignment.

Most Common Diagnosis Codes

DRG 079

- 482.1, *Pseudomonas*
- 482.41, *S. Aureus*
- 482.83, Gram-negative organisms
- 507.0, Pneumonia due to aspiration of food or vomitus

DRG 089

- 486, Pneumonias, not otherwise specified

Step 5: Issues Summarized

If one of the diagnosis codes chosen as the principal diagnosis for the record under review is one of the diagnoses most likely to be assigned for a targeted DRG, it is essential to validate that your medial record documentation will support the assignment of the targeted DRG.

For example, code 482.83 is listed as the principal diagnosis in the medical record being reviewed. Locate 482.83 and review the physician documentation issues (DOC), ICD-9-CM coding guidelines (CG), and the AHA's *Coding Clinic for ICD-9-CM* guidelines (AHA CC), to ensure coding compliance and accurate DRG assignment. A partial excerpt of the text is provided as an example on the following page.

482.83   Gram-negative organisms

AHA CC: A culture of expectorated sputum may be of limited value in the diagnosis of the agent causing acute pneumonia, especially when antibiotics have previously been administered. In the absence of confirmatory cultures (e.g., the culture and smear reveal several organisms, none of which can be identified as the causative agent, the sputum was not obtainable or sputum reveals no growth or normal flora) review the medical record documentation for the following factors:

- a debilitated, chronically ill, or aged patient
- worsening of cough, dyspnea, reduction of oxygen level
- fever
- purulent sputum
- patchy infiltration on chest x-ray (in addition to those previously noted densities caused by a primary underlying disease)
- elevated leukocyte count or a normal count in aged and debilitated patients

If these conditions exist in the patient and the physician documents a diagnosis of gram-negative pneumonia, probable gram-negative pneumonia or mixed bacterial pneumonia, assign code 482.8, pneumonia due to other specified bacteria, with the additional code of 041.8. [*Coding Clinic*, 3Q, '88, 11]

AHA CC: If the results of the sputum culture with gram-stain show the presence of gram-negative bacteria, but the physician documents only pneumonia in the final diagnosis statement, do not assign code 482.83. A gram-stain does not constitute conclusive evidence of gram-negative pneumonia. The physician must document in the medical record a final diagnosis of gram-negative pneumonia before code 482.83 is assigned. [*Coding Clinic*, 2Q, '98, 5, effective with discharges July 1, 1998]

AHA CC: An abnormal finding on a sputum gram stain is not necessarily indicative of a bacterial pathogen and, therefore, should not be coded as a specified cause of bacterial pneumonia without definitive sputum cultures and further chart documentation. Use code 482.9, bacterial pneumonia unspecified, if the physician documents that the patient had a bacterial pneumonia without further specification. Code 486, pneumonia, organism unspecified, is used if the physician does not specify an etiology. [*Coding Clinic*, 1Q, '94, 17, effective with discharges January 1, 1994, and *Coding Clinic*, 2Q, '98, 3,4, effective with discharges July 1, 1998]

AHA CC: If these conditions exist in the patient and the physician documents a diagnosis of gram-negative pneumonia, probable gram-negative pneumonia or mixed bacterial pneumonia, assign code 482.8, pneumonia due to other specified bacteria, with the additional code of 041.8. [*Coding Clinic*, 3Q, '88, 11]

AHA CC: If the results of the sputum culture laboratory report provide evidence of a gram-negative type of bacteria but no specific organism is stated and the physician documents in the medical record that the cause or probable cause of the pneumonia is this organism, code 482.83 may be assigned. [*Coding Clinic*, M-A, '85, 3]

AHA CC: *Do not* assign a code indicating bacterial pneumonia unless the medical record documentation supports the presence of a bacterial organism. *Do not* assume that pneumonia not specified as viral or bacterial is bacterial. [*Coding Clinic*, 3Q, '94, 10, effective with discharges July 1, 1994]

DOC: Use this code when the physician documents a diagnosis of pneumonia due to *Proteus*, pneumonia due to *Serratia marcascens,* pneumonia due to *Bacterium anitratum*, or pneumonia due to *Herellea*.

Note that there are four elements under discussion, physician documentation issues, ICD-9-CM coding guidelines, and *Coding Clinic for ICD-9-CM* coding guidelines specific to code under discussion. When relevant, the *Coding Clinic* sections are subdivided into citations that are code specific and citations that are related to the topic, but in which the code under discussion is not specifically mentioned. The specific citations are always listed first, followed by the related citations under each section.

Note: It is crucial to follow the coding guidelines that were effective for the date of discharge of the case. Guideline changes are published with effective dates of discharge. When reviewing the coding guidelines provided, note the "effective with discharge" date and choose the appropriate coding advice applicable to the case under audit.

It is understood that the following three statements are applicable to every code in the book:

- The listing of the diagnosis is the responsibility of the attending physician. If there is a diagnosis listed for which no supporting documentation appears in the body of the medical record, consult with the physician before assigning a code. *Do not* report conditions for which there is no supporting documentation. [*AHIMA Practice Brief on Data Quality*]
- When a diagnosis documented at the time of discharge is qualified as "probable," "suspected," "likely," "?," "possible," or "still to be ruled out," code it as if it existed or was established. Medical record documentation would show a diagnostic workup, arrangements for further workup or observation, and initial therapeutic approach that conform most closely to the established diagnosis. [*Coding Clinic*, M-A, '85, 3]
- *Do not* arbitrarily report a diagnosis code on the basis of test results alone. The medical record must provide adequate documentation to support the principal diagnosis. Check with the physician and have him or her document in the body of the medical record the significance of the test results. [*AHIMA Practice Brief on Data Quality*]

Step 6: Assignment of the Most Appropriate DRG

The coding and documentation guidelines are provided to assist you in determining whether the information in your medical records supports your ICD-9-CM codes and DRG assignment. Having reviewed the comparison and explanation of the requirements for ICD-9-CM codes for the targeted DRG pair to uncover possible coding and documentation errors, you can now determine whether a particular DRG assignment is valid.

Key Fields for Coder Abstracting

Abstracting Basics

Chart abstraction is an important practice in coding departments to compile pertinent information for each patient upon discharge for data collection and billing. Using the medical record as the source document, the coding staff key information into an abstracting system either through free text entry or drop-down menu. Typically there is automated data collection interface from the billing system to the coding abstracting system for important information such as demographics, payment source data, admission and discharge dates. An interface from the admissions system to the abstract allows the coding staff to validate the patient information is correct using the medical record as the source document. An interface from the abstracting system to the billing system also allows critical information to flow for accurate DRG payment as obtained by the coding staff using the medical record as the source document.

The role of the coding staff in the revenue cycle flow is critical to obtaining appropriate reimbursement. Primarily, the most important function of the coding staff is to ensure the most accurate and complete medical record information is available for abstraction. Using a standard record format and ensuring the record is in an orderly fashion will facilitate the abstraction process. Secondly, in providing raw data for billing, the coding staff must ensure the key fields for reimbursement are abstracted correctly based on the medical record documentation. Abstraction is not only critical for reimbursement but information collected is also used to make vital decisions within the health care facility, including patient care, clinical research, medical education, and may be used for external analysis such as benchmarking and outcomes comparisons.

Coding staff who are properly trained in identifying the essential information for abstraction as well as applying appropriate policies and procedures for interpretation should perform the abstracting function. Specific definitions, when available, should be utilized to facilitate consistency. Errors or inconsistency in interpretation from one coding abstractor to another could lead to inaccurate reimbursement and data.

Standard Abstracting Elements

The National Committee on Vital and Health Statistics (NCVHS) in its advisory capacity to the Department of Health and Human Services (HHS) defined standards for a uniform reporting of hospital discharge data in 1972. Originally as adopted in 1979 these data elements became known as the UHDDS and consisted of 14 key data items. The bolded elements represent the original data items originally defined in 1972 as part of the UHDDS.

Key Data Elements
1. **Personal/Unique Identifier**
2. **Date of Birth**
3. **Gender**
4. **Race and Ethnicity**
5. **Residence**
6. Living/Residential Arrangement
7. Marital Status

8.   Self-Reported Health Status
9.   Functional Status
10. Years of Schooling
11. Patient's Relationship to Subscriber/Person Eligible for Entitlement
12. Current or Most Recent Occupation/Industry
13. Type of Encounter
14. **Admission Date (inpatient)**
15. **Discharge Date (inpatient)**
16. Date of Encounter (ambulatory and physician services)
17. **Facility Identification**
18. Type of Facility/Place of Encounter
19. **Provider Identification (ambulatory)**
20. Provider Location or Address (ambulatory)
21. **Attending Physician Identification (inpatient)**
22. Operating Physician Identification (inpatient)
23. Provider Specialty
24. **Principal Diagnosis (inpatient)**
25. **Primary Diagnosis (inpatient)**
26. **Other Diagnoses (inpatient)**
27. Qualifier for Other Diagnoses (inpatient)
28. **Patient's Stated Reason for Visit or Chief Complaint (ambulatory)**
29. Physician's Tentative Diagnosis (ambulatory)
30. **Diagnosis Chiefly Responsible for Services Provided (ambulatory)**
31. **Other Diagnoses (ambulatory)**
32. External Cause of Injury
33. Birth Weight of Newborn (inpatient)
34. **Principal Procedure (inpatient)**
35. **Other Procedures (inpatient)**
36. **Dates of Procedures (inpatient)**
37. Services (ambulatory)
38. Medications Prescribed
39. Medications Dispensed (pharmacy)
40. **Disposition of Patient (inpatient)**
41. **Disposition (ambulatory)**
42. **Patient's Expected Sources of Payment**
43. Injury Related to Employment
44. Total Billed Charges

Not all fields listed above are abstracted by coding staff, each facility may have a different abstracting protocol based on internal and external data collection needs. Typically coding staff are primarily responsible for the key fields involving DRG assignment. Facilities will be required to gather several other data elements effective October 2003 for the HIPAA transactions standards guidelines.

Key Fields for DRG Reimbursement

DRGs are assigned using the principal diagnosis; up to eight additional diagnoses; the principal procedure and up to five additional procedure codes; and age, sex, and discharge status. One DRG is assigned to each inpatient stay and diagnoses and procedure codes are designated by ICD-9-CM codes. A case is assigned to one of 25 MDCs based on its principal diagnosis.

Upon chart abstraction from the medical record, the coding staff begins to assign key fields driving DRG reimbursement such as those mentioned above. This critical information is entered into the abstracting system, which may reside within the billing system or may be a separate information system, which interfaces with the billing system.

The uniform bill known as the UB-92, also called the HCFA-1450, was developed and approved for use in 1992. This form serves the needs of many payers in the electronic claims submission. Hospitals, skilled nursing facilities (SNFs) and other providers, such as home health practitioners use the UB-92 to bill Medicare. Other major third-party payers have substantially adopted Medicare UB-92 guidelines. The UB-92 claim form contains 86 data elements. A particular payer may not need some data elements. In determining the data elements to be included on the billing form, the National Uniform Billing Committee (NUBC) and state billing committees (SUBCs) attempt to balance the needs of the payer organizations with the hospital's and other provider's burden of providing information. The data elements and design of the UB-92 and its electronic media format are determined by the NUBC and the SUBCs.

A sample UB-92 and input data elements critical to appropriate DRG payment is provided in the following table.

Table 1.1.   Sample UB-92

		6 Statement Covers Period		4 Type of Bill	
		From	**Through**		
14 Birthdate	**15 Sex**			**22 Discharge Status**	
42 Rev. Co.	**43 Description**	**45 Serv. Date**	**46 Serv.Units**	**47 Total Charges**	**50 Payer**
67-75. Prin./Sec. Diag. CD		**76. Adm.Diag.CD.**		**80-81. Prin./Sec. Proc CD**	

The direct interface from the abstracting system to the billing system helps populate the UB-92 fields driving DRG reimbursement. A sample of fields for coding abstracting and definitions used to assign each field accurately is provided in table 1.2. Coding staff are accountable for the accurate assignment of each field and facilities must ensure the interface from the abstracting system to the billing system transmits properly. One way to verify accuracy is to review the UB-92 after billing. Reconciling the UB-92 information against the information in the abstracting system can help verify the accurate transmission of DRG reimbursement fields.

How to Verify Transfer of Codes From Medical Records to UB-92

Even if hospitals submit their claims electronically and do not maintain a hard copy backup of the claim form, there is a backup "document." Always verify that the "claim" reviewed replicates the actual claim that was transmitted to Medicare. Knowing where to find the key data elements on the electronic screen or printout is important.

To compare information on the UB-92 to the medical record either

- request that the billing department provide a print out of the electronic claim
- obtain training on the electronic billing system (this may be a different system from the patient accounting system) so that easy retrieval and review the electronic claim on-line is possible
- review the patient account file on-line if the claim is billed directly from the patient accounting system

Table 1.2. Sample Abstract Screen Showing Key Fields for DRG Payment

The fields highlighted are those directly related to DRG assignment.	
Patient Information	
Name:_____	Medical Record Number: _____
Birth Date: _____	Sex:_____
Age in Years: _____	
Patient Stay Information	
Account Number: _____	Primary Payer:_____
Admit Date: _____	Discharge Date:_____
Discharge Status: _____	Length of Stay: _____
Codes	
Admit Diagnosis:_____	
Principal Diagnosis: _____	Secondary Diagnoses: _____
Principal Procedure:_____	Secondary Procedures:_____

Table 1.3. Sample Field Definitions for Abstraction

Field Name	Length	Description
Patient Information		
Patient name	31	Name of patient.
Medical record number	17	Patient's medical record number.
Birth date	10	Patient's birth date in mm/dd/yyyy format. Used for age calculation. The date must be after 01/01/1850.
Age in years	3	Patient's age in years. Valid values: 0-124.
Sex	1	Patient's gender. Unknown, Male, Female
Patient Stay Information		
Account number	17	Patient account number.
Primary payer	2	Primary payer for the service provided. Select from the list of values: 01 Medicare 06 Blue Cross 02 Medicaid 07 Insur Co 03 Title V 08 Self Pay 04 Other Govt 09 Other 05 Work Comp 10 No charge
Admit date	10	Date of admission to the facility. Format: mm/dd/yyyy. The admit and birth dates are used for calculation of patient age; the admit and discharge dates are used for calculation of length of stay (LOS).
Discharge date	10	Discharge date from the facility. Format: mm/dd/yyyy. The discharge and admit dates are used for automatic calculation of LOS.
Discharge status	2	Status of discharge. Select from the following list of values: 01 Home or self-care 02 Discharge/transfer to another short term hospital 03 Discharge/transfer to skilled nursing facility (SNF) 04 Discharge/transfer to an intermediate care facility (ICF) 05 Discharge/transfer to another type of facility 06 Care of home health service 07 Left against medical advice 08 Home IV service 20 Expired 30 Still a patient 50 Hospice—Home 51 Hospice—Medical Facility 61 Swing bed 62 Rehab facility/rehab unit 63 Long term care hospital 71 Outpatient services—other facility 72 Outpatient services—this facility

Key Fields for Coder Abstracting

Table 1.3. Sample Field Definitions for Abstraction (continued)

Field Name	Length	Description
Length of stay (LOS)	3	Number of days the patient was in the facility. Calculated LOS takes precedence over entered LOS. LOS is calculated based on admit and discharge dates.
Codes		
Admit diagnosis	6	Enter an ICD-9-CM diagnosis code representing condition identified by the physician at the time of the patient's admission requiring hospitalization.
Diagnoses PDX (principal diagnosis) and secondary diagnoses 2-9	6	Enter an ICD-9-CM diagnosis code(s). Only diagnoses codes up to five digits are accepted. The principal diagnosis is the condition established after study to be chiefly responsible for this admission. Even though another diagnosis may be more severe than the principal diagnosis, enter the principal diagnosis. Entering any other diagnosis may result in incorrect assignment of a DRG and cause you to be incorrectly paid under PPS. Secondary diagnoses: Enter the full ICD-9-CM codes for up to eight additional conditions if they coexisted at the time of admission or developed subsequently, and which had an effect upon the treatment or the length of stay. Do not duplicate the principal diagnosis listed as an additional or secondary diagnosis.
Procedures PP (principal procedure) and secondary procedures 2-6	7	Enter ICD-9-CM procedure code(s). Only procedure codes up to four digits are accepted. Enter the full ICD-9-CM, volume 3, procedure code, including all four digits where applicable, for the definitive treatment rather than for diagnostic or exploratory purposes or that was necessary to take care of a complication. It is also the procedure most closely related to the principal diagnosis. For this purpose, surgery includes incision, excision, amputation, introduction, repair, destructions, endoscopy, suture, and manipulation. Show the date of the principal procedure numerically as mmddyy in the "date" portion. Secondary procedures: Enter the full ICD-9-CM, volume 3, procedure codes, including all four digits where applicable, for up to five significant procedures other than the principle procedure. Show the date of each procedure numerically as mmddyy in the "date" portion. Do not repeat procedures unless you do them more than once.

Code Edits

Many payers, including Medicare and Medicaid, have implemented software code edits to help identify coding errors and inconsistencies with clinical data and coding. CMS maintains these edits internally within their Medicare DRG Grouper called the Medicare Code Editor (MCE) software. These edits may indirectly affect reimbursement by stopping payment of the claim until the returned claim to the provider is corrected. The edits are directly related to diagnosis and procedure codes abstracted by coding staff. Therefore, it is important that the correction of these edits involves the coding staff to ensure a claims resubmission is based upon appropriate coding guidelines and hospital policy and procedure. Information in the medical record should be the source from which corrections are made.

The following are examples of edits related to coding errors:

- Invalid ICD-9-CM code—the code listed is not valid or is missing a digit. DRG 470, Ungroupable, may be assigned based on the invalid code selection.
- Age conflict—some diagnoses are unlikely for specific ages (e.g., a two year old with prostate cancer). Codes are assigned to four age categories: newborn (age of 0), pediatric (ages 0–17), maternity (ages 12–55), and adult (ages 15–124).
- Sex conflict—some codes are specific to gender, this edit indicates such a diagnosis inconsistent with the gender of the patient, for example prostate cancer reported for a female patient.

Compliance Issues Related to Abstracting

QIOs (formerly known as PROs) are required by CMS to improve quality of care for beneficiaries by ensuring that beneficiary care meets professionally recognized standards of health care; to protect the integrity of the Medicare Trust Fund; and to protect beneficiaries. The QIOs are currently functioning under the seventh statement of work (SOW, formerly known as the scope of work). The seventh statement of work includes a component called the Hospital Payment Monitoring Review Program (formerly known as PEPP). One of the requirements of this program is that the QIOs produce national and statewide error rates for coding and medical necessity for estimating the payment error rate for inpatient PPS services. The payment error rate will be monitored and reported for each state. CMS will provide Clinical Data Abstraction Centers (CDACs) with a random sample of PPS discharges. The CDACs will perform a review of the cases and those cases that fail will be referred to the QIOs. The QIOs will review 100 percent of the cases referred by the CDACs and calculate error rates. In addition, under the seventh SOW, the QIOs will review services provided to Medicare beneficiaries to determine whether the services support the validity and diagnosis of medical information supplied by providers. As a result of this review the QIO may make an initial determination that may result in denial of payment and/or DRG changes. The QIOs will also monitor hospital coding patterns by conducting hospital profiling and trend monitoring. The QIOs will develop proposals to address any potentially significant aberrant coding patterns.

With regards to coding and DRG assignment, the coding abstracting process is vulnerable to risk areas identified by the OIG and QIO reviews, and the following should be monitored for accuracy:

- selection of principal diagnosis
- selection of secondary diagnoses and procedures (especially those that affect the DRG)
- selection of the discharge status
- sequencing
- code assignment, to the highest level of specificity
- medical record documentation support for billed codes
- admission and discharge dates
- age

Effective monitoring may lead to identification of root causes of problems such as

- lack of coder experience
- lack of appropriate coding resources
- unclear or lack of policies and procedures
- failure of the coder to review the entire medical record
- lack of complete medical record information

- misinterpretation of regulations by coder

The area of discharge status assignment has been under increased scrutiny by the QIO and OIG, and continues under the new QIO Seventh Statement of Work. Coding staffs role in the abstracting of these fields should be defined in policies and procedures as well as reviewed periodically to internally identify errors and proactively implement education.

Qualified Discharges Considered Transfer Cases

A discharge is defined as a situation in which a patient leaves an acute care (prospective payment) hospital after receiving complete acute care treatment. A transfer is defined as any situation where the beneficiary is admitted to another IPPS hospital on the same date that he or she is discharged from an IPPS hospital, even if the patient left against medical advice from the first hospital. Patients are considered discharged from the hospital, under the transfer payment definition, if they are transferred to a facility excluded from the PPS. Due to the high volume of discharges to subacute care (prospective payment exempt) facilities for certain DRGs, CMS has selected 29 DRGs to be paid as transfer cases instead of discharge cases. These are termed "qualified discharges" and must meet the following criteria:

- The hospital stay is classified to one of the 29 selected DRGs and one of the following occurs upon discharge:
  — the individual is admitted to a hospital or hospital unit that is not a PPS hospital
  — the individual is admitted to a skilled nursing facility
  — the individual is provided home health services if the services relate to the condition or diagnosis for which inpatient hospital services were provided within three days after discharge

The following DRGs are included under the expanded transfer definition, and payment for these cases is made under the current transfer methodology (twice the per diem rate for the first day and the per diem rate for each subsequent day):

012	Degenerative Nervous System Disorders
014	Intracranial Hemorrhage and Stroke with Infarction
024	Seizure and Headache Age >17 with CC
025	Seizure and Headache Age >17 without CC
088	Chronic Obstructive Pulmonary Disease
089	Simple Pneumonia and Pleurisy Age > 17 with CC
090	Simple Pneumonia and Pleurisy Age >17 without CC
113	Amputation for Circulatory System Disorders Except Upper Limb and Toe
121	Circulatory Disorders with AMI and Major Complication, Discharged Alive
122	Circulatory Disorders with AMI Without Major Complications Discharged Alive
127	Heart Failure & Shock
130	Peripheral Vascular Disorders with CC
131	Peripheral Vascular Disorders without CC
236	Fractures of Hip and Pelvis
239	Pathological Fractures and Musculoskeletal and Connective Tissue Malignancy
277	Cellulitis Age >17 with CC
278	Cellulitis Age >17 without CC
294	Diabetes Age >35
296	Nutritional and Miscellaneous Metabolic Disorders Age >17 with CC
297	Nutritional and Miscellaneous Metabolic Disorders Age >17 without CC

320   Kidney and Urinary Tract Infectious Age >17 with CC

321   Kidney and Urinary Tract Infections Age >17 without CC

395   Red Blood Cell Disorders Age >17

429   Organic Disturbances and Mental Retardation

468   Extensive O.R. Procedure Unrelated to Principal Diagnosis

483   Tracheotomy with Mechanical Ventilation 96 + Hours or Principal Diagnosis Except Face, Mouth, and Neck Diagnoses

The following DRGs are included under the expanded transfer definition, and payment for these cases is made based on 50 percent of the full DRG payment plus the single per diem for the first day of the stay and 50 percent of the per diem rate for each subsequent day of the stay:

209   Major Joint and Limb Reattachment Procedures of Lower Extremity

210   Hip and Femur Procedures Except Major Joint Procedures, Age Greater Than 17 With CC

211   Hip and Femur Procedures Except Major Joint Procedures, Age Greater Than 17 Without CC

DRG Assignment Tutorial

Importance of Accurate DRG Assignment

DRGs serve three main purposes: to determine hospital reimbursement based on severity of illness, to evaluate the quality of care and to evaluate the utilization of services consumed. Since all cases in a DRG are similar clinically, comparative analysis of treatment protocols, related conditions, or demographic distribution can be done internally and externally. Critical pathways are designed around DRGs to focus the efficient delivery of care. National or regional benchmarking and outcomes analysis is being launched by many managed care organizations using the DRG clinical framework. Hospital report cards and physician profiles are being developed using outcome data for public distribution to patients and other health care plans and organizations.

A collaborative approach to coding for DRG assignment is the key to successful accuracy and reimbursement of DRG payment. The relationship between the health information coding staff and all clinical staff documenting in the medical record must be interactive and complementary to engage more complete, compliant, and accurate medical record documentation of each patients condition. The result will improve clarity for an increased level of coding specificity, thus, yielding appropriate DRG assignment practices.

DRGs are assigned using the principal diagnosis; up to eight additional diagnoses; the principal procedure and up to five additional procedure codes; and age, sex, and discharge status. One DRG is assigned to each inpatient stay. Diagnoses and procedures are designated by ICD-9-CM codes. The following describes the typical decision process used to assign a DRG to a case.

A case is assigned to one of 25 major MDCs based on its principal diagnosis. DRG assignment is based upon the following considerations:

- principal and secondary diagnosis and procedure codes
- sex
- age
- discharge status
- presence or absence of CCs
- birthweight for neonates

Each MDC is organized into one of two sections surgical or medical. The surgical section classifies all surgical conditions based upon operating room procedures. The medical section classifies all diagnostic conditions based upon diagnosis codes. MDCs are mutually exclusive. The majority are organized by major body system and/or are associated with a particular medical specialty.

Why Coding Accuracy Is Not Enough

How Reporting Principal and Secondary Codes Can Affect Payment

Experts agree that health information personnel can have a major impact on a hospitals financial health. Studies have shown that optimal sequencing can increase reimbursement, often by thousands of dollars.

In one study, consultants discovered that nearly half of the patient records that were analyzed fell into DRGs scattered throughout MDC 5, Diseases and Disorders of the Circulatory System. Often, hospitals failed to receive optimum payment because a CC condition was omitted or the principal and secondary diagnoses were incorrectly sequenced. These shortfalls could be due directly to coder error. However, with qualified coding staff, the most likely source of error is physician documentation. Health information professionals play a key role in hospitals financial health. The coders role in educating the physician regarding appropriate coding guidelines, sequencing, and establishment of final diagnosis upon discharge can have a tremendous effect on accuracy of payment.

The following examples demonstrate situations where adequate payment had not been received. In each of the following cases, another DRG, more precisely reflecting treatment and resulting in higher payment, should have been assigned:

- A patient who underwent cardiac catheterization had severe chest pain and was treated with Nitrostat. The original DRG was 125. When the attending physician was asked and agreed to add unstable angina as a secondary diagnosis to the diagnostic profile, the discharge was reassigned to DRG 124. The average national payment increase from DRG 125 to 124 is $1501.38.

- A patient who was admitted for chronic ischemic heart disease was treated with Procainamide for arrhythmia. Paroxysmal ventricular tachycardia was documented on the admission and discharge summary. The original DRG was 132 for ischemic heart disease; when paroxysmal ventricular tachycardia was sequenced as the principal diagnosis, the DRG was changed to DRG 138. The average national payment increase from DRG 132 to 138 is $848.59.

- A physicians notes documented that a patients blood sugar fluctuated to a high of 300. The patient was treated with Micronase to control increased blood sugar. When the physician was asked and agreed to document out of control diabetes, code 250.02 was added. The original DRG 151 assignment was changed to DRG 150 with the addition of a CC, increasing payment by approximately $6,870.35.

DRG Surgical Hierarchy

The surgical hierarchy reflects the relative resources requirement of the various surgical procedures of each MDC. The hierarchy is based upon variables such as principal diagnosis, surgical class, age, complications and comorbidities.

Arranging the surgical DRGs in this manner allows for the assignment of patients with multiple procedures related to the principal diagnosis to a surgical DRG that best reflects the resources used in that care of that patient. Since patients can be assigned only one surgical class for each inpatient stay, patients with multiple procedures related to the principal diagnosis are assigned to the highest surgical DRG in the MDC assigned according to the principal diagnosis. Coding staff must understand this concept in order to sequence and obtain the proper DRG assignment for reimbursement.

The Roadblocks to Effective Coding Programs

Many factors lead to the confusion that surrounds coding. Coding experts do not always agree about the proper application of coding rules. By some industry experts, coding is described as an art, not an exact science. To achieve accurate payment, coding staffs must agree upon their individual coding guidelines and be sure that the guidelines are compatible with information published by the AHA's *Coding Clinic for ICD-9-CM*. Supervisors must sometimes disagree with practicing guidelines due to various payer requirements. QIOs (formerly known as PROs) should follow the AHA's *Coding Clinic for ICD-9-CM*, as it is CMS's official ICD-9-CM coding source.

Lack of knowledge regarding clinical issues can affect code assignment. The clinical differences among DRGs may not be recognized by the health information coder because of lack of education in DRGs and failure to recognize missing documentation.

Adequate resources and training are critical to successful coding practices. Essential tools include code books, AHA's *Coding Clinic for ICD-9-CM*, *Physician's Desk Reference*, anatomy and physiology books, medical dictionary, and hospital-approved abbreviation list. Education in anatomy and physiology and medical terminology creates the foundation for coding education.

Health information coders roles and responsibilities have not always been well defined. The following questions must be considered:

- Who identifies patterns in DRG payment?
- Who ensures optimal DRG assignment for each record?
- Who plans and implements DRG education?

The Components of DRG Coding and Management

The DRG Coding and Management Team

Goals

DRG coding and management goals include the following:

- ensure the facility is receiving the reimbursement it is entitled to by assigning the best DRG for each case
- ensure accurate DRG payments by improving the hospitals case mix
- become a revenue-controlling department
- go through successful QIO (formerly known as PRO) review
- avoid QIO (formerly known as PRO) intensified review

The Members of the DRG Assignment Team

The team management strategy for accurate DRG payments is critical to turning your coding department into a revenue controlling center. The lead players are the coders, the coding supervisor, the attending physician and the health information manager.

Coder

The coder, who must be an expert in the coding process, ensures appropriate DRG assignment.

The coder's responsibilities include

- coding accurately and completely
- understanding the variables used in DRG assignment
- understanding clinical differences in DRGs
- understanding how to review the record for accurate payment

The coder's relationships are

- serving as a liaison for reconciling physician documentation
- serving as a resource for identifying documentation patterns that may jeopardize appropriate payment

Coding Supervisor

The coding supervisor serves as quality control for the DRG coding and management team. The coding supervisor ensures coding integrity and ensures DRG integrity. The coding supervisor also serves as the trainer to new and current coding staff.

The coding supervisor's responsibilities include

- evaluating and reporting on the effectiveness of the current coding operation and DRG assignments
- developing and maintaining coding policies and procedures
- verifying adherence to corporate compliance policies

- organizing regular coding continuing education

The coding supervisor's relationships are

- serving as coding instructor/trainer of the coding staff
- serving as a liaison for educating the medical staff on documentation issues affecting code assignment
- serving as liaison for educating ancillary departments in appropriate documentation/ resource needs
- identifying and reporting trends to the health information manager

Health Information Manager

The health information manager, who is manager of the DRG coding and management team, is pivotal to the whole payment scheme. The health information manager monitors, analyzes and interprets case mix management reports.

The health information manager's responsibilities include

- understanding case mix management
- understanding how to identify patterns in DRG payment to increase revenues where appropriate, or decrease where required
- developing reports showing the department as a revenue controlling center
- preparing reports from QIO (formerly known as PRO) reviews

The health information manager's relationships are

- working with the entire coding/DRG team to maintain a satisfactory case mix
- reporting results to the chief executive officer (CEO), showing the department is revenue controlling
- working with the QIO (formerly known as PRO)

The supporting roles include the physician, the nursing department, and the ancillary services department.

Physician

The physician documents why a patient receives services.

The physician's responsibilities include

- understanding and adhering to DRG documentation requirements, in order to select the most appropriate DRG
- providing assistance to the health information personnel on QIO (formerly known as PRO) issues

The physician works closely with the coder to reconcile the following documentation problems:

- Because DRG assignment is based on documentation in the medical record, the record should be comprehensive and complete.
- The physician should document all diagnoses, procedures, complications, and comorbidities, as well as abnormal test results. Any suspected conditions and what was done to investigate or evaluate them should also be documented in a timely manner.
- All dictation, signatures, etc., should be completed in the medical record as patient care is provided and should be legible.
- The information should be readable and well documented.

The information should be documented properly. With complete information in the medical record, coders will be able to properly analyze, code, and report the required information. This ensures that proper payment is received. For example, if the physician documents that a patient with a skull fracture was in a coma for less than one hour, DRG 28 is assigned. If the physician documents that the coma lasted for more than one hour, DRG 27 is assigned, with a resulting payment difference.

Nursing Department
The nursing department has the responsibility of understanding DRG documentation requirements for services rendered the patient, such as identification of infectious processes that may go undocumented by the attending physician. Additionally, the nursing department is responsible for documenting problems that could affect a patient's stay. The nursing department helps lead players understand what clues to look for in nursing records.

Ancillary Service Department
The ancillary service department serves as a resource to the DRG coding and management team.

The ancillary service department's responsibilities include

- developing indicators for abnormal lab values/actions of commonly used drugs
- ensuring ancillary reports are available in timely manner

The ancillary service department also works closely with lead players to provide a better understanding of ancillary reports.

Four Steps to Assigning the Most Appropriate DRG

Step 1: Carefully consider the assigned DRG that results from your coding operation.

Many DRGs have nearly identical diagnoses and procedures. The coder should first analyze the detailed descriptions of similar DRGs, since they contain information that could result in different payment levels.

Step 2: Compare the assigned DRG with similar DRGs to determine the differences.

Once similar DRGs have been identified, finding the DRG with the highest level of payment is easy. The DRG with the highest RW will be the highest paying DRG.

Step 3: Check the record for documentation that supports any of the differences among DRGs.

For example, the following can effect a DRG change: abnormal ancillary report findings and documentation of treatment for the condition(s).

To become an effective DRG coder, it is important to

- Recognize and react to clues in the record.
  A common barrier to accurate payment is incomplete or less than thorough documentation by the attending physician. To combat this, check to see if the diagnoses listed match the treatment provided. Find documentation to determine whether the highest paying DRG can be selected. This involves review of the **entire** medical record by
  — reviewing the history and physical, emergency room record, and discharge summary
  — reviewing the physician progress notes and nursing notes
  — reviewing the physician orders and medication records
  — reviewing all ancillary reports
- Look for abnormal results and any medications prescribed. Look for conditions that are not documented. For example, an investigation of the laboratory values might review that the patient had a urine culture. The results of the culture could show a greater than 100,000 colony growth of an organism called *E. Coli*. This abnormal finding should alert the coder to a urinary tract infection (UTI). Next, see if the physician documented a UTI in the medical record. If not, examine the medication record for signs that the patient was treated for this condition. The prescription of Septra, Cipro, or Bactrim would indicate the physician is treating a UTI.

Step 4: Obtain physician approval.

If a potential additional diagnosis is suspected, the coder must ask the attending physician to verify that the condition exists, and add documentation to the record to support the diagnosis.

A review of each step, with accompanying documentation, follows.

Step 1: Carefully consider the assigned DRG that results from your coding operation.

Step 2: Compare the assigned DRG with similar DRGs to determine the differences. Note the differences on the worksheet below.

Exhibit 1: Worksheet: Comparing DRGs

DRG	Description	RW
DRG 195	Cholecystectomy **with CDE with CC**	3.0613
DRG 196	Cholecystectomy **with CDE** without CC	1.6117
DRG 197	Cholecystectomy Except by Laparoscope wiithout CDE **with CC**	2.5547
DRG 198	Cholecystectomy Except by Laparoscope without CDE without CC	1.1831

Step 3: Check the record for documentation that supports any of the differences among DRGs

Exhibit 2: MDC 7 Diseases and Disorders of the Hepatobiliary System and Pancreas

DRG 198	**Cholecystectomy Except by Laparoscope Without CDE Without CC**	**RW 1.1831**

Potential DRGs

193	**Biliary Tract Procedure with CC** Except Only Cholecystectomy with or without CDE	RW 3.4211
194	**Biliary Tract Procedure** without CC Except Only Cholecystectomy with or without CDE	RW 1.6030
195	Cholecystectomy **with CDE with CC**	RW 3.0613
196	Cholecystectomy **with CDE** without CC	RW 1.6117
197	Cholecystectomy Except by Laparoscope without CDE **with CC**	RW 2.5547
493	**Laparoscopic** Cholecystectomy without CDE **with CC**	RW 1.8302

DRG	Principal Dx/Procedure	Codes	Tips
193	Another biliary tract procedure	*51.3	■ Anastomosis of gallbladder or bile duct
	CC condition	See CC section.	■ Post-op ileus
194	Another biliary tract procedure	*51.3	■ Anastomosis of gallbladder or bile duct
195	Common bile duct exploration	51.51	■ Limited to exploration of common duct
	AND CC condition	See CC section.	■ Post-op ileus
196	Common bile duct exploration	51.51	■ Limited to exploration of common duct
197	CC condition	See CC section.	■ Post-op ileus
493	Laparoscopic cholecystectomy *AND* CC condition	51.23 See CC section.	● By laser ■ Post-op ileus

Step 4: Obtain physician approval.

DRG Documentation Clarification Form

	Patient Name:_____
	Medical Record Number:_____
	Discharge Date:_____
Dear DR._____,	
_____	
_____	
_____	
_____	
_____	
Principal diagnosis—that condition established after study to be chiefly responsible for causing admission of the patient to the hospital for care.	
Secondary diagnoses—any condition which affected the patients care, required treatment, monitoring, work-up or evaluation.	

Developing Target DRGs

What is a target DRG?

A target DRG is a DRG with a potential for undercoding or overcoding that is frequently assigned in a hospital.

Enhancing Record Review Skills

The following steps describe how to identify inappropriate DRG assignments and inappropriate payments:

Step 1. Identify assigned DRG.

Step 2. Identify similar DRGs.

Step 3. Compare assigned DRG with similar DRGs.

Step 4. Review the record for documentation that may indicate missing information.

Step 5. Obtain physician approval and additional documentation to support any change.

Step 6. Recognize patterns in inaccurate DRG payments.

Exhibit 3: Differences in DRG Payment

Compare the differences in DRG payment for the DRGs found in the MDC 5, Circulatory System.

DRG	Relative Weight	Payment*
121	1.6169	$7098.19
122	1.0297	$4520.38
123	1.5645	$6868.16
124	1.4367	$6307.11
125	1.0947	$4805.73
140	0.5305	$2328.90
*Based on the average hospital rate of $4,390.		

Exercise: Comparing DRGs 125 and 122

DRG 122   Circulatory Disorders with Acute Myocardial Infarction without Major Complications, Discharged Alive

DRG 125   Circulatory Disorders Except Acute Myocardial Infarction with Cardiac Catheterization without Complex Diagnosis

DRGs in MDC 5 are frequently assigned. Exhibit 3 shows the differing RWs. In reviewing the description of the DRGs, perform the following exercise.

Assume that you have coded the patient's chart and assigned the case to DRG 125.

List the types of documentation you might find in the chart to reassign the case into DRG 122.

1._____

2._____

3._____

Exhibit 4: MDC 5 Diseases and Disorders of the Circulatory System

DRG 125	Circulatory Disorders Except AMI with Cardiac Catheterization without Complex Diagnosis	RW 1.0947

Potential DRGs

121	Circulatory Disorders with AMI and Major Complications, Discharged Alive	RW 1.6169
124	Circulatory Disorders Except AMI with Cardiac Catheterization & Complex Diagnosis	RW 1.4367

DRG	Principal Dx/Procedure	Codes	Tips
121 ⬇YIELD	AMI, initial episode of care *AND* Major Complications *AND* Discharge status, alive	410.0–410.9 (with fifth digit of 1)	■ Describes an acute event, if multiple sites or subsequent sites identified for infarction documented, code all sites. ◆ Non-Q wave codes to subendocardial (410.7x)
124 ⬇YIELD	Circulatory principal diagnosis: Hypertensive heart disease with heart failure	402.91	■ Due to hypertension, hypertensive heart disease, cardiomegaly, cardiopathy, heart failure
	Acute ischemic heart disease without MI	*411	■ Impending infarction, Dresslers syndrome, unstable angina, preinfarction angina
	Post-MI syndrome (Dresslers syndrome)	411.0	
	Unstable angina	411.1	
	Coronary insufficiency	411.89	
	Acute pericarditis	*420.9	■ Pericarditis, NOS
	Endocarditis	*421	
	Acute myocarditis	*422	
	Cardiomyopathy	425.4, 425.5, 425.7, 425.9	■ Secondary cardiomyopathies; code primary disease as well
	Cardiac arrest	427.5	■ Cardiorespiratory arrest
	CHF, unspecified	428.0	
	Left heart failure	428.1	
	Failure, heart, systolic	*428.2	
	Failure, heart, diastolic, acute	*428.3	
	Failure, heart, combined systolic and diastolic	*428.4	
	Shock	785.50	

Results of Review

Comment	Original DRG	Revised DRG
Documentation shows congestive heart failure Report code 428.0 to reflect the current condition	125	124

Exhibit 5: MDC 5 Diseases and Disorders of the Circulatory System

DRG 122	Circulatory Disorders with AMI and without Major Complication, Discharged Alive	RW 1.0297

Potential DRGs

110	Major Cardiovascular Procedures with CC	RW 4.0492
111	Major Cardiovascular Procedures without CC	RW 2.4797
115	Permanent Cardiac Pacemaker Implant with AMI, Heart Failure or Shock	RW 3.5465
121	Circulatory Disorders with AMI and Major Complications, Discharged Alive	RW 1.6169
123	Circulatory Disorders with AMI, Expired	RW 1.5645

DRG	Principal Dx/Procedures	Codes	Tips
110	Major cardiovascular procedure AND CC conditions	37.61 See CC section.	◆ Balloon pulsation device inserted for mechanical circulation assistance. Not to be confused with a heart assist system (37.62–37.66)
111	Major cardiovascular procedure	37.61	◆ Balloon pulsation device inserted for mechanical circulation assistance. Not to be confused with a heart assist system (37.62–37.66)
115	Permanent cardiac pacemaker implant	37.70–37.76, 37.80–37.87	
121 ▽	AMI, initial episode of care AND Complex diagnosis:	410.0–410.9 (with fifth digit of 1)	■ Describes an acute event, if multiple sites or subsequent sites identified for infarction documented, code all sites. ◆ Non-Q wave codes to subendocardial (410.7x)
	Rheumatic heart failure	398.91	■ If physician documents both congestive failure as and rheumatic or rheumatic heart failure, use this code and 396.3.
	Primary pulmonary hypertension	416.0	● Idiopathic pulmonary arteriosclerosis
	Subarachnoid hemorrhage	430	
	Intracerebral hemorrhage	431	
	Nontraumatic extradural hemorrhage	432.0	
	Subdural hemorrhage	432.9	
	Occluded basilar artery with cerebral infarction	433.01	
121 ▽	Occluded carotid artery with cerebral infarction	433.11	
	Occluded vertebral artery with cerebral infarction	433.21	
	Occluded multiple and bilateral precerebral artery with cerebral infarction	433.31	
	Occluded specified precerebral artery with cerebral infarction	433.81	
	Cerebral thrombosis	434.00	
	Cerebral thrombosis with cerebral infarction	434.01	
	Cerebral embolism with cerebral infarction	434.11	
	Cerebral artery occlusion	434.90	
	Occluded precerebral artery NOS with cerebral infarction	433.91	
	Cerebral artery occlusion with cerebral infarction	434.91	
	CVA NOS	436	■ Always use solo; documentation will state CVA and no additional etiology.

DRG 122 (continued)

DRG	Principal Dx/Procedures	Codes	Tips
121 ⟨YIELD⟩ cont.	Pneumococcal pneumonia	481	■ If presence of pneumococcal pneumonia and pneumococcal septicemia (038.2) confirmed in record, code both entities.
	Other bacterial pneumonia (all fourth & fifth digits except 482.84)	482.xx	■ Mixed bacterial pneumonia NOS
	Pneumonia due to other specified organism (all fourth digits)	483.x	
	Pneumonia in infectious diseases classified elsewhere (all fourth digits)	484.x	
	Bronchopneumonia, organism unspecified	485	■ Lobular pneumonia, pleurobroncho-pneumonia, hemorrhagic pneumonia
	Pneumonia, organism unspecified	486	
	Influenza with pneumonia	487.0	
	Pneumonitis due to solids and liquids (all fourth digits)	507.x	■ If both aspiration and bacterial pneumonia are documented, code both.
	Pulmonary collapse	518.0	■ Atelectasis, postoperative complication must be documented by physician as such based on workup and physician findings.
	Pulmonary insufficiency following trauma and surgery	518.5	■ ARDS, shock lung
	Acute respiratory failure	518.81	
	Chronic respiratory failure	518.83	
	Acute and chronic respiratory failure	518.84	
	Decubitus ulcer	707.0	■ If ulcer is staged as superficial or advanced in progress notes this is, irrelevant to ICD-9-CM assignment.
	Infection and inflammatory reaction due to vascular device, implant and graft	996.62	■ If physician documents sepsis (present on admission) causing an infected access device, 996.62 must be the principal Dx with *038 as additional.
123	Discharge status, expired		

Results of Review

Comment	Original DRG	Revised DRG
Documentation shows an episode of paroxsymal tachycardia, report 427.1	122	121

Developing a Working Relationship with the Physician

Once the coder has identified possible missing information, the next step is to ask the attending physician to verify that the condition exists.

Problem: Missing or lack of specific information.

Solution: Approach physician to reconcile documentation.

Road Blocks: Problems may arise in reconciling the information with the physician.

- Coders may not be used to dealing directly with the medical staff.
- Physicians may respond with coders are trying to diagnose patients.
- Physicians may also respond with the hospital is just trying to get more money out of the government.
- Ineffective communication between physicians and coding staff may make it difficult to resolve differences.

Benefit: Appropriate payment for all services.

Learning to Be Proactive Concerning QIO Practices

- QIOs (formerly known as PROs) have their own criteria.
- DRG validations are subject to the individual QIO (formerly known as PRO) interpretation.
- DRG assignments/coding guidelines must conform to QIO (formerly known as PRO) requirements.

Pulling it all Together

Implementing the Team Strategy

The Steps

Step 1: Develop an action plan.

Step 2: Establish case mix information.
Consider the following:
- monthly monitoring of case mix
- fluctuations in case mix

Step 3: Develop target DRGs for the following:
- validation
- education

Step 4: Identify patterns in DRG payment. Recognize trends in potential revenue loss.

Step 5: Enhance record review skills for coding staff. Teach coding staff how to
- recognize missing diagnoses
- reconcile documentation with physician staff

Step 6: Develop communication channels with medical staff and ancillary departments by providing
- in-service education for ancillary departments
- one-on-one physician education

Step 7: Identify what the QIO (formerly known as PRO) expects and how to deal with disagreements.

Step 8: Report the results. Demonstrate the financial impact of the coding/DRG program. Share the data with administration, finance, departmental managers, and coding staff.

The Action Plan

Effective planning is essential to implement the DRG team management strategy. The tasks, the roles, and the responsibilities of each team member must be defined, and the timetable for implementation clearly specified. The following is a sample action plan.

DRG Assignment Tutorial

Exhibit 6: Sample Action Plan (partial)

DRG Team management
Medical Record Department
XYZ Hospital
Prepared by: Health Information Manager

Task	Responsible Party	Time for Completion	Status
Translate the building blocks into an action plan	Health Information Manager	4 weeks	completed
Develop target DRG list that represents potential revenue loss for the hospital	Manager/Coding Supervisor	2 weeks	in progress
Begin coding and DRG assignment training	Coding Supervisor/ Coders		
Evaluate what DRGs the QIOs (formerly known as PROs) are focusing on	Manager/Coding Supervisor		
Revise coding guideline manual	Coding Supervisor/ Coders		

Training the Coding Staff

One of the most important parts of a successful DRG team management strategy is training the coding staff to understand the purpose of the strategy, and the necessary steps to accomplish the goal.

Basic Training Elements

Basic training elements must teach the coding staff to

- Understand the relationship between case mix and DRGs.
- Identify missing record information. Coders will analyze the medical record by reviewing the physicians overall management of the patient to identify resource consumption as areas of emphasis.
- Respond to record clues. Coders will use unusual results to
  — Substantiate a previously noted diagnosis. A clinical condition may explain an abnormal result.
  — Add a diagnosis or procedure not already documented. The coder will have to ask the physician to add this diagnosis prior to code assignment.
- Understand and be able to distinguish the clinical differences among DRGs.

Suggestions for Coder Education

To accurately assign DRGs, initiate and intensify medical record coding training and record investigative skills.

Monthly Inservice Programs with Ancillary and Nursing Personnel

Monthly inservice programs should be held with ancillary and nursing personnel.

Who	Why
Laboratory technicians/ director	To better understand abnormal laboratory values and their indications.
Pharmacist	To discuss new drugs and commonly used drugs and their action.
Infection control nurse	To assist in recognition of infectious processes that may go undocumented by the attending physician.
Dietician	Identification of treatment for malnutrition.

Periodic Record Reabstraction

Periodic reabstracting of selected records is recommended to compare coding results and DRG assignments. Coders often times must code without the final summary. Reviewing the chart after the final summary has been completed can offer insight into documentation issues. If the physician adds information to the final summary not documented anywhere else in the record, this information can change the DRG. These documentation issues should be tracked and addressed.

DRG Changes Identified by the QIO (formerly known as PRO)

Review all records identified by the QIO (formerly known as PRO) as an error. Use these records as an educational tool.

The Importance of Training to the Success of the DRG Team Management Strategy

Training all team members is an integral step in successfully implementing the DRG team management strategy. Cross-departmental coordination and training facilitates the accomplishment of the DRG strategy. The article below illustrates the benefits of a cross-departmental and intradepartmental training approach.

After reviewing the computerized Medicare case mix reports, administrators realized that the hospital had a low Medicare case mix. They hired a national consulting company to review charts of Medicare patients discharged during the preceding 60 days for diagnosis sequencing, complication, or comorbidity omissions, and incomplete physician documentation. This review provided a basis for developing coder and physician training programs that would be adopted by the hospital.

After this review, the hospital started a three-month training program for coders that covered the coding and documentation issues identified in the initial audit. For immediate feedback on the accuracy of their DRG assignments, the coders received individual assistance in reviewing current charts.

As a result of the training, coding procedures at the hospital were changed. Instead of reviewing only a sample number of Medicare charts for accuracy and optimal billing, the coding supervisor began to review all Medicare charts. In a one-year period, the hospital estimates that its payments increased by more than $2.3 million.

Concurrent Review Offers Additional DRG Team Management Services

To maintain its increased case mix, the hospital administration decided to designate a nursing unit as a test site for concurrent review. Additional goals were to decrease the patient length of stay, improve cash flow, and assist physicians in completing charts. Coders concurrently followed a patient from admission to discharge, the chart was up to date and ready for code assignment and billing.

According to the medical record department supervisor, communication between the coders, unit nurses, utilization review nurses, and social workers has improved. Prior to concurrent review, the coders rarely talked with the health care staff about the patients progress. Now they do. The hospital administration is now planning to expand concurrent review to other nursing units.

Keeping Staff Current

On going education is the key to keeping the coding staff current. Education could occur in the following multiple ways:

- Time should be designated each quarter for the coding staff to review and discuss the most recent AHA's *Coding Clinic for ICD-9-CM*.
- Attend seminars, audioconferences, and/or teleconferences.

- Choose one topic per month and develop and offer an education training session on the topic. For example, educate on the clinical aspects of respiratory failure and the proper code assignment. If possible, seek assistance from the medical staff on the clinical aspects of the diagnosis and ask for an inservice.
- Work with ancillary department personnel to assist in the understanding of different tests and diagnoses. For example, schedule a meeting with the medical nutritionist to discuss parameters for diagnosing malnutrition.

Evaluating the Results

The Steps
- Compare new case mix to old.
- Report the bottom line: DRG impact statement.

Compare New Case Mix to Old
Case Mix is essential to achieving optimal payment. The first step in evaluating the results of the DRG team management strategy is to review the case mix index and the payment for each month the strategy was in place. To facilitate this review, complete a worksheet each month.

Exhibit 8: Worksheet: Case Mix Record (student worksheet)

Last month's case mix:	_____			
This month's case mix:	_____			
Difference in case mix:	_____			
(difference in case mix)	x	(your hospital rate)	=	(+/- in average resource in $)
(difference in average resource used per pt.)	x	(#pts. discharged this month)	=	(revenue impact from change in case mix)
Projected Annual Dollar Impact				
(monthly revenue impact)	x	12 months	=	(annualized dollar impact)

Example of Case Mix Impact

Last month's case mix:	1.3209			
This months case mix:	1.3769			
Difference in case mix:	0.056			
0.056 (difference in case mix)	x	$3,100 (your hospital rate)	=	+ $174 (+/- in average resource in $)
+ $174 (difference in average resource used per pt.)	x	300 (#pts. discharged this month)	=	$52,200 (revenue impact from change in case mix)
Projected Annual Dollar Impact				
$52,200 (monthly revenue impact)	x	12 months	=	$626,400 (annualized dollar impact)

Exhibit 9: Worksheet: Tracking Your Case Mix

Month	Case Mix	Year-to-Date
January		
February		
March		
April		
May		
June		
July		
August		
September		
October		
November		
December		

Factors Producing Fluctuation in Monthly Case Mix Index

The fluctuations in case mix may be due to the following factors:

Patients
Case complexity/severity
Demographics
Referral patterns
Seasonal influences

Hospitals
Preadmission screening
UR & QA
Formal educational process

External Environment
Regulatory requirements
QIO (formerly known as PRO) review
Workload
JCAHO review
Reward structure

Coders
Knowledge:
    Formal training
    Experience
Motivation:
    Work load
    Job stress
    Philosophy of coding
Process:
    DRG-relevant coding
    Concurrent coding

Physicians
Knowledge
    Specialty
    Clinical experience
    Special service programs
    Recording skills
    Cognizance of reporting rules
    Case-specific feedback
    Formal educational programs
    Documentation practices
    Motivations
    Staff by-laws
    Professional (peer) pressure
    QIO & JCAHO pressure
    Hospital administrative pressure
    Helpful encouragement
    Competitive demands

Process
    Relevant problem detection
    Establish clinical relevance
    Communications/logistics
    Completeness and promptness
    Systematic feedback

Reporting the Results

Team Responsibilities

Each member of the medical record team has a responsibility in the reporting process.

The coder prepares the DRG coding log, a monthly report that
- lists review of records with resulting DRG change
- shows revenue affected from coding process

The coding supervisor prepares the DRG revenue profile, a monthly report that
- summarizes DRG changes
- shows percentage of changes in DRGs
- lists total increased and decreased revenues by DRG
- identifies DRGs that may require further education

The DRG Impact Statement is a monthly report that
- lists current case mix, impact, and projected annual revenues
- shows total increased and decreased revenues from DRG coding program

Samples of each report follow.

Sample Report—Coder's DRG Log

The following is a completed sample of the DRG log kept by coders

Prepared by: K. Jones, Coder
Reporting Month: October 2003

DRG LOG

Medical Record #	Old DRG	RW	Payment*	DRG	New R.W.	Payment*	Reason for Change
1234	090	0.6147	$2,698.53	089	1.0463	$4,593.26	CC
1776	089	1.0463	$4,593.26	079	1.5974	$7,012.59	Omitted organism
3456	141	0.7473	$3,280.65	024	1.0121	$4,443.12	Sequence of Pdx
4567	122	1.0297	$4,520.38	121	1.6169	$7,098.19	Cardiovascular complications
5678	125	1.0947	$4,805.73	124	1.4367	$6,307.11	Complex diagnosis

*Based on average hospital rate of $4,390

Supervisor Reports

The following is a sample of the DRG revenue profile maintained by the coding supervisor.

Exhibit 11: DRG Revenue Profile

Monthly DRG Revenue Profile

Reporting month:	October 2003
Monthly report submitted by:	S. Smith, coding supervisor
Total # discharges:	300
# DRG discharges reviewed:	30
Total additional DRG revenues:	$21,579.95

DRG Trends

Old DRG	New DRG	# Changed	Total Variance	Reason for Change
090	089	4	$7,578.92	Omitted CC
089	079	3	7,257.99	Omitted organism
125	124	2	3,002.76	Complex diagnosis
122	121	1	2,577.81	Cardiovascular complication
141	024	1	1,162.47	Sequence
		11	$21,579.95	

The next report prepared by the supervisor is the monthly impact report. This report summarizes the status of the records.

Exhibit 13: Monthly Impact Report (completed sample)

TO: Health Information Manager

FROM: Coding Supervisor

Month: October 2003

Number of Records Reviewed: 30

Number of Records Referred: 14   47 percent of total

Number of Records Upgrade: 11   37 percent of total

Number of Records Decreased: 0

Method of Upgrading = Type of Change

  1. Sequencing of Principal: 1

  2. Additions: 9

  3. Other (specify, etc.): 1 Billing Department error

Average increase per case: $1,961.81

Average decrease per case: $0

Total increase for month: $21,579.95

Total decrease for month: $0

Conclusions: This month shows a 7% increase in the number of cases referred, and a 27 percent increase in the amount of increased payment over September.

Reports From the Health Information Manager to the Chief Executive Officer (CEO)/Chief Financial Officer (CFO)

The first reporting responsibility of the health information manager is to record fluctuations in the hospital's case mix.

The reports prepared by the coders and coding supervisor are used to report the case mix changes. These changes may be reported in a graphic representation, which clearly illustrates the trend of the case mix between months and over a designated time period.

Exhibit 15: Case Mix Comparison

Hospital X

2003–2004

  The Medicare case mix index reached a record high of 1.6162 in August 2003. This represents an increase of 0.1161 from the July 2003 figure.

  The cumulative 2003 Medicare case mix index is 1.4605, compared with the 2003 cumulative case mix index of 1.3382. This represents an increase of 0.1223.

  Coding education and up-front coding audits will remain a priority in an effort to maintain a high case mix index.

Using the case mix comparison, the health information manager may prepare a DRG increase and loss statement for the CEO/CFO.

Exhibit 16: Sample Report (completed sample)

DRG INCREASE STATEMENT	
HEALTH INFORMATION MANAGEMENT DEPARTMENT	
Month of September	
To: CEO/CFO	
FROM: Health information manager	
Operating expenses:	
Salaries	$15,000
Equipment/supplies	$ 387
Professional supplies	
Fees	$ 1,095
Hotel	$ 600
Transportation	$ 1,200
Food	$ 400
Revenues:	
	Case Mix
Last month's case mix	1.1593
Current case mix	1.2153
Case Mix difference	.056
Revenue attributable to case mix	
Fluctuation due to DRG Increase + $50,400	
Departmental profit/loss attributable to DRG organization + $31,718	

The Medicare case mix, or case mix index, measures the cost of a hospitals Medicare patient mix in relation to the cost of all Medicare patients. A low case mix may be indicative of coders not assigning a DRG that reflects hospital resources used to treat patients or potential documentation issues affecting accurate code assignment.

Why Concentrate on Case Mix?

Hospital payment under the IPPS depends largely on the DRGs assigned to Medicare cases. Higher weighted DRGs generate higher payments; as the case mix goes up, hospital payments should increase proportionally. Since Medicare accounts for a substantial portion of most hospital patients (typically 40 percent to 60 percent), it is worthwhile to concentrate on the case mix.

Small movements in the case mix can mean substantial gains or losses in income. For example, in the average 200 to 300 bed hospital with 2,750 annual Medicare discharges, if the case mix increases by one tenth of a point over the period of a year, a facility can expect to earn $700,000 to $1.21 million in additional income.

Important points about case mix include

- Higher weighted DRGs generate higher payments.
- As case mix goes up, payment goes up.
- Medicare normally accounts for 40 to 60 percent of hospital revenue.
- Even small moves in case mix mean substantial gains in payment.

Potential revenue impact on the hospital is great.

How to Calculate Your Case Mix

Case mix can be calculated by averaging the DRG RWs for all Medicare patients. Case mix is based upon the RWs assigned to DRGs. These RWs compare the average resources used in DRGs. Case mix is calculated as the sum of all DRG RWs divided by the number of Medicare cases. The following steps demonstrate case mix calculation.

Step 1: Figure the number of cases per DRG and the total weight of those cases.

Example:

DRG	No. of cases		RW per case	=	Total Weight
131	1	x	0.5676		0.5676
130	8	x	0.9505		7.6040
125	5	x	1.0947		5.4735
210	7	x	1.8477		12.9339
211	2	x	1.2544		2.5088
122	10	x	1.0297		10.2970
306	15	x	1.2257		18.3855
426	12	x	0.5087		6.1044
311	3	x	0.6258		1.8774
	63				65.7521

Step 2:   Divide the total weight of all DRGs by the total number of cases to obtain the CMI.

Example: 65.7521 / 63 = 1.044 (CMI)

Step 3:   Determine the average DRG payment by multiplying the case mix number by the hospital base rate.

Example: 1.044 x $4,390.00 (hospital base rate) = $4,583.16.

Relationship of Case Mix to Revenue

The relationship of case mix to revenue is illustrated in the following exhibit.

Exhibit 18: Hospital Average Payment (based on 4,400 discharges)

Medicare Case mix	Hospital Base Rate	Hospital Average Payment	Annual Revenue
1.32	$4,390	$5,795	$25,498,000
1.35	$4,390	$5,927	$26,078,800
1.49	$4,390	$6,541	$28,780,840
1.50	$4,390	$6,585	$28,974,000

Why Is Case Mix Rising?

We have seen an overall rise in the CMI from the initiation of the IPPS. The Prospective Payment Commission (ProPAC) states that three factors are pushing the case mix higher: (1) treatment patterns, (2) technology, and (3) coding.

The average DRG weight for Medicare discharges has increased as more patients in lower-weighted DRGs are shifted out of the inpatient setting and treated on an ambulatory basis. ProPAC notes that increases in the Medicare CMI between 1981 and 1984 are chiefly the result of this movement.

As technology changes, patients are being treated with more resource-intensive procedures. For example, the growth in coronary artery bypass surgery has contributed to an increase in the national case mix.

More complete and accurate coding is also responsible for an increase in the national case mix. An increase in the case mix does not reflect an actual increase in resource use, but increases payment by identifying factors that allow cases to be reassigned to a higher weighted DRG.

Of these factors, only coding can be directly influenced by hospitals.

How Your Case Mix Compares with Other Area Hospitals

Enter the state or regional numbers on the following worksheet. Enter your hospital's figures. Compare your hospitals case mix to the indicator for your region.

Worksheet Case Mix Comparisons

Use this worksheet to compare your hospital's case mix to the standard for your state or region.

Specific	State/Regional	Hospital	Difference
Case mix			
Avg. LOS (days)			
Avg. Medicare LOS (days)			

How Case Mix Is Improved

A hospitals ability to improve case mix is related primarily to physician documentation and medical record coding. One of the best ways to try to improve case mix is to determine whether CCs are present.

Tools for Data Quality: Focus on Inpatient Documentation for Coding

Introduction

Ingenix, Inc's. "tools for data quality" is a comprehensive source of information that can help the health care professional obtain accurate coding according to the latest federal rules and regulations.

These tools are based on various sources, all of which incorporate the latest information available from the CMS. The sources include *DRG Expert*, the AHA's *Coding Clinic for ICD-9-CM* publications, *3M's DRGs Definitions Manual*, and UHDDS definitions.

These tools promote accurate reimbursement because they help the coder understand how to read and review the medical record for documentation. The coder learns how to select and sequence diagnoses and procedures, identify conditions that can affect payment, and assign optimum diagnosis-related groups in accordance with the latest CMS regulations.

Health information managers can benefit from the information by using it to establish and follow consistent policies and procedures. The tools help coding supervisors monitor the quality of coding and DRG assignment and train coders and other staff in coding.

In todays health care environment, health information management isn't the only department that can contribute to optimum reimbursement. In addition to coders, the tools are designed to serve utilization review personnel, concurrent review staff, DRG coordinators and nursing staff.

The tools are divided into the following sections:

- definitions of the basic medical and reimbursement terms needed to assign proper ICD-9-CM codes
- guidelines for record review of documentation
- guidelines for selecting the principal diagnosis
- guidelines for sequencing the secondary diagnosis codes
- guidelines for selecting the principal procedure
- optimization techniques and investigative review

The information contained in the tools forms the basic infrastructure that underlies coding today. Following these rules and guidelines will help the health care professional obtain optimal reimbursement, in full accordance with federal rules and regulations.

Definitions

Principal diagnosis*
The condition established after study to be chiefly responsible for occasioning the patients admission to the hospital for care.

Other (additional) diagnoses*
All conditions that coexist at the time of admission, that develop subsequently or that affect the treatment received and/or the length of stay. Diagnoses related to an earlier episode of care that have no bearing on the current hospital stay are to be excluded.

Complication⁺
A condition that arises during the hospital stay that prolongs the length of stay at least one day in approximately 75 percent of cases.

Comorbid condition⁺
A pre-existing condition that, because of its presence with a specific diagnosis, causes an increase in length of stay by at least one day in approximately 75 percent of cases.

Principal procedure*
A procedure performed for definitive treatment rather than for diagnostic or exploratory purposes, or if necessary to take care of a complication. If two procedures appear to be principal, the one most closely related to the principal diagnosis should be selected as the principal procedure.

Secondary procedure(s)
Procedures performed in addition to the principal procedure during the patients stay.

Diagnosis-related groups (DRGs)
A patient classification scheme that provides a means of relating the type of patients a hospital treats to the costs incurred by the hospital.

---

*Definition is taken from the uniform hospital discharge data set.

⁺Complications/comorbid conditions are termed "CCs."

Guidelines for Record Review of Documentation

The entire medical record should be reviewed when coding. All reports should be reviewed and findings and treatment correlated with the diagnoses that are identified.

History and Physical

Review the reason for admission by examining symptoms, signs and physicians initial impression, and correlate with the treatment plan and principal diagnosis. The medical service or specialty unit to which the patient was admitted may also help determine the principal diagnosis. Scan the history and physical to identify conditions that could be comorbid and coexisting at the time of admission. The history may document conditions such as previous myocardial infarctions, pacemaker in situ, dialysis status, stoma status, organ or tissue transplants, history of cancer, or chronic conditions such as hypertension, diabetes mellitus, chronic bronchitis, renal failure, COPD and cardiac conditions.

Progress Notes

Carefully review the progress notes. At the time of coding, they may be the sole documentation source to detect

- complications that arose during the hospitalization
- a secondary diagnosis for which the patient was treated
- procedures performed during the hospital stay that were performed outside the operating room

Remember that an excisional (surgical) debridement may be done anywhere in the hospital as long as a surgical instrument was used to debride the area.

Emergency Room Report

If present, this document should be reviewed to identify signs and symptoms that can be correlated with other diagnoses that could be designated as principal diagnoses. Also, vital signs and laboratory and x-ray findings may be documented, which can help substantiate principal and secondary diagnoses.

Consultation Report

Read these reports to detect additional diagnoses or clarifications of the principal diagnosis. Review for complications for which the patient might have been treated. In general, consultations use additional hospital resources and may validate the addition of certain secondary sources.

Operative Report

Review the operative report to identify additional procedures that might not be documented in the title of the operative procedure. Sometimes biopsies, lysis of adhesions or other additional procedures are performed during the same operative episode. Look for the presence of iatrogenic complications, such as intraoperative lacerations, that may have occurred during the course of surgery. If joint replacement surgery is performed bilaterally, code the procedure twice.

Pre- and Postoperative Anesthesia Report

Review the pre- and postoperative anesthesia report for any preoperative conditions, complications during surgery or complications occurring immediately after surgery.

Diagnoses such as COPD, chronic atrial fibrillation or asthma, which may not be under active treatment but affect the anesthesiologists management of the patient, should be coded.

Pathology Report

Review this report to confirm or obtain more detailed information about the postoperative diagnosis. If the procedure was performed to check for a malignancy, review the pathology report to see if there were any metastatic sites, and code accordingly.

When the pathology report and the attending physicians list of final diagnoses appear to be in conflict, the attending physician must be consulted for clarification.

All pertinent diagnoses documented in the pathology report that relate to the surgical procedure(s) preformed should be coded.

Physicians Orders

Review physicians orders for a treatment plan, and correlate with the principal diagnosis and additional diagnoses. If the order included routine treatment for chronic conditions, such as diabetes and CHF, review the record for documentation. Ask the physician for additional documentation if medication and treatment, such as antibiotic usage and blood transfusions, reflect conditions that are not documented.

Physicians orders are the primary documentation source for correlating patient management and resource consumption with diagnoses and procedures.

Nurses Notes

Review nurses notes to identify any problems (e.g., for surgical patients, watch for wound appearance, drainage, redness, swelling, infection, etc., minor procedures and treatment the patient may have had). Ask for physician documentation of conditions that were found and treated, including conditions for which resources were required for investigation while the patient was in the hospital. The following are conditions that might be identified:

- decubitus ulcers (documentation of skin conditions and breakdown, excisional debridements performed)
- urinary retention requiring a straight catheterization or Foley catheter
- postoperative complications, such as nausea, vomiting, temperature elevation, urinary retention and wound infections
- telemetry readings (e.g., combination heart blocks, atrial fibrillation, ventricular fibrillation)
- hypotension in myocardial infarctions (cardiovascular complication)
- blood transfusion reactions
- hallucinations in a previously normal patient
- seizures

Medication Record

Review the medication record for documentation of medications given to the patient, and correlate with the diagnoses identified. Ideally, a diagnosis should relate to each medication administered.

Laboratory Reports

Review the laboratory reports for abnormal findings. Documentation of normal ranges of laboratory tests for your facility are helpful. It is beneficial for the coder to determine which disease process the physician is ruling in or out by relating it to the laboratory tests ordered. Look especially at the serum electrolyte report for increased or decreased sodium and potassium. Correlate this information with the physicians orders and progress notes for the treatment plan.

Never code a diagnosis on the basis of abnormal laboratory values alone. Use abnormal laboratory values as a trigger for more intense chart review and ask the physician for clarification.

Radiology Reports

Review the radiology reports for abnormal findings. Chest x-ray reports may document conditions such as chronic pulmonary disease, bronchiectasis and abnormal infiltrates in the lungs. Documentation in the x-ray report may indicate adverse reactions that may be a CC. Such reactions may include respiratory insufficiency from an allergic reaction to intravenous pyelogram (IVP) dye or any other reaction to a procedure performed in x-ray.

Never code a diagnosis on the basis of radiological interpretations alone. Use the abnormal radiological interpretations as a trigger for more intense chart review and ask the physician for clarification.

Respiratory Therapy Notes

Review the respiratory therapy notes for conditions for which the patient is receiving therapy. Coexisting conditions include:

- atelectasis, postoperative or otherwise
- chronic obstructive lung disease
- bronchiolectasis
- coal workers pneumonoconiosis (black lung disease)
- bacterial or aspiration pneumonitis/pneumonia
- respiratory insufficiency
- respiratory failure
- chronic mucopurulent bronchitis

Also review the respiratory therapy notes for any changes in treatments (e.g., discontinuation of ventilator, treatment with continuous positive airway pressure [CPAP], etc.)

Seek additional documentation from the physician if any potential diagnoses are identified.

Physical Therapy Notes

Review physical therapy (PT) notes for CCs, other conditions or additional procedures. Such conditions might be

- pathological fractures
- torticollis
- pyogenic arthritis
- juvenile rheumatoid arthritis
- brachial neuritis (radicular syndrome of upper limbs) and cervical radiculitis
- residuals of a cardiovascular accident (CVA), such as hemiparesis. (These types of conditions can help to validate a prolonged length of stay or the severity of the illness.)
- postlaminectomy syndrome
- excisional debridements performed in PT by a physician

Seek additional documentation from the physician if any potential diagnoses are identified.

Social Service Notes

Conditions that are long standing or that may have developed while the patient was in the hospital are important to document. Conditions that require posthospital management and may increase the length of stay include

- alcoholism
- high-risk pregnancies
- mechanical ventilation dependence
- renal dialysis status
- organ or tissue replacement (except skin, cornea and bone)
- COPD

Dietary Notes

Review notes for specific dietary needs that indicate the treatment of conditions such as

- malnutrition (supplemental feedings, such as Ensure, correction of fluid and electrolyte abnormalities, and hyperalimentation therapy)
- cachexia
- cholelithiasis/cholesystitis
- protein deficiency anemia
- other specified nutritional anemias (e.g., scorbutic anemia)
- acute gastritis
- diabetes mellitus (insulin dependent or out of control)
- vitamin K deficiency

Pharmacy Notes

Review pharmacy notes for drug sensitivity, which may indicate adverse effects of drugs. Some examples are

- urinary retention when related to drug usage
- urticaria/hives, allergic
- toxic side effects of certain drugs (e.g., renal manifestations)
- drug-related hallucinations;
- brief psychotic states secondary to drug reactions
- palpitations

It is helpful to know which drugs these side effects are related to and what conditions are managed with specific drugs. For instance, the drugs below are used to manage the conditions described:

- quinidine-arrhythmia
- septra-urinary tract infections
- aminoglycosides-resistant infections
- digoxin-congestive heart failure
- theophylline-asthma, COPD

Discharge Summary

If available, review the discharge summary and compare it with the diagnoses found throughout the medical record. If information is found within the discharge summary that is not found within the body of the record, the physician should be educated on the need of concurrent documentation. The discharge summary should be a summation of what is already documented in the medical record.

Guidelines for Selecting the Principal Diagnosis

Steps for Selecting the Principal Diagnosis

The selection of principal diagnosis will always be determined by the circumstances leading to acute care hospitalization.

First, look for the reason for admission, such as symptoms, complaints and the suspected, probable or rule out diagnoses to be studied by the physician. Second, review the treatment rendered, such as medications prescribed, tests ordered and procedures performed. Third, correlate the treatment with each possible or probable principal diagnosis. Finally, select the principal diagnosis according to the UHDDS definitions and the following guidelines.

Coexisting Conditions

When two or more conditions coexist at the time of admission and are treated equally, select the most resource-intensive condition as the principal diagnosis, indicated by the DRG with the highest RW.

Example: The patient presented on admission with congestive heart failure with coexisting pneumonia. Both were treated with IV medication during the patients hospital stay.

Principal diagnosis: pneumonia

Suspected Condition

A diagnosis described as possible, probable, suspected or in other inconclusive terms may be designated as the principal diagnosis when it remains the final diagnosis after study and meets the UHDDS definition of principal diagnosis.

Example: An 80-year-old female presented with fever, shaking, chills, and cough that had lasted two days. The complete blood count (CBC) showed a white blood cell count (WBC) of 16,000. The chest x-ray showed slight haziness in the right middle lobe. Blood/sputum cultures were negative. The patient was given two antibiotics (a cephalosporin and an aminiglycoside), oxygen and intravenous (IV) fluids, and she gradually improved. The physician treated the patient for pneumonia even though the culture evidence was absent. This is a clinical pneumonia.

Principal diagnosis: probable pneumonia right lobe

Unclear diagnosis

When a patient presents with symptoms, the cause of the symptoms may be unclear. Probable causes of and treatment for the symptom should be researched and documented in the medial record.

Example: The patient presented with syncope and disorientation. Possible causes of the syncope could be bradycardia or other arrhythmias, severe anemia, transient ischemic attack (TIA), electrolyte imbalance or a low blood sugar level.

Principal diagnosis: Consult with the physician to clarify the cause(s) before assigning the principal diagnosis.

Symptoms

If a symptom or abnormal sign is stated in the medical record as the reason for admission but its cause is identified after study, assign the code for the cause as the principal diagnosis. Do not code a symptom when it is inherent in the expected disease process.

Example: A patient was admitted with abdominal pain, but acute appendicitis was confirmed. Do not code the symptom.

Principal diagnosis: acute appendicitis

A symptom may be designated as a principal diagnosis in only the following three instances:

- When no definitive diagnosis has been established (etiology unknown)
  Example: A patient was admitted with abdominal pain. The gastrointestinal (GI) series, ultrasound and oral cholecystogram were negative. No definitive diagnosis was established.
  Principal diagnosis: abdominal pain, etiology unknown
- When the symptom is a manifestation of an adverse reaction to a drug used therapeutically
  Example: A patient was admitted with nausea and vomiting due to a toxic effect of digitalis (digitalis toxicity).
  Principal diagnosis: nausea and vomiting
  Secondary diagnosis: digitalis toxicity (E code)

- When a symptom is followed by contrasting or comparative diagnoses, the symptom should be sequenced first. Each contrasting or comparative diagnosis should be coded as a suspected (secondary) condition.
  Example: The patients final diagnosis was hematuria due to acute pyelonephritis versus renal calculi.
  Principal diagnosis: Hematuria
  Secondary diagnoses: acute pyelonephritis, renal calculi

Contrasting or Comparative Diagnoses

For contrasting or comparative diagnoses, the conditions are coded and sequenced according to the details on admission. If no further ruling identifies the principal diagnosis, either may be chosen. You may choose the most resource-intensive diagnosis (highest paying DRG) as the principal diagnosis.

Example: The patients final diagnosis was cholelithiasis versus ulcer.

Principal diagnosis: cholelithiasis

Secondary diagnosis: ulcer

Late effect

When the residual condition is the reason for admission, it is sequenced as the principal diagnosis. The cause of the late effect is listed as a late effect secondary diagnosis. When a residual is not identified, the cause of the late effect is the principal diagnosis.

Example: A patient was admitted because of scarring due to a previous third-degree burn.

Principal diagnosis: scarring

Secondary diagnosis: late effect of burn

Multiple injuries

If a patient has multiple injuries, the injury the attending physician identifies as the most resource-intensive is the principal diagnosis.

Example: After an automobile accident, a patient was admitted with facial lacerations, which were sutured, a closed fracture of the left tibia, which was casted, a fractured rib and a pneumothorax. Chest tubes were inserted for drainage and to reinflate the lung. The physician determined that the pneumothorax was the most severe injury.

Principal diagnosis: pneumothorax

Secondary diagnoses: fractured rib, fractured tibial shaft, closed, and facial lacerations.

Rule out or R/O

If ruled out or R/O is noted at the end of the diagnosis statement, do not code the conditions.

If rule out or R/O is noted at the beginning of the diagnosis statement, the suspected condition can be sequenced as the principal diagnosis. See the guidelines for "Suspected Condition."

Example: The patients final diagnosis was R/O kidney stones.

Principal diagnosis: kidney stones

Manifestation Codes

Never use a manifestation code as a principal diagnosis. (Manifestation codes are italicized in the ICD-9-CM code book.) The underlying disease is reported as the principal diagnosis.

Example: The patients final diagnosis was diabetic cataract.

Principal diagnosis: diabetes with ophthalmic manifestation

Secondary diagnosis: diabetic cataract

Classification of External Causes of Injury and Poisoning (E Codes)

Never use codes E800–E999 to designate the principal diagnosis.

E codes may be used to classify environmental events, circumstances and other conditions as the cause of injury and other adverse effects. E codes are used in addition to a code from the main classification. Use of E codes is optional except for codes E930–E949, which identify substances used therapeutically as the cause of adverse effects.

Example: Patient was admitted to the hospital after falling on the ice and fracturing her hip.

Principal diagnosis: fracture of hip

Secondary diagnosis: fall from slipping on ice (E code)

Classification of Factors Influencing Health Status and Contact with Health Services (V codes)

Certain V codes that represent the reason for admission to the hospital are assigned as principal diagnoses. Conditions that coexist at the time of admission are coded and sequenced following the V code.

Example: A patient was admitted to the hospital for chemotherapy for cancer of the liver.

Principal diagnosis: admission for chemotherapy (V code)

Secondary diagnosis: cancer of the liver

Multiple Burns

The principal diagnosis will be the burn site of the greatest severity. Code burns in the following priority list order:

- deep necrosis of underlying tissues with loss of a body part (deep third or fourth degree)
- deep necrosis of underlying tissues without loss of a body part (deep third or fourth degree)
- full-thickness skin loss (third degree)
- blisters, epidermal loss (second degree)
- erythema (first degree)
- unspecified degree of burn

Original Treatment Plan Not Carried Out

The principal diagnosis will be the condition, which after study occasioned an acute-care level of hospitalization, even though diagnostic and treatment plans were not carried out, for any reason.

Example: A patient is admitted for abdominal pain, etiology unknown. After less than 24 hours on the medical unit, the patient refuses scheduled exploratory laparotomy.

Principal diagnosis: Abdominal pain

Secondary diagnosis: surgical or other procedure not carried out because of patients decision (V code)

Guidelines for Reporting Secondary Diagnosis Codes

For reporting purposes the definition of other diagnoses is interpreted in addition conditions that affect patient care in terms of requiring

- clinical evaluation
- therapeutic treatment
- diagnostic procedures
- extended length of stay
- increased nursing care and/or monitoring

©2003 Ingenix, Inc.

As a generalization, other diagnoses that should be reported are conditions affecting patient management and/or consuming hospital resources.

Guidelines for Sequencing Secondary Diagnostic Codes

Correct sequencing of secondary diagnostic codes is of the utmost importance.

- CCs always should be sequenced in the nos. 2 through 9 positions on the UB-92, thereby taking precedence over non-CC diagnoses and ensuring proper DRG assignment.
- The CC exclusion list always should be consulted when sequencing secondary diagnosis codes.

(Note: This should not affect sequencing in the nos. 2 through 9 positions if the condition is documented and treated.)

Guidelines for Selecting the Principal Procedure

When there is more than one possible principal procedure, sequence the one most closely related to the principal diagnosis first.

Sequence therapeutic procedures first, even if the therapeutic procedure does not relate to the principal diagnosis. A therapeutic rather than a diagnostic procedure is the principal procedure, no matter how closely related the diagnostic procedure is to the principal diagnosis.

When two or more therapeutic procedures are equally related to the principal diagnosis, sequence the procedure that took place in the operating room first. If both were performed in the operating room, sequence the procedure involving tissue removal first.

The UHDDS states that all significant procedures must be reported. A significant procedure is one that

- is surgical in nature
- carries a procedural risk
- carries an anesthetic risk
- requires specialized training

All procedures affecting the determination of payment must be reported.

Coding Techniques and Investigative Review

The following conditions and specific DRGs lend themselves to coding potential. When different types of conditions change to specific DRGs, they are listed at the end of the description of each condition.

MDC 4: Respiratory System

Condition–Pneumonia
Tentative DRGs: 089, 090, 091
Potential DRGs: 079, 081

Investigative Review–Aspiration Pneumonia
The patient may present with a history of nausea and vomiting and/or choking on foods or fluids. This condition is most frequently seen in elderly bedridden patients and those in nursing homes. A history of recurrent pneumonia, previous cerebrovascular accident (CVA) with dysphagia or a patient with a feed tube are "red flags" for suspected aspiration pneumonia. Documentation may indicate a sudden marked elevation of temperature, marked increase in white blood cell count and infiltrate in left lower lobe.

Investigative Review—Bacterial Pneumonia

When physicians admit patients to the hospital with a diagnosis of pneumonia, they usually will order a sputum culture. Review the culture and sensitivity for growth of one of the following resistant organisms:

- *Klebsiella pneumoniae (482.0)*
- *Salmonella* (003.22)
- Gram-negative (482.83)
- *Staphylococcus* (482.4X)
- *E. coli* (482.82)
- *Psueudomonas* (482.1)
- *Proteus* (482.83)
- Other specified bacteria (*Citrobacter, Serratia, Legionella*, etc.) (482.89)

If an organism is identified in the sputum cultures, the physician MUST identify the organism as the causative agent in relation to the pneumonia.

Condition—Acute and simple chronic bronchitis

Tentative DRGs: 096, 097

Potential DRG: 088

Investigative Review—Acute bronchitis and COPD

Patients with an underlying COPD who are admitted with acute bronchitis are assigned code 491.21, obstructive chronic bronchitis with acute exacerbation. No code is necessary for acute bronchitis (466.0). However, if the patient is admitted with another acute lung condition, which causes an exacerbation of his or her chronic obstructive bronchitis, such as viral pneumonia (480.9) with acute exacerbation of chronic obstructive bronchitis (491.21), both codes may be used. The selection of principal diagnosis will depend on the circumstances of the admission.

Condition—Any respiratory diagnosis as principal diagnosis

Tentative DRGs: 078–102

Potential DRGs: 475, 482, 483

Investigative Review—Mechanical Ventilator Support

Carefully review the medical record (progress, radiological, respiratory therapy, and nurses notes) for documentation indicating that the patient was being maintained on ventilator support, and no OR procedure or tracheostomy was performed during the hospital stay. Patients with a respiratory system principal diagnosis with no surgical system principal diagnosis with no surgical procedure or tracheostomy and mechanical ventilation (96.70–96.72) will continue to group to DRG 475.

Investigative Review—Tracheostomies

Carefully review the medical record (progress, radiological, respiratory therapy, and nurses notes) for documentation indicating that the patient had a temporary (31.1), mediastinal (31.21) or other permanent (31.29) tracheostomy. Determine whether the patient was treated for a condition/disorder of the mouth, larynx or pharynx. These cases will group to DRG 482. Cases that do not include a mouth, larynx, or pharynx condition will group to the high-weighted DRG 483.

(DRGs 078-102 to DRGs 482 and 483)

MDC 5: Circulatory System

Condition –Myocardial infarction without major complication
Tentative DRG: 122
Potential DRG: 121

Investigative Review—Major Complication
Review the emergency room record, progress notes, blood pressure record, and nurses notes for documentation of a valid major complication.

Condition–Angina pectoris
Tentative DRG: 140
Potential DRG: 138

Investigative Review—Cardiac Arrhythmia
When a patient is admitted with chest pain, the most common diagnosis assigned is angina pectoris. However, in certain stances there can be an underlying cause for the angina other than arteriosclerotic heart disease (ASHD).

If the patient had a history of and was admitted with cardiac arrhythmia (tachycardia, atrial fibrillation) and required control of the arrhythmia, which in turn produced the angina, then the arrhythmias should be sequenced as the principal diagnosis, with the angina pectoris as the secondary diagnosis. Medications to look for are quinidine and other cardiac regulators and antiarrhythmic drugs.

Condition–Circulatory disorders with cardiac catheterization without complex diagnosis
Tentative DRG: 125
Potential DRG: 124

Investigative Review—Complex Diagnosis
These diagnoses may be sequenced as principal or secondary.

Review the history and physical, transfer summary, special ancillary reports and progress notes for documentation of
- unstable angina (411.1)
- congestive cardiomyopathy (425.4)
- congestive heart failure (428.0)
- cardiogenic shock (785.51)
- any other condition designated as a complex diagnosis

Condition/Procedure–Percutaneous cardiovascular procedures
Tentative DRGs: 516, 517, 518
Potential DRG: 106

Investigative Review—Coronary Bypass Surgery
Review cardiac lab reports for percutaneous procedures (35.96, 36.01, 36.05) performed along with bypass surgery.

Condition–Coronary bypass without cardiac catheterization
Tentative DRG: 107
Potential DRG: 106

Investigative Review—Cardiac Catheterization
Review the operative report and cardiac lab reports for cardiac catheterization (37.21, 37.22, 37.23) performed in conjunction with bypass surgery.

MDC 6: Digestive System

Condition–Gastroenteritis
Tentative DRGs: 182, 183, 184
Potential DRGs: 174, 175, 176, 179, 296, 297

Investigative Review—Dehydration
If a patient was admitted with dehydration due to nausea, vomiting and diarrhea and was found to have gastroenteritis, review the record for treatment directed toward the dehydration. The dehydration can be used as the principal diagnosis when the physicians plans included rehydration at the time of admission. Look for IV fluids being administered at a rate greater than 100 cc per hour for initial rehydration.
(DRGs 182, 183, 184 to DRGs 296, 297)

Investigative Review—Severe Gastritis with Gastrointestinal Bleeding
Gastrointestinal bleeding may be sequenced as the principal diagnosis if it is addressed and aggressively treated (e.g., esophagogastroduodenoscopy, medication treatment). Review the record for documentation of treatment given. Note that category 535 now carries a fifth digit to identify any gastrointestinal bleeding associated with gastritis and/or duodenitis.

Code 578.X may be sequenced as the principal diagnosis only when the etiology of the bleeding is unknown.
(DRG 182, 183, 184 to DRGs 174, 175)

Investigative Review—Erosive Gastritis with Obstruction or Perforation
Review the discharge summary and progress notes for evidence of erosive gastritis with evidence of obstruction or perforation (531.10, 531.11, 531.31, 531.50, 531.51, 531.71, 531.91).

Investigative Review—Regional Enteritis
Documentation in the medical record of regional enteritis or idiopathic proctocolitis can result in optimization.
(DRGs 182, 183, 184 to DRG 179)

Condition–Uncomplicated peptic ulcer
Tentative DRGs: 177, 178
Potential DRG:176

Investigative Review—Complicated Peptic Ulcer
Review the pathology report for acute appendicitis with peritoneal abscess, peritonitis or malignant neoplasm of appendix.
(DRGs 166, 167 to DRGs 164, 165)

Investigative Review—Peritoneal Adhesiolysis
Review the operative report for documentation indicating that lysis of adhesions was performed because of obstruction due to the adhesions or that the adhesions increased the difficulty of the procedure.
(DRG 166 to DRG 150)

Condition—Cholecystitis with total cholecystectomy with common duct exploration (CDE) with CC
Tentative DRG: 195
Potential DRG: 193

Investigative Review—Other Billing Tract Procedures
Review the operative notes for any valid biliary tract procedures, such as anastomosis, cholecystostomy or dilation of sphincter of Oddi, and anesthesia record or progress notes to ensure that all procedures performed were coded appropriately. Also, review the operative report for documentation that a partial cholecystectomy was performed, as this will impact payment.

Condition—Total cholecystectomy except by laparoscope without common duct exploration with CC
Tentative DRG: 197
Potential DRG: 195

Investigative Review—Common Bile Duct Exploration
Review the operative report to see if a common bile duct exploration was performed.

MDC 9: Integumentary System

Condition—Cellulitis
Tentative DRGs: 277, 278, 279
Potential DRGs: 271, 263, 264

Investigative Review—Skin Ulcer
When there is documentation of a decubitus ulcer (707.0) or other chronic skin ulcer (707.1x–707.9) in addition to cellulitis, both conditions should be coded. The selection of principal diagnosis depends upon the circumstances of the admission. If the focus of the admission is limited to therapy of the cellulitis, it is designated the principal diagnosis; but in many cases treatment will be directed toward the chronic ulcer with debridements and/or skin grafting in which case, the chronic ulcer may be the principal diagnosis. Note that gangrenous cellulitis is coded to 785.4, gangrene, and the ulcer would be sequenced first (principal diagnosis).

Note that in an infected open wound may also be described as an ulcer. These wounds should be classified as open wounds, complicated, in chapter 17 of the ICD-9-CM code book.

(DRGs 277, 278, 279 to DRG 271)

Investigative Review—Surgical Debridement
Excisional (surgical) debridements are performed to remove necrotic skin. This excision is performed using a sharp instrument (scalpel), rather than chemical debriders or whirlpool debridement. Check the record, particularly in the progress notes, for documentation of surgical debridement.

(DRGs 277, 278, 279 to DRGs 263, 264)

Condition-Ulcer
Tentative DRG: 271
Potential DRGs: 263, 264

Investigative Review—Surgical Debridement
Excisional (surgical) debridements are performed to remove necrotic skin. This excision is performed using a sharp instrument (scalpel), rather than chemical debriders or whirlpool debridement. Check the record, particularly in the progress notes, for documentation of surgical debridement.

The following list shows some of the most common diagnoses for which debridements are performed:

- decubitus ulcer
- cellulitis
- stasis ulcer
- burns
- diabetic ulcer
- arteriosclerotic ulcers

DRG Decision Trees

Typical DRG Structure for a Major Diagnostic Category

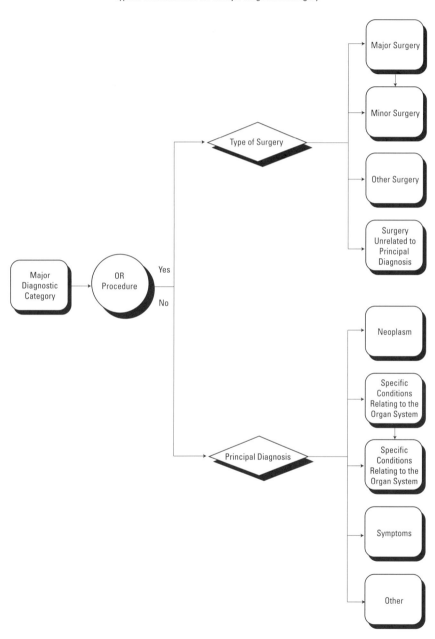

DRG Decision Trees

Major Diagnostic Category 1
Diseases and Disorders of the Nervous System

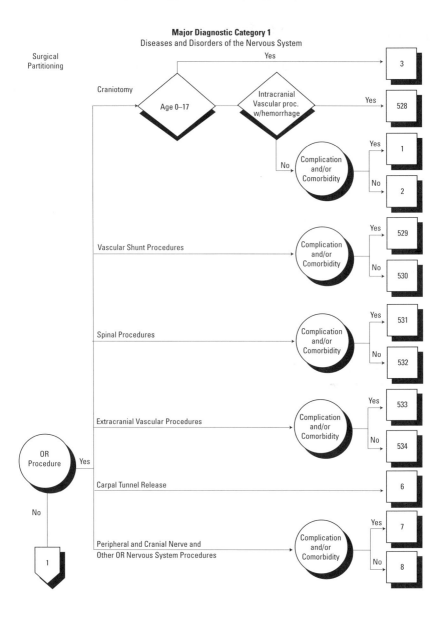

Surgical
Partitioning

Yes → 3

Craniotomy

Age 0–17

Intracranial Vascular proc. w/hemorrhage — Yes → 528

No → Complication and/or Comorbidity
- Yes → 1
- No → 2

Vascular Shunt Procedures → Complication and/or Comorbidity
- Yes → 529
- No → 530

Spinal Procedures → Complication and/or Comorbidity
- Yes → 531
- No → 532

Extracranial Vascular Procedures → Complication and/or Comorbidity
- Yes → 533
- No → 534

OR Procedure — Yes

Carpal Tunnel Release → 6

Peripheral and Cranial Nerve and Other OR Nervous System Procedures → Complication and/or Comorbidity
- Yes → 7
- No → 8

No → 1

Major Diagnostic Category 1
Diseases and Disorders of the Nervous System

Medical
Partitioning

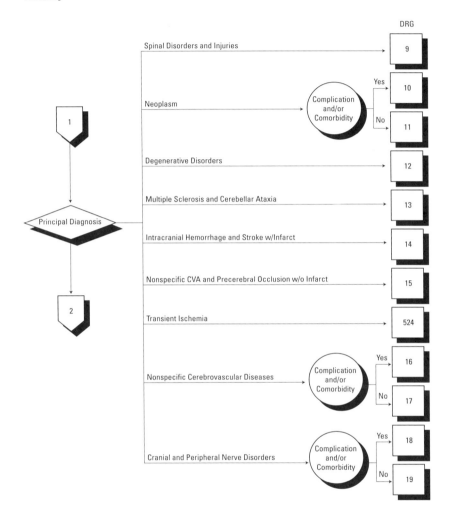

Major Diagnostic Category 1
Diseases and Disorders of the Nervous System

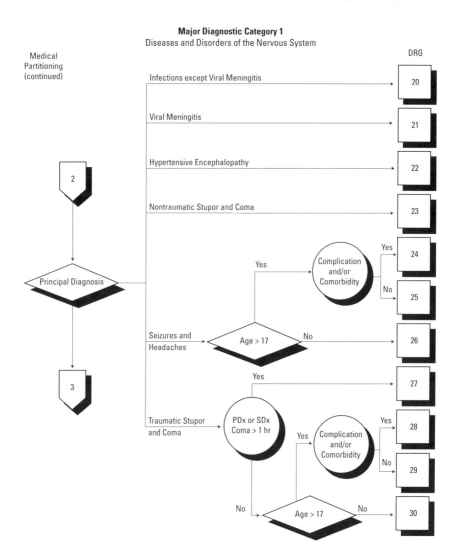

PDx = Principal Diagnosis
SDx = Secondary Diagnosis

Major Diagnostic Category 1
Diseases and Disorders of the Nervous System

Medical
Partitioning
(continued)

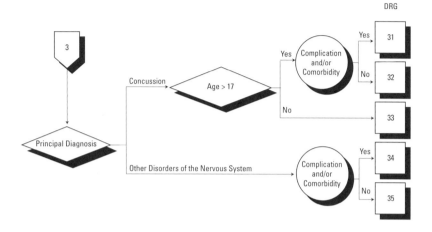

Major Diagnostic Category 2
Diseases and Disorders of the Eye

Surgical
Partitioning

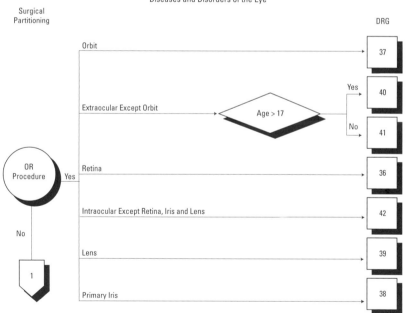

DRG Decision Trees

Major Diagnostic Category 2
Diseases and Disorders of the Eye

Medical
Partitioning

DRG

©2003 Ingenix, Inc.

Major Diagnostic Category 3
Diseases and Disorders of the Ear, Nose, Mouth, and Throat

Surgical
Partitioning

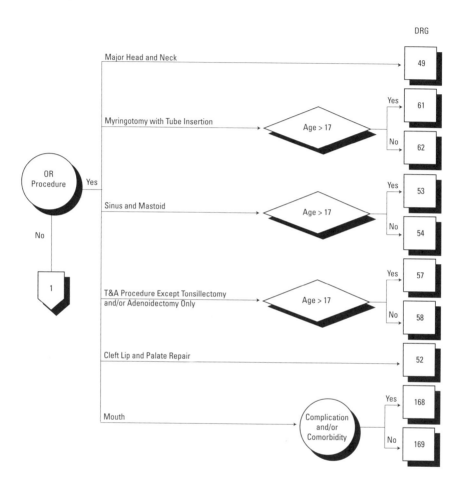

Major Diagnostic Category 3
Diseases and Disorders of the Ear, Nose, Mouth, and Throat

Surgical
Partitioning
(continued)

DRG

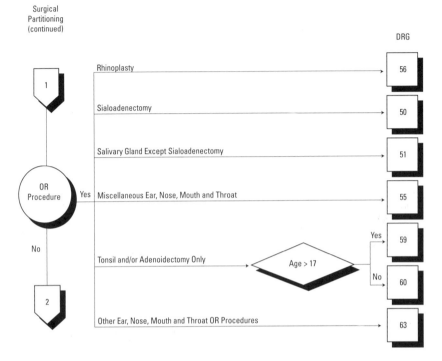

Rhinoplasty	56
Sialoadenectomy	50
Salivary Gland Except Sialoadenectomy	51
Miscellaneous Ear, Nose, Mouth and Throat	55
Tonsil and/or Adenoidectomy Only — Age > 17 — Yes	59
Tonsil and/or Adenoidectomy Only — Age > 17 — No	60
Other Ear, Nose, Mouth and Throat OR Procedures	63

Major Diagnostic Category 3
Diseases and Disorders of the Ear, Nose, Mouth, and Throat

Medical
Partitioning

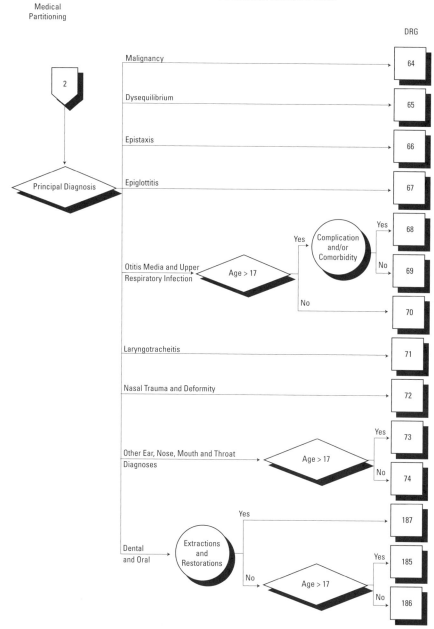

Major Diagnostic Category 4
Diseases and Disorders of the Respiratory System

Surgical
Partitioning

DRG

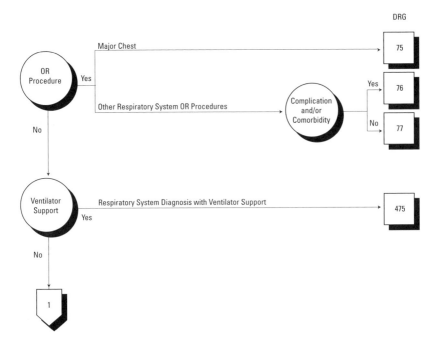

Major Diagnostic Category 4

Diseases and Disorders of the Respiratory System

Medical
Partitioning

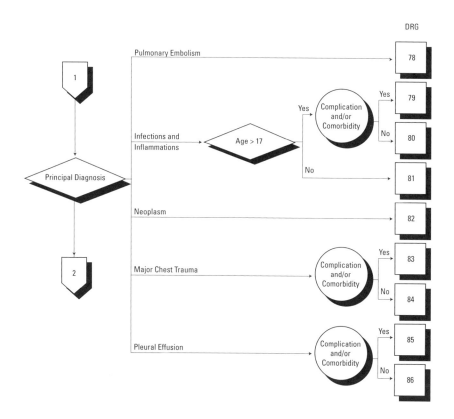

DRG Decision Trees

Major Diagnostic Category 4
Diseases and Disorders of the Respiratory System

Medical
Partitioning
(continued)

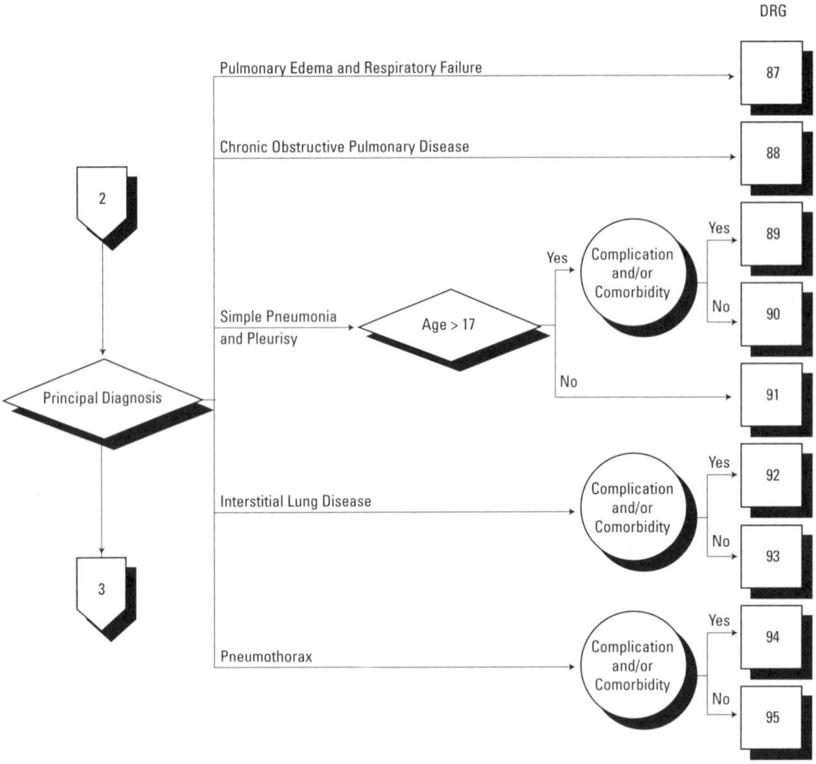

DRG

Pulmonary Edema and Respiratory Failure → 87

Chronic Obstructive Pulmonary Disease → 88

2

Simple Pneumonia and Pleurisy → Age > 17

Yes → Complication and/or Comorbidity
- Yes → 89
- No → 90

No → 91

Principal Diagnosis

Interstitial Lung Disease → Complication and/or Comorbidity
- Yes → 92
- No → 93

3

Pneumothorax → Complication and/or Comorbidity
- Yes → 94
- No → 95

Major Diagnostic Category 4
Diseases and Disorders of the Respiratory System

Medical
Partitioning
(continued)

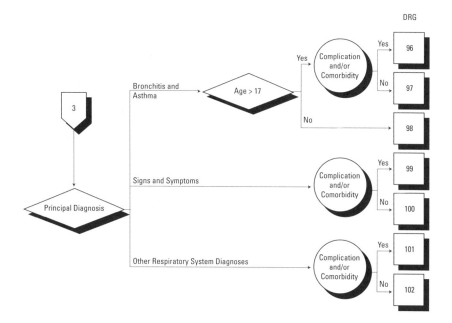

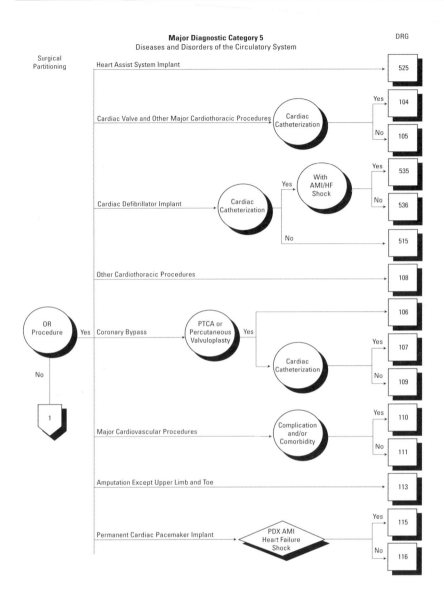

Major Diagnostic Category 5
Diseases and Disorders of the Circulatory System

Major Diagnostic Category 5
Diseases and Disorders of the Circulatory System

Surgical
Partitioning
(continued)

DRG

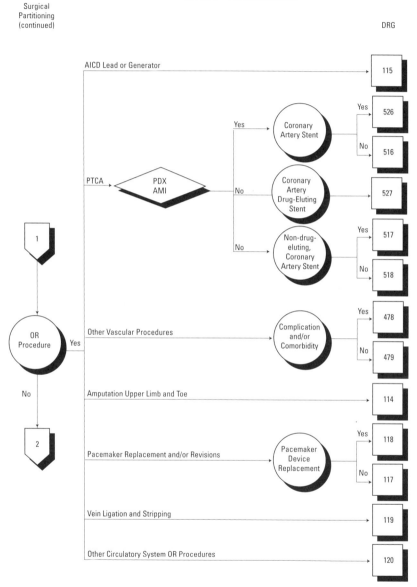

Major Diagnostic Category 5
Diseases and Disorders of the Circulatory System

Medical
Partitioning

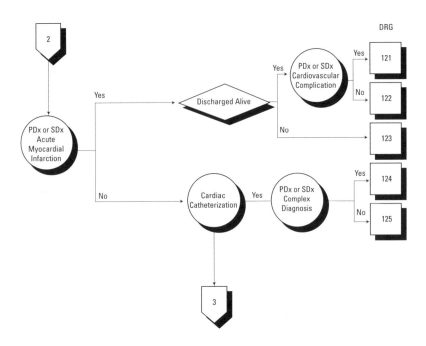

DRG

PDx = Principal Diagnosis
SDx = Secondary Diagnosis

Major Diagnostic Category 5
Diseases and Disorders of the Circulatory System

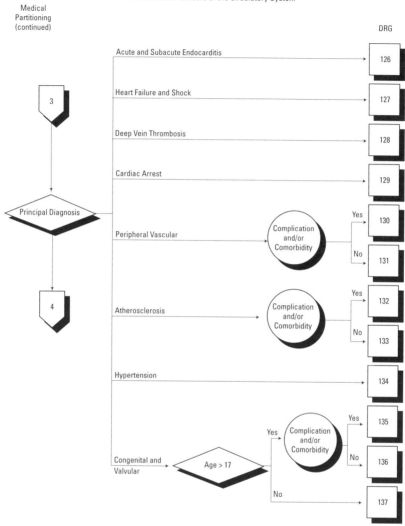

Medical
Partitioning
(continued)

DRG

Acute and Subacute Endocarditis → 126

3

Heart Failure and Shock → 127

Deep Vein Thrombosis → 128

Cardiac Arrest → 129

Principal Diagnosis

Peripheral Vascular → Complication and/or Comorbidity → Yes 130 / No 131

4

Atherosclerosis → Complication and/or Comorbidity → Yes 132 / No 133

Hypertension → 134

Congenital and Valvular → Age > 17 → Yes → Complication and/or Comorbidity → Yes 135 / No 136
No → 137

Major Diagnostic Category 5
Diseases and Disorders of the Circulatory System

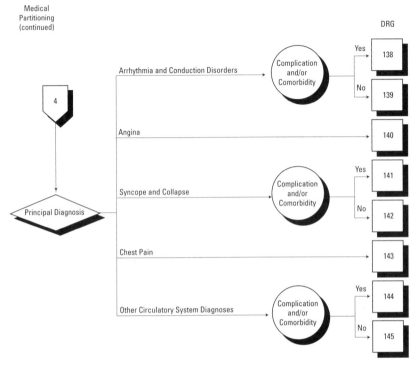

Medical Partitioning (continued)

DRG

4

Principal Diagnosis

Arrhythmia and Conduction Disorders → Complication and/or Comorbidity → Yes → 138 / No → 139

Angina → 140

Syncope and Collapse → Complication and/or Comorbidity → Yes → 141 / No → 142

Chest Pain → 143

Other Circulatory System Diagnoses → Complication and/or Comorbidity → Yes → 144 / No → 145

Major Diagnostic Category 6
Diseases and Disorders of the Digestive System

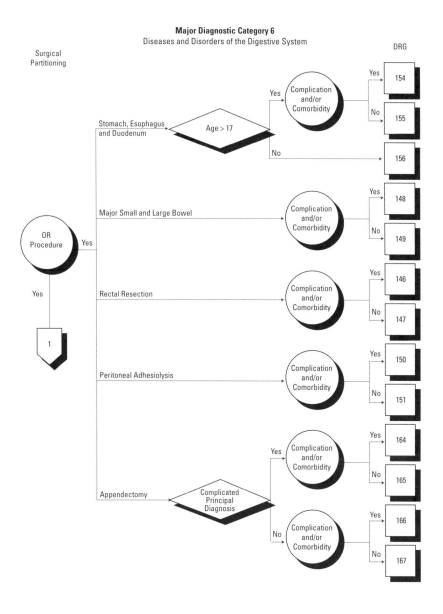

Major Diagnostic Category 6
Diseases and Disorders of the Digestive System

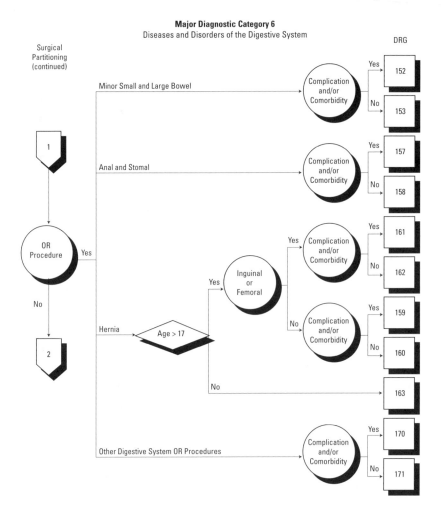

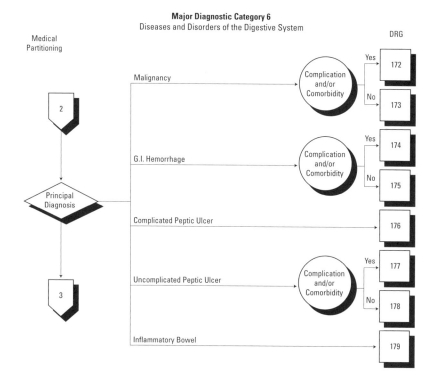

Major Diagnostic Category 6
Diseases and Disorders of the Digestive System

Major Diagnostic Category 6
Diseases and Disorders of the Digestive System

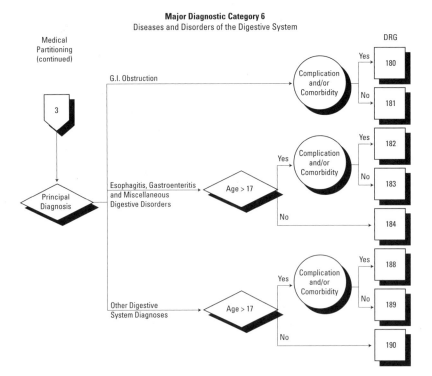

Major Diagnostic Category 7
Diseases and Disorders of the Hepatobiliary System and Pancreas

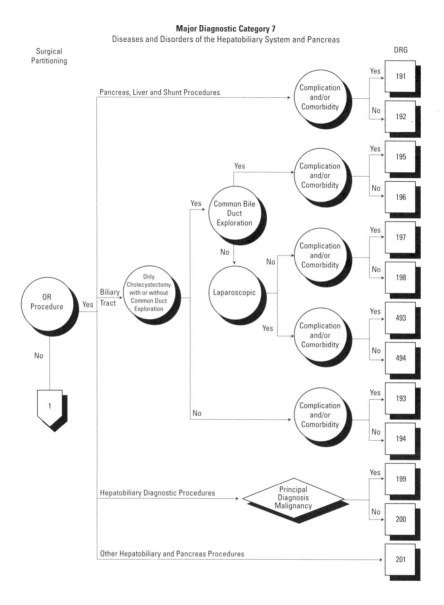

Surgical Partitioning

DRG

Pancreas, Liver and Shunt Procedures → Complication and/or Comorbidity — Yes → 191 / No → 192

Biliary Tract → Only Cholecystectomy with or without Common Duct Exploration:
- Yes → Common Bile Duct Exploration:
  - Yes → Complication and/or Comorbidity — Yes → 195 / No → 196
  - No → Laparoscopic:
    - No → Complication and/or Comorbidity — Yes → 197 / No → 198
    - Yes → Complication and/or Comorbidity — Yes → 493 / No → 494
- No → Complication and/or Comorbidity — Yes → 193 / No → 194

Hepatobiliary Diagnostic Procedures → Principal Diagnosis Malignancy — Yes → 199 / No → 200

Other Hepatobiliary and Pancreas Procedures → 201

OR Procedure — Yes (to Biliary Tract) / No → 1

Major Diagnostic Category 7
Diseases and Disorders of the Hepatobiliary System and Pancreas

Medical
Partitioning

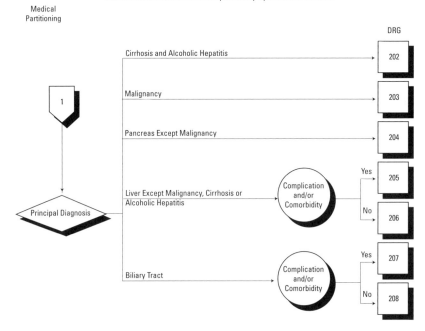

DRG

Cirrhosis and Alcoholic Hepatitis — 202

Malignancy — 203

Pancreas Except Malignancy — 204

Liver Except Malignancy, Cirrhosis or Alcoholic Hepatitis — Complication and/or Comorbidity — Yes 205 / No 206

Biliary Tract — Complication and/or Comorbidity — Yes 207 / No 208

Principal Diagnosis

1

Major Diagnostic Category 8
Diseases and Disorders of the Musculoskeletal System and Connective Tissue

Surgical
Partitioning

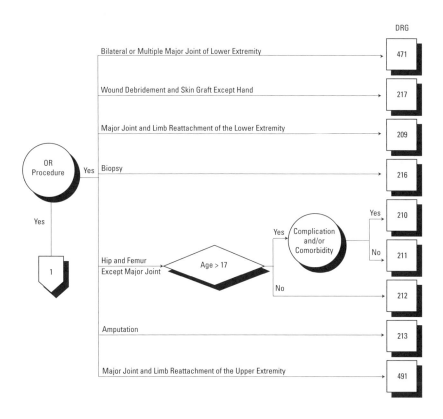

DRG Decision Trees

Major Diagnostic Category 8
Diseases and Disorders of the Musculoskeletal System and Connective Tissue

Surgical
Partitioning
(continued)

DRG

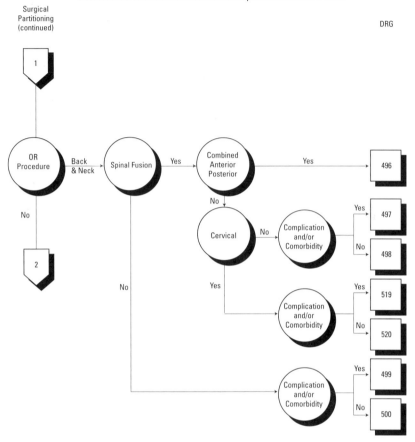

Major Diagnostic Category 8
Diseases and Disorders of the Musculoskeletal System and Connective Tissue

DRG

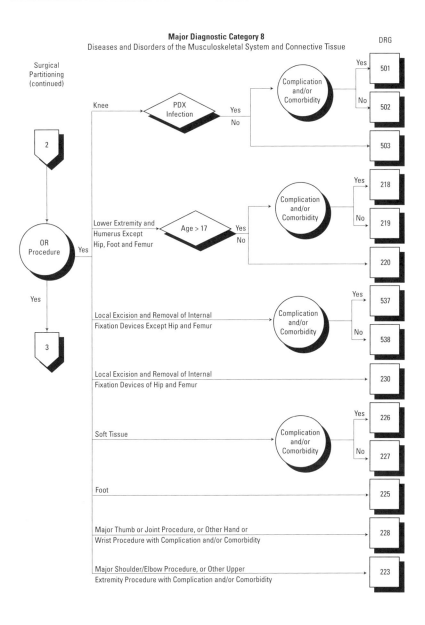

Surgical
Partitioning
(continued)

Major Diagnostic Category 8
Diseases and Disorders of the Musculoskeletal System and Connective Tissue

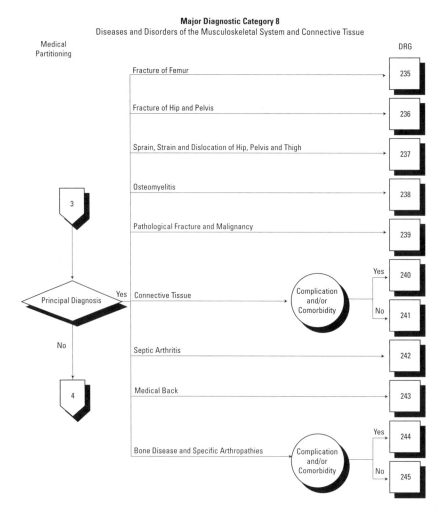

Medical
Partitioning

DRG

Major Diagnostic Category 8
Diseases and Disorders of the Musculoskeletal System and Connective Tissue

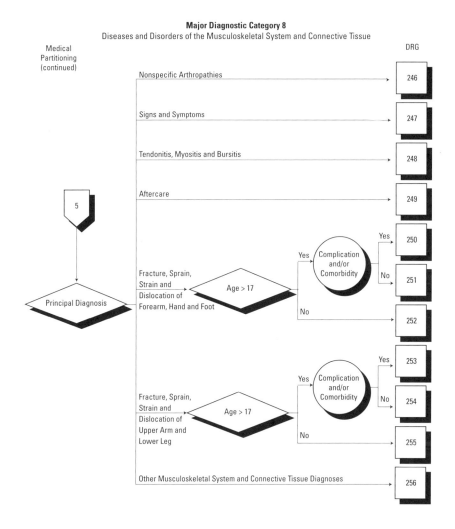

Major Diagnostic Category 9
Diseases and Disorders of the Skin, Subcutaneous Tissue and Breast

Surgical
Partitioning

DRG

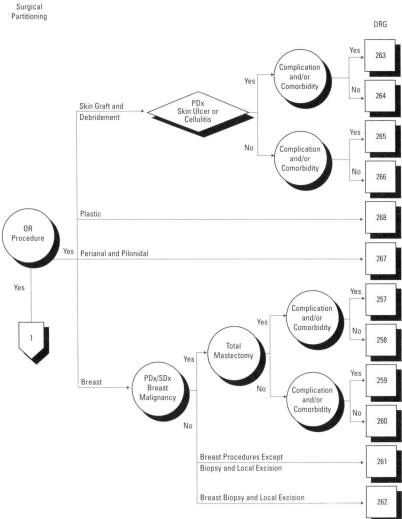

Major Diagnostic Category 9
Diseases and Disorders of the Skin, Subcutaneous Tissue asnd Breast

Surgical
Partitioning
(continued)

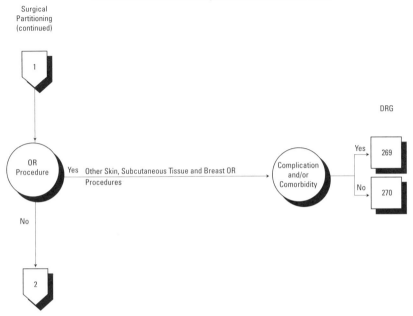

DRG

Major Diagnostic Category 9
Diseases and Disorders of the Skin, Subcutaneous Tissue and Breast

Medical
Partitioning

DRG

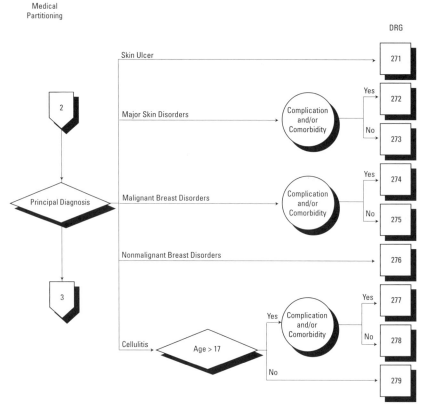

Major Diagnostic Category 9
Diseases and Disorders of the Skin, Subcutaneous Tissue and Breast

Medical
Partitioning
(continued)

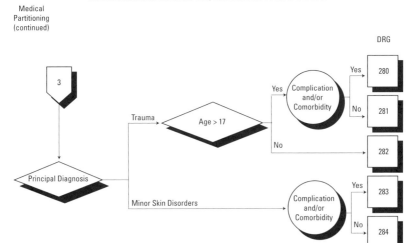

Major Diagnostic Category 10
Endocrine, Nutritional and Metabolic Diseases and Disorders

Surgical
Partitioning

DRG

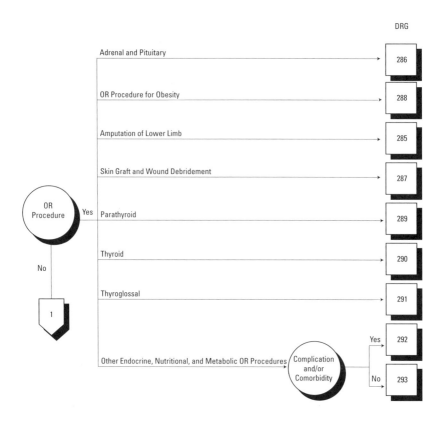

Major Diagnostic Category 10
Endocrine, Nutritional and Metabolic Diseases and Disorders

Medical
Partitioning

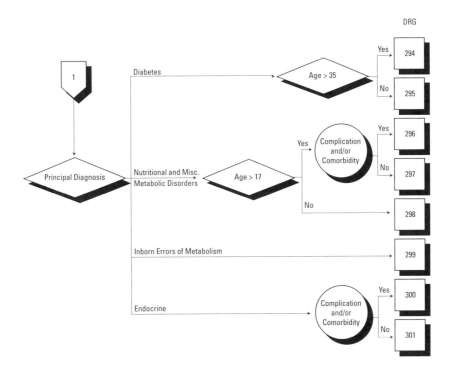

Major Diagnostic Category 11
Diseases and Disorders of the Kidney and Urinary Tract

Surgical
Partitioning

DRG

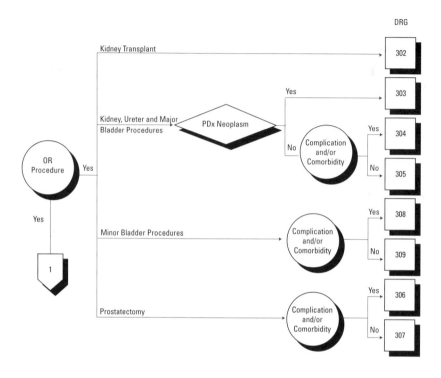

Kidney Transplant → 302

Yes → 303

Kidney, Ureter and Major Bladder Procedures — PDx Neoplasm — Yes → 303

No — Complication and/or Comorbidity — Yes → 304

No → 305

OR Procedure — Yes

Yes

1

Minor Bladder Procedures — Complication and/or Comorbidity — Yes → 308

No → 309

Prostatectomy — Complication and/or Comorbidity — Yes → 306

No → 307

PDx = Principal Diagnosis

Major Diagnostic Category 11

Diseases and Disorders of the Kidney and Urinary Tract

Surgical
Partitioning
(continued)

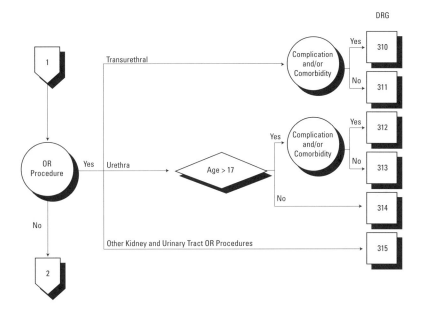

Major Diagnostic Category 11
Diseases and Disorders of the Kidney and Urinary Tract

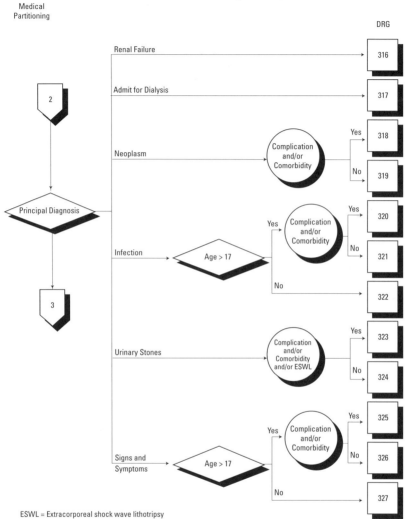

ESWL = Extracorporeal shock wave lithotripsy

Major Diagnostic Category 11
Diseases and Disorders of the Kidney and Urinary Tract

Medical
Partitioning
(continued)

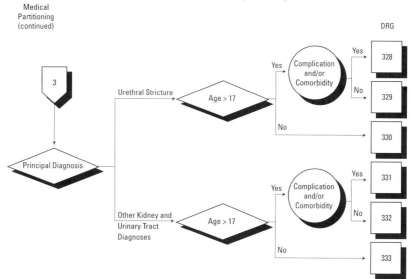

Major Diagnostic Category 12
Diseases and Disorders of the Male Reproductive System

Surgical
Partitioning

DRG

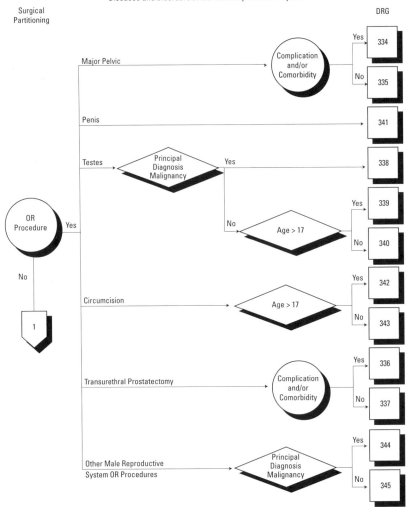

Major Diagnostic Category 12
Diseases and Disorders of the Male Reproductive System

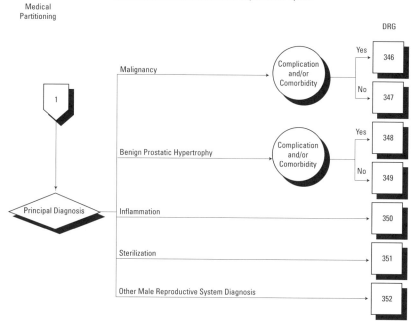

DRG Decision Trees

Major Diagnostic Category 13
Diseases and Disorders of the Female Reproductive System

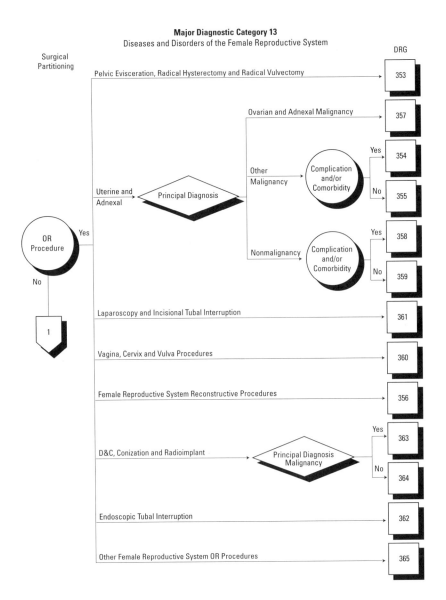

Major Diagnostic Category 13
Diseases and Disorders of the Female Reproductive System

Medical
Partitioning

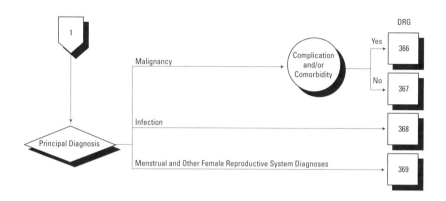

DRG Decision Trees

Major Diagnostic Category 14
Pregnancy, Childbirth and Puerperium

Surgical and Medical
Partitioning

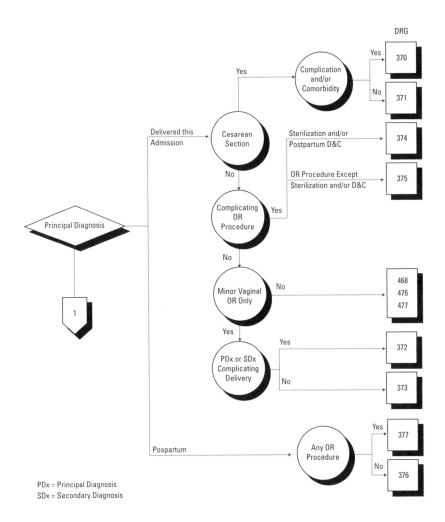

PDx = Principal Diagnosis
SDx = Secondary Diagnosis

Major Diagnostic Category 14
Pregnancy, Childbirth and Puerperium

Surgical and Medical
Partitioning
(continued)

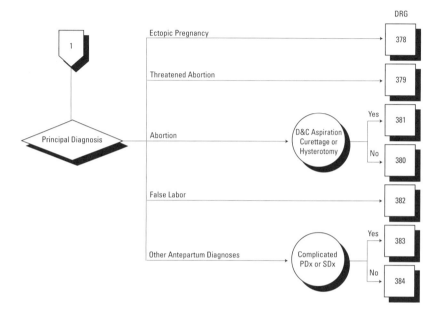

PDx = Principal Diagnosis
SDx = Secondary Diagnosis

Major Diagnostic Category 15
Newborns and Other Neonates with Conditions Originating in the Perinatal Period

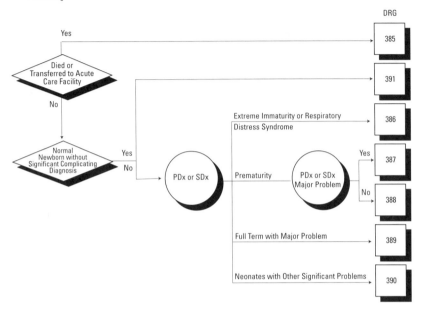

Surgical and Medical
  Partitioning

DRG

PDx = Principal Diagnosis
SDx = Secondary Diagnosis

Major Diagnostic Category 16
Diseases and Disorders of the Blood and Blood Forming Organs and Immunological Disorders

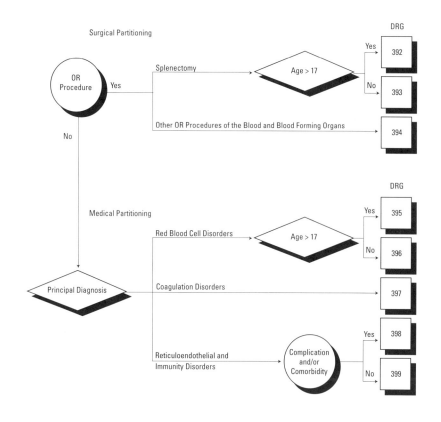

Major Diagnostic Category 17
Myeloproliferative Diseases and Disorders, Poorly Differentiated Neoplasms

Medical and Surgical
Partitioning

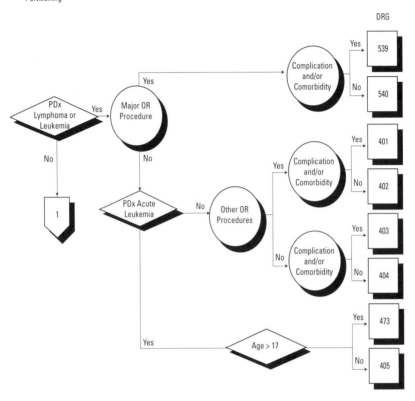

PDx = Principal Diagnosis

Major Diagnostic Category 17
Myeloproliferative Diseases and Disorders, Poorly Differentiated Neoplasms

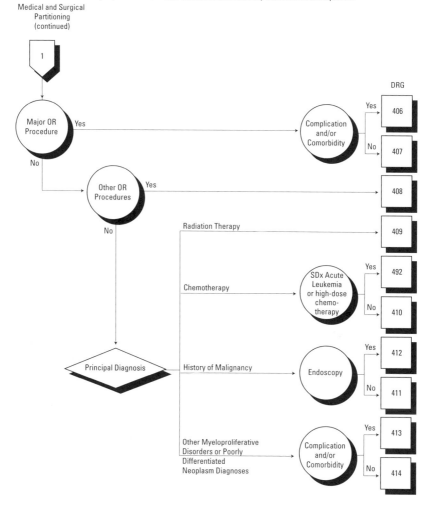

SDx = Secondary Diagnosis

Major Diagnostic Category 18
Infectious and Parasitic Disease (Systemic or Unspecified Sites)

Surgical Partitioning

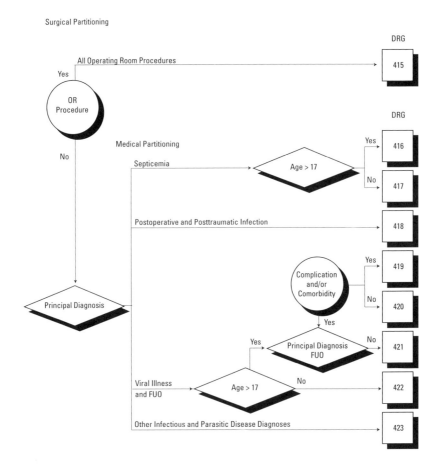

Major Diagnostic Category 19
Mental Diseases and Disorders

Surgical Partitioning

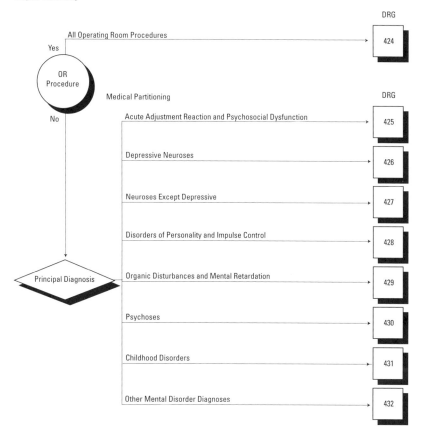

DRG

All Operating Room Procedures → 424
Yes

OR
Procedure

No

Medical Partitioning

DRG

Acute Adjustment Reaction and Psychosocial Dysfunction → 425

Depressive Neuroses → 426

Neuroses Except Depressive → 427

Disorders of Personality and Impulse Control → 428

Principal Diagnosis   Organic Disturbances and Mental Retardation → 429

Psychoses → 430

Childhood Disorders → 431

Other Mental Disorder Diagnoses → 432

Major Diagnostic Category 20
Alcohol/Drug Use and Alcohol/Drug Induced Organic Mental Disorders

Surgical and Medical
Partitioning

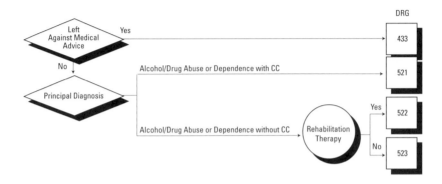

Major Diagnostic Category 21
Injuries, Poisonings and Toxic Effects of Drugs

Surgical
Partitioning

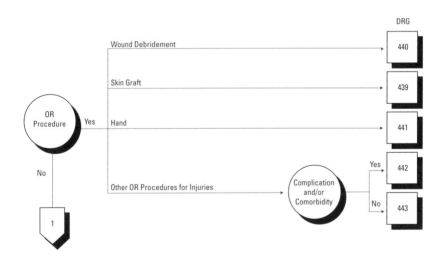

Major Diagnostic Category 21
Injuries, Poisonings and Toxic Effects of Drugs

Medical
Partitioning

DRG

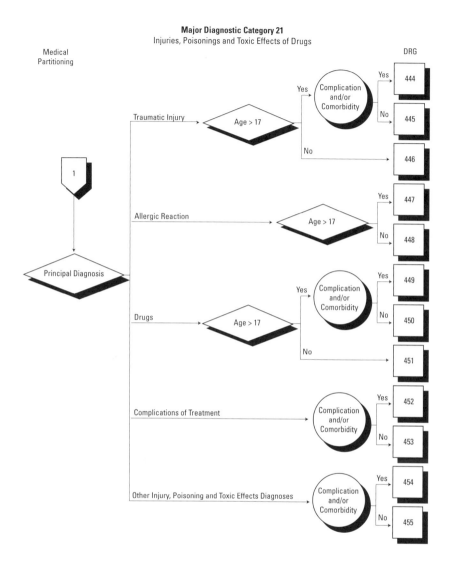

Major Diagnostic Category 22
Burns

Medical and Surgical
Partitioning

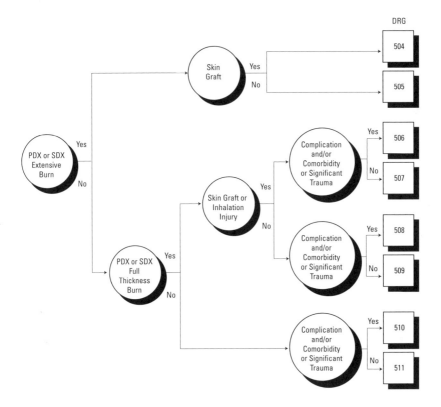

Major Diagnostic Category 23
Factors Influencing Health Status and Other Contacts with Health Services

Surgical Partitioning

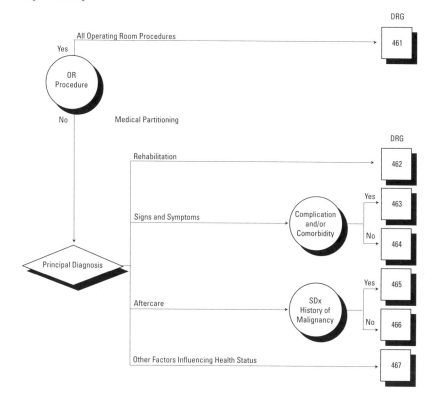

SDx = Secondary Diagnosis

Major Diagnostic Category 24
Multiple Significant Trauma

Patients are assigned to MDC 24 based on both the principal and secondary diagnoses. Patients are assigned to MDC 24 with a principal diagnosis of trauma and at least two significant trauma diagnosis codes (either as principal or secondaries) from different body site categories.

There are eight different body site categories as follows:

1. Significant head trauma
2. Significant chest trauma
3. Significant abdominal trauma
4. Significant kidney trauma
5. Significant trauma of the urinary system
6. Significant trauma of the pelvis or spine
7. Significant trauma of the upper limb
8. Significant trauma of the lower limb

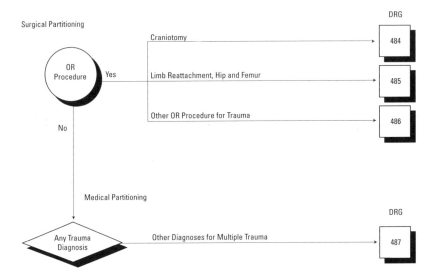

Major Diagnostic Category 25
Human Immunodeficiency Virus (HIV) Infections

Patients assigned to MDC 25 must have a principal diagnosis of an HIV
infection or a principal diagnosis of a significant HIV related condition
and a secondary diagnosis of an HIV infection.

Surgical and Medical Partitioning

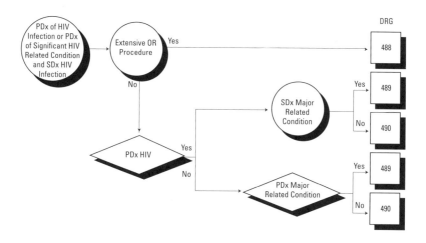

PDx = Principal Diagnosis
SDx = Secondary Diagnosis

Major Diagnostic Category PRE

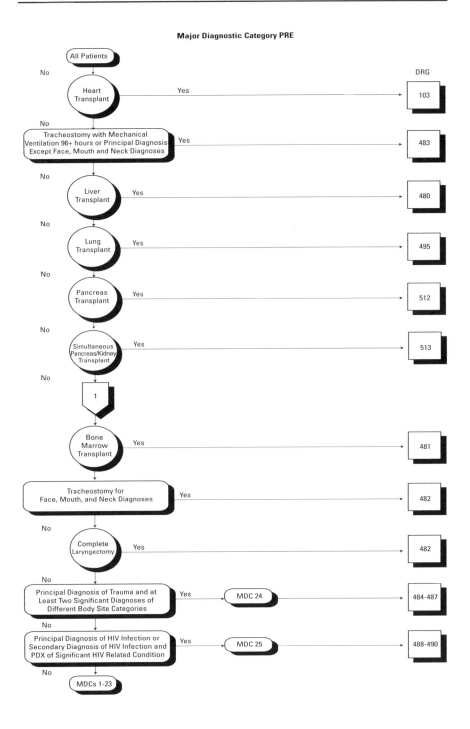

Optimizing Tips

Numeric Listing of DRGs included in this section

Optimizing Tips

Nervous System, MDC 1

Craniotomy, Age > 17 with CC   RW 3.6186   **DRG 001**

Potential DRGs

483	Tracheostomy with Mech Vent 96+ Hours or Principal Diagnosis Except Face, Mouth and Neck Diagnoses	RW	16.7762
484	Craniotomy for **Multiple Significant Trauma**	RW	5.4179
528	Intracranial Vascular Procedure **with a Principal Diagnosis of Hemorrhage**	RW	7.2205

DRG	Principal Dx/Procedure	Codes	Tips
483	Tracheostomy with mechanical ventilation 96+ hours or principal diagnosis except face, mouth, and neck diagnoses	31.1, 31.21, 31.29, 96.72	■ A minitracheostomy is coded as a temporary tracheostomy. ■ Tracheostomy carried out elsewhere prior to admission or in ambulance prior to arrival should not be reported as a current procedure. ● Tracheostomy procedure may be performed either at the bedside and documented in the progress notes or in the operating room and documented in an operative note.
484	Craniotomy for multiple significant trauma		■ Craniotomy and principal diagnosis of trauma and at least two injuries (assigned either as principal or secondary) that are defined as significant trauma from different body site categories located under DRG 487
528	Craniotomy *AND* Cerebral hemorrhages	*01.2, *02.0 430-*432	◆ Acute disorders

Craniotomy Age > 17 without CC   RW 2.0850   **DRG 002**

Potential DRGs

001	Craniotomy Age > 17 **with CC**	RW	3.6186
483	**Tracheostomy** with **Mech Vent 96+ Hours or Principal Diagnosis Except for Face, Mouth & Neck Diagnoses**	RW	16.7762
484	Craniotomy for **Multiple Significant Trauma**	RW	5.4179
528	Intracranial Vascular Procedure **with a Principal Diagnosis of Hemorrhage**	RW	7.2205

DRG	Principal Dx/Procedure	Codes	Tips
001	Craniotomy *AND* patient's age > 17 *AND* CC condition	See CC section.	
483	Tracheostomy with mechanical ventilation 96+ hours or principal diagnosis except face, mouth, and neck diagnoses	31.1, 31.21, 31.29, 96.72	■ A minitracheostomy is coded as a temporary tracheostomy. ■ Tracheostomy carried out elsewhere prior to admission or in ambulance prior to arrival should not be reported as a current procedure. ● Tracheostomy procedure may be performed either at the bedside and documented in the progress notes or in the operating room and documented in an operative note.

Nervous System, MDC 1

DRG 002 (continued)

DRG	Principal Dx/Procedure	Codes	Tips
484	Craniotomy for multiple significant trauma		■ Craniotomy and principal diagnosis of trauma and at least two injuries (assigned either as principal or secondary) that are defined as significant trauma from different body site categories located under DRG 487
528	Craniotomy *AND* Cerebral hemorrhages	*01.2, *02.0 430-*432	◆ Acute disorders

DRG 003   Craniotomy, Age 0-17   RW 1.9753

Potential DRGs

001	Craniotomy **Age > 17 with CC**	RW	3.6186
002	Craniotomy **Age > 17** without CC	RW	2.0850
483	**Tracheostomy with Mech Vent 96+ Hours or Principal Diagnosis Except For Face, Mouth & Neck Diagnoses**	RW	16.7762
484	**Craniotomy For Multiple Significant Trauma**	RW	5.4179
528	Intracranial Vascular Procedure **with a Principal Diagnosis of Hemorrhage**	RW	7.2205

DRG	Principal Dx/Procedure	Codes	Tips
001	Patient's age > 17 *AND* CC condition	See CC section.	
002	Patient's age > 17		
483	Tracheostomy with mechanical ventilation 96+ hours or principal diagnosis except face, mouth, and neck diagnoses	31.1, 31.21, 31.29, 96.72	■ A minitracheostomy is coded as a temporary tracheostomy. ■ Tracheostomy carried out elsewhere prior to admission or in ambulance prior to arrival should not be reported as a current procedure. ● Tracheostomy procedure may be performed either at the bedside and documented in the progress notes or in the operating room and documented in an operative note.
484	Craniotomy for multiple significant trauma		■ Craniotomy and principal diagnosis of trauma and at least two injuries (assigned either as principal or secondary) that are defined as significant trauma from different body site categories located under DRG 487
528	Craniotomy *AND* Cerebral hemorrhages	*01.2, *02.0 430-*432	◆ Acute disorders

DRG 006   Carpal Tunnel Release

No Potential DRGs

DRG 007   Peripheral and Cranial Nerve and Other Nervous System Procedures with CC

No Potential DRGs

■ Coding Tip   ● Documentation Tip   ◆ Encoder Tip   ▧ Targeted DRG

Peripheral and Cranial Nerve and Other Nervous System Procedures without CC

RW 1.5453 **DRG 008**

Potential DRGs
007   Peripheral & Cranial Nerve & Other Nervous System Procedures **with CC**   RW   2.6519

DRG	Principal Dx/Procedure	Codes	Tips
007	CC condition	See CC section.	

Spinal Disorders & Injuries

RW 1.4214 **DRG 009**

Potential DRGs
487   Other Multiple Significant Trauma   RW   2.0057

DRG	Principal Dx/Procedure	Codes	Tips
487	Other multiple significant trauma		■ Principal diagnosis of trauma and at least two injuries (assigned either as principal or secondary) that are defined as significant trauma from different body site categories located under DRG 487

Nervous System Neoplasms with CC

DRG 010

No Potential DRGs

Nervous System Neoplasms without CC

RW 0.8571 **DRG 011**

Potential DRGs
010   Nervous System Neoplasms **with CC**   RW   1.2448

DRG	Principal Dx/Procedure	Codes	Tips
010	Nervous system neoplasm, primary or secondary, malignant or benign *AND* CC condition	*191, *192, *225, 198.3, 198.4, 239.6 See CC section.	

Degenerative Nervous System Disorders

DRG 012

No Potential DRGs

Multiple Sclerosis & Cerebellar Ataxia

RW 0.8176 **DRG 013**

Potential DRGs
007   Peripheral & Cranial Nerve & Other Nervous System Procedures **with CC**   RW   2.6519
008   Peripheral & Cranial Nerve & Other Nervous System Procedures **without CC**   RW   1.5453

DRG	Principal Dx/Procedure	Codes	Tips
007	Insertion of infusion pump and other central and peripheral nervous system procedures *AND* CC condition	86.06 and other therapeutic and diagnostic nervous system categories See CC section.	■ 86.06 code limited to self-contained infusion pumps surgically implanted into the patient, insertion only
008	Insertion of infusion pump and other central and peripheral nervous system procedures	86.06 and other therapeutic and diagnostic nervous system categories	■ 86.06 code limited to self-contained infusion pumps surgically implanted into the patient, insertion only

---

■ Coding Tip   ● Documentation Tip   ◆ Encoder Tip   ▼ Targeted DRG

DRG 014▽ Intracranial Hemorrhage and Stroke with Infarction
RW 1.2682

Potential DRGs
005	Extracranial Vascular Procedures	RW	0.0000
027	**Traumatic** Stupor & Coma, Coma > 1 Hour	RW	1.3370
442	Other O.R. Procedures **for Injuries** with CC	RW	2.4200
528	**Intracranial Vascular Procedure** with a Principal Diagnosis of Hemorrhage	RW	7.2205

DRG	Principal Dx/Procedure	Codes	Tips
005	Endarterectomy of jugular vein	38.12	■ Use code 38.12 if procedure is documented as "re-do," code as new endarterectomy.
	Excision of aneurysm of carotid artery or jugular vein with anastomosis	38.32	■ Includes reconnection of involved vessel after excision.
	angioplasty of carotid artery	39.50	■ Includes PTA of noncoronary vessel
027	Head trauma diagnosis *AND* Diagnosis of coma > 1 hr	*800, *801, *803, *804, *851–*854	● Physician must document length of time of loss of consciousness.
442	Operations on intracranial or other vessels of head and neck for injuries *AND* CC condition	900.00–900.9 and other operating room procedures for injuries See CC section.	
528	Craniotomy *AND* Cerebral hemorrhages	*01.2, *02.0 430–*432	◆ Acute disorders

DRG 015▽ Nonspecific Cerebrovascular and Precerebral Occlusion without Infarction
RW 0.9677

Potential DRGs
005	Extracranial Vascular Procedures	RW	0.0000
007	Peripheral & Cranial Nerve & Other Nervous System Procedures **with CC**	RW	2.6519
008	Peripheral & Cranial Nerve & Other Nervous System Procedures **without CC**	RW	1.5453
014	**Intracranial Hemorrhage and Stroke with Infarction**	RW	1.2943
016	Nonspecific **Cerebrovascular Disorders with CC**	RW	1.2618

DRG	Principal Dx/Procedure	Codes	Tips
005	Endarterectomy of jugular vein	38.12	■ Use code 38.12 if procedure is documented as "re-do," code as new endarterectomy
	Excision of aneurysm of carotid artery or jugular vein with anastomosis	38.32	■ Includes reconnection of involved vessel after excision
	angioplasty of carotid artery	39.50	■ Includes PTA of noncoronary vessel
007	Insertion of cardiac pacemaker with leads *AND* CC condition	37.70–37.76 See CC section.	■ Insertion/replacement of leads must be in combination with insertion/replacement of pacemaker.
008	Insertion of cardiac pacemaker with leads	37.70–37.76	■ Insertion/replacement of leads must be in combination with insertion/replacement of pacemaker.

■ Coding Tip   ● Documentation Tip   ◆ Encoder Tip   ▽ Targeted DRG

(continued) ▽DRG 015

DRG	Principal Dx/Procedure	Codes	Tips
014 ▽	Cerebral hemorrhages Cerebral thrombosis w/cerebral infarction Cerebral embolism w/cerebral infarction Cerebral artery occlusion w/cerebral infarction	430–*432 434.01 434.11 434.91	◆ Acute disorders ■ fifth digit for presence of cerebral infarction should be coded only when documented for current admission, not previous episode of care. ■ Acute event, code also documented neurological deficits. Use to code lacunar infarct.
016	Central nervous system disorders Cerebral atherosclerosis Cerebral insufficiency Encephalopathy *AND* CC condition	349.9 437.0 437.9 438.3 See CC section.	◆ Nonacute, chronic or unspecific disorders.

Nonspecific Cerebrovascular Disorders with CC   RW 1.2618 **DRG 016**

Potential DRGs
014	Intracranial Hemorrhage and Stroke with Infarction	RW	1.2682
528	Intracranial Vascular Procedure with a Principal Diagnosis of Hemorrhage	RW	7.2205

DRG	Principal Dx/Procedure	Codes	Tips
014 ▽	Cerebral hemorrhages Cerebral thrombosis w/cerebral infarction Cerebral embolism w/cerebral infarction Cerebral artery occlusion w/cerebral infarction	430–*432 434.01 434.11 434.91	◆ Acute disorders ■ Fifth digit for presence of cerebral infarction should be coded only when documented for current admission, not previous episode of care. ■ Acute event, code also documented neurological deficits. Use to code lacunar infarct.
528	Craniotomy *AND* Cerebral hemorrhages	*01.2, *02.0 430-*432	◆ Acute disorders

Nonspecific Cerebrovascular Disorders without CC   RW 0.6991 **DRG 017**

Potential DRGs
014	Intracranial Hemorrhage and Stroke with Infarction	RW	1.2682
016	Nonspecific Cerebrovascular Disorders with CC	RW	1.2618
528	Intracranial Vascular Procedure with a Principal Diagnosis of Hemorrhage	RW	7.2205

DRG	Principal Dx/Procedure	Codes	Tips
014 ▽	Cerebral hemorrhages Cerebral thrombosis w/cerebral infarction Cerebral embolism w/cerebral infarction Cerebral artery occlusion w/cerebral infarction	430–*432 434.01 434.11 434.91	◆ Acute disorders ■ Fifth digit for presence of cerebral infarction should be coded only when documented for current admission, not previous episode of care. ■ Acute event, code also documented neurological deficits. Use to code lacunar infarct.

■ Coding Tip	● Documentation Tip	◆ Encoder Tip	▽ Targeted DRG

Nervous System, MDC 1

DRG 017   (continued)

DRG	Principal Dx/Procedure	Codes	Tips
016	Central nervous system disorders Cerebral atherosclerosis Cerebral insufficiency Encephalopathy *AND* CC condition	349.9 437.0 437.9 438.3 See CC section.	◆ Nonacute, chronic or unspecific disorders.
528	Craniotomy *AND* Cerebral hemorrhages	*01.2, *02.0 430-*432	◆ Acute disorders

DRG 018   Cranial and Peripheral Nerve Disorders with CC

No Potential DRGs

DRG 019   Cranial and Peripheral Nerve Disorders   RW 0.7041
without CC

Potential DRGs
018   Cranial & Peripheral Nerve Disorders with CC   RW   1.0026

DRG	Principal Dx/Procedure	Codes	Tips
018	CC condition	See CC section.	

DRG 020   Nervous System Infection Except Viral Meningitis

No Potential DRGs

DRG 021   Viral Meningitis   RW 1.5138

Potential DRGs
020   **Nervous System Infection** Except Viral Meningitis   RW   2.7394

DRG	Principal Dx/Procedure	Codes	Tips
020	Salmonella meningitis Syphilitic (neurosyphilitic) meningitis Tuberculous meningitis Candidal meningitis Coccidioidal meningitis Bacterial meningitis NOS Pneumococcal meningitis Streptococcal meningitis Staphylococcal meningitis Meningitis NOS	003.21 094.2–094.3 *013 112.83 114.2 *320 320.1 320.2 320.3 *322	■ Code candidial meningitis by site identified. ● Aseptic meningitis with no virus or other organism documented classifies to *322.

■ Coding Tip   ● Documentation Tip   ◆ Encoder Tip   ᵂ Targeted DRG

Hypertensive Encephalopathy

RW 1.0737 **DRG 022**

Potential DRGs

014	Intracranial Hemorrhage and Stroke with Infarction	RW	1.2682
528	Intracranial Vascular Procedure with a Principal Diagnosis of Hemorrhage	RW	7.2205

DRG	Principal Dx/Procedure	Codes	Tips
014 ⛛	Cerebral hemorrhages Cerebral thrombosis w/cerebral infarction	430–*432 434.01	◆ Acute disorders ■ Fifth digit for presence of cerebral infarction should be coded only when documented for current admission, not previous episode of care.
	Cerebral embolism w/cerebral infarction	434.11	
	Cerebral artery occlusion w/cerebral infarction	434.91	■ Acute event, code also documented neurological deficits. Use to code lacunar infarct.
528	Craniotomy *AND* Cerebral hemorrhages	 430-*432	◆ Acute disorders

Nontraumatic Stupor & Coma

RW 0.8239 **DRG 023**

Potential DRGs

001	Craniotomy Age > 17 **with CC**	RW	3.6186
002	**Craniotomy** Age > 17 without CC	RW	2.0850
027	Traumatic Stupor & Coma, **Coma > 1 Hour**	RW	1.3370
028	Traumatic Stupor & Coma, **Coma 1 Hour**, Age > 17 with CC	RW	1.3386
528	**Intracranial Vascular Procedure with a Principal Diagnosis of Hemorrhage**	RW	7.2205

DRG	Principal Dx/Procedure	Codes	Tips
001	Craniotomy *AND* Patient's age > 17 *AND* CC condition	 See CC section.	
002	Patient's age > 17	*01.2, 02.0*	
027	Traumatic stupor or coma w/coma > 1 hour	*800, *801, *803, *804, *850–*854	● Physician must document length of time of loss of consciousness.
028	Traumatic stupor or coma w/coma < 1 hour *AND* Patient's age > 17 *AND* CC condition	 See CC section.	● Mental confusion/disorientation may occur w/o loss of consciousness; physician must document length of time of loss of consciousness.
528	Craniotomy *AND* Cerebral hemorrhages	*01.2, *02.0 430-*432	◆ Acute disorders

---

■ Coding Tip	● Documentation Tip	◆ Encoder Tip	⛛ Targeted DRG

Nervous System, MDC 1

DRG 024 Seizure & Headache, Age > 17 with CC RW 1.0121

Potential DRGs

010	Nervous System Neoplasms **with CC**	RW	1.2448
014	**Intracranial Hemorrhage and Stroke with Infarction**	RW	1.2682

DRG	Principal Dx/Procedure	Codes	Tips
010	Nervous system neoplasm, primary or secondary, malignant or benign *AND* CC condition	*191, *192, *225, 198.3, 198.4, 239.6 See CC section.	● Seizure work up for, or attributed to, nervous system neoplasm
014 ▽	Cerebral hemorrhages Cerebral thrombosis w/cerebral infarction Cerebral embolism w/cerebral infarction Cerebral artery occlusion w/cerebral infarction	430–*432 434.01 434.11 434.91	◆ Acute disorders ■ Fifth digit for presence of cerebral infarction should be coded only when documented for current admission, not previous episode of care. ■ Acute event, code also documented neurological deficits. Use to code lacunar infarct.

DRG 025 Seizure & Headache, Age > 17 without CC RW 0.6109

Potential DRGs

010	Nervous System Neoplasms **with CC**	RW	1.2448
014	**Intracranial Hemorrhage and Stroke with Infarction**	RW	1.2682
024	Seizure & Headache, Age > 17 **with CC**	RW	1.0121
026	Seizure & Headache, **Age 0–17**	RW	1.3730

DRG	Principal Dx/Procedure	Codes	Tips
010	Seizure workup for, or attributed to, nervous system neoplasm, primary or secondary, malignant or benign *AND* CC condition	*191, *192, *225, 198.3, 198.4, 239.6 See CC section.	
014 ▽	Cerebral hemorrhages Cerebral thrombosis w/cerebral infarction Cerebral embolism w/cerebral infarction Cerebral artery occlusion w/cerebral infarction	430–*432 434.01 434.11 434.91	◆ Acute disorders ■ Fifth digit for presence of cerebral infarction should be coded only when documented for current admission, not previous episode of care. ■ Acute event, code also documented neurological deficits. Use to code lacunar infarct.
024	CC condition	See CC section.	
026	Patient's age 0–17		

DRG 026 Seizure & Headache, Age 0–17 RW 1.3730

Potential DRGs

010	Nervous System Neoplasms **with CC**	RW	1.2448
011	**Nervous System Neoplasms** without CC	RW	0.8571
014	**Intracranial Hemorrhage and Stroke with Infarction**	RW	1.2682

DRG	Principal Dx/Procedure	Codes	Tips
010	Seizure workup for, or attributed to, nervous system neoplasm, primary or secondary, malignant or benign *AND* CC condition	*191, *192, *225, 198.3, 198.4, 239.6 See CC section.	
011	Seizure workup for, or attributed to, nervous system neoplasm, primary or secondary, malignant or benign	*191, *192, *225, 198.3, 198.4, 239.6	

■ Coding Tip   ● Documentation Tip   ◆ Encoder Tip   ▽ Targeted DRG

(continued) **DRG 026**

DRG	Principal Dx/Procedure	Codes	Tips
014 ▽YIELD/	Cerebral hemorrhages	430–*432	◆ Acute disorders
	Cerebral thrombosis w/cerebral infarction	434.01	■ Fifth digit for presence of cerebral infarction should be coded only when documented for current admission, not previous episode of care.
	Cerebral embolism w/cerebral infarction	434.11	
	Cerebral artery occlusion w/cerebral infarction	434.91	■ Acute event, code also documented neurological deficits. Use to code lacunar infarct.

Traumatic Stupor & Coma, Coma > 1 Hour   RW 1.3370   **DRG 027**

Potential DRGs

001	**Craniotomy** Age > 17 **with CC**	RW	3.6186
002	**Craniotomy** Age > 17 **without CC**	RW	2.0850
028	Traumatic Stupor & Coma, Coma < 1 Hour, Age > 17 **with CC**	RW	1.3386
484	**Craniotomy for Multiple Significant Trauma**	RW	5.4179
486	Other **O.R. Procedures for Multiple Significant Trauma**	RW	4.8793
487	Other Multiple Significant Trauma	RW	2.0057
528	**Intracranial Vascular Procedure with a Principal Diagnosis of Hemorrhage**	RW	7.2205

DRG	Principal Dx/Procedure	Codes	Tips
001	Craniotomy *AND* Patient's age > 17 *AND* CC condition	See CC section.	
002	Craniotomy *AND* Patient's age > 17	*01.2, *02.0	
028	Traumatic stupor or coma w/coma < 1 hour *AND* Patient's age > 17 *AND* CC condition	See CC section.	● Mental confusion/disorientation may occur w/o loss of consciousness; physician must document length of time of loss of consciousness.
484	Craniotomy for multiple significant trauma		■ Craniotomy and principal diagnosis of trauma and at least two injuries (assigned either as principal or secondary) that are defined as significant trauma from different body site categories located under DRG 487
486	Other O.R. procedures for multiple significant trauma		■ Principal diagnosis of trauma and at least two injuries (assigned either as principal or secondary) that are defined as significant trauma from different body site categories located under DRG 487 *AND* O.R. procedure other than craniotomy or limb reattachment, hip and femur procedures
487	Other multiple significant trauma		■ Principal diagnosis of trauma and at least two injuries (assigned either as principal or secondary) that are defined as significant trauma from different body site categories located under DRG 487
528	Craniotomy *AND* Cerebral hemorrhages	*01.2, *02.0 430-*432	◆ Acute disorders

■ Coding Tip   ● Documentation Tip   ◆ Encoder Tip   ▽YIELD/ Targeted DRG

Nervous System, MDC 1

DRG 028   Traumatic Stupor & Coma, Coma < 1   RW 1.3386
Hour, Age > 17 with CC

Potential DRGs
001	Craniotomy Age >17 with CC	RW	3.6186
002	Craniotomy Age > 17 without CC	RW	2.0850
484	Craniotomy For Multiple Significant Trauma	RW	5.4179
486	Other O.R. Procedures for Multiple Significant Trauma	RW	4.8793
487	Other Multiple Significant Trauma	RW	2.0057
528	Intracranial Vascular Procedure with a Principal Diagnosis of Hemorrhage	RW	7.2205

DRG	Principal Dx/Procedure	Codes	Tips
001	Craniotomy *AND* Patient's age > 17 *AND* CC condition	See CC section.	
002	Craniotomy *AND* Patient's age > 17	*01.2, *02.0	
484	Craniotomy for multiple significant trauma		■ Craniotomy and principal diagnosis of trauma and at least two injuries (assigned either as principal or secondary) that are defined as significant trauma from different body site categories located under DRG 487
486	Other O.R. procedures for multiple significant trauma		■ Principal diagnosis of trauma and at least two injuries (assigned either as principal or secondary) that are defined as significant trauma from different body site categories located under DRG 487 *AND* O.R. procedure other than craniotomy or limb reattachment, hip and femur procedures
487	Other multiple significant trauma		■ Principal diagnosis of trauma and at least two injuries (assigned either as principal or secondary) that are defined as significant trauma from different body site categories located under DRG 487
528	Craniotomy *AND* Cerebral hemorrhages	*01.2, *02.0 430-*432	◆ Acute disorders

---

■ Coding Tip   ● Documentation Tip   ◆ Encoder Tip   ⒲ Targeted DRG

Traumatic Stupor & Coma, Coma < 1 Hour, RW 0.7087   **DRG 029**
Age > 17 without CC

Potential DRGs

001	Craniotomy Age > 17 with CC	RW	3.6186
002	Craniotomy Age > 17 without CC	RW	2.0850
027	Traumatic Stupor & Coma, Coma > 1 Hour	RW	1.3370
028	Traumatic Stupor & Coma, Coma < 1 Hour, Age > 17 with CC	RW	1.3386
484	Craniotomy for Multiple Significant Trauma	RW	5.4179
486	Other O.R. Procedures for Multiple Significant Trauma	RW	4.8793
487	Other Multiple Significant Trauma	RW	2.0057
528	Intracranial Vascular Procedure with a Principal Diagnosis of Hemorrhage	RW	7.2205

DRG	Principal Dx/Procedure	Codes	Tips
001	Craniotomy *AND* Patient's age > 17 *AND* CC condition	See CC section.	
002	Craniotomy *AND* Patient's age > 17	*01.2, *02.0	
027	Head trauma diagnosis *AND* Diagnosis of coma > 1 hour	*800, *801, *803, *804, *850–*854	● Physician must document length of time of loss of consciousness.
028	Traumatic stupor or coma w/coma < 1 hour *AND* Patient's age > 17 *AND* CC condition	See CC section.	● Mental confusion/disorientation may occur w/o loss of consciousness; physician must documention length of time of loss of consciousness.
484	Craniotomy for multiple significant trauma		■ Craniotomy and principal diagnosis of trauma and at least two injuries (assigned either as principal or secondary) that are defined as significant trauma from different body site categories located under DRG 487
486	Other O.R. procedures for multiple significant trauma		■ Principal diagnosis of trauma and at least two injuries (assigned either as principal or secondary) that are defined as significant trauma from different body site categories located under DRG 487 *AND* O.R. procedure other than craniotomy or limb reattachment, hip and femur procedures
487	Other multiple significant trauma		■ Principal diagnosis of trauma and at least two injuries (assigned either as principal or secondary) that are defined as significant trauma from different body site categories located under DRG 487
528	Craniotomy *AND* Cerebral hemorrhages	*01.2, *02.0 430–*432	◆ Acute disorders

---

■ Coding Tip   ● Documentation Tip   ◆ Encoder Tip   ▽ Targeted DRG

Nervous System, MDC 1

DRG 030 Traumatic Stupor & Coma, Coma < 1 Hour, Age 0-17

RW 0.3341

Potential DRGs

001	Craniotomy Age > 17 **with CC**	RW	3.6186
002	**Craniotomy** Age > 17 **without CC**	RW	2.0850
027	Traumatic Stupor & Coma, **Coma > 1 Hour**	RW	1.3370
028	Traumatic Stupor & Coma, Coma < 1 Hour, Age > 17 **with CC**	RW	1.3386
029	Traumatic Stupor & Coma, Coma < 1 Hour, **Age > 17 without CC**	RW	0.7087
484	**Craniotomy for Multiple Significant Trauma**	RW	5.4179
486	Other **O.R. Procedures for Multiple Significant Trauma**	RW	4.8793
487	Other **Multiple Significant Trauma**	RW	2.0057
528	**Intracranial Vascular Procedure with a Principal Diagnosis of Hemorrhage**	RW	7.2205

DRG	Principal Dx/Procedure	Codes	Tips
001	Craniotomy *AND* Patient's age > 17 *AND* CC condition	See CC section.	
002	Craniotomy *AND* Patient's age > 17	*01.2, *02.0	
027	Head trauma diagnosis *AND* Diagnosis of coma > 1 hour	*800, *801, *803, *804, *850–*854	● Physician must document length of time of loss of consciousness.
028	Traumatic stupor or coma w/coma < 1 hour *AND* Patient's age > 17 *AND* CC condition	See CC section.	● Mental confusion/disorientation may occur w/o loss of consciousness; physician must document length of time of loss of consciousness.
029	Cerebral contusion, cerebral laceration, skull fracture *AND* Evidence of a loss of consciousness < 1 hour *AND* Patient's age > 17		
484	Craniotomy for multiple significant trauma		■ Craniotomy and principal diagnosis of trauma and at least two injuries (assigned either as principal or secondary) that are defined as significant trauma from different body site categories located under DRG 487
486	Other O.R. procedures for multiple significant trauma		■ Principal diagnosis of trauma and at least two injuries (assigned either as principal or secondary) that are defined as significant trauma from different body site categories located under DRG 487 *AND* O.R. procedure other than craniotomy or limb reattachment, hip and femur procedures
487	Other multiple significant trauma		■ Principal diagnosis of trauma and at least two injuries (assigned either as principal or secondary) that are defined as significant trauma from different body site categories located under DRG 487

■ Coding Tip   ● Documentation Tip   ◆ Encoder Tip   ▧ Targeted DRG

(continued) **DRG 030**

528	Craniotomy *AND* Cerebral hemorrhages	*01.2, *02.0 430–*432	◆ Acute disorders

Concussion, Age > 17 with CC — RW 0.9117 **DRG 031**

Potential DRGs

001	**Craniotomy** Age > 17 **with CC**	RW	3.6186
002	**Craniotomy** Age > 17 **without CC**	RW	2.0850
027	**Traumatic Stupor & Coma, Coma > 1 Hour**	RW	1.3370
028	**Traumatic Stupor & Coma, Coma < 1 Hour**, Age > 17 **with CC**	RW	1.3386
484	**Craniotomy for Multiple Significant Trauma**	RW	5.4179
486	Other **O.R. Procedures for Multiple Significant Trauma**	RW	4.8793
487	Other Multiple Significant Trauma	RW	2.0057
528	**Intracranial Vascular Procedure with a Principal Diagnosis of Hemorrhage**	RW	7.2205

DRG	Principal Dx/Procedure	Codes	Tips
001	Craniotomy *AND* Patient's age > 17 *AND* CC condition	See CC section.	
002	Craniotomy *AND* Patient's age > 17	*01.2, *02.0	
027	Head trauma diagnosis *AND* Diagnosis of coma > 1 hour	*800, *801, *803, *804, *850–*854	● Physician must document length of time of loss of consciousness.
028	Traumatic stupor or coma w/coma < 1 hour *AND* Patient's age > 17 *AND* CC condition	See CC section.	● Mental confusion/disorientation may occur w/o loss of consciousness; physician must document length of time of loss of consciousness.
484	Craniotomy for multiple significant trauma		■ Craniotomy and principal diagnosis of trauma and at least two injuries (assigned either as principal or secondary) that are defined as significant trauma from different body site categories located under DRG 487
486	Other O.R. procedures for multiple significant trauma		■ Principal diagnosis of trauma and at least two injuries (assigned either as principal or secondary) that are defined as significant trauma from different body site categories located under DRG 487 *AND* O.R. procedure other than craniotomy or limb reattachment, hip and femur procedures
487	Other multiple significant trauma		■ Principal diagnosis of trauma and at least two injuries (assigned either as principal or secondary) that are defined as significant trauma from different body site categories located under DRG 487
528	Craniotomy *AND* Cerebral hemorrhages	*01.2, *02.0 430–*432	◆ Acute disorders

---

■ Coding Tip   ● Documentation Tip   ◆ Encoder Tip   ▼ Targeted DRG

DRG 032 Concussion Age > 17 without CC
RW 0.5684

Potential DRGs

001	Craniotomy Age > 17 with CC	RW	3.6186
002	Craniotomy Age > 17 without CC	RW	2.0850
027	Traumatic Stupor & Coma, Coma > 1 Hour	RW	1.3370
028	Traumatic Stupor & Coma, Coma < 1 Hour, Age > 17with CC	RW	1.3386
029	Traumatic Stupor & Coma, Coma < 1 Hour, Age > 17 without CC	RW	0.7087
031	Concussion, Age > 17 with CC	RW	0.9117
484	Craniotomy for Multiple Significant Trauma	RW	5.4179
486	Other O.R. Procedures for Multiple Significant Trauma	RW	4.8793
487	Other Multiple Significant Trauma	RW	2.0057
528	Intracranial Vascular Procedure with a Principal Diagnosis of Hemorrhage	RW	7.2205

DRG	Principal Dx/Procedure	Codes	Tips
001	Craniotomy *AND* Patient's age > 17 *AND* CC condition	See CC section.	
002	Craniotomy *AND* Patient's age > 17	*01.2, *02.0	
027	Head trauma diagnosis *AND* Diagnosis of coma > 1 hour	*800, *801, *803, *804, *850–*854	● Physician must document length of time of loss of consciousness.
028	Traumatic stupor or coma w/coma < 1 hour *AND* Patient's age > 17 *AND* CC condition	See CC section.	● Mental confusion/disorientation may occur w/o loss of consciousness; physician must document length of time of loss of consciousness.
029	Cerebral contusion, cerebral laceration, skull fracture *AND* Evidence of a loss of consciousness < 1 hour *AND* Patient's age > 17		
031	CC condition	See CC section.	● Postconcussion syndrome (310.2) occurs following a concussion, when documented consult with the physician to determine if concussion is current stage or post syndrome.
484	Craniotomy for multiple significant trauma		■ Craniotomy and principal diagnosis of trauma and at least two injuries (assigned either as principal or secondary) that are defined as significant trauma from different body site categories located under DRG 487
486	Other O.R. procedures for multiple significant trauma		■ Principal diagnosis of trauma and at least two injuries (assigned either as principal or secondary) that are defined as significant trauma from different body site categories located under DRG 487 *AND* O.R. procedure other than craniotomy or limb reattachment, hip and femur procedures
487	Other multiple significant trauma		■ Principal diagnosis of trauma and at least two injuries (assigned either as principal or secondary) that are defined as significant trauma from different body site categories located under DRG 487
528	Craniotomy *AND* Cerebral hemorrhages	*01.2, *02.0 430–*432	◆ Acute disorders

---

■ Coding Tip   ● Documentation Tip   ◆ Encoder Tip   ▽ Targeted DRG

Concussion, Age 0–17
RW 0.2098 **DRG 033**

Potential DRGs

001	**Craniotomy** Age > 17 with CC	RW	3.6186
002	**Craniotomy** Age > 17 without CC	RW	2.0850
003	**Craniotomy** Age 0–17	RW	1.9753
027	Traumatic Stupor & Coma,**Coma > 1 Hour**	RW	1.3370
028	Traumatic Stupor & Coma,**Coma < 1 Hour, Age > 17 with CC**	RW	1.3386
029	Traumatic Stupor & Coma, **Coma < 1 Hour, Age > 17 without CC**	RW	0.7087
030	**Traumatic Stupor & Coma, Coma < 1 Hour,** Age 0–17	RW	0.3341
031	Concussion, **Age > 17 with CC**	RW	0.9117
032	Concussion, **Age > 17 without CC**	RW	0.5684
484	**Craniotomy for Multiple Significant Trauma**	RW	5.4179
486	Other **O.R. Procedures for Multiple Significant Trauma**	RW	4.8793
487	Other Multiple Significant Trauma	RW	2.0057
528	**Intracranial Vascular Procedure with a Principal Diagnosis of Hemorrhage**	RW	7.2205

DRG	Principal Dx/Procedure	Codes	Tips
001	Craniotomy *AND* Patient's age > 17 *AND* CC condition	See CC section.	
002	Craniotomy *AND* Patient's age > 17	*01.2, *02.0	
003	Craniotomy *AND* Patient's age 0–17		
027	Head trauma diagnosis *AND* Diagnosis of coma > 1 hour	*800, *801, *803, *804, *850–*854	● Physician must document length of time of loss of consciousness.
028	Traumatic stupor or coma w/coma < 1 hour *AND* Patient's age > 17 *AND* CC condition	See CC section.	● Mental confusion/disorientation may occur w/o loss of consciousness; physician must document length of time of loss of consciousness.
029	Cerebral contusion, cerebral laceration, skull fracture *AND* Evidence of a loss of consciousness < 1 hour *AND* Patient's age > 17		
030	Cerebral contusion, cerebral laceration, skull fracture *AND* Evidence of a loss of consciousness < 1 hour	*800, *803, *804, *851	● Physician must document length of time of loss of consciousness.
031	Patient's age > 17 *AND* CC condition	See CC section.	● Postconcussion syndrome (310.2) occurs following a concussion, when documented consult with the physician to determine if concussion is current stage or post syndrome.
032	Patient's age > 17		● Postconcussion syndrome (310.2) occurs following a concussion, when documented consult with the physician to determine if concussion is current stage or post syndrome.
484	Craniotomy for multiple significant trauma		■ Craniotomy and principal diagnosis of trauma and at least two injuries (assigned either as principal or secondary) that are defined as significant trauma from different body site categories located under DRG 487

■ Coding Tip ● Documentation Tip ◆ Encoder Tip ▼ Targeted DRG

Nervous System, MDC 1

DRG 033   (continued)

DRG	Principal Dx/Procedure	Codes	Tips
486	Other O.R. procedures for multiple significant trauma		■ Principal diagnosis of trauma and at least two injuries (assigned either as principal or secondary) that are defined as significant trauma from different body site categories located under DRG 487 *AND* O.R. procedure other than craniotomy or limb reattachment, hip and femur procedures
487	Other multiple significant trauma		■ Principal diagnosis of trauma and at least two injuries (assigned either as principal or secondary) that are defined as significant trauma from different body site categories located under DRG 487
528	Craniotomy *AND* Cerebral hemorrhages	*01.2, *02.0 430-*432	◆ Acute disorders

DRG 034   Other Disorders of Nervous System with CC   RW 0.9931

Potential DRGs

009	Spinal Disorders & Injuries	RW	1.4214
487	Other Multiple Significant Trauma	RW	2.0057

DRG	Principal Dx/Procedure	Codes	Tips
009	Paralysis due to spinal cord injury	*806, 907.2, *952	
487	Other multiple significant trauma		■ Principal diagnosis of trauma and at least two injuries (assigned either as principal or secondary) that are defined as significant trauma from different body site categories located under DRG 487

DRG 035   Other Disorders of Nervous System without CC   RW 0.6355

Potential DRGs

009	Spinal Disorders & Injuries	RW	1.4214
034	Other Disorders of Nervous System **with CC**	RW	0.9931
487	Other Multiple Significant Trauma	RW	2.0057

DRG	Principal Dx/Procedure	Codes	Tips
009	Paralysis due to spinal cord injury	*806, 907.2, *952	
034	CC condition	See CC section.	
487	Other multiple significant trauma		■ Principal diagnosis of trauma and at least two injuries (assigned either as principal or secondary) that are defined as significant trauma from different body site categories located under DRG 487

■ Coding Tip   ● Documentation Tip   ◆ Encoder Tip   ▼ Targeted DRG

Transient Ischemia   RW 0.7320 **DRG 524**

Potential DRGs

014	**Intracranial Hemorrhage and Stroke with Infarction**	RW	1.2682
015	Nonspecific CVA & Precerebral Occlusion without Infarction	RW	0.9677
528	Intracranial Vascular Procedure **with a Principal Diagnosis of Hemorrhage**	RW	7.2205

DRG	Principal Dx/Procedure	Codes	Tips
014	Cerebral hemorrhages Cerebral thrombosis w/cerebral infarction Cerebral embolism w/cerebral infarction Cerebral artery occlusion w/cerebral infarction	430- *432 434.01 434.11 434.91	◆ Acute disorders ■ Fifth digit for presence of cerebral infarction should be coded only when documented for current admission, not previous episode of care. ■ Acute event, code also documented neurological deficits. Use to code lacunar infarct.
015	Precerebral occlusions/stenosis wthout infarction Cerebral thrombosis/embolism/ unspecified occlusion without infarction Acute, but ill-defined CVA	*433 (fifth digit of 0 only) *434 (fifth digit of 0 only) 436	■ Fifth digit for presence of cerebral infarction should be coded only when documented for current admission, not previous episode of care.
528	Craniotomy *AND* Cerebral hemorrhages	*01.2, *02.0 430–*432	◆ Acute disorders

Ventricular Shunt Procedures with CC   RW 2.2529 **DRG 529**

Potential DRGs

001	**Craniotomy** Age > 17 with CC	RW	3.6186
528	**Intracranial Vascular Procedure** with Principal Diagnosis of Hemorrhage	RW	7.2205

DRG	Principal Dx/Procedure	Codes	Tips
001	Craniotomy *AND* Patient's age > 17 *AND* CC condition	022 See CC section.	
528	Craniotomy *AND* Cerebral hemorrhages	 430–*432	◆ Acute disorders

Ventricular Shunt Procedures without CC   RW 1.2017 **DRG 530**

Potential DRGs

001	**Craniotomy** Age > 17 with CC	RW	3.6186
528	**Intracranial Vascular Procedure** with Principal Diagnosis of Hemorrhage	RW	7.2205
529	Ventricular Shunt Procedures **with CC**	RW	2.2529

DRG	Principal Dx/Procedure	Codes	Tips
001	Craniotomy *AND* Patient's age > 17 *AND* CC condition	022 See CC section.	
528	Craniotomy *AND* Cerebral hemorrhages	 430–*432	◆ Acute disorders
529	Ventricular shunt procedure *AND* CC condition	*02.3, 02.42, 02.43 See CC section.	

■ Coding Tip   ● Documentation Tip   ◆ Encoder Tip   ▽ Targeted DRG

DRG 531   Spinal Procedures with CC

No Potential DRGs
Page 139

DRG 532   Spinal Procedures without CC   RW 1.4482

Potential DRGs
531   Spinal Procedures with CC   RW   3.0552

DRG	Principal Dx/Procedure	Codes	Tips
531	Spinal procedure *AND* CC condition	See CC section.	

DRG 533   Extracranial Vascular Procedures with CC

No Potential DRGs

DRG 534   Extracranial Vascular Procedures   RW 1.0748
              without CC

Potential DRGs
533   Extracranial Vascular Procedures with CC   RW   1.6678

DRG	Principal Dx/Procedure	Codes	Tips
533	Extracranial procedure *AND* CC condition	See CC section.	

Eye, MDC 2

DRG 036   Retinal Procedures   RW 0.6298

Potential DRGs
040   Extraocular Procedures Except Orbits, Age >17   RW   0.8937

DRG	Principal Dx/Procedure	Codes	Tips
040	Extraocular procedures, Age > 17	*10, *11.2, *11.3, *11.4, *15	● Excision of granuloma of conjunctiva; important to note number of muscles involved on each eye, as well as, whether unilateral or bilateral involvement

DRG 037   Orbital Procedures

No Potential DRGs

DRG 038   Primary Iris Procedures

No Potential DRGs

■ Coding Tip   ● Documentation Tip   ◆ Encoder Tip   ▽ Targeted DRG

Lens Procedures with or without Vitrectomy

RW 0.6285 **DRG 039**

Potential DRGs

477   Nonextensive O.R. Procedure Unrelated to Principal Diagnosis   RW   1.8873

DRG	Principal Dx/Procedure	Codes	Tips
477	Principal diagnosis unrelated to the O.R. procedure (e.g., cardiac diagnosis, other non-eye-related facial injury)		

Extraocular Procedures Except Orbit, Age > 17

RW 0.8937 **DRG 040**

Potential DRGs

037   Orbital Procedures   RW   1.0575

DRG	Principal Dx/Procedure	Codes	Tips
037	Orbital procedures (involving the eyeball or facial bone)	*16.0, *16.3, *16.4, *16.5, 16.6, *16.7, *16.8, 76.46, 76.79	

Extraocular Procedures Except Orbit, Age 0–17

RW 0.3401 **DRG 041**

Potential DRGs

037   Orbital Procedures   RW   1.0575
040   Extraocular Procedures Except Orbit, Age > 17   RW   0.8937

DRG	Principal Dx/Procedure	Codes	Tips
037	Orbital procedures (involving the eyeball or facial bone)	*16.0, *16.3, *16.4, *16.5, 16.6, *16.7, *16.8, 76.46, 76.79	
040	Patient's age > 17		

Intraocular Procedures Except Retina, Iris & Lens

RW 0.7064 **DRG 042**

Potential DRGs

036   Retinal Procedures   RW   0.6298

DRG	Principal Dx/Procedure	Codes	Tips
036	Retinal procedures	*14.4, *14.5	● Vitrectomy with scleral buckling; repair of retinal detachment

---

■ Coding Tip   ● Documentation Tip   ◆ Encoder Tip   ▽ Targeted DRG

Eye, MDC 2

DRG 043   Hyphema   RW 0.5382

Potential DRGs

046	Other Disorders of the Eye, Age > 17 **with CC**	RW	0.7936
047	Other Disorders of the Eye, Age > 17 **without CC**	RW	0.5317
134	Hypertension	RW	0.5954

DRG	Principal Dx/Procedure	Codes	Tips
046	Orbital hemorrhage Open wound, eyeball *AND* CC condition	376.32 *871 950.0 See CC section.	● Corneal laceration, corneoscleral laceration ◆ Traumatic with optic nerve injury
047	Orbital hemorrhage Open wound, eyeball	376.32 *871 950.0	● Corneal laceration, corneoscleral laceration ◆ Traumatic with optic nerve injury
134	Hypertension	401.0, 401.9, 404.90, *405	● Hypertension must be directly linked as cause of hyphema

DRG 044   Acute Major Eye Infections   RW 0.6597

Potential DRGs

046	Other Disorders of the Eye, Age > 17 **with CC**	RW	0.7936

DRG	Principal Dx/Procedure	Codes	Tips
046	Tuberculosis, eye Herpes virus, ophthalmic complications Gonococcal, infection, eye Histoplasmosis, retinitis Toxoplasmosis, ophthalmic *AND* CC condition	*017.3 *053.2, *054.4 *098.4 115.02, 115.12, 115.92 130.1, 130.2 See CC section.	◆ Key terms: chronic infection, uveitis, retinitis, excluding acute endophthal-mitis

DRG 045   Neruological Eye Disorders

No Potential DRGs

DRG 046   Other Disorders of the Eye Age > 17 with CC

No Potential DRGs

DRG 047   Other Disorders of the Eye, Age > 17   RW 0.5317
without CC

Potential DRGs

044	**Acute Major Eye Infections**	RW	0.6597
046	Other Disorders of the Eye, Age > 17 **with CC**	RW	0.7936

DRG	Principal Dx/Procedure	Codes	Tips
044	Acute dacryoadenitis Acute dacryocystitis	375.01 375.32	
046	CC condition	See CC section.	

Other Disorders of the Eye, Age 0–17   RW 0.2996   **DRG 048**

Potential DRGs

| 044 | Acute Major Eye Infections | RW | 0.6597 |
| 046 | Other Disorders of the Eye, **Age > 17 with CC** | RW | 0.7936 |

DRG	Principal Dx/Procedure	Codes	Tips
044	Acute dacryoadenitis Acute dacryocystitis	375.01 375.32	
046	Patient's age > 17 *AND* CC condition	See CC section.	

Ear, Nose, Mouth, and Throat, MDC 3

Major Head & Neck Procedures   RW 1.7277   **DRG 049**

Potential DRGs

| 482 | **Tracheostomy** For Face, Mouth and Neck Diagnoses | RW | 3.4803 |

DRG	Principal Dx/Procedure	Codes	Tips
482	Tracheostomy	31.1, 31.21, 31.29	■ A minitracheostomy is coded as a temporary tracheostomy. ■ Tracheostomy carried out elsewhere prior to admission or in ambulance prior to arrival should not be reported as a current procedure. ● Tracheostomy procedure may be performed either at the bedside and documented in the progress notes or in the operating room and documented in an operative note.

Sialoadenectomy   RW 0.8317   **DRG 050**

Potential DRGs

| 049 | Major Head & Neck Procedures | RW | 1.7277 |

DRG	Principal Dx/Procedure	Codes	Tips
049	Radical neck dissection	40.40, 40.41, 40.42	◆ Key terms: modified/complete/radical neck dissection, bilateral, unilateral.

Salivary Gland Procedures Except Sialoadenectomy   **DRG 051**

No Potential DRGs

Cleft Lip and Palate Repair   **DRG 052**

No Potential DRGs

Sinus and Mastoid Procedures Age >17   **DRG 053**

No Potential DRGs

Sinus and Mastoid Procedures Age 0–17   **DRG 054**

No Potential DRGs

■ Coding Tip   ● Documentation Tip   ◆ Encoder Tip   ▽ Targeted DRG

145

Ear, Nose, Mouth, and Throat, MDC 3

DRG 055   Miscellaneous Ear, Nose, Mouth and Throat Procedures

No Potential DRGs

DRG 056   Rhinoplasty   RW 0.9233

Potential DRGs
053   Sinus & Mastoid Procedures, Age >17   RW   1.2520

DRG	Principal Dx/Procedure	Codes	Tips
053	Major sinus procedure	*20.4, *22.3 *22.7	◆ Key terms: diagnostic, endoscopic, ethmoidectomy, sinusectomy, mastoidectomy, antrotomy

DRG 057   Tonsil & Adenoid Procedures Except   RW 1.1029 Tonsillectomy and/or Adenoidectomy Only, Age > 17

Potential DRGs
No information available at this time for optimizing payment.
*Ensure accurate DRG assignment, see below:

Peritonsillar I&D 28.0
Tonsil/adenoid biopsy 28.11
Tonsil/adenoid diagnostic operations NEC 28.19
Excision, tonsil tag 28.4
Excision, lingual tonsi 28.5
Hemorrhage control, post T&A 28.7
Removal, tonsil/adenoid foreign body 28.91
Excision, lesion, tonsil/adenoid 28.92

Tonsil/adenoid operations NEC 28.99
OR
Tonsillectomy 28.2
Tonsillectomy with adenoidectomy 28.3
Adenoidectomy 28.6
AND
Any other OR procedure

DRG 058   Tonsil & Adenoid Procedures Except   RW 0.2757 Tonsillectomy and/or Adenoidectomy Only, Age 0–17

Potential DRGs
057   Tonsil & Adenoid Procedures Except Tonsillectomy and/or Adenoidectomy   RW   1.1029
Only, **Age > 17**

DRG	Principal Dx/Procedure	Codes	Tips
057	Patient's age > 17		

DRG 059   Tonsillectomy and/or Adenoidectomy   RW 0.9557 Only, Age > 17

Potential DRGs
057   **Tonsil & Adenoid Procedures** Except Tonsillectomy and/or Adenoidectomy   RW   1.1029
Only, Age > 17

DRG	Principal Dx/Procedure	Codes	Tips
057	Patient's age > 17		

Tonsillectomy and/or Adenoidectomy Only, Age 0–17
RW 0.2099 **DRG 060**

Potential DRGs

057	Tonsil & Adenoid Procedures **Except Tonsillectomy and/or Adenoidectomy Only, Age > 17**	RW	1.1029
058	Tonsil & Adenoid Procedures **Except Tonsillectomy and/or Adenoidectomy Only, Age 0–17**	RW	0.2757
059	Tonsillectomy and/or Adenoidectomy, **Age > 17**	RW	0.9557

DRG	Principal Dx/Procedure	Codes	Tips
057	Tonsillectomy &/or Adenoidectomy *AND* Any Other Operating Procedure	28.0, *28.1, 28.4, 28.5, 28.7, *28.9	
058	Tonsillectomy &/or Adenoidectomy *AND* Any Other Operating Procedure	28.0, *28.1, 28.4, 28.5, 28.7, *28.9	
059	Patient's age > 17		

Myringotomy with Tube Insertion, Age > 17
DRG 061

No Potential DRGs

Myringotomy with Tube Insertion, Age 0–17
RW 0.2973 **DRG 062**

Potential DRGs

| 061 | Myringotomy with Tube Insertion, **Age > 17** | RW | 1.2334 |

DRG	Principal Dx/Procedure	Codes	Tips
061	Patient's age > 17		

Other Ear, Nose, Mouth & Throat O.R. Procedures
RW 1.3759 **DRG 063**

Potential DRGs

| 482 | **Tracheostomy** for Face, Mouth and Neck Diagnoses | RW | 3.4803 |

DRG	Principal Dx/Procedure	Codes	Tips
482	Tracheostomy	31.1, 31.21, 31.29	■ A minitracheostomy is coded as a temporary tracheostomy. ■ Tracheostomy carried out elsewhere prior to admission or in ambulance prior to arrival should not be reported as a current procedure. ● Tracheostomy procedure may be performed either at the bedside and documented in the progress notes or in the operating room and documented in an operative note.

■ Coding Tip   ● Documentation Tip   ◆ Encoder Tip   ▽ Targeted DRG

DRG 064   Ear, Nose, Mouth & Throat Malignancy   RW 1.3089

Potential DRGs

482   **Tracheostomy** for Face, Mouth and Neck Diagnoses   RW   3.4803

DRG	Principal Dx/Procedure	Codes	Tips
482	Tracheostomy	31.1, 31.21, 31.29	■ A minitracheostomy is coded as a temporary tracheostomy. ■ Tracheostomy carried out elsewhere prior to admission or in ambulance prior to arrival should not be reported as a current procedure. ● Tracheostomy procedure may be performed either at the bedside and documented in the progress notes or in the operating room and documented in an operative note.

DRG 065   Dysequilibrium   RW 0.5748

Potential DRGs

018   Cranial & Peripheral Nerve Disorders with CC   RW   1.0026

DRG	Principal Dx/Procedure	Codes	Tips
018	Unspecified disorder CNS *AND* CC condition	337.9 See CC section.	■ Code 780.4 dizziness and giddiness could be a symptom of other disease processes listed under DRG 018

DRG 066   Epistaxis   RW 0.5811

Potential DRGs

063   **Other Ear, Nose, Mouth & Throat O.R. Procedures**   RW   1.3759
072   Nasal Trauma and Deformity   RW   0.6954
101   Other Respiratory System Diagnoses **with CC**   RW   0.8654
134   **Hypertension**   RW   0.5954
487   Other Multiple Significant Trauma   RW   2.0057

DRG	Principal Dx/Procedure	Codes	Tips
063	O.R. procedure surgical control of epistaxis	21.04, 21.09	◆ Key terms: ligation of arteries, excision of mucosa, skin grafting of septum, other specified
072	Nasal trauma and deformity	802.0, 802.1, 873.20	
101	Complication, surgical, respiratory *AND* CC condition	997.3 See CC section.	
134	Hypertension (the cause of the epistaxis)	401.0, 402.00, 404.00, *405	■ Hypertension must be directly linked as cause of epistaxis; see guidelines for hypertension coding.
487	Other multiple significant trauma		■ Craniotomy and principal diagnosis of trauma and at least two injuries (assigned either as principal or secondary) that are defined as significant trauma from different body site categories located under DRG 487

DRG 067   Epiglottitis

No Potential DRGs

■ Coding Tip   ● Documentation Tip   ◆ Encoder Tip   ▽ Targeted DRG

Otitis Media & Upper Respiratory Infection, Age > 17 with CC

RW 0.6531 **DRG 068**

Potential DRGs

067 Epiglottitis   RW   0.7780

DRG	Principal Dx/Procedure	Codes	Tips
067	Acute epiglottitis	*464.3	◆ Key terms: acute, viral, unspecified ● Identify site of infection of supraglottis structures.

Otitis Media & Upper Respiratory Infection, Age > 17 without CC

RW 0.4987 **DRG 069**

Potential DRGs

067 Epiglottitis   RW   0.7780
068 Otitis Media & Upper Respiratory Infection, Age > 17 **with CC**   RW   0.6531
071 Laryngotracheitis   RW   0.7065

DRG	Principal Dx/Procedure	Codes	Tips
067	Acute epiglottitis	*464.3	◆ Key terms: acute, viral, unspecified ● Identify site of infection of supraglottis structures.
068	CC condition	See CC section.	
071	Acute laryngotracheitis	*464.2	◆ Key terms: laryngitis, croup, spasmodic, acute, bacterial ● Identify site of infection of supraglottis structures.

Otitis Media & Upper Respiratory Infection, Age 0–17

RW 0.3188 **DRG 070**

Potential DRGs

067 Epiglottitis   RW   0.7780
068 Otitis Media & Upper Respiratory Infection, **Age > 17 with CC**   RW   0.6531
069 Otitis Media & Upper Respiratory Infection, **Age > 17** without CC   RW   0.4987
071 Laryngotracheitis   RW   0.7065

DRG	Principal Dx/Procedure	Codes	Tips
067	Acute epiglottitis	*464.3	◆ Key terms: acute, viral, unspecified. ● Identify site of infection of supraglottis structures.
068	Patient's age > 17 *AND* CC condition	See CC section.	
069	Patient's age > 17		
071	Acute laryngotracheitis	*464.2	◆ Key terms: laryngitis, croup, spasmodic, acute, bacterial ● Identify site of infection of supraglottis structures.

■ Coding Tip   ● Documentation Tip   ◆ Encoder Tip   ▽ Targeted DRG

Ear, Nose, Mouth, and Throat, MDC 3

DRG 071   Laryngotracheitis   RW 0.7065

Potential DRGs

067   Epiglottitis   RW   0.7780

DRG	Principal Dx/Procedure	Codes	Tips
067	Acute epiglottitis	*464.3	◆ Key terms: acute, viral, unspecified ● Identify site of infection of supraglottis structures.

DRG 072   Nasal Trauma & Deformity   RW 0.6954

Potential DRGs

055   Nasal procedures   RW   0.9247
056   Rhinoplasty   RW   0.9233
063   Other Ear, Nose, Mouth & Throat O.R. Procedures   RW   1.3759

DRG	Principal Dx/Procedure	Codes	Tips
055	Nasal procedures	21.4, 21.5, 21.6x, 21.72, 21.82, 21.89, 21.99	
056	Rhinoplasty, septoplasty or nasal reconstruction	21.83, 21.87, 21.88	
063	Any other ear, nose, mouth and throat O.R. procedure not listed for DRGs 049–062		

DRG 073   Other Ear, Nose, Mouth & Throat   RW 0.8184
          Diagnoses, Age > 17

Potential DRGs

484   Craniotomy for Multiple Significant Trauma   RW   5.4179
486   Other O.R. Procedures for Multiple Significant Trauma RW   4.8793
487   Other Multiple Significant Trauma   RW   2.0057

DRG	Principal Dx/Procedure	Codes	Tips
484	Craniotomy for multiple significant trauma		■ Craniotomy and principal diagnosis of trauma and at least two injuries (assigned either as principal or secondary) that are defined as significant trauma from different body site categories located under DRG 487
486	Other O.R. procedures for multiple significant trauma		■ Principal diagnosis of trauma and at least two injuries (assigned either as principal or secondary) that are defined as significant trauma from different body site categories located under DRG 487 **AND** O.R. procedure other than craniotomy or limb reattachment, hip and femur procedures
487	Other multiple significant trauma		■ Principal diagnosis of trauma and at least two injuries (assigned either as principal or secondary) that are defined as significant trauma from different body site categories located under DRG 487

■ Coding Tip   ● Documentation Tip   ◆ Encoder Tip   ▼ Targeted DRG

Other Ear, Nose, Mouth & Throat Diagnoses, Age 0-17

RW 0.3380   **DRG 074**

Potential DRGs

073	Other Ear, Nose, Mouth & Throat Diagnoses, **Age >17**	RW	0.8184
484	**Craniotomy for Multiple Significant Trauma**	RW	5.4179
486	**Other O.R. Procedures for Multiple Significant Trauma**	RW	4.8793
487	Other Multiple Significant Trauma	RW	2.0057

DRG	Principal Dx/Procedure	Codes	Tips
073	Patient's age > 17		
484	Craniotomy for multiple significant trauma		■ Craniotomy and principal diagnosis of trauma and at least two injuries (assigned either as principal or secondary) that are defined as significant trauma from different body site categories located under DRG 487
486	Other O.R. procedures for multiple significant trauma		■ Principal diagnosis of trauma and at least two injuries (assigned either as principal or secondary) that are defined as significant trauma from different body site categories located under DRG 487 *AND* O.R. procedure other than craniotomy or limb reattachment, hip and femur procedures
487	Other multiple significant trauma		■ Principal diagnosis of trauma and at least two injuries (assigned either as principal or secondary) that are defined as significant trauma from different body site categories located under DRG 487

Mouth Procedures with CC

RW 1.3158   **DRG 168**

Potential DRGs

049	**Major Head & Neck Procedures**	RW	1.7277

DRG	Principal Dx/Procedure	Codes	Tips
049	Cochlear device procedures	20.96–20.98	
	Glossectomy, complete or radical	25.3, 25.4	
	Wide excision or destruction of lesion or tissue of bony palate	27.32	
	Laryngectomy, partial	30.29	
	Radical neck dissection, unilateral or bilateral	40.41, 40.42	
	Mandibulectomy, total or partial	76.31, 76.41	

■ Coding Tip   ● Documentation Tip   ◆ Encoder Tip   ▽ Targeted DRG

DRG 169   Mouth Procedures without CC   RW 0.7525

Potential DRGs

049	Major Head & Neck Procedures	RW	1.7277
168	Mouth Procedures **with CC**	RW	1.3158

DRG	Principal Dx/Procedure	Codes	Tips
049	Cochlear device procedures Glossectomy, complete or radical Wide excision or destruction of lesion or tissue of bony palate Laryngectomy, partial Radical neck dissection, unilateral or bilateral Mandibulectomy, total or partial	20.96–20.98 25.3, 25.4 27.32, 30.29 40.41, 40.42 76.31, 76.41	
168	CC condition	See CC section.	

DRG 185   Dental & Oral Disorders Except Extractions & Restorations, Age > 17

No Potential DRGs

DRG 186   Dental & Oral Disorders Except Extractions & Restorations, Age 0–17   RW 0.3236

Potential DRGs

185	Dental & Oral Disorders Except Extractions & Restorations, **Age > 17**	RW	0.8685

DRG	Principal Dx/Procedure	Codes	Tips
185	Patient's age > 17		

DRG 187   Dental Extractions & Restorations

No Potential DRGs

Respiratory System, MDC 4

DRG 075   Major Chest Procedures   RW 3.0437

Potential DRGs

483	Tracheostomy with Mech Vent 96+ Hours or Principal Diagnosis Except Face, Mouth and Neck Diagnoses	RW	16.7762

DRG	Principal Dx/Procedure	Codes	Tips
483	Tracheostomy *AND* Mechanical ventilation 96+ hours	31.1, 31.21, 31.29 96.72	■ A minitracheostomy is coded as a temporary tracheostomy. ■ Tracheostomy carried out elsewhere prior to admission or in ambulance prior to arrival should not be reported as a current procedure. ● Tracheostomy procedure may be performed either at the bedside and documented in the progress notes or in the operating room and documented in an operative note.

Other Respiratory System O.R. Procedures with CC   RW 2.8184   **DRG 076**

Potential DRGs
075	Major Chest Procedures	RW	3.0437
475	Respiratory System Diagnosis with Ventilator Support	RW	3.6000
483	Tracheostomy with Mech Vent 96+ Hours or Principal Diagnosis Except Face, Mouth and Neck Diagnoses	RW	16.7762

DRG	Principal Dx/Procedure	Codes	Tips
075 ▽YIELD	Open bronchial biopsy Open lung biopsy	33.25 33.28	■ Thoroscopic wedge open/incisional biopsy of lung, if wedge resection is for treatment code 32.29.
475	Resp Dx and continuous mechanical ventilation	486, 491.21, 507.0, 518.81	■ Aspiration pneumonia: code both aspiration and bacterial pneumonia if documented. ● Arterial blood gas determinations are supportive; do not base definitive dx on clinical findings. ■ Mech ventilation used during surgery is not coded unless MD documents unexpected extended period of time following surgery.
483	Tracheostomy *AND* Mechanical ventilation 96+ hours	31.1, 31.21, 31.29 96.72	■ A minitracheostomy is coded as a temporary tracheostomy. ■ Tracheostomy carried out elsewhere prior to admission or in ambulance prior to arrival should not be reported as a current procedure. ● Tracheostomy procedure may be performed either at the bedside and documented in the progress notes or in the operating room and documented in an operative note.

Other Respiratory System O.R. Procedures without CC   RW 1.2378   **DRG 077**

Potential DRGs
075	Major Chest Procedures	RW	3.0437
076	Other Respiratory System O.R. Procedures **with CC**	RW	2.8184
475	Respiratory Diagnosis with Continuous Mechanical Ventilation	RW	3.6000
483	Tracheostomy with Mech Vent 96+ Hours or Principal Diagnosis Except Face, Mouth and Neck Diagnoses	RW	16.7762

DRG	Principal Dx/Procedure	Codes	Tips
075	Open bronchial biopsy, open lung biopsy	33.25, 33.28	■ Thoroscopic wedge open/incisional biopsy of lung, if wedge resection is for treatment code 32.29.
076	CC condition	See CC section.	
475 ▽YIELD	Resp Dx and continuous mechanical ventilation	486, 491.21, 507.0, 518.81	■ Aspiration pneumonia: code both aspiration and bacterial pneumonia if documented. ● Arterial blood gas determinations are supportive; do not base definitive dx on clinical findings. ■ Mech ventilation used during surgery is not coded unless MD documents unexpected extended period of time following surgery.

■ Coding Tip   ● Documentation Tip   ◆ Encoder Tip   ▽ Targeted DRG

Respiratory System, MDC 4

DRG 077 (continued)

DRG	Principal Dx/Procedure	Codes	Tips
483	Tracheostomy *AND* Mechanical ventilation 96+ hours	31.1, 31.21, 31.29 96.72	■ A minitracheostomy is coded as a temporary tracheostomy. ■ Tracheostomy carried out elsewhere prior to admission or in ambulance prior to arrival should not be reported as a current procedure. ● Tracheostomy procedure may be performed either at the bedside and documented in the progress notes or in the operating room and documented in an operative note.

DRG 078 Pulmonary Embolism   RW 1.2731

Potential DRGs

075	Major Chest Procedures	RW	3.0437
076	Other Respiratory System OR Procedures with CC	RW	2.8184
121	Circulatory Disorders **with AMI and Major Complications**, Discharged Alive	RW	1.6169
387	Prematurity **with Major Problems**	RW	3.1203
475	Respiratory System Diagnosis **with Ventilator Support**	RW	3.6000
483	**Tracheostomy with Mech Vent 96+ Hours or Principal Diagnosis Except Face, Mouth and Neck Diagnoses**	RW	16.7762

DRG	Principal Dx/Procedure	Codes	Tips
075	Pulmonary embolectomy	38.05	■ Embolectomy or thrombectomy of superior vena cava, subclavian vein, pulmonary (artery)(vein)
076	Plication and ligation procedures *AND* CC condition	38.7 See CC section.	■ Percutaneous insertion of vena cava sieve or umbrella, ligation, or plication
121 ▽	AMI, initial episode of care *AND* MAJOR COMPLICATIONS: Rheumatic heart failure Primary pulmonary hypertension Subarachnoid hemorrhage Intracerebral hemorrhage Nontraumatic extradural hemorrhage Subdural hemorrhage Unspecified intracranial hemorrhage Occluded basilar artery with cerebral infarction Occluded carotid artery with cerebral infarction Occluded vertebral artery with cerebral infarction Occluded multiple and bilateral precerebral artery with cerebral infarction Occluded specified precerebral artery with cerebral infarction Occluded precerebral artery NOS with cerebral infarction Cerebral thrombosis Cerebral thrombosis with cerebral infarction Cerebral embolism Cerebral embolism with cerebral infarction Cerebral artery occlusion	 398.91 416.0 430 431 432.0 432.1 432.9 433.01 433.11 433.21 433.31 433.81 433.91 434.00 434.01 434.10 434.11 434.90	

■ Coding Tip   ● Documentation Tip   ◆ Encoder Tip   ▽ Targeted DRG

DRG	Principal Dx/Procedure	Codes	Tips
121 cont.	Cerebral artery occlusion with cerebral infarction	434.91	
	CVA NOS	436	
	Pneumococcal pneumonia	481	
	Other bacterial pneumonia (all fourth and fifth digits except 482.84)		
	Pneumonia due to other specified organism	482.xx	
	Pneumonia in infectious diseases classified elsewhere (all fourth digits)	483.x	
	Bronchopneumonia, organism unspecified	484.x	
	Pneumonia, organism unspecified	485	
	Influenza with pneumonia	486	
	Pneumonitis due to solids and liquids (all fourth digits)	487.0 507.x	
	Pulmonary collapse	518.0	
	Pulmonary insufficiency following trauma and surgery	518.5	
	Acute respiratory failure	518.81	
	Chronic respiratory failure	518.83	
	Acute and chronic respiratory failure	518.84	
	Decubitus ulcer	707.0	
	Infection and inflammatory reaction due to vascular device, implant or graft	996.62	
	Other complications due to other cardiac device, implant and graft	996.72	
387	Premature newborn **WITH** Major problems:	765.0, 765.08, 765.06, *765.1, 765.07	
	Pulmonary embolism	415.11, 415.19	
475 ⟨ᵛᴱᴸᴼ⟩	Continuous mechanical ventilation	96.70–96.79	◆ Key terms: IMV, PEEP, PSV, endotracheal respiratory assistance
483	Tracheostomy *AND* Mechanical ventilation 96+ hours	31.1, 31.21, 31.29 96.72	■ A minitracheostomy is coded as a temporary tracheostomy. ■ Tracheostomy carried out elsewhere prior to admission or in ambulance prior to arrival should not be reported as a current procedure. ● Tracheostomy procedure may be performed either at the bedside and documented in the progress notes or in the operating room and documented in an operative note.

DRG 079 Respiratory Infections & Inflammations, RW 1.5974
Age > 17 with CC

Potential DRGs

475	Respiratory System Diagnosis **with Ventilator Support**	RW	3.6000
483	**Tracheostomy with Mech Vent 96+ Hours or Principal Diagnosis**	RW	16.7762
	Except Face, Mouth and Neck Diagnoses		
489	**HIV with Major Related Condition**	RW	1.8603

DRG	Principal Dx/Procedure	Codes	Tips
475 ▽	Continuous mechanical ventilation	96.70–96.79	◆ Key terms: IMV, PEEP, PSV, endotracheal respiratory assistance
483	Tracheostomy *AND* Mechanical ventilation 96+ hours	31.1, 31.21, 31.29 96.72	■ A minitracheostomy is coded as a temporary tracheostomy. ■ Tracheostomy carried out elsewhere prior to admission or in ambulance prior to arrival should not be reported as a current procedure. ● Tracheostomy procedure may be performed either at the bedside and documented in the progress notes or in the operating room and documented in an operative note.
489	Dx of HIV *AND* Opportunistic lung infection	042 112.4	◆ AIDS; ARV; ARC; HIV infection, symptomatic; HIV-2 associated with AIDS

DRG 080 Respiratory Infections & Inflammations, RW 0.8400
Age > 17 without CC

Potential DRGs

079	Respiratory Infections & Inflammations, Age > 17 **with CC**	RW	1.5974
475	Respiratory System Diagnosis **with Ventilator Support**	RW	3.6000
483	**Tracheostomy with Mech Vent 96+ Hours or Principal Diagnosis**	RW	16.7762
	Except Face, Mouth and Neck Diagnoses		
489	**HIV with Major Related Condition**	RW	1.8603

DRG	Principal Dx/Procedure	Codes	Tips
079 ▽	CC condition	See CC section.	
475 ▽	Continuous mechanical ventilation	96.70–96.79	◆ Key terms: IMV, PEEP, PSV, endotracheal respiratory assistance
483	Tracheostomy *AND* Mechanical ventilation 96+ hours	31.1, 31.21, 31.29 96.72	■ A minitracheostomy is coded as a temporary tracheostomy. ■ Tracheostomy carried out elsewhere prior to admission or in ambulance prior to arrival should not be reported as a current procedure. ● Tracheostomy procedure may be performed either at the bedside and documented in the progress notes or in the operating room and documented in an operative note.
489	Dx of HIV *AND* Opportunistic lung infection	042 112.4	

■ Coding Tip	● Documentation Tip	◆ Encoder Tip	▽ Targeted DRG

Respiratory Infections & Inflammations, Age 0–17   RW 1.5300   **DRG 081**

Potential DRGs
079   Respiratory Infections & Inflammations, **Age > 17 with CC**   RW   1.5974
475   Respiratory System Diagnosis **with Ventilator Support**   RW   3.6000
483   **Tracheostomy with Mech Vent 96+ Hours or Principal Diagnosis Except Face, Mouth and Neck Diagnoses**   RW   16.7762
489   **HIV with Major Related Condition**   RW   1.8603

DRG	Principal Dx/Procedure	Codes	Tips
079 🔻	Patient's age > 17 *AND* CC condition	See CC section.	
475 🔻	Continuous mechanical ventilation	96.70–96.79	◆ Key terms: IMV, PEEP, PSV, endotracheal respiratory assistance
483	Tracheostomy *AND* Mechanical ventilation 96+ hours	31.1, 31.21, 31.29 96.72	■ A minitracheostomy is coded as a temporary tracheostomy. ■ Tracheostomy carried out elsewhere prior to admission or in ambulance prior to arrival should not be reported as a current procedure. ● Tracheostomy procedure may be performed either at the bedside and documented in the progress notes or in the operating room and documented in an operative note.
489	Dx of HIV *AND* Opportunistic lung infection	042 112.4	

Respiratory Neoplasms   RW 1.3724   **DRG 082**

Potential DRGs
076   Other Respiratory System OR Procedures **with CC**   RW   2.8184
475   Respiratory System Diagnosis **with Ventilator Support**   RW   3.6000
483   **Tracheostomy with Mech Vent 96+ Hours or Principal Diagnosis Except Face, Mouth and Neck Diagnoses**   RW   16.7762

DRG	Principal Dx/Procedure	Codes	Tips
076	Brachytherapy radioactive implant *AND* CC condition	92.27 See CC section.	■ Bronchoscopy with placement of catheter for radiotherapy; do not code bronch approach ◆ Intracavitary; interstitial; intravascular
475 🔻	Continuous mechanical ventilation	96.70–96.79	◆ Key terms: IMV, PEEP, PSV, endotracheal respiratory assistance
483	Tracheostomy *AND* Mechanical ventilation 96+ hours	31.1, 31.21, 31.29 96.72	■ A minitracheostomy is coded as a temporary tracheostomy. ■ Tracheostomy carried out elsewhere prior to admission or in ambulance prior to arrival should not be reported as a current procedure. ● Tracheostomy procedure may be performed either at the bedside and documented in the progress notes or in the operating room and documented in an operative note.

Respiratory System, MDC 4

DRG 083   Major Chest Trauma with CC   RW 0.9620

Potential DRGs

475	Respiratory System Diagnosis **with Ventilator Support**	RW 3.6000
483	**Tracheostomy with Mech Vent 96+ Hours or Principal Diagnosis Except Face, Mouth and Neck Diagnoses**	RW 16.7762
484	Craniotomy for **Multiple Significant Trauma**	RW 5.4179
486	**Other O.R. Procedures for Multiple Significant Trauma**	RW 4.8793
487	Other Multiple Significant Trauma	RW 2.0057

DRG	Principal Dx/Procedure	Codes	Tips
475 ▽	Continuous mechanical ventilation	96.70–96.79	◆ Key terms: IMV, PEEP, PSV, endotracheal respiratory assistance
483	Tracheostomy *AND* Mechanical ventilation 96+ hours	31.1, 31.21, 31.29 96.72	■ A minitracheostomy is coded as a temporary tracheostomy. ■ Tracheostomy carried out elsewhere prior to admission or in ambulance prior to arrival should not be reported as a current procedure. ● Tracheostomy procedure may be performed either at the bedside and documented in the progress notes or in the operating room and documented in an operative note.
484	Craniotomy for multiple significant trauma		■ Craniotomy and principal diagnosis of trauma and at least two injuries (assigned either as principal or secondary) that are defined as significant trauma from different body site categories located under DRG 487
486	Other O.R. procedures for multiple significant trauma		■ Principal diagnosis of trauma and at least two injuries (assigned either as principal or secondary) that are defined as significant trauma from different body site categories located under DRG 487 *AND* O.R. procedure other than craniotomy or limb reattachment, hip and femur procedures
487	Other multiple significant trauma		■ Principal diagnosis of trauma and at least two injuries (assigned either as principal or secondary) that are defined as significant trauma from different body site categories located under DRG 487

DRG 084   Major Chest Trauma without CC   RW 0.5371

Potential DRGs

083	Major Chest Trauma **with CC**	RW 0.9620
475	Respiratory System Diagnosis **with Ventilator Support**	RW 3.6000
483	**Tracheostomy with Mech Vent 96+ Hours or Principal Diagnosis Except Face, Mouth and Neck Diagnoses**	RW 16.7762
484	Craniotomy for **Multiple Significant Trauma**	RW 5.4179
486	**Other O.R. Procedures for Multiple Significant Trauma**	RW 4.8793
487	Other Multiple Significant Trauma	RW 2.0057

DRG	Principal Dx/Procedure	Codes	Tips
083	CC condition	See CC section.	
475 ▽	Continuous mechanical ventilation	96.70–96.79	◆ Key terms: IMV, PEEP, PSV, endotracheal respiratory assistance

---

■ Coding Tip   ● Documentation Tip   ◆ Encoder Tip   ▽ Targeted DRG

(continued) DRG 084

DRG	Principal Dx/Procedure	Codes	Tips
483	Tracheostomy *AND* Mechanical ventilation 96+ hours	31.1, 31.21, 31.29 96.72	■ A minitracheostomy is coded as a temporary tracheostomy. ■ Tracheostomy carried out elsewhere prior to admission or in ambulance prior to arrival should not be reported as a current procedure. ● Tracheostomy procedure may be performed either at the bedside and documented in the progress notes or in the operating room and documented in an operative note.
484	Craniotomy for multiple significant trauma		■ Craniotomy and principal diagnosis of trauma and at least two injuries (assigned either as principal or secondary) that are defined as significant trauma from different body site categories located under DRG 487
486	Other O.R. procedures for multiple significant trauma		■ Principal diagnosis of trauma and at least two injuries (assigned either as principal or secondary) that are defined as significant trauma from different body site categories located under DRG 487 *AND* O.R. procedure other than craniotomy or limb reattachment, hip and femur procedures
487	Other multiple significant trauma		■ Principal diagnosis of trauma and at least two injuries (assigned either as principal or secondary) that are defined as significant trauma from different body site categories located under DRG 487

Pleural Effusion with CC   RW 1.1927 **DRG 085**

Potential DRGs

475	Respiratory System Diagnosis **with Ventilator Support**	RW 3.6000
483	**Tracheostomy with Mech Vent 96+ Hours or Principal Diagnosis Except Face, Mouth and Neck Diagnoses**	RW 16.7762

DRG	Principal Dx/Procedure	Codes	Tips
475 ▽	Continuous mechanical ventilation	96.70–96.79	◆ Key terms: IMV, PEEP, PSV, endotracheal respiratory assistance
483	Tracheostomy *AND* Mechanical ventilation 96+ hours	31.1, 31.21, 31.29 96.72	■ A minitracheostomy is coded as a temporary tracheostomy. ■ Tracheostomy carried out elsewhere prior to admission or in ambulance prior to arrival should not be reported as a current procedure. ● Tracheostomy procedure may be performed either at the bedside and documented in the progress notes or in the operating room and documented in an operative note.

DRG 086   Pleural Effusion without CC   RW 0.6864

Potential DRGs

075	Major Chest Procedures	RW	3.0437
077	Other Respiratory System O.R. Procedures **without CC**	RW	1.2378
082	Respiratory Neoplasms	RW	1.3724
085	Pleural Effusion **with CC**	RW	1.1927
127	**Heart Failure & Shock**	RW	1.0265
475	**Respiratory System Diagnosis with Ventilator Support**	RW	3.6000
483	**Tracheostomy with Mech Vent 96+ Hours or Principal Diagnosis Except Face, Mouth and Neck Diagnoses**	RW	16.7762

DRG	Principal Dx/Procedure	Codes	Tips
075	Pleurodesis	34.6	◆ Surgical abrasion, scarification of pleura
077	Transpleural thoracoscopy	34.21	◆ Diagnostic; omit when considered approach
082	Respiratory neoplasm	*162, *163, 197.0, 197.2, 212.9	◆ Malignant pleural effusion
085	CC condition	See CC section.	
127 ⟁	CHF (sequence as principal diagnosis when associated with pleural effusion)	*428	◆ PE commonly seen as part of congestive heart failure disease process; when evaluated and treated report as additional diagnosis ■ End-stage congestive heart failure, compensated heart failure, decompensated heart failure, heart failure NOS
475 ⟁	Continuous mechanical ventilation	96.70–96.79	◆ Key terms: IMV, PEEP, PSV, endotracheal respiratory assistance
483	Tracheostomy *AND* Mechanical ventilation 96+ hours	31.1, 31.21, 31.29 96.72	■ A minitracheostomy is coded as a temporary tracheostomy. ■ Tracheostomy carried out elsewhere prior to admission or in ambulance prior to arrival should not be reported as a current procedure. ● Tracheostomy procedure may be performed either at the bedside and documented in the progress notes or in the operating room and documented in an operative note.

■ Coding Tip   ● Documentation Tip   ◆ Encoder Tip   ⟁ Targeted DRG

Pulmonary Edema & Respiratory Failure   RW 1.3430 ▽**DRG 087**

Potential DRGs

475	Respiratory System Diagnosis **with Ventilator Support**	RW	3.6000
483	**Tracheostomy with Mech Vent 96+ Hours or Principal Diagnosis**	RW	16.7762
	Except Face, Mouth and Neck Diagnoses		

DRG	Principal Dx/Procedure	Codes	Tips
475 ▽YIELD	Continuous mechanical ventilation	96.70–96.79	◆ Key terms: IMV, PEEP, PSV, endotracheal respiratory assistance
483	Tracheostomy *AND* Mechanical ventilation 96+ hours	31.1, 31.21, 31.29 96.72	■ A minitracheostomy is coded as a temporary tracheostomy. ■ Tracheostomy carried out elsewhere prior to admission or in ambulance prior to arrival should not be reported as a current procedure. ● Tracheostomy procedure may be performed either at the bedside and documented in the progress notes or in the operating room and documented in an operative note.

Chronic Obstructive Pulmonary Disease   RW 0.9031 ▽**DRG 088**

Potential DRGs

087	Pulmonary Edema & **Respiratory Failure**	RW	1.3430
127	**Heart Failure** & Shock	RW	1.0265
475	Respiratory System Diagnosis **with Ventilator Support**	RW	3.6000
483	**Tracheostomy with Mech Vent 96+ Hours or Principal Diagnosis**	RW	16.7762
	Except Face, Mouth and Neck Diagnoses		

DRG	Principal Dx/Procedure	Codes	Tips
087 ▽YIELD	Respiratory failure	518.81, 518.83, 518.84	◆ COPD generic term; common cause of failure. Look for failure as acute exacerbation or underlying cause of admission per MD documentation.
127 ▽YIELD	CHF (sequence as principal diagnosis when associated with pleural effusion)	*428	◆ PE commonly seen as part of congestive heart failure disease process; when evaluated and treated report as additional diagnosis ■ End-stage congestive heart failure, compensated heart failure, decompensated heart failure, heart failure NOS
475 ▽YIELD	Continuous mechanical ventilation	96.70–96.79	◆ Key terms: IMV, PEEP, PSV, endotracheal respiratory assistance
483	Tracheostomy *AND* Mechanical ventilation 96+ hours	31.1, 31.21, 31.29 96.72	■ A minitracheostomy is coded as a temporary tracheostomy. ■ Tracheostomy carried out elsewhere prior to admission or in ambulance prior to arrival should not be reported as a current procedure. ● Tracheostomy procedure may be performed either at the bedside and documented in the progress notes or in the operating room and documented in an operative note.

■ Coding Tip   ● Documentation Tip   ◆ Encoder Tip   ▽ Targeted DRG

DRG 089▽ Simple Pneumonia & Pleurisy, Age > 17   RW 1.0463
with CC

Potential DRGs

079	Respiratory Infections & Inflammations, Age > 17 with CC	RW	1.5974
082	Respiratory Neoplasms	RW	1.3724
416	Septicemia, Age > 17	RW	1.5918
475	Respiratory System Diagnosis with Ventilator Support	RW	3.6000
483	Tracheostomy with Mech Vent 96+ Hours or Principal diagnosis Except Face, Mouth and Neck Diagnoses	RW	16.7762
489	HIV with Major Related Condition	RW	1.8603

DRG	Principal Dx/Procedure	Codes	Tips

079 ▽	Cause of pneumonia:
	  Salmonella
	  Klebsiella pneumoniae
	  Pseudomonas
	  Proteus
	  Staphylococcus
	  Aspiration
	AND
	CC condition
		003.22
		482.0
		482.1
		482.83
		482.40
		*507
		
		See CC section.	

082	Respiratory neoplasm	*162, *163, 197.0, 197.2, 212.9	◆ Malignant pleural effusion (197.2)
416 ▽	Septicemia	*038	■ Septicemia with pneumonia; code both. ● If sepsis is documented, it may be coded in absence of positive blood cultures.
475 ▽	Continuous mechanical ventilation	96.70–96.79	◆ Key terms: IMV, PEEP, PSV, endotracheal respiratory assistance
483	Tracheostomy *AND* Mechanical ventilation 96+ hours	31.1, 31.21, 31.29 96.72	■ A minitracheostomy is coded as a temporary tracheostomy. ■ Tracheostomy carried out elsewhere prior to admission or in ambulance prior to arrival should not be reported as a current procedure. ● Tracheostomy procedure may be performed either at the bedside and documented in the progress notes or in the operating room and documented in an operative note.
489	Opportunistic lung infection (e.g., pneumocystosis candidiasis of lung) *WITH* Diagnosis of HIV	112.4 042	

■ Coding Tip   ● Documentation Tip   ◆ Encoder Tip   ▽ Targeted DRG

Simple Pneumonia & Pleurisy, Age > 17 without CC

RW 0.6147 **DRG 090**

Potential DRGs

079	Respiratory Infections & Inflammations, Age > 17 with CC	RW	1.5974
080	Respiratory Infections & Inflammations, Age > 17 without CC	RW	0.8400
081	Respiratory Infections & Inflammations, Age 0–17	RW	1.5300
082	Respiratory Neoplasms	RW	1.3724
089	Simple Pneumonia & Pleurisy, Age > 17 with CC	RW	1.0463
127	Heart Failure & Shock	RW	1.0265
416	Septicemia, Age > 17	RW	1.5918
475	Respiratory System Diagnosis with Ventilator Support	RW	3.6000
483	Tracheostomy with Mech Vent 96+ Hours or Principal Diagnosis Except Face, Mouth and Neck Diagnoses	RW	16.7762
489	HIV with Major Related Condition	RW	1.8603

DRG	Principal Dx/Procedure	Codes	Tips
079 ▽	Cause of pneumonia: *Salmonella* *Klebsiella pneumoniae* *Pseudomonas* *Proteus* *Staphylococcus* Aspiration AND CC condition	003.22 482.0 482.1 482.83 482.40 *507 See CC section.	
080	Cause of pneumonia: *Salmonella* *Klebsiella pneumoniae* *Pseudomonas* *Staphylococcus* *Proteus* Aspiration AND Patient's age > 17	003.22 482.0 482.1 482.40 482.83 *507	■ If both aspiration and bacterial pneumonia are documented, code both.
081	Cause of pneumonia: *Salmonella* *Klebsiella pneumoniae* *Pseudomonas* *Staphylococcus* *Proteus* Aspiration AND Patient's age > 17	003.22 482.0 482.1 482.40 482.83 *507	■ If both aspiration and bacterial pneumonia are documented, code both.
082	Respiratory neoplasm	*162, *163, 197.0, 197.2, 212.9	◆ Malignant pleural effusion (code 197.2)
089 ▽	CC condition	See CC section.	
127 ▽	CHF (sequence as principal diagnosis when associated with pleural effusion)	*428	◆ PE commonly seen as part of CHF disease process; when evaluated and treated report as additional diagnosis ■ End-stage congestive heart failure, compensated heart failure, decompensated heart failure, heart failure NOS
416 ▽	Septicemia	*038	■ Septicemia with pneumonia; code both. ● If sepsis is documented, it may be coded in absence of positive blood cultures.

■ Coding Tip　　　● Documentation Tip　　　◆ Encoder Tip　　　▽ Targeted DRG

　　　163

Respiratory System, MDC 4

DRG 090 (continued)

DRG	Principal Dx/Procedure	Codes	Tips
475 ⟨YIELD⟩	Continuous mechanical ventilation	96.70–96.79	◆ Key terms: IMV, PEEP, PSV, endotracheal respiratory assistance
483	Tracheostomy AND Mechanical ventilation 96+ hours	31.1, 31.21, 31.29 96.72	■ A minitracheostomy is coded as a temporary tracheostomy. ■ Tracheostomy carried out elsewhere prior to admission or in ambulance prior to arrival should not be reported as a current procedure. ● Tracheostomy procedure may be performed either at the bedside and documented in the progress notes or in the operating room and documented in an operative note.
489	Opportunistic lung infection (e.g., pneumocystosis candidiasis of lung) WITH Diagnosis of HIV	112.4 042	

DRG 091 Simple Pneumonia & Pleurisy, Age 0–17   RW 0.7408

Potential DRGs

079	Respiratory Infections & Inflammations, Age > 17 with CC	RW	1.5974
080	Respiratory Infections & Inflammations, Age > 17 without CC	RW	0.8400
081	Respiratory Infections & Inflammations, Age 0–17	RW	1.5300
082	Respiratory Neoplasm	RW	1.3724
089	Simple Pneumonia & Pleurisy, Age > 17 with CC	RW	1.0463
475	Respiratory System Diagnosis with Ventilator Support	RW	3.6000
483	Tracheostomy with Mech Vent 96+ Hours or Principal Diagnosis Except Face, Mouth and Neck Diagnoses	RW	16.7762
489	HIV with Major Related Condition	RW	1.8603

DRG	Principal Dx/Procedure	Codes	Tips
079 ⟨YIELD⟩	Cause of pneumonia: Salmonella Klebsiella pneumoniae Pseudomonas Proteus Staphylococcus Aspiration AND CC condition	003.22 482.0 482.1 482.83 482.40 *507 See CC section.	■ If both aspiration and bacterial pneumonia are documented, code both.
080	Cause of pneumonia: Salmonella Klebsiella pneumoniae Pseudomonas Staphylococcus Proteus Aspiration AND Patient's age > 17	003.22 482.0 482.1 482.40 482.83 *507	■ If both aspiration and bacterial pneumonia are documented, code both.
081	Cause of pneumonia: Salmonella Klebsiella pneumoniae Pseudomonas Staphylococcus Proteus Aspiration AND Patient's age > 17	003.22 482.0 482.1 482.40 482.83 *507	■ If both aspiration and bacterial pneumonia are documented, code both.

■ Coding Tip   ● Documentation Tip   ◆ Encoder Tip   ⟨YIELD⟩ Targeted DRG

©2003 Ingenix, Inc.

(continued)   DRG 091

DRG	Principal Dx/Procedure	Codes	Tips
082	Respiratory neoplasm	*162, *163, 197.0, 197.2, 212.9	◆ Malignant pleural effusion
089 ▽	CC condition	See CC section.	
475 ▽	Continuous mechanical ventilation	96.70–96.79	◆ Key terms: IMV, PEEP, PSV, endotracheal respiratory assistance
483	Tracheostomy AND Mechanical ventilation 96+ hours	31.1, 31.21, 31.29 96.72	■ A minitracheostomy is coded as a temporary tracheostomy. ■ Tracheostomy carried out elsewhere prior to admission or in ambulance prior to arrival should not be reported as a current procedure. ● Tracheostomy procedure may be performed either at the bedside and documented in the progress notes or in the operating room and documented in an operative note.
489	Opportunistic lung infection (e.g., pneumocystosis candidiasis of lung) WITH Diagnosis of HIV	112.4 042	

Interstitial Lung Disease with CC   RW 1.2024   DRG 092

Potential DRGs

075	**Major Chest Procedures**	RW	3.0437
076	Other Respiratory System OR Procedures **with CC**	RW	2.8184
475	Respiratory System Diagnosis **with Ventilator Support**	RW	3.6000
483	**Tracheostomy with Mech Vent 96+ Hours or Principal Diagnosis Except Face, Mouth and Neck Diagnoses**	RW	16.7762

DRG	Principal Dx/Procedure	Codes	Tips
075	Open lung biopsy Destruction lung lesion	33.28 32.29	
076	Closed endoscopic lung biopsy Transpleural thoracoscopy AND CC condition	33.27 34.21 See CC section.	
475 ▽	Continuous mechanical ventilation	96.70–96.79	◆ Key terms: IMV, PEEP, PSV, endotracheal respiratory assistance
483	Tracheostomy AND Mechanical ventilation 96+ hours	31.1, 31.21, 31.29 96.72	■ A minitracheostomy is coded as a temporary tracheostomy. ■ Tracheostomy carried out elsewhere prior to admission or in ambulance prior to arrival should not be reported as a current procedure. ● Tracheostomy procedure may be performed either at the bedside and documented in the progress notes or in the operating room and documented in an operative note.

■ Coding Tip   ● Documentation Tip   ◆ Encoder Tip   ▽ Targeted DRG

Respiratory System, MDC 4

DRG 093   Interstitial Lung Disease without CC   RW 0.7176

Potential DRGs

092	Interstitial Lung Disease **with CC**	RW 1.2024
475	Respiratory System Diagnosis **with Ventilator Suppor**	RW 3.6000
483	**Tracheostomy with Mech Vent 96+ Hours or Principal Diagnosis**	RW 16.7762
	Except Face, Mouth and Neck Diagnoses	

DRG	Principal Dx/Procedure	Codes	Tips
092	CC condition	See CC section.	
475 ▽	Continuous mechanical ventilation	96.70–96.79	◆ Key terms: IMV, PEEP, PSV, endotracheal respiratory assistance
483	Tracheostomy *AND* Mechanical ventilation 96+ hours	31.1, 31.21, 31.29 96.72	■ A minitracheostomy is coded as a temporary tracheostomy. ■ Tracheostomy carried out elsewhere prior to admission or in ambulance prior to arrival should not be reported as a current procedure. ● Tracheostomy procedure may be performed either at the bedside and documented in the progress notes or in the operating room and documented in an operative note.

DRG 094   Pneumothorax with CC   RW 1.1340

Potential DRGs

475	Respiratory System Diagnosis **with Ventilator Support**	RW 3.6000
483	**Tracheostomy with Mech Vent 96+ Hours or Principal Diagnosis**	RW 16.7762
	Except Face, Mouth and Neck Diagnoses	
484	**Craniotomy for Multiple Significant Trauma**	RW 5.4179
486	**Other O.R. Procedures for Multiple Significant Trauma**	RW 4.8793
487	Other Multiple Significant Trauma	RW 2.0057

DRG	Principal Dx/Procedure	Codes	Tips
475 ▽	Continuous mechanical ventilation	96.70–96.79	◆ Key terms: IMV, PEEP, PSV, endotracheal respiratory assistance
483	Tracheostomy *AND* Mechanical ventilation 96+ hours	31.1, 31.21, 31.29 96.72	■ A minitracheostomy is coded as a temporary tracheostomy. ■ Tracheostomy carried out elsewhere prior to admission or in ambulance prior to arrival should not be reported as a current procedure. ● Tracheostomy procedure may be performed either at the bedside and documented in the progress notes or in the operating room and documented in an operative note.
484	Craniotomy for multiple significant trauma		■ Craniotomy and principal diagnosis of trauma and at least two injuries (assigned either as principal or secondary) that are defined as significant trauma from different body site categories located under DRG 487

Respiratory System, MDC 4

(continued) **DRG 094**

DRG	Principal Dx/Procedure	Codes	Tips
486	Other O.R. procedures for multiple significant trauma		■ Principal diagnosis of trauma and at least two injuries (assigned either as principal or secondary) that are defined as significant trauma from different body site categories located under DRG 487 *AND* O.R. procedure other than craniotomy or limb reattachment, hip and femur procedures
487	Other multiple significant trauma		■ Principal diagnosis of trauma and at least two injuries (assigned either as principal or secondary) that are defined as significant trauma from different body site categories located under DRG 487

Pneumothorax without CC RW 0.6166 **DRG 095**

Potential DRGs

094	Pneumothorax **with CC**	RW 1.1340
475	Respiratory System Diagnosis **with Ventilator Support**	RW 3.6000
483	Tracheostomy with Mech Vent 96+ Hours or Principal Diagnosis Except Face, Mouth and Neck Diagnoses	RW 16.7762
484	Craniotomy for Multiple Significant Trauma	RW 5.4179
486	Other O.R. Procedures for Multiple Significant Trauma	RW 4.8793
487	Other Multiple Significant Trauma	RW 2.0057

DRG	Principal Dx/Procedure	Codes	Tips
094	CC condition	See CC section.	
475 ▽	Continuous mechanical ventilation	96.70–96.79	◆ Key terms: IMV, PEEP, PSV, endotracheal respiratory assistance
483	Tracheostomy *AND* Mechanical ventilation 96+ hours	31.1, 31.21, 31.29 96.72	■ A minitracheostomy is coded as a temporary tracheostomy. ■ Tracheostomy carried out elsewhere prior to admission or in ambulance prior to arrival should not be reported as a current procedure. ● Tracheostomy procedure may be performed either at the bedside and documented in the progress notes or in the operating room and documented in an operative note.
484	Craniotomy for multiple significant trauma		■ Craniotomy and principal diagnosis of trauma and at least two injuries (assigned either as principal or secondary) that are defined as significant trauma from different body site categories located under DRG 487
486	Other O.R. procedures for multiple significant trauma		■ Principal diagnosis of trauma and at least two injuries (assigned either as principal or secondary) that are defined as significant trauma from different body site categories located under DRG 487 *AND* O.R. procedure other than craniotomy or limb reattachment, hip and femur procedures

---

■ Coding Tip ● Documentation Tip ◆ Encoder Tip ▽ Targeted DRG

DRG 095   (continued)

DRG	Principal Dx/Procedure	Codes	Tips
487	Other multiple significant trauma		■ Principal diagnosis of trauma and at least two injuries (assigned either as principal or secondary) that are defined as significant trauma from different body site categories located under DRG 487

DRG 096▽   Bronchitis & Asthma, Age > 17 with CC   RW 0.7464

Potential DRGs

079	**Respiratory Infections & Inflammations**, Age > 17 **with CC**	RW	1.5974
087	Pulmonary Edema & **Respiratory Failure**	RW	1.3430
088	**Chronic Obstructive Pulmonary Disease**	RW	0.9031
089	**Simple Pneumonia** & Pleurisy, Age > 17 **with CC**	RW	1.0463
475	Respiratory System Diagnosis **with Ventilator Support**	RW	3.6000
483	**Tracheostomy with Mech Vent 96+ Hours or Principal Diagnosis Except Face, Mouth and Neck Diagnoses**	RW	16.7762

DRG	Principal Dx/Procedure	Codes	Tips
079 ▽	Cause of pneumonia: *Salmonella* *Klebsiella pneumoniae* *Pseudomonas* *Staphylococcus* *E. coli* *Proteus* Aspiration AND Patient's age >17	003.22 482.0 482.1 482.40 482.82 482.83 *507	■ If both aspiration and bacterial pneumonia are documented, code both.
087 ▽	Respiratory failure	518..81, 518.83, 518.84	◆ COPD generic term; common cause of failure. Look for failure as acute exacerbation or underlying cause of admission per MD documentation.
088 ▽	Acute exacerbation chronic obstructive bronchitis	491.21	■ 491.21 If pneumonia is also documented, code it.
089 ▽	Pneumonia	481, 482.2, 482.3, 486	■ 481 If presence of pneumococcal pneumonia and pneumococcal septicemia confirmed in record, code both entities.
475 ▽	Continuous mechanical ventilation	96.70–96.79	◆ Key terms: IMV, PEEP, PSV, endotracheal respiratory assistance
483	Tracheostomy AND Mechanical ventilation 96+ hours	31.1, 31.21, 31.29 96.72	■ A minitracheostomy is coded as a temporary tracheostomy. ■ Tracheostomy carried out elsewhere prior to admission or in ambulance prior to arrival should not be reported as a current procedure. ● Tracheostomy procedure may be performed either at the bedside and documented in the progress notes or in the operating room and documented in an operative note.

■ Coding Tip   ● Documentation Tip   ◆ Encoder Tip   ▽ Targeted DRG

Bronchitis & Asthma, Age > 17 without CC   RW 0.5505   **DRG 097**

Potential DRGs

080	Respiratory Infections & Inflammations, Age > 17 without CC	RW	0.8400
087	Pulmonary Edema & **Respiratory Failure**	RW	1.3430
088	**Chronic Obstructive Pulmonary Disease**	RW	0.9031
089	**Simple Pneumonia** & Pleurisy, Age > 17 **with CC**	RW	1.0463
090	**Simple Pneumonia** & Pleurisy, Age > 17 **without CC**	RW	0.6147
096	Bronchitis & Asthma, Age > 17**with CC**	RW	0.7464
475	Respiratory System Diagnosis **with Ventilator Support**	RW	3.6000
483	**Tracheostomy with Mech Vent 96+ Hours or Principal Diagnosis Except Face, Mouth and Neck Diagnoses**	RW	16.7762

DRG	Principal Dx/Procedure	Codes	Tips
080	Cause of pneumonia: *Salmonella* *Klebsiella pneumoniae* *Pseudomonas* *Staphylococcus* *Proteus* Aspiration *AND* Patient's age >17	003.22 482.0 482.1 482.40 482.82 482.83 *507	■ If both aspiration and bacterial pneumonia are documented, code both.
087 ▽	Respiratory failure	518..81, 518.83, 518.84	◆ COPD generic term; common cause of failure. Look for failure as acute exacerbation or underlying cause of admission per MD documentation.
088 ▽	Acute exacerbation chronic obstructive bronchitis	491.21	■ 491.21 If pneumonia is also documented, code it.
089 ▽	Pneumonia *AND* CC condition	481, 482.2, 282.3, 486 See CC section.	■ 481 If presence of pneumococcal pneumonia and pneumococcal septicemia confirmed in record, code both entities.
090	Pneumonia	481, 482.2, 282.3, 486	■ 481 If presence of pneumococcal pneumonia and pneumococcal septicemia confirmed in record, code both entities.
096 ▽	CC condition	See CC section.	
475 ▽	Continuous mechanical ventilation	96.70–96.79	◆ Key terms: IMV, PEEP, PSV, endotracheal respiratory assistance
483	Tracheostomy *AND* Mechanical ventilation 96+ hours	31.1, 31.21, 31.29, 96.72	■ A minitracheostomy is coded as a temporary tracheostomy. ■ Tracheostomy carried out elsewhere prior to admission or in ambulance prior to arrival should not be reported as a current procedure. ● Tracheostomy procedure may be performed either at the bedside and documented in the progress notes or in the operating room and documented in an operative note.

■ Coding Tip   ● Documentation Tip   ◆ Encoder Tip   ▽ Targeted DRG

DRG 098   Bronchitis & Asthma, Age 0-17   RW 0.9662

Potential DRGs

081	Respiratory Infections & Inflammations, Age 0-17	RW	1.5300
087	Pulmonary Edema & **Respiratory Failure**	RW	1.3430
088	**Chronic Obstructive Pulmonary Disease**	RW	0.9031
089	Simple Pneumonia & Pleurisy, Age > 17 with CC	RW	1.0463
096	Bronchitis & Asthma, **Age > 17 with CC**	RW	0.7464
475	**Respiratory System Diagnosis with Ventilator Support**	RW	3.6000
483	**Tracheostomy with Mech Vent 96+ Hours or Principal Diagnosis** **Except Face, Mouth and Neck Diagnoses**	RW	16.7762

DRG	Principal Dx/Procedure	Codes	Tips
081	Cause of pneumonia: 　*Salmonella* 　*Klebsiella pneumoniae* 　*Pseudomonas* 　*Staphylococcus* 　*Proteus* 　Aspiration *AND* Patient's age 0-17	003.22 482.0 482.1 482.40 482.82 482.83 *507	■ If both aspiration and bacterial pneumonia are documented, code both.
087 ⟱	Respiratory failure	518..81, 518.83, 518.84	◆ COPD generic term; common cause of failure. Look for failure as acute exacerbation or underlying cause of admission per MD documentation.
088 ⟱	Acute exacerbation chronic obstructive bronchitis	491.21	■ 491.21 If pneumonia is also documented, code it.
089 ⟱	Pneumonia *AND* CC condition	481, 482.2, 282.3, 486 See CC section.	■ 481 If presence of pneumococcal pneumonia and pneumococcal septicemia confirmed in record, code both entities.
096 ⟱	CC condition	See CC section.	
475 ⟱	Continuous mechanical ventilation	96.70–96.79	◆ Key terms: IMV, PEEP, PSV, endotracheal respiratory assistance
483	Tracheostomy *AND* Mechanical ventilation 96+ hours	31.1, 31.21, 31.29 96.72	■ A minitracheostomy is coded as a temporary tracheostomy. ■ Tracheostomy carried out elsewhere prior to admission or in ambulance prior to arrival should not be reported as a current procedure. ● Tracheostomy procedure may be performed either at the bedside and documented in the progress notes or in the operating room and documented in an operative note.

■ Coding Tip   ● Documentation Tip   ◆ Encoder Tip   ⟱ Targeted DRG

Respiratory Signs & Symptoms with CC   RW 0.7032   **DRG 099**

Potential DRGs

087	Pulmonary Edema & **Respiratory Failure**	RW	1.3430
101	Other Respiratory System Diagnoses **with CC**	RW	0.8654
475	Respiratory System Diagnosis **with Ventilator Support**	RW	3.6000
483	**Tracheostomy with Mech Vent 96+ Hours or Principal Diagnosis Except Face, Mouth and Neck Diagnoses**	RW	16.7762

DRG	Principal Dx/Procedure	Codes	Tips
087 ▽	Respiratory failure	518.81, 518.83, 518.84	◆ COPD generic term; common cause of failure. Look for failure as acute exacerbation or underlying cause of admission per MD documentation.
101	1 or 2 fractured ribs *AND* CC condition	See CC section.	■ Key terms: closed, unspecified
475 ▽	Continuous mechanical ventilation	96.70–96.79	◆ Key terms: IMV, PEEP, PSV, endotracheal respiratory assistance
483	Tracheostomy *AND* Mechanical ventilation 96+ hours	31.1, 31.21, 31.29 96.72	■ A minitracheostomy is coded as a temporary tracheostomy. ■ Tracheostomy carried out elsewhere prior to admission or in ambulance prior to arrival should not be reported as a current procedure. ● Tracheostomy procedure may be performed either at the bedside and documented in the progress notes or in the operating room and documented in an operative note.

Respiratory Signs & Symptoms without CC   RW 0.5222   **DRG 100**

Potential DRGs

087	Pulmonary Edema & **Respiratory Failure**	RW	1.3430
099	Respiratory Signs & Symptoms **with CC**	RW	0.7032
101	Other Respiratory System Diagnoses **with CC**	RW	0.8654
102	Other Respiratory System Diagnoses **without CC**	RW	0.5437
475	Respiratory System Diagnosis **with Ventilator Support**	RW	3.6000
483	**Tracheostomy with Mech Vent 96+ Hours or Principal Diagnosis Except Face, Mouth and Neck Diagnoses**	RW	16.7762

DRG	Principal Dx/Procedure	Codes	Tips
087 ▽	Respiratory failure	518..81, 518.83, 518.84	◆ COPD generic term; common cause of failure. Look for failure as acute exacerbation or underlying cause of admission per MD documentation.
099	See CC section.	See CC section.	
101	1 or 2 fractured ribs *AND* CC condition	See CC section.	■ Key terms: closed, unspecified
102	1 or 2 fractured ribs	807.00, 807.01, 807.02	
475 ▽	Continuous mechanical ventilation	96.70–96.79	◆ Key terms: IMV, PEEP, PSV, endotracheal respiratory assistance

---

■ Coding Tip   ● Documentation Tip   ◆ Encoder Tip   ▽ Targeted DRG

DRG 100   (continued)

DRG	Principal Dx/Procedure	Codes	Tips
483	Tracheostomy *AND* Mechanical ventilation 96+ hours	31.1, 31.21, 31.29, 96.72	■ A minitracheostomy is coded as a temporary tracheostomy. ■ Tracheostomy carried out elsewhere prior to admission or in ambulance prior to arrival should not be reported as a current procedure. ● Tracheostomy procedure may be performed either at the bedside and documented in the progress notes or in the operating room and documented in an operative note.

DRG 101   Other Respiratory System Diagnoses with CC   RW 0.8654

Potential DRGs

083	Major Chest Trauma with CC	RW	0.9620
087	Pulmonary Edema & **Respiratory Failure**	RW	1.3430
475	Respiratory System Diagnosis **with Ventilator Support**	RW	3.6000
483	**Tracheostomy with Mech Vent 96+ Hours or Principal Diagnosis Except Face, Mouth and Neck Diagnoses**	RW	16.7762
484	**Craniotomy for Multiple Significant Trauma**	RW	5.4179
486	**Other O.R. Procedures for Multiple Significant Trauma**	RW	4.8793
487	Other Multiple Significant Trauma	RW	2.0057

DRG	Principal Dx/Procedure	Codes	Tips
083	Fracture of rib, open Fracture of ribs (more than two), closed	807.1 807.03	
087 ⬇	Respiratory failure	518..81, 518.83, 518.84	◆ COPD generic term; common cause of failure. Look for failure as acute exacerbation or underlying cause of admission per MD documentation.
475 ⬇	Continuous mechanical ventilation	96.70–96.79	◆ Key terms: IMV, PEEP, PSV, endotracheal respiratory assistance
483	Tracheostomy *AND* Mechanical ventilation 96+ hours	31.1, 31.21, 31.29 96.72	■ A minitracheostomy is coded as a temporary tracheostomy. ■ Tracheostomy carried out elsewhere prior to admission or in ambulance prior to arrival should not be reported as a current procedure. ● Tracheostomy procedure may be performed either at the bedside and documented in the progress notes or in the operating room and documented in an operative note.
484	Craniotomy for multiple significant trauma		■ Craniotomy and principal diagnosis of trauma and at least two injuries (assigned either as principal or secondary) that are defined as significant trauma from different body site categories located under DRG 487

■ Coding Tip   ● Documentation Tip   ◆ Encoder Tip   ⬇ Targeted DRG

(continued)   **DRG 101**

DRG	Principal Dx/Procedure	Codes	Tips
486	Other O.R. procedures for multiple significant trauma		■ Principal diagnosis of trauma and at least two injuries (assigned either as principal or secondary) that are defined as significant trauma from different body site categories located under DRG 487 *AND* O.R. procedure other than craniotomy or limb reattachment, hip and femur procedures
487	Other multiple significant trauma		■ Principal diagnosis of trauma and at least two injuries (assigned either as principal or secondary) that are defined as significant trauma from different body site categories located under DRG 487

Other Respiratory System Diagnoses without CC   RW 0.5437   **DRG 102**

Potential DRGs

083	**Major Chest Trauma with CC**	RW	0.9620
087	**Pulmonary Edema & Respiratory Failure**	RW	1.3430
101	Other Respiratory System Diagnoses **with CC**	RW	0.8654
475	**Respiratory System Diagnosis with Ventilator Support**	RW	3.6000
483	**Tracheostomy with Mech Vent 96+ Hours or Principal Diagnosis Except Face, Mouth and Neck Diagnoses**	RW	16.7762
484	**Craniotomy for Multiple Significant Trauma**	RW	5.4179
486	**Other O.R. Procedures for Multiple Significant Trauma**	RW	4.8793
487	Other Multiple Significant Trauma	RW	2.0057

DRG	Principal Dx/Procedure	Codes	Tips
083	Fracture of rib, open Fracture of ribs (more than two), closed	807.1 807.03	
087 🔻	Respiratory failure	518..81, 518.83, 518.84	◆ COPD generic term; common cause of failure. Look for failure as acute exacerbation or underlying cause of admission per MD documentation.
101	CC condition	See CC section.	
475 🔻	Continuous mechanical ventilation	96.70–96.79	◆ Key terms: IMV, PEEP, PSV, endotracheal respiratory assistance
483	Tracheostomy *AND* Mechanical ventilation 96+ hours	31.1, 31.21, 31.29 96.72	■ A minitracheostomy is coded as a temporary tracheostomy. ■ Tracheostomy carried out elsewhere prior to admission or in ambulance prior to arrival should not be reported as a current procedure. ● Tracheostomy procedure may be performed either at the bedside and documented in the progress notes or in the operating room and documented in an operative note.
484	Craniotomy for multiple significant trauma		■ Craniotomy and principal diagnosis of trauma and at least two injuries (assigned either as principal or secondary) that are defined as significant trauma from different body site categories located under DRG 487

■ Coding Tip   ● Documentation Tip   ◆ Encoder Tip   🔻 Targeted DRG

Respiratory System, MDC 4

DRG 102 (continued)

DRG	Principal Dx/Procedure	Codes	Tips
486	Other O.R. procedures for multiple significant trauma		■ Principal diagnosis of trauma and at least two injuries (assigned either as principal or secondary) that are defined as significant trauma from different body site categories located under DRG 487 AND O.R. procedure other than craniotomy or limb reattachment, hip and femur procedures
487	Other multiple significant trauma		■ Principal diagnosis of trauma and at least two injuries (assigned either as principal or secondary) that are defined as significant trauma from different body site categories located under DRG 487

DRG 474 Invalid DRG

No Potential DRGs

DRG 475 Respiratory System Diagnosis with Ventilator Support

RW 3.6000

Potential DRGs

483   Tracheostomy with Mech Vent 96+ Hours or Principal Diagnosis Except Face, Mouth and Neck Diagnoses   RW   16.7762

DRG	Principal Dx/Procedure	Codes	Tips
483	Tracheostomy AND Mechanical ventilation 96+ hours	31.1, 31.21, 31.29 96.72	■ A minitracheostomy is coded as a temporary tracheostomy. ■ Tracheostomy carried out elsewhere prior to admission or in ambulance prior to arrival should not be reported as a current procedure. ● Tracheostomy procedure may be performed either at the bedside and documented in the progress notes or in the operating room and documented in an operative note.

Circulatory System, MDC 5

Cardiac Valve and Other Major Cardiothoracic Procedures with Cardiac Catheterization DRG 104

No Potential DRGs

Cardiac Valve and Other Major Cardiothoracic Procedures without Cardiac Catheterization RW 5.7088 DRG 105

Potential DRGs

104   Cardiac Valve and Other Major Cardiothoracic Procedures **with Cardiac**   RW   7.9351
Catheterization

DRG	Principal Dx/Procedure	Codes	Tips
104	Cardiac catheterization	37.21, 37.22, 37.23	■ The passage of catheter in heart chambers does not constitute a diagnostic cardiac catheterization. Procedure includes invasive recording of intracardiac and intravascular pressures, tracings, blood sampling, and cardiac output.
	Cardiac electrophysiology study	37.26	■ EPS, programmed electrical stimulation, ICD, implantable stimulation and pacing/recording studies excluding Bundle of HIS recording (37.29)
	Angiocardiography	88.52, 88.58	■ Arteriography by Sones, Judkins, or Ricketts and Abrams techniques, direct selective arteriography

Coronary Bypass with PTCA DRG 106

No Potential DRGs

Coronary Bypass with Cardiac Catheterization RW 5.3751 DRG 107

Potential DRGs

105   **Cardiac Valve** and **Other Major Cardiothoracic Procedures** without   RW   5.7088
Cardiac Catheterization
106   **Coronary Bypass with PTCA**   RW   7.2936
108   Other Cardiothoracic Procedures   RW   5.3656
535   **Cardiac Defibrillator Implant with Cardiac Catheterization** with Acute   RW   8.1560
Myocardial Infarction/Heart Failure/Shock
536   **Cardiac Defibrillator Implant with Cardiac Catheterization** without Acute   RW   6.2775
Myocardial Infarction/Heart Failure/Shock

DRG	Principal Dx/Procedure	Codes	Tips
105	Cardiac valve procedure	*35.1, *35.2	■ Annuloplasty is included in the valvuloplasty operation

---

■ Coding Tip   ● Documentation Tip   ◆ Encoder Tip   ▽ Targeted DRG

Circulatory System, MDC 5

DRG 107 (continued)

DRG	Principal Dx/Procedure	Codes	Tips
106	Percutaneous valvuloplasty	35.96	■ PTCA with infusion of thrombolytic agent; coronary atherectomy; PTCA, NOS; balloon angioplasty of coronary vessel ■ Percutaneous coronary angioplasty 36.01, 36.02, 36.05 ■ Balloon angioplasty of coronary artery w/infusion of thrombolytic agent ◆ Would be assigned regardless if performed on bypass graft site or native vessels
108	Open chest coronary artery angioplasty	36.03	■ Coronary endarterectomy w/patch graft ◆ May be performed on same vessels during a CABG or on vessels not bypassed during a CABG. Only code separately when performed on separate vessels, considered integral to CABG at the same vessel.
	OR Other revascularization of heart (e.g., by arterial implant)	36.2	■ Indirect heart revascularization, NOS
535	Implantation or replacement of automatic cardioverter/defibrillator, total system (AICD)	37.94	■ Implantation of defibrillator with leads; formation of pocket; obtaining defibrillator threshold measurements
	Implantation of automatic cardioverter/ defibrillator lead(s) only	37.95	
	Implantation of automatic cardioverter/ defibrillator pulse generator only	37.96	
	Replacement of automatic cardioverter/ defibrillator lead(s) only	37.97	
	Replacement of automatic cardioverter/ defibrillator pulse generator only	37.98	
	Cardiac catheterization	37.21, 37.22, 37.23	■ The passage of catheter in heart chambers does not constitute a diagnostic cardiac catheterization. Procedure includes invasive recording of intracardiac and intravascular pressures, tracings, blood sampling, and cardiac output.
	Cardiac electrophysiology study	37.26	■ EPS, programmed electrical stimulation, ICD, implantable stimulation and pacing/recording studies excluding bundle of HIS recording (37.29)
	Angiocardiography	88.52–88.58	■ Arteriography by Sones, Judkins, or Ricketts and Abrams techniques, direct selective arteriography
	AMI, initial episode of care	410.0-410.9 (with fifth digit of 1)	■ Describes an acute event, if multiple sites or subsequent sites identified for infarction documented, code all sites. ◆ Non-Q wave codes to subendocardial (410.7x)
	CHF	*428	◆ PE commonly seen as part of CHFdisease process; when evaluated and treated report as additional diagnosis ■ End-stage congestive heart failure, compensated heart failure, decompensated heart failure, heart failure NOS
	Shock	785.50, 785.51	

(continued)   **DRG 107**

DRG	Principal Dx/Procedure	Codes	Tips
536	Implantation or replacement of automatic cardioverter/defibrillator, total system (AICD)	37.94	■ Implantation of defibrillator with leads; formation of pocket; obtaining defibrillator threshold measurements
	Implantation of automatic cardioverter/ defibrillator lead(s) only	37.95	
	Implantation of automatic cardioverter/ defibrillator pulse generator only	37.96	
	Replacement of automatic cardioverter/ defibrillator lead(s) only	37.97	
	Replacement of automatic cardioverter/ defibrillator pulse generator only	37.98	
	Cardiac catheterization	37.21, 37.22, 37.23	■ The passage of catheter in heart chambers does not constitute a diagnostic cardiac catheterization. Procedure includes invasive recording of intracardiac and intravascular pressures, tracings, blood sampling, and cardiac output.
	Cardiac electrophysiology study	37.26	■ EPS, programmed electrical stimulation, ICD, implantable stimulation and pacing/recording studies excluding bundle of HIS recording (37.29)
	Angiocardiography	88.52–88.58	■ Arteriography by Sones, Judkins, or Ricketts and Abrams techniques, direct selective arteriography

Other Cardiothoracic Procedures   RW 5.3656   **DRG 108**

Potential DRGs

104	**Cardiac Valve** and **Other Major Cardiothoracic Procedures** with Cardiac Catheterization	RW	7.9351
105	**Cardiac Valve** and **Other Major Cardiothoracic Procedures** without Cardiac Catheterization	RW	5.7088
535	**Cardiac Defibrillator Implant with Cardiac Catheterization** with Acute Myocardial Infarction/Heart Failure/Shock	RW	8.1560
536	**Cardiac Defibrillator Implant with Cardiac Catheterization** without Acute Myocardial Infarction/Heart Failure/Shock	RW	6.2775

DRG	Principal Dx/Procedure	Codes	Tips
104	Cardiac catheterization	37.21, 37.22, 37.23	■ The passage of catheter in heart chambers does not constitute a diagnostic cardiac catheterization. Procedure includes invasive recording of intracardiac and intravascular pressures, tracings, blood sampling, and cardiac output.
	Cardiac electrophysiology study	37.26	■ EPS, programmed electrical stimulation, ICD, implantable stimulation and pacing/recording studies excluding bundle of HIS recording (37.29)
	Angiocardiography	88.52–88.58	■ Arteriography by Sones, Judkins, or Ricketts and Abrams techniques, direct selective arteriography
105	Cardiac valve procedure	*35.1, *35.2	■ Annuloplasty is included in the valvuloplasty operation

---

■ Coding Tip   ● Documentation Tip   ◆ Encoder Tip   Ⓣ Targeted DRG

DRG 108   (continued)

DRG	Principal Dx/Procedure	Codes	Tips
535	Implantation or replacement of automatic cardioverter/defibrillator, total system (AICD)	37.94	■ Implantation of defibrillator with leads; formation of pocket; obtaining defibrillator threshold measurements
	Implantation of automatic cardioverter/ defibrillator lead(s) only	37.95	
	Implantation of automatic cardioverter/ defibrillator pulse generator only	37.96	
	Replacement of automatic cardioverter/ defibrillator lead(s) only	37.97	
	Replacement of automatic cardioverter/ defibrillator pulse generator only	37.98	
	Cardiac catheterization	37.21, 37.22, 37.23	■ The passage of catheter in heart chambers does not constitute a diagnostic cardiac catheterization. Procedure includes invasive recording of intracardiac and intravascular pressures, tracings, blood sampling, and cardiac output.
	Cardiac electrophysiology study	37.26	■ EPS, programmed electrical stimulation, ICD, implantable stimulation and pacing/recording studies excluding bundle of HIS recording (37.29)
	Angiocardiography	88.52–88.58	■ Arteriography by Sones, Judkins, or Ricketts and Abrams techniques, direct selective arteriography
	AMI, initial episode of care	410.0-410.9 (with fifth digit of 1)	■ Describes an acute event, if multiple sites or subsequent sites identified for infarction documented, code all sites. ◆ Non-Q wave codes to subendocardial (410.7x)
	CHF	*428	◆ PE commonly seen as part of CHF disease process; when evaluated and treated report as additional diagnosis ■ End-stage congestive heart failure, compensated heart failure, decompensated heart failure, heart failure NOS
	Shock	785.50, 785.51	

(continued) **DRG 108**

DRG	Principal Dx/Procedure	Codes	Tips
536	Implantation or replacement of automatic cardioverter/defibrillator, total system (AICD)	37.94	■ Implantation of defibrillator with leads; formation of pocket; obtaining defibrillator threshold measurements
	Implantation of automatic cardioverter/ defibrillator lead(s) only	37.95	
	Implantation of automatic cardioverter/ defibrillator pulse generator only	37.96	
	Replacement of automatic cardioverter/ defibrillator lead(s) only	37.97	
	Replacement of automatic cardioverter/ defibrillator pulse generator only	37.98	
	Cardiac catheterization	37.21, 37.22, 37.23	■ The passage of catheter in heart chambers does not constitute a diagnostic cardiac catheterization. Procedure includes invasive recording of intracardiac and intravascular pressures, tracings, blood sampling, and cardiac output.
	Cardiac electrophysiology study	37.26	■ EPS, programmed electrical stimulation, ICD, implantable stimulation and pacing/recording studies excluding bundle of HIS recording (37.29)
	Angiocardiography	88.52–88.58	■ Arteriography by Sones, Judkins, or Ricketts and Abrams techniques, direct selective arteriography

Coronary Bypass without PTCA or Cardiac Catheterization   RW 3.9401   **DRG 109**

Potential DRGs

104	**Cardiac Valve** and **Other Major Cardiothoracic Procedures** with Cardiac Catheterization	RW	7.9351
105	**Cardiac Valve** and **Other Major Cardiothoracic Procedures** without Cardiac Catheterization	RW	5.7088
106	Coronary Bypass **with PTCA**	RW	7.2936
107	Coronary Bypass **with Cardiac Catheterization**	RW	5.3751
108	Other Cardiothoracic Procedures	RW	5.3656

DRG	Principal Dx/Procedure	Codes	Tips
104	Cardiac valve procedure	*35.1, *35.2	■ Annuloplasty is included in the valvuloplasty operation
	Cardiac catheterization	37.21, 37.22, 37.23	■ The passage of catheter in heart chambers does not constitute a diagnostic cardiac catheterization. Procedure includes invasive recording of intracardiac and intravascular pressures, tracings, blood sampling, and cardiac output.
	Cardiac electrophysiology study	37.26	■ EPS, programmed electrical stimulation, ICD, implantable stimulation and pacing/recording studies excluding bundle of HIS recording (37.29)
	Angiocardiography	88.52–88.58	■ Arteriography by Sones, Judkins, or Ricketts and Abrams techniques, direct selective arteriography
105	Cardiac valve procedure	*35.1, *35.2	■ Annuloplasty is included in the valvuloplasty operation

---

■ Coding Tip   ● Documentation Tip   ◆ Encoder Tip   ▽ Targeted DRG

179

Circulatory System, MDC 5

DRG 109 (continued)

DRG	Principal Dx/Procedure	Codes	Tips
106	Percutaneous valvuloplasty	35.96	■ PTCA with infusion of thrombolytic agent; coronary atherectomy; PTCA, NOS; balloon angioplasty of coronary vessel
	Percutaneous coronary angioplasty	36.01, 36.02, 36.05	■ Balloon angioplasty of coronary artery w/infusion of thrombolytic agent
107	Cardiac catheterization	37.21 37.22 37.23	■ The passage of catheter in heart chambers does not constitute a diag-nostic cardiac catheterization. Procedure includes invasive recording of intracar-diac and intravascular pressures, tracings, blood sampling, and cardiac output.
	Angiocardiography	88.52, 88.58	■ Arteriography by Sones, Judkins, or Ricketts and Abrams techniques, direct selective arteriograph
108	Open chest coronary artery angioplasty	36.03	■ Endarterectomy with patch graft; thromboendarterectomy with patch graft ◆ May be performed on same vessels during a CABG or on vessels not bypassed during a CABG. Only code separately when performed on separate vessels, considered integral to CABG at the same vessel

DRG 110 Major Cardiovascular Procedures with CC RW 4.0492

Potential DRGs

104	**Cardiac Valve** and **Other Major Cardiothoracic Procedures** with Cardiac Catheterization	RW	7.9351
105	**Cardiac Valve** and **Other Major Cardiothoracic Procedures** without Cardiac Catheterization	RW	5.7088
108	Other Cardiothoracic Procedures	RW	5.3656
535	**Cardiac Defibrillator Implant with Cardiac Catheterization** with Acute Myocardial Infarction/Heart Failure/Shock	RW	8.1560
536	**Cardiac Defibrillator Implant with Cardiac Catheterization** without Acute Myocardial Infarction/Heart Failure/Shock	RW	6.2775

DRG	Principal Dx/Procedure	Codes	Tips
104	Cardiac valve procedure Cardiac catheterization	*35.1, *35.2 37.21, 37.22, 37.23	■ Annuloplasty is included in the valvuloplasty operation ■ The passage of catheter in heart chambers does not constitute a diagnostic cardiac catheterization. Procedure includes invasive recording of intracardiac and intravascular pressures, tracings, blood sampling, and cardiac output.
	Cardiac electrophysiology study	37.26	■ EPS, programmed electrical stimulation, ICD, implantable stimulation and pacing/recording studies excluding bundle of HIS recording (37.29)
	Angiocardiography	88.52–88.58	■ Arteriography by Sones, Judkins, or Ricketts and Abrams techniques, direct selective arteriography
105	Cardiac valve procedure	*35.1, *35.2	■ Annuloplasty is included in the valvuloplasty operation

■ Coding Tip   ● Documentation Tip   ◆ Encoder Tip   ⓦ Targeted DRG

©2003 Ingenix, Inc.

(continued) **DRG 110**

DRG	Principal Dx/Procedure	Codes	Tips
108	Cardiotomy	37.10, 37.11	■ Cardiolysis; incision of atrium, endocardium, myocardium, or ventricle
535	Implantation or replacement of automatic cardioverter/defibrillator, total system (AICD)	37.94	■ Implantation of defibrillator with leads; formation of pocket; obtaining defibrillator threshold measurements
	Implantation of automatic cardioverter/defibrillator lead(s) only	37.95	
	Implantation of automatic cardioverter/defibrillator pulse generator only	37.96	
	Replacement of automatic cardioverter/defibrillator lead(s) only	37.97	
	Replacement of automatic cardioverter/defibrillator pulse generator only	37.98	
	Cardiac catheterization	37.21, 37.22, 37.23	■ The passage of catheter in heart chambers does not constitute a diagnostic cardiac catheterization. Procedure includes invasive recording of intracardiac and intravascular pressures, tracings, blood sampling, and cardiac output.
	Cardiac electrophysiology study	37.26	■ EPS, programmed electrical stimulation, ICD, implantable stimulation and pacing/recording studies excluding bundle of HIS recording (37.29)
	Angiocardiography	88.52–88.58	■ Arteriography by Sones, Judkins, or Ricketts and Abrams techniques, direct selective arteriography
	AMI, initial episode of care	410.0-410.9 (with fifth digit of 1)	■ Describes an acute event, if multiple sites or subsequent sites identified for infarction documented, code all sites. ◆ Non-Q wave codes to subendocardial (410.7x)
	CHF	*428	◆ PE commonly seen as part of CHFdisease process; when evaluated and treated report as additional diagnosis ■ End-stage congestive heart failure, compensated heart failure, decompensated heart failure, heart failure NOS
	Shock	785.50, 785.51	

Circulatory System, MDC 5

DRG 110 (continued)

DRG	Principal Dx/Procedure	Codes	Tips
536	Implantation or replacement of automatic cardioverter/defibrillator, total system (AICD)	37.94	■ Implantation of defibrillator with leads; formation of pocket; obtaining defibrillator threshold measurements
	Implantation of automatic cardioverter/defibrillator lead(s) only	37.95	
	Implantation of automatic cardioverter/defibrillator pulse generator only	37.96	
	Replacement of automatic cardioverter/defibrillator lead(s) only	37.97	
	Replacement of automatic cardioverter/defibrillator pulse generator only	37.98	
	Cardiac catheterization	37.21, 37.22, 37.23	■ The passage of catheter in heart chambers does not constitute a diagnostic cardiac catheterization. Procedure includes invasive recording of intracardiac and intravascular pressures, tracings, blood sampling, and cardiac output.
	Cardiac electrophysiology study	37.26	■ EPS, programmed electrical stimulation, ICD, implantable stimulation and pacing/recording studies excluding bundle of HIS recording (37.29)
	Angiocardiography	88.52–88.58	■ Arteriography by Sones, Judkins, or Ricketts and Abrams techniques, direct selective arteriography

DRG 111 Major Cardiovascular Procedures without CC   RW 2.4797

Potential DRGs

104	**Cardiac Valve** and **Other Major Cardiothoracic Procedures** with Cardiac Catheterization	RW	7.9351
105	**Cardiac Valve** and **Other Major Cardiothoracic Procedures** without Cardiac Catheterization	RW	5.7088
108	Other Cardiothoracic Procedures	RW	5.3656
110	Major Cardiovascular Procedures **with CC**	RW	4.0492
535	**Cardiac Defibrillator Implant with Cardiac Catheterization** with Acute Myocardial Infarction/Heart Failure/Shock	RW	8.1560
536	**Cardiac Defibrillator Implant with Cardiac Catheterization** without Acute Myocardial Infarction/Heart Failure/Shock	RW	6.2775

DRG	Principal Dx/Procedure	Codes	Tips
104	Cardiac valve procedure	*35.1, *35.2	■ Annuloplasty is included in the valvuloplasty operation
	Cardiac catheterization	37.21, 37.22, 37.23	■ The passage of catheter in heart chambers does not constitute a diagnostic cardiac catheterization. Procedure includes invasive recording of intracardiac and intravascular pressures, tracings, blood sampling, and cardiac output.
	Cardiac electrophysiology study	37.26	■ EPS, programmed electrical stimulation, ICD, implantable stimulation and pacing/recording studies excluding bundle of HIS recording (37.29)
	Angiocardiography	88.52–88.58	■ Arteriography by Sones, Judkins, or Ricketts and Abrams techniques, direct selective arteriography
105	Cardiac valve procedure	*35.1, *35.2	■ Annuloplasty is included in the valvuloplasty operation

---

■ Coding Tip   ● Documentation Tip   ◆ Encoder Tip   ▽ Targeted DRG

DRG	Principal Dx/Procedure	Codes	Tips
108	Cardiotomy	37.10, 37.11	■ Cardiolysis; incision of atrium, endocardium, myocardium, or ventricle
110	CC condition	See CC section.	
535	Implantation or replacement of automatic cardioverter/defibrillator, total system (AICD)	37.94	■ Implantation of defibrillator with leads; formation of pocket; obtaining defibrillator threshold measurements
	Implantation of automatic cardioverter/defibrillator lead(s) only	37.95	
	Implantation of automatic cardioverter/defibrillator pulse generator only	37.96	
	Replacement of automatic cardioverter/defibrillator lead(s) only	37.97	
	Replacement of automatic cardioverter/defibrillator pulse generator only	37.98	
	Cardiac catheterization	37.21, 37.22, 37.23	■ The passage of catheter in heart chambers does not constitute a diagnostic cardiac catheterization. Procedure includes invasive recording of intracardiac and intravascular pressures, tracings, blood sampling, and cardiac output.
	Cardiac electrophysiology study	37.26	■ EPS, programmed electrical stimulation, ICD, implantable stimulation and pacing/recording studies excluding bundle of HIS recording (37.29)
	Angiocardiography	88.52–88.58	■ Arteriography by Sones, Judkins, or Ricketts and Abrams techniques, direct selective arteriography
	AMI, initial episode of care	410.0-410.9 (with fifth digit of 1)	■ Describes an acute event, if multiple sites or subsequent sites identified for infarction documented, code all sites. ◆ Non-Q wave codes to subendocardial (410.7x)
	CHF	*428	◆ PE commonly seen as part of CHFdisease process; when evaluated and treated report as additional diagnosis ■ End-stage congestive heart failure, compensated heart failure, decompensated heart failure, heart failure NOS
	Shock	785.50, 785.51	

■ Coding Tip   ● Documentation Tip   ◆ Encoder Tip   ▽ Targeted DRG

Circulatory System, MDC 5

DRG 111   (continued)

DRG	Principal Dx/Procedure	Codes	Tips
536	Implantation or replacement of automatic cardioverter/defibrillator, total system (AICD)	37.94	■ Implantation of defibrillator with leads; formation of pocket; obtaining defibrillator threshold measurements
	Implantation of automatic cardioverter/ defibrillator lead(s) only	37.95	
	Implantation of automatic cardioverter/ defibrillator pulse generator only	37.96	
	Replacement of automatic cardioverter/ defibrillator lead(s) only	37.97	
	Replacement of automatic cardioverter/ defibrillator pulse generator only	37.98	
	Cardiac catheterization	37.21, 37.22, 37.23	■ The passage of catheter in heart chambers does not constitute a diagnostic cardiac catheterization. Procedure includes invasive recording of intracardiac and intravascular pressures, tracings, blood sampling, and cardiac output.
	Cardiac electrophysiology study	37.26	■ EPS, programmed electrical stimulation, ICD, implantable stimulation and pacing/recording studies excluding bundle of HIS recording (37.29)
	Angiocardiography	88.52–88.58	■ Arteriography by Sones, Judkins, or Ricketts and Abrams techniques, direct selective arteriography

DRG 112   Invalid DRG

No Potential DRGs

DRG 113   Amputation for Circulatory System Disorders Except Upper Limb and Toe

No Potential DRGs

DRG 114   Upper Limb & Toe Amputation for Circulatory System Disorders   RW 1.6436

Potential DRGs

285   Amputation of Lower Limb for Endocrine, Nutritional & Metabolic Disorders RW   2.0825

DRG	Principal Dx/Procedure	Codes	Tips
285	Diabetic osteomyelitis	*250.8, 731.8	◆ Hypoglycemic shock

---

■ Coding Tip   ● Documentation Tip   ◆ Encoder Tip   ^(WB) Targeted DRG

Permanent Pacemaker Implant with AMI, Heart Failure or Shock, or AICD Lead or Generator Procedure

RW 3.5465 **DRG 115**

Potential DRGs

515	Cardiac Defibrillator Implant without Cardiac Catheterizaton	RW	5.3366
535	Cardiac Defibrillator Implant with Cardiac Catheterization with Acute Myocardial Infarction/Heart Failure/Shock	RW	8.1560
536	Cardiac Defibrillator Implant with Cardiac Catheterization without Acute Myocardial Infarction/Heart Failure/Shock	RW	6.2775

DRG	Principal Dx/Procedure	Codes	Tips
515	Implantation or replacement of automatic cardioverter/defibrillator, total system (AICD)	37.94	■ Implantation of defibrillator with leads; formation of pocket; obtaining defibrillator threshold measurements
	Implantation of automatic cardioverter/defibrillator lead(s) only	37.95	
	Implantation of automatic cardioverter/defibrillator pulse generator only	37.96	
	Replacement of automatic cardioverter/defibrillator lead(s) only	37.97	
	Replacement of automatic cardioverter/defibrillator pulse generator only	37.98	
535	Implantation or replacement of automatic cardioverter/defibrillator, total system (AICD)	37.94	■ Implantation of defibrillator with leads; formation of pocket; obtaining defibrillator threshold measurements
	Implantation of automatic cardioverter/defibrillator lead(s) only	37.95	
	Implantation of automatic cardioverter/defibrillator pulse generator only	37.96	
	Replacement of automatic cardioverter/defibrillator lead(s) only	37.97	
	Replacement of automatic cardioverter/defibrillator pulse generator only	37.98	
	Cardiac catheterization	37.21, 37.22, 37.23	■ The passage of catheter in heart chambers does not constitute a diagnostic cardiac catheterization. Procedure includes invasive recording of intracardiac and intravascular pressures, tracings, blood sampling, and cardiac output.
	Cardiac electrophysiology study	37.26	■ EPS, programmed electrical stimulation, ICD, implantable stimulation and pacing/recording studies excluding bundle of HIS recording (37.29)
	Angiocardiography	88.52–88.58	■ Arteriography by Sones, Judkins, or Ricketts and Abrams techniques, direct selective arteriography
	AMI, initial episode of care	410.0-410.9 (with fifth digit of 1)	■ Describes an acute event, if multiple sites or subsequent sites identified for infarction documented, code all sites. ◆ Non-Q wave codes to subendocardial (410.7x)
	CHF	*428	◆ PE commonly seen as part of CHF disease process; when evaluated and treated report as additional diagnosis ■ End-stage congestive heart failure, compensated heart failure, decompensated heart failure, heart failure NOS
	Shock	785.50, 785.51	

■ Coding Tip   ● Documentation Tip   ◆ Encoder Tip   ▽ Targeted DRG

DRG 115 (continued)

DRG	Principal Dx/Procedure	Codes	Tips
536	Implantation or replacement of automatic cardioverter/defibrillator, total system (AICD)	37.94	■ Implantation of defibrillator with leads; formation of pocket; obtaining defibrillator threshold measurements
	Implantation of automatic cardioverter/ defibrillator lead(s) only	37.95	
	Implantation of automatic cardioverter/ defibrillator pulse generator only	37.96	
	Replacement of automatic cardioverter/ defibrillator lead(s) only	37.97	
	Replacement of automatic cardioverter/ defibrillator pulse generator only	37.98	
	Cardiac catheterization	37.21, 37.22, 37.23	■ The passage of catheter in heart chambers does not constitute a diagnostic cardiac catheterization. Procedure includes invasive recording of intracardiac and intravascular pressures, tracings, blood sampling, and cardiac output.
	Cardiac electrophysiology study	37.26	■ EPS, programmed electrical stimulation, ICD, implantable stimulation and pacing/recording studies excluding bundle of HIS recording (37.29)
	Angiocardiography	88.52–88.58	■ Arteriography by Sones, Judkins, or Ricketts and Abrams techniques, direct selective arteriography

DRG 116 Other Cardiac Pacemaker Implantation RW 2.3590

Potential DRGs

105	**Cardiac Valve** and **Other Major Cardiothoracic Procedures** without Cardiac Catheterization	RW	5.7088
108	Other Cardiothoracic Procedures	RW	5.3656
110	Major Cardiovascular Procedures **with CC**	RW	4.0492
111	Major Cardiovascular Procedures **without CC**	RW	2.4797
115	Permanent Cardiac Pacemaker Implant **with AMI, Heart Failure or Shock**	RW	3.5465
515	**Cardiac Defibrillator Implant** without Cardiac Catheterizaton	RW	5.3366
535	**Cardiac Defibrillator Implant with Cardiac Catheterization** with Acute Myocardial Infarction/Heart Failure/Shock	RW	8.1560
536	**Cardiac Defibrillator Implant with Cardiac Catheterization** without Acute Myocardial Infarction/Heart Failure/Shock	RW	6.2775

DRG	Principal Dx/Procedure	Codes	Tips
105	Cardiac valve procedure	*35.1, *35.2	■ Annuloplasty is included in the valvuloplasty operation
108	Open chest coronary artery angioplasty	36.03	■ Endarterectomy with patch graft; thromboendarterectom y with patch graft ◆ May be performed on same vessels during a CABG or on vessels not bypassed during a CABG. Only code separately when performed on separate vessels, considered integral to CABG at the same vessel
110	Major cardiovascular procedure (e.g., closed heart valvotomy) *AND* CC condition	*35.0 See CC section.	■ Sternotomy, thoracotomy as operative approach
111	Major cardiovascular procedure without CC (e.g., closed heart valvotomy)	*35.0	■ Sternotomy, thoracotomy as operative approach

---

■ Coding Tip ● Documentation Tip ◆ Encoder Tip ▼ Targeted DRG

DRG	Principal Dx/Procedure	Codes	Tips
115	Hypertensive heart disease with heart failure	402.01, 402.11, 402.91	■ Due to hypertension, hypertensive heart disease, cardiomegaly, cardiopathy, heart failure
	Hypertensive heart & renal disease with heart failure	404.11, 404.13, 404.91	■ Cardiorenal disease, cardiovascular renal disease
	AMI, initial episode of care	410.0–410.9 (with fifth digit of 1)	
	Congestive heart failure, unspecified	428.0	■ CHF, decompensated
	Heart failure NOS	428.9	
	Shock, cardiogenic or unspecified	785.50, 785.51	◆ ALTE for newborns; near miss SIDS
	AND AICD lead or generator procedure	37.70–37.76, 37.80–37.87	
515	Implantation or replacement of automatic cardioverter/defibrillator, total system (AICD)	37.94	■ Implantation of defibrillator with leads; formation of pocket; obtaining defibrillator threshold measurements
	Implantation of automatic cardioverter/defibrillator lead(s) only	37.95	
	Implantation of automatic cardioverter/defibrillator pulse generator only	37.96	
	Replacement of automatic cardioverter/defibrillator lead(s) only	37.97	
	Replacement of automatic cardioverter/defibrillator pulse generator only	37.98	
535	Implantation or replacement of automatic cardioverter/defibrillator, total system (AICD)	37.94	■ Implantation of defibrillator with leads; formation of pocket; obtaining defibrillator threshold measurements
	Implantation of automatic cardioverter/defibrillator lead(s) only	37.95	
	Implantation of automatic cardioverter/defibrillator pulse generator only	37.96	
	Replacement of automatic cardioverter/defibrillator lead(s) only	37.97	
	Replacement of automatic cardioverter/defibrillator pulse generator only	37.98	
	Cardiac catheterization	37.21, 37.22, 37.23	■ The passage of catheter in heart chambers does not constitute a diagnostic cardiac catheterization. Procedure includes invasive recording of intracardiac and intravascular pressures, tracings, blood sampling, and cardiac output.
	Cardiac electrophysiology study	37.26	■ EPS, programmed electrical stimulation, ICD, implantable stimulation and pacing/recording studies excluding bundle of HIS recording (37.29)
	Angiocardiography	88.52–88.58	■ Arteriography by Sones, Judkins, or Ricketts and Abrams techniques, direct selective arteriography
	AMI, initial episode of care	410.0-410.9 (with fifth digit of 1)	■ Describes an acute event, if multiple sites or subsequent sites identified for infarction documented, code all sites. ◆ Non-Q wave codes to subendocardial (410.7x)

Circulatory System, MDC 5

DRG 116 (continued)

535 cont.	CHF	*428	◆ PE commonly seen as part of CHFdisease process; when evaluated and treated report as additional diagnosis ■ End-stage congestive heart failure, compensated heart failure, decompensated heart failure, heart failure NOS
	Shock	785.50, 785.51	
536	Implantation or replacement of automatic cardioverter/defibrillator, total system (AICD)	37.94	■ Implantation of defibrillator with leads; formation of pocket; obtaining defibrillator threshold measurements
	Implantation of automatic cardioverter/ defibrillator lead(s) only	37.95	
	Implantation of automatic cardioverter/ defibrillator pulse generator only	37.96	
	Replacement of automatic cardioverter/ defibrillator lead(s) only	37.97	
	Replacement of automatic cardioverter/ defibrillator pulse generator only	37.98	
	Cardiac catheterization	37.21, 37.22, 37.23	■ The passage of catheter in heart chambers does not constitute a diagnostic cardiac catheterization. Procedure includes invasive recording of intracardiac and intravascular pressures, tracings, blood sampling, and cardiac output.
	Cardiac electrophysiology study	37.26	■ EPS, programmed electrical stimulation, ICD, implantable stimulation and pacing/recording studies excluding bundle of HIS recording (37.29)
	Angiocardiography	88.52–88.58	■ Arteriography by Sones, Judkins, or Ricketts and Abrams techniques, direct selective arteriography

DRG 117 Cardiac Pacemaker Revision Except Device Replacement   RW 1.3951

Potential DRGs

115	**Permanent Cardiac Pacemaker Implant** with AMI, Heart Failure or Shock	RW	3.5465
116	**Other Cardiac Pacemaker Implantation**	RW	2.3590
118	Cardiac Pacemaker **Device Replacement**	RW	1.6089
515	**Cardiac Defibrillator Implant** without Cardiac Catheterizaton	RW	5.3366
535	**Cardiac Defibrillator Implant with Cardiac Catheterization** with Acute Myocardial Infarction/Heart Failure/Shock	RW	8.1560
536	**Cardiac Defibrillator Implant with Cardiac Catheterization** without Acute Myocardial Infarction/Heart Failure/Shock	RW	6.2775

DRG	Principal Dx/Procedure	Codes	Tips
115	Hypertensive heart disease with heart failure	402.01, 402.11, 402.91	■ Due to hypertension, hypertensive heart disease, cardiomegaly, cardiopathy, heart failure
	Hypertensive heart & renal disease with heart failure	404.11, 404.13, 404.91	■ Cardiorenal disease, cardiovascular renal disease
	AMI, initial episode of care	410.0–410.9 (with fifth digit of 1)	
	Congestive heart failure, unspecified	428.0	■ CHF, decompensated
	Heart failure NOS	428.9	
	Shock, cardiogenic or unspecified	785.50, 785.51	◆ ALTE for newborns; near miss SIDS
	AND AICD lead or generator procedure	37.70–37.76, 37.80–37.87	

■ Coding Tip   ● Documentation Tip   ◆ Encoder Tip   ▽ Targeted DRG

©*2003 Ingenix, Inc.*

DRG	Principal Dx/Procedure	Codes	Tips
116	Permanent cardiac pacemaker implantation (original insertion)	37.80–37.87, 37.95–37.98	
118	Replacement of pacemaker device only	37.80, 37.85–37.87	
515	Implantation or replacement of automatic cardioverter/defibrillator, total system (AICD)	37.94	■ Implantation of defibrillator with leads; formation of pocket; obtaining defibrillator threshold measurements
	Implantation of automatic cardio-verter/defibrillator lead(s) only	37.95	
	Implantation of automatic cardioverter/defibrillator pulse generator only	37.96	
	Replacement of automatic cardio-verter/defibrillator lead(s) only	37.97	
	Replacement of automatic cardioverter/defibrillator pulse generator only	37.98	
535	Implantation or replacement of automatic cardioverter/defibrillator, total system (AICD)	37.94	■ Implantation of defibrillator with leads; formation of pocket; obtaining defibrillator threshold measurements
	Implantation of automatic cardioverter/defibrillator lead(s) only	37.95	
	Implantation of automatic cardioverter/defibrillator pulse generator only	37.96	
	Replacement of automatic cardioverter/defibrillator lead(s) only	37.97	
	Replacement of automatic cardioverter/defibrillator pulse generator only	37.98	
	Cardiac catheterization	37.21, 37.22, 37.23	■ The passage of catheter in heart chambers does not constitute a diagnostic cardiac catheterization. Procedure includes invasive recording of intracardiac and intravascular pressures, tracings, blood sampling, and cardiac output.
	Cardiac electrophysiology study	37.26	■ EPS, programmed electrical stimulation, ICD, implantable stimulation and pacing/recording studies excluding bundle of HIS recording (37.29)
	Angiocardiography	88.52–88.58	■ Arteriography by Sones, Judkins, or Ricketts and Abrams techniques, direct selective arteriography
	AMI, initial episode of care	410.0-410.9 (with fifth digit of 1)	■ Describes an acute event, if multiple sites or subsequent sites identified for infarction documented, code all sites. ◆ Non-Q wave codes to subendocardial (410.7x)
	CHF	*428	◆ PE commonly seen as part of CHF disease process; when evaluated and treated report as additional diagnosis ■ End-stage congestive heart failure, compensated heart failure, decompensated heart failure, heart failure NOS
	Shock	785.50, 785.51	

Circulatory System, MDC 5

DRG 117   (continued)

DRG	Principal Dx/Procedure	Codes	Tips
536	Implantation or replacement of automatic cardioverter/defibrillator, total system (AICD)	37.94	■ Implantation of defibrillator with leads; formation of pocket; obtaining defibrillator threshold measurements
	Implantation of automatic cardioverter/ defibrillator lead(s) only	37.95	
	Implantation of automatic cardioverter/ defibrillator pulse generator only	37.96	
	Replacement of automatic cardioverter/ defibrillator lead(s) only	37.97	
	Replacement of automatic cardioverter/ defibrillator pulse generator only	37.98	
	Cardiac catheterization	37.21, 37.22, 37.23	■ The passage of catheter in heart chambers does not constitute a diagnostic cardiac catheterization. Procedure includes invasive recording of intracardiac and intravascular pressures, tracings, blood sampling, and cardiac output.
	Cardiac electrophysiology study	37.26	■ EPS, programmed electrical stimulation, ICD, implantable stimulation and pacing/recording studies excluding bundle of HIS recording (37.29)
	Angiocardiography	88.52–88.58	■ Arteriography by Sones, Judkins, or Ricketts and Abrams techniques, direct selective arteriography

*Ensure accurate DRG assignment.
The only procedures in DRG 117 are:
37.74 Insertion or replacement of epicardial lead into epicardium
37.75 Revision of lead
37.76 Replacement of transvenous atrial &/or ventricular leads
37.77 Removal of lead without replacement
37.79 Revision or relocation of pacemaker pocket
37.89 Revision or removal of pacemaker device

DRG 118   Cardiac Pacemaker Device Replacement   RW 1.6089

Potential DRGs

115	**Permanent Cardiac Pacemaker Implant** with AMI, Heart Failure or Shock, or AICD Lead or Generator Procedure	RW	3.5465
116	**Other Cardiac Pacemaker Implantation**	RW	2.3590
515	**Cardiac Defibrillator Implant** without Cardiac Catheterizaton	RW	5.3366
535	**Cardiac Defibrillator Implant with Cardiac Catheterization** with Acute Myocardial Infarction/Heart Failure/Shock	RW	8.1560
536	**Cardiac Defibrillator Implant with Cardiac Catheterization** without Acute Myocardial Infarction/Heart Failure/Shock	RW	6.2775

DRG	Principal Dx/Procedure	Codes	Tips
115	Hypertensive heart disease with heart failure	402.01, 402.11, 402.91	■ Due to hypertension, hypertensive heart disease, cardiomegaly, cardiopathy, heart failure
	Hypertensive heart & renal disease with heart failure	404.11, 404.13, 404.91	■ Cardiorenal disease, cardiovascular renal disease
	AMI, initial episode of care	410.0–410.9 (with fifth digit of 1)	
	Congestive heart failure, unspecified	428.0	■ CHF, decompensated
	Heart failure NOS	428.9	
	Shock, cardiogenic or unspecified	785.50, 785.51	◆ ALTE for newborns; near miss SIDS
	AND	37.70–37.76,	
	AICD lead or generator procedure	37.80–37.87	

■ Coding Tip   ● Documentation Tip   ◆ Encoder Tip   ▽ Targeted DRG

(continued)   DRG 118

DRG	Principal Dx/Procedure	Codes	Tips
116	Permanent cardiac pacemaker implantation (original insertion)	37.80–37.87, 37.95–37.98	
515	Implantation or replacement of automatic cardioverter/defibrillator, total system (AICD)	37.94	■ Implantation of defibrillator with leads; formation of pocket; obtaining defibrillator threshold measurements
	Implantation of automatic cardio-verter/defibrillator lead(s) only	37.95	
	Implantation of automatic cardioverter/defibrillator pulse generator only	37.96	
	Replacement of automatic cardio-verter/defibrillator lead(s) only	37.97	
	Replacement of automatic cardioverter/defibrillator pulse generator only	37.98	
535	Implantation or replacement of automatic cardioverter/defibrillator, total system (AICD)	37.94	■ Implantation of defibrillator with leads; formation of pocket; obtaining defibrillator threshold measurements
	Implantation of automatic cardioverter/defibrillator lead(s) only	37.95	
	Implantation of automatic cardioverter/defibrillator pulse generator only	37.96	
	Replacement of automatic cardioverter/defibrillator lead(s) only	37.97	
	Replacement of automatic cardioverter/defibrillator pulse generator only	37.98	
	Cardiac catheterization	37.21, 37.22, 37.23	■ The passage of catheter in heart chambers does not constitute a diagnostic cardiac catheterization. Procedure includes invasive recording of intracardiac and intravascular pressures, tracings, blood sampling, and cardiac output.
	Cardiac electrophysiology study	37.26	■ EPS, programmed electrical stimula-tion, ICD, implantable stimulation and pacing/recording studies excluding bundle of HIS recording (37.29)
	Angiocardiography	88.52–88.58	■ Arteriography by Sones, Judkins, or Ricketts and Abrams techniques, direct selective arteriography
	AMI, initial episode of care	410.0-410.9 (with fifth digit of 1)	■ Describes an acute event, if multiple sites or subsequent sites identified for infarction documented, code all sites. ◆ Non-Q wave codes to subendocardial (410.7x)
	CHF	*428	◆ PE commonly seen as part of CHFdisease process; when evaluated and treated report as additional diagnosis ■ End-stage congestive heart failure, compensated heart failure, decompensated heart failure, heart failure NOS
	Shock	785.50, 785.51	

■ Coding Tip   ● Documentation Tip   ◆ Encoder Tip   ⬡ Targeted DRG

©2003 *Ingenix, Inc.*

Circulatory System, MDC 5

DRG 118 (continued)

DRG	Principal Dx/Procedure	Codes	Tips
536	Implantation or replacement of automatic cardioverter/defibrillator, total system (AICD)	37.94	■ Implantation of defibrillator with leads; formation of pocket; obtaining defibrillator threshold measurements
	Implantation of automatic cardioverter/ defibrillator lead(s) only	37.95	
	Implantation of automatic cardioverter/ defibrillator pulse generator only	37.96	
	Replacement of automatic cardioverter/ defibrillator lead(s) only	37.97	
	Replacement of automatic cardioverter/ defibrillator pulse generator only	37.98	
	Cardiac catheterization	37.21, 37.22, 37.23	■ The passage of catheter in heart chambers does not constitute a diagnostic cardiac catheterization. Procedure includes invasive recording of intracardiac and intravascular pressures, tracings, blood sampling, and cardiac output.
	Cardiac electrophysiology study	37.26	■ EPS, programmed electrical stimulation, ICD, implantable stimulation and pacing/recording studies excluding bundle of HIS recording (37.29)
	Angiocardiography	88.52–88.58	■ Arteriography by Sones, Judkins, or Ricketts and Abrams techniques, direct selective arteriography

DRG 119 Vein Ligation and Stripping
No Potential DRGs

DRG 120 Other Circulatory System Operating Room Procedures
No Potential DRGs

DRG 121▼ Circulatory Disorders with AMI and Major Complications, Discharged Alive
RW 1.6169

Potential DRGs

110	**Major Cardiovascular Procedures** with CC	RW	4.0492
111	**Major Cardiovascular Procedures** without CC	RW	2.4797
115	**Permanent Cardiac Pacemaker Implant** with AMI, Heart Failure or Shock	RW	3.5465

DRG	Principal Dx/Procedure	Codes	Tips
110	Major cardiovascular procedure *AND* CC condition	37.61, 37.64 See CC section.	◆ Balloon pulsation device inserted for mechanical circulation assistance. Not to be confused with a heart assist system (37.62–37.66) ■ Be sure to review the operative report for code 37.64 Removal of heart assist system. Code 37.64 has recently been moved to DRGs 110 & 111.
111	Major cardiovascular procedure	37.61, 37.64	◆ Balloon pulsation device inserted for mechanical circulation assistance. Not to be confused with a heart assist system (37.62–37.66) ■ Be sure to review the operative report for code 37.64 Removal of heart assist system. Code 37.64 has recently been moved to DRGs 110 & 111.

(continued) ▽DRG 121

DRG	Principal Dx/Procedure	Codes	Tips
115	Permanent cardiac pacemaker implant	37.70–37.76, 37.80–37.87	

Circulatory Disorders with AMI and without Major Complications, Discharged Alive
RW 1.0297 ▽DRG 122

Potential DRGs

110	Major Cardiovascular Procedures with CC	RW	4.0492
111	Major Cardiovascular Procedures without CC	RW	2.4797
115	Permanent Cardiac Pacemaker Implant with AMI, Heart Failure or Shock	RW	3.5465
121	Circulatory Disorders with AMI and Major Complications, **Discharged Alive**	RW	1.6169
123	Circulatory Disorders with AMI, **Expired**	RW	1.5645

DRG	Principal Dx/Procedure	Codes	Tips
110	Major cardiovascular procedure *AND* CC condition	37.61, 37.64 See CC section.	◆ Balloon pulsation device inserted for mechanical circulation assistance. Not to be confused with a heart assist system (37.62–37.66) ■ Be sure to review the operative report for code 37.64 Removal of heart assist system. Code 37.64 has recently been moved to DRGs 110 & 111.
111	Major cardiovascular procedure	37.61, 37.64	◆ Balloon pulsation device inserted for mechanical circulation assistance. Not to be confused with a heart assist system (37.62–37.66) ■ Be sure to review the operative report for code 37.64 Removal of heart assist system. Code 37.64 has recently been moved to DRGs 110 & 111.
115	Permanent cardiac pacemaker implant	37.70–37.76, 37.80–37.87	
121 ▽	AMI, initial episode of care *AND* Major complication diagnosis:	410.0–410.9 (with fifth digit of 1)	■ Describes an acute event, if multiple sites or subsequent sites identified for infarction documented, code all sites. ◆ Non-Q wave codes to subendocardial (410.7x)
	Rheumatic heart failure	398.91	■ If physician documents both congestive failure as and rheumatic or rheumatic heart failure, use this code and 396.3.
	Primary pulmonary hypertension	416.0	● Idiopathic pulmonary arteriosclerosis
	Cardiac dysrythmias	*427	
	Heart failure	*428	
	Subarachnoid hemorrhage	430	
	Intracerebral hemorrhage	431	
	Nontraumatic extradural hemorrhage	432.0	
	Subdural hemorrhage	432.9	
	Occluded basilar artery with cerebral infarction	433.01	
	Occluded carotid artery with cerebral infarction	433.11	
	Occluded vertebral artery with cerebral infarction	433.21	
	Occluded multiple and bilateral precerebral artery with cerebral infarction	433.31	

■ Coding Tip   ● Documentation Tip   ◆ Encoder Tip   ▽ Targeted DRG

DRG 122▽ (continued)

DRG	Principal Dx/Procedure	Codes	Tips
121 ▽ cont.	Occluded specified precerebral artery with cerebral infarction	434.00 434.01	
	Cerebral thrombosis		
	Cerebral thrombosis with cerebral infarction	434.11	
	Cerebral embolism with cerebral infarction	434.90 433.91	
	Cerebral artery occlusion		
	Occluded precerebral artery NOS with cerebral infarction	434.91	
	Cerebral artery occlusion with cerebral infarction	436	■ Always use solo; documentation will state CVA and no additional etiology.
	CVA NOS	481	■ If presence of pneumococcal pneumonia and pneumococcal septicemia (038.2) confirmed in record, code both entities.
	Pneumococcal pneumonia		
		482.xx	■ Mixed bacterial pneumonia NOS
	Other bacterial pneumonia (all fourth & fifth digits except 482.84)	483.x	
	Pneumonia due to other specified organism (all fourth digits)	484.x	
	Pneumonia in infectious diseases classified elsewhere (all fourth digits)	485	■ Lobular pneumonia, pleurobroncho-pneumonia, hemorrhagic pneumonia
	Bronchopneumonia, organism unspecified	486 487.0	
	Pneumonia, organism unspecified	507.x	■ If both aspiration and bacterial pneumonia are documented, code both.
	Influenza with pneumonia		
	Pneumonitis due to solids and liquids (all fourth digits)	518.0	■ Atelectasis, postoperative complication must be documented by physician as such based on workup and physician findings.
	Pulmonary collapse		
		518.5	■ ARDS, shock lung
	Pulmonary insufficiency following trauma and surgery	518.81 518.83	
	Acute respiratory failure	518.84	
	Chronic respiratory failure	707.0	■ If ulcer is staged as superficial or advanced in progress notes this is, irrelevant to ICD-9-CM assignment.
	Acute and chronic respiratory failure		
	Decubitus ulcer		
		996.62	■ If physician documents sepsis (present on admission) causing an infected access device, 996.62 must be the principal Dx with *038 as additional.
	Infection and inflammatory reaction due to vascular device, implant and graft		
123	Discharge status, expired		

Circulatory Disorders with AMI, Expired   RW 1.5645   **DRG 123**

Potential DRGs

| 115 | Permanent Cardiac Pacemaker Implant with AMI, Heart Failure or Shock | RW | 3.5465 |
| 121 | Circulatory Disorders with AMI and Major Complications, **Discharged Alive** | RW | 1.6169 |

DRG	Principal Dx/Procedure	Codes	Tips
115	Permanent cardiac pacemaker implant	37.70–37.76, 37.80–37.87	
121 ▽YIELD	AMI, initial episode of care *AND* Major Complication *AND* Discharge status, alive	410.0–410.9 (with fifth digit of 1)	■ Describes an acute event, if multiple sites or subsequent sites identified for infarction documented, code all sites. ◆ Non-Q wave codes to subendocardial (410.7x)

Circulatory Disorders Except AMI with   RW 1.4367   ▽**DRG 124**
Cardiac Catheterization & Complex
Diagnosis Potential DRGs

| 121 | Circulatory Disorders with AMI and Major Complications, Discharged Alive | RW | 1.6169 |
| 126 | Acute & Subacute Endocarditis | RW | 2.5418 |

DRG	Principal Dx/Procedure	Codes	Tips
121 ▽YIELD	AMI, initial episode of care *AND* Major Complications *AND* Discharge status, alive	410.0–410.9 (with fifth digit of 1)	■ Describes an acute event, if multiple sites or subsequent sites identified for infarction documented, code all sites. ◆ Non-Q wave codes to subendocardial (410.7x)
126	Acute or subacute endocarditis	421.0, 421.1, 421.9	◆ SBE, infective aneurysm, malignant endocarditis ◆ Key terms bacterial, constructive, infectious, pneumococci, septic, streptococcal, meningiococcal, candidal.

Circulatory Disorders Except AMI with   RW 1.0947   ▽**DRG 125**
Cardiac Catheterization without Complex
Diagnosis

Potential DRGs

| 121 | Circulatory Disorders with **AMI** and **Major Complications, Discharged Alive** | RW | 1.6169 |
| 124 | Circulatory Disorders Except AMI with Cardiac Catheterization & **Complex Diagnosis** | RW | 1.4367 |

DRG	Principal Dx/Procedure	Codes	Tips
121 ▽YIELD	AMI, initial episode of care *AND* Major Complications *AND* Discharge status, alive	410.0–410.9 (with fifth digit of 1)	■ Describes an acute event, if multiple sites or subsequent sites identified for infarction documented, code all sites. ◆ Non-Q wave codes to subendocardial (410.7x)

■ Coding Tip   ● Documentation Tip   ◆ Encoder Tip   ▽ Targeted DRG

Circulatory System, MDC 5

DRG 125▽ (continued)

DRG	Principal Dx/Procedure	Codes	Tips
124 ▽	Complex diagnosis: Hypertensive heart disease with heart failure	402.91	■ Due to hypertension, hypertensive heart disease, cardiomegaly, cardiopathy, heart failure
	Acute ischemic heart disease without MI	*411	■ Impending infarction, Dresslers syndrome, unstable angina, preinfarction angina
	Post-MI syndrome (Dresslers syndrome)	411.0	
	Unstable angina	411.1	
	Coronary insufficiency	411.89	
	Acute pericarditis	*420.9	■ Pericarditis, NOS
	Endocarditis	*421	
	Acute myocarditis	*422	
	Cardiomyopathy	425.4, 425.5, 425.7, 425.9	■ Secondary cardiomyopathies; code primary disease as well
	Cardiac arrest	427.5	■ Cardiorespiratory arrest
	Heart failure	*428	
	Failure, heart, systolic	*428.2	
	Failure, heart, diastolic, acute	*428.3	
	Failure, heart, combined systolic and diastolic	*428.4	
	Shock	785.50	

DRG 126   Acute and Subacute Endocarditis
No Potential DRGs

DRG 127▽ Heart Failure & Shock   RW 1.0265
Potential DRGs

078	**Pulmonary Embolism**	RW	1.2731
079	Respiratory Infections & Inflammations, Age > 17 **with CC**	RW	1.5974
089	**Simple Pneumonia** & Pleurisy, Age > 17 **with CC**	RW	1.0463
110	Major Cardiovascular Procedures **with CC**	RW	4.0492
111	**Major Cardiovascular Procedures** without CC	RW	2.4797
120	Other Circulatory System O.R. Procedures	RW	2.3164
121	Circulatory Disorders with **AMI** and **Major Complications, Discharged Alive**	RW	1.6169
123	Circulatory Disorder with **AMI**, **Expired**	RW	1.5645
124	Circulatory Disorders Except AMI **with Cardiac Catheterization** **& Complex Diagnosis**	RW	1.4367

DRG	Principal Dx/Procedure	Codes	Tips
078	Pulmonary embolism	*415.1	
079 ▽	Respiratory infections and inflammations, age >17 with CC	003.22	
	Pneumonia due to *Salmonella* Pneumonia due to *Klebsiella pneumoniae*	482.0	■ Bacterial pneumonia should be assigned based on physician documentation. ◆ Nonessential modifiers may be gram negative or gram posititive, seek physician consultation.
		482.1	
	Pneumonia due to *Pseudomonas*	482.40	
	Pneumonia due to *Staphylococcus*	482.83	
	Pneumonia due to *Proteus*	*507	■ If both aspiration and bacterial pneumonia are documented, code both.
	Aspiration pneumonia		

■ Coding Tip   ● Documentation Tip   ◆ Encoder Tip   ▽ Targeted DRG

(continued) ⏷DRG 127

DRG	Principal Dx/Procedure	Codes	Tips
089 ⏷	Simple pneumonia and pleurisy, Age > 17 with CC Pneumonia, NOS	486 See CC section.	◆ May be caused by bacteria, viruses, parasites, and other organisms.
110	Major cardiovascular procedure with CC	37.61, 37.64 See CC section.	◆ Balloon pulsation device inserted for mechanical circulation assistance. Not to be confused with a heart assist system (37.62–37.66) ■ Be sure to review the operative report for code 37.64 Removal of heart assist system. Code 37.64 has recently been moved to DRGs 110 & 111.
111	Major cardiovascular procedure	37.61, 37.64	◆ Balloon pulsation device inserted for mechanical circulation assistance. Not to be confused with a heart assist system (37.62–37.66) ■ Be sure to review the operative report for code 37.64 Removal of heart assist system. Code 37.64 has recently been moved to DRGs 110 & 111.
120	Insertion of an arteriovenous fistula, cutaneoperitoneal fistula or vessel-to-vessel cannula for renal dialysis	39.27, 39.93	◆ Internal formation of AV shunt code 39.27. External vessel-to-vessel shunt (ex, Scribner) code 39.93.
121 ⏷	AMI, initial episode of care AND Major Complications AND Discharge status, alive	410.0–410.9 (with fifth digit of 1)	■ Describes an acute event, if multiple sites or subsequent sites identified for infarction documented, code all sites. ◆ Non-Q wave codes to subendocardial (410.7x)
123	AMI, initial episode of care AND Discharge status, expired	410.0–410.9 (with fifth digit of 1)	■ Code all sites of MI documented in the medical record; see guidelines for coding myocardial infarctions.
124 ⏷	Circulatory principal diagnosis excluding AMI AND Cardiac catheterization	37.21–37.23, 88.52–88.58	● Written report of diagnostic cardiac catheterization required to use with 89.63 or 89.64.

Deep Vein Thrombophlebitis   RW 0.7285 ⏷DRG 128

Potential DRGs

130	Peripheral Vascular Disorders with CC	RW	0.9505
478	Other Vascular Procedures with CC	RW	2.3743

DRG	Principal Dx/Procedure	Codes	Tips
130 ⏷	Phlebitis and thrombophlebitis of other sites AND CC condition	451.0, 451.82, 451.89, 451.9, 453.1 See CC section.	● Physician should be queried when documentation of DVT does not further qualify as thrombophlebitis/phlebitis. ◆ Include terms superficial lower extremities (other than femoral), upper extremities, unspecified sites, or other specified veins.
478	Plication of vena cava	38.7	

Cardiac Arrest, Unexplained   DRG 129

No Potential DRGs

■ Coding Tip	● Documentation Tip	◆ Encoder Tip	⏷ Targeted DRG

Circulatory System, MDC 5

DRG 130▽ Peripheral Vascular Disorders with CC   RW 0.9505

Potential DRGs

078	Pulmonary Embolism	RW	1.2731
478	Other Vascular Procedures **with CC**	RW	2.3743

DRG	Principal Dx/Procedure	Codes	Tips
078	Pulmonary embolism	*415.1	
478	Angioplasty or atherectomy of noncoronary vessel *OR* Endarterectomy of upper/lower limb *OR* Excision or clipping of aneurysm	39.50 38.13, 38.18 38.33, 38.38, 38.43, 38.48, 39.51	■ PTA of noncoronary vessel ■ Endarterectomy w/patch graft

DRG 131   Peripheral Vascular Disorders without CC   RW 0.5676

Potential DRGs

078	Pulmonary Embolism	RW	1.2731
128	Deep Vein Thrombosis	RW	0.7285
130	Peripheral Vascular Disorders **with CC**	RW	0.9505

DRG	Principal Dx/Procedure	Codes	Tips
078	Pulmonary embolism	*415.1	
128	Phlebitis and thrombophlebitis of lower extremities	451.2	● Physician should be queried when documentation of DVT does not further qualify as thrombophlebitis/phlebitis.
	Phlebitis and thrombophlebitis of iliac vein	451.81	
	Embolism and thrombosis of vena cava	453.2	
130 ▽	CC condition	See CC section.	

DRG 132▽ Atherosclerosis with CC   RW 0.6422

Potential DRGs

138	Cardiac Arrhythmia & **Conduction Disorders** with CC	RW	0.8355

DRG	Principal Dx/Procedure	Codes	Tips
138 ▽	Atrial fibrillation	427.31	
	Atrial flutter	427.32	■ If diagnosis stated as holiday heart, syndrome, code both acute alcohol ingestion and arrhythmia. The principal diagnosis would be the condition that necessitated admission.
	Ventricular fibrillation	*427.4	
	Ventricular flutter		
	Premature beats	*427.6	
	Cardiac dysrhythmia	427.9	

Atherosclerosis without CC   RW 0.5559   **DRG 133**

Potential DRGs
132 Atherosclerosis **with CC**   RW   0.6422
138 Cardiac Arrhythmia & Conduction Disorders with CC   RW   0.8355

DRG	Principal Dx/Procedure	Codes	Tips
132	CC condition	See CC section.	◆ Angina often present with CAD
138	Atrial fibrillation	427.31	
	Atrial flutter	427.32	■ If diagnosis stated as holiday heart, syndrome, code both acute alcohol ingestion and arrhythmia. The principal diagnosis would be the condition that necessitated admission.
	Ventricular fibrillation	*427.4	
	Ventricular flutter		
	Premature beats	*427.6	
	Cardiac dysrhythmia	427.9	

Hypertension   RW 0.5954   **DRG 134**

Potential DRGs
121 Circulatory Disorders with AMI and **Major Complications**, Discharged Alive   RW   1.6169
122 Circulatory Disorders with AMI and **without Major Complications**, Discharged Alive   RW   1.0297
127 **Heart Failure & Shock**   RW   1.0265
316 **Renal Failure**   RW   1.2987
331 **Other Kidney & Urinary Tract Diagnoses** Age >17 with CC   RW   1.0618

DRG	Principal Dx/Procedure	Codes	Tips
121	AMI, initial episode of care *AND* Major Complications *AND* Discharge status, alive	410.0–410.9 (with fifth digit of 1)	■ Describes an acute event, if multiple sites or subsequent sites identified for infarction documented, code all sites. ◆ Non-Q wave codes to subendocardial (410.7x)
122	AMI, initial episode of care	410.0–410.9 (with fifth digit of 1)	■ Code all sites of MI documented in the medical record; see guidelines for coding myocardial infarctions.
127	Hypertensive heart disease with heart failure	402.01, 402.11, 402.91	■ See guidelines on coding hypertensive disease; hypertensive heart disease must be documented; it may not be inferred.
316	Hypertensive renal disease with renal failure	403.91	● Hypertensive heart disease must be documented; it may not be inferred.
331	Hypertensive renal disease without renal failure *AND* Patient's age > 17 *AND* CC condition	403.90 See CC section.	

Cardiac Congenital & Valvular Disorders,   RW 0.9282   **DRG 135**
Age > 17 with CC

Potential DRGs
126 **Acute & Subacute Endocarditis**   RW   2.5418

DRG	Principal Dx/Procedure	Codes	Tips
126	Acute or subacute endocarditis	421.0	◆ SBE, infective aneurysm, malignant endocarditis ◆ Key terms: bacterial, constructive, infectious, pneumococci, septic, streptococcal, meningiococcal, candidal

■ Coding Tip   ● Documentation Tip   ◆ Encoder Tip   ▽ Targeted DRG

DRG 136 Cardiac Congenital & Valvular Disorders, RW 0.5740
Age > 17 without CC

Potential DRGs

126	Acute & Subacute Endocarditis	RW	2.5418
135	Cardiac Congenital & Valvular Disorders, Age > 17 **with CC**	RW	0.9282
137	Cardiac Congenital & Valvular Disorders, **Age 0–17**	RW	0.8243

DRG	Principal Dx/Procedure	Codes	Tips
126	Acute or subacute endocarditis	421.0	◆ SBE, infective aneurysm, malignant endocarditis ◆ Key terms: bacterial, constructive, infectious, pneumococci, septic, streptococcal, meningiococcal, candidal.
135	CC condition	See CC section.	
137	Patient's age 0–17		

DRG 137 Cardiac Congenital & Valvular RW 0.8243
Disorders, Age 0–17

Potential DRGs

126	Acute & Subacute Endocarditis<	RW	2.5418
135	Cardiac Congenital & Valvular Disorders, Age > 17 **with CC**	RW	0.9282

DRG	Principal Dx/Procedure	Codes	Tips
126	Acute or subacute endocarditis	421.0	◆ SBE, infective aneurysm, malignant endocarditis ◆ Key terms: bacterial, constructive, infectious, pneumococci, septic, streptococcal, meningiococcal, candidal.
135	Patient's age 0–17 *AND* CC condition	See CC section.	

DRG 138▽ Cardiac Arrhythmia & Conduction RW 0.8355
Disorders with CC

Potential DRGs

121	Circulatory Disorders with AMI and **Major Complications**, Discharged Alive	RW	1.6169
122	Circulatory Disorders with AMI and **without Major Complications**, Discharged Alive	RW	1.0297
127	Heart Failure & Shock	RW	1.0265

DRG	Principal Dx/Procedure	Codes	Tips
121 ▽	AMI, initial episode of care *AND* Major Complications *AND* Discharge status, alive	410.0–410.9 (with fifth digit of 1)	■ Describes an acute event, if multiple sites or subsequent sites identified for infarction documented, code all sites. ◆ Non-Q wave codes to subendocardial (410.7x)
122 ▽	AMI, initial episode of care	410.0–410.9 (with fifth digit of 1)	■ *410 Code all sites of MI documented in the medical record.
127 ▽	Heart failure, unspecified	*428	■ Use code 428.0 to describe decompensated CHF. ■ See guidelines on coding hypertensive disease; hypertensive heart disease must be documented; it may not be inferred.
	Hypertensive heart disease with heart failure	402.91	
	Hypertensive heart and renal disease with heart failure	404.91	

Cardiac Arrhythmia & Conduction Disorders without CC

RW 0.5160 **DRG 139**

Potential DRGs

121	Circulatory Disorders with AMI and **Major Complications**, Discharged Alive	RW	1.6169
122	Circulatory Disorders with AMI and **without Major Complications**, Discharged Alive	RW	1.0297
127	**Heart Failure & Shock**	RW	1.0265
138	Cardiac Arrhythmia & Conduction Disorders **with CC**	RW	0.8355

DRG	Principal Dx/Procedure	Codes	Tips
121 ▽	AMI, initial episode of care *AND* Major Complications *AND* Discharge status, alive	410.0–410.9 (with fifth digit of 1)	■ Describes an acute event, if multiple sites or subsequent sites identified for infarction documented, code all sites. ◆ Non-Q wave codes to subendocardial (410.7x)
122 ▽	AMI, initial episode of care	410.0–410.9 (with fifth digit of 1)	■ *410 Code all sites of MI documented in the medical record.
127 ▽	Heart failure, unspecified	*428	■ Use code 428.0 to describe decompensated CHF. ■ See guidelines on coding hypertensive disease; hypertensive heart disease must be documented; it may not be inferred.
	Hypertensive heart disease with heart failure	402.91	
	Hypertensive heart and renal disease with heart failure	404.91	
138 ▽	CC condition	See CC section.	

Angina Pectoris

RW 0.5305 ▽**DRG 140**

Potential DRGs

121	Circulatory Disorders with AMI and **Major Complications**, Discharged Alive	RW	1.6169
122	Circulatory Disorders with AMI and **without Major Complications**, Discharged Alive	RW	1.0297
127	**Heart Failure & Shock**	RW	1.0265
132	Atherosclerosis with CC	RW	0.6422
138	Cardiac Arrhythmia & Conduction Disorders **with CC**	RW	0.8355
143	Chest Pain	RW	0.5480
144	**Other Circulatory System Diagnoses** with CC	RW	1.2260

DRG	Principal Dx/Procedure	Codes	Tips
121 ▽	AMI, initial episode of care *AND* Major Complications *AND* Discharge status, alive	410.0–410.9 (with fifth digit of 1)	■ Describes an acute event, if multiple sites or subsequent sites identified for infarction documented, code all sites. ◆ Non-Q wave codes to subendocardial (410.7x)
122 ▽	AMI, initial episode of care	410.0–410.9 (with fifth digit of 1)	■ *410 Code all sites of MI documented in the medical record.
127 ▽	Heart failure, unspecified	*428	■ Use code 428.0 to describe decompensated CHF. ■ Hypertensive heart disease must be documented; it may not be inferred.
	Hypertensive heart disease with heart failure	402.91	
	Hypertensive heart and renal disease with heart failure	404.91	
132 ▽	Angina due to or associated with chronic heart disease (e.g., ASHD) *AND* CC condition	414.0x / See CC section.	■ Sequence 414.0x as principal diagnosis

■ Coding Tip   ● Documentation Tip   ◆ Encoder Tip   ▽ Targeted DRG

Circulatory System, MDC 5

DRG 140🔻 (continued)

DRG	Principal Dx/Procedure	Codes	Tips
138 🔻	Cardiac arrhythmia (e.g., SVT, atrial fibrillation) Conduction disorder AND CC condition	427.0, *427.3, *426 See CC section.	■ If diagnosis stated as holiday heart, syndrome, code both acute alcohol ingestion and arrhythmia. The principal diagnosis would be the condition that necessitated admission.
143	Chest pain	*786.5	
144	Cardiac neurosis	306.2	● Must be documented by cardiologist.

DRG 141 Syncope & Collapse with CC RW 0.7473

Potential DRGs

015	Nonspecific Cerebrovascular and Precerebral Occlusion without Infarction	RW	0.9677
138	**Cardiac Arrhythmia & Conduction Disorders** with CC	RW	0.8355
144	**Other Circulatory System Diagnoses with CC**	RW	1.2260
294	**Diabetes**, Age > 35	RW	0.7800
296	**Nutritional & Miscellaneous Metabolic Disorders**, Age > 17 with CC	RW	0.8639

DRG	Principal Dx/Procedure	Codes	Tips
015 🔻	Nonspecific cerebrovascular and precerebral occlusion without infarction	433.00, 433.90, 434.00	
138 🔻	Cardiac arrhythmia Conduction disorder	427.0, *427.3, *426	■ If diagnosis stated as holiday heart, syndrome, code both acute alcohol ingestion and arrhythmia. The principal diagnosis would be the condition that necessitated admission.
144	Syncope or collapse due to other circulatory system disorders	458.1, 458.8, 458.9	◆ Hypopiesis
294	Diabetes mellitus (out of control) AND Patient's age greater than 35	*250.0, *250.2	◆ 250.20: NIDDM is usually found in this population.
296 🔻	Metabolic disorder AND Patient's age greater than 17 AND CC condition	*276 See CC section.	■ IV hydration should be ordered for correct coding. If patient admitted with gastroenteritis and dehydration, w/IV hydration ordered, which necessitated the admission, 276.5 is the principal Dx.

DRG 142 Syncope & Collapse without CC RW 0.5761

Potential DRGs

015	Nonspecific Cerebrovascular and Precerebral Occlusion without Infarction	RW	0.9677
138	**Cardiac Arrhythmia & Conduction Disorders** with CC	RW	0.8355
141	Syncope & Collapse **with CC**	RW	0.7473
144	**Other Circulatory System Diagnoses with CC**	RW	1.2260
145	**Other Circulatory System Diagnoses without CC**	RW	0.5787
296	**Nutritional & Miscellaneous Metabolic Disorders**, Age > 17 with CC	RW	0.8639

DRG	Principal Dx/Procedure	Codes	Tips
015 🔻	Nonspecific cerebrovascular and precerebral occlusion without infarction	433.00, 433.90, 434.00	
138 🔻	Cardiac arrhythmia Conduction disorder	427.0, *427.3, *426	■ If diagnosis stated as holiday heart, syndrome, code both acute alcohol ingestion and arrhythmia. The principal diagnosis would be the condition that necessitated admission.

■ Coding Tip　　● Documentation Tip　　◆ Encoder Tip　　🔻 Targeted DRG

©2003 Ingenix, Inc.

(continued) **DRG 142**

DRG	Principal Dx/Procedure	Codes	Tips
141	CC condition	See CC section.	
144	Syncope or collapse due to other circulatory system disorders	458.1, 458.8, 458.9	◆ Hypopiesis
145	Hypotension	458.1, 458.8, 458.9	◆ Hypopiesis
296 〽	Metabolic disorder *AND* Patient's age > 17 *AND* CC condition	*276 See CC section.	■ IV hydration should be ordered for correct coding. If patient admitted with gastroenteritis and dehydration, w/IV hydration ordered, which necessitated the admission, 276.5 is the principal Dx.

Chest Pain   RW 0.5480 〽**DRG 143**

Potential DRGs

099	**Respiratory Signs & Symptoms with CC**	RW	0.7032
121	Circulatory Disorders with AMI and **Major Complications**, Discharged Alive	RW	1.6169
122	Circulatory Disorders with AMI and **without Major Complications**, Discharged Alive	RW	1.0679
127	Heart Failure and Shock	RW	1.0265
132	Atherosclerosis **with CC**	RW	0.6422
138	**Cardiac Arrhythmia & Conduction Disorders** with CC	RW	0.8355
144	Other Circulatory System Diagnoses **with CC**	RW	1.2260
182	**Esophagitis, Gastroenteritis & Miscellaneous Digestive Disorders** Age >17 **with CC**	RW	0.8223
183	**Esophagitis, Gastroenteritis & Miscellaneous Digestive Disorders** Age >17 **without CC**	RW	0.5759

DRG	Principal Dx/Procedure	Codes	Tips
099	Chest wall pain, Pleuritic pain *AND* CC condition	*786.0, 786.52 See CC section.	◆ Key terms: chest wall, pleuritic, anterior, respiration.
121 〽	AMI, initial episode of care *AND* Major Complications *AND* Discharge status, alive	410.0–410.9 (with fifth digit of 1)	■ Describes an acute event, if multiple sites or subsequent sites identified for infarction documented, code all sites. ◆ Non-Q wave codes to subendocardial (410.7x)
122 〽	AMI, initial episode of care	410.0–410.9 (with fifth digit of 1)	■ *410 Code all sites of MI documented in the medical record.
127 〽	Heart failure, unspecified Hypertensive heart disease with heart failure Hypertensive heart and renal disease with heart failure	*428 402.91 404.91	■ Use code 428.0 to describe decompensated CHF. ■ Hypertensive heart disease must be documented; it may not be inferred.
132 〽	Angina due to or associated with chronic heart disease (e.g., ASHD) *AND* CC condition	414.0x See CC section.	■ ASHD
138 〽	Cardiac arrhythmia (e.g., SVT, atrial fibrillation) Conduction disorder *AND* CC condition	427.0, *427.3, *426 See CC section.	■ If diagnosis stated as holiday heart, syndrome, code both acute alcohol ingestion and arrhythmia. The principal diagnosis would be the condition that necessitated admission

---

■ Coding Tip   ● Documentation Tip   ◆ Encoder Tip   〽 Targeted DRG

Circulatory System, MDC 5

DRG 143▽ (continued)

DRG	Principal Dx/Procedure	Codes	Tips
144	Syncope or collapse due to other circulatory system disorders with CC (e.g., hypotension)	458.1, 458.8, 458.9	
182 ▽	Reflux esophagitis Esophageal reflux Dyspepsia Hiatal hernia *AND* CC condition	530.11 530.81 536.8 553.3 See CC section.	■ Query physician for etiology of noncardiac chest pain
183	Reflux esophagitis Esophageal reflux Dyspepsia Hiatal hernia	530.11 530.81 536.8 553.3	■ Query physician for etiology of noncardiac chest pain

DRG 144   Other Circulatory System Diagnoses with CC   RW 1.2260

Potential DRGs

121	Circulatory Disorders with AMI and Major Complications, Discharged Alive	RW	1.6169
484	Craniotomy for **Multiple Significant Trauma**	RW	5.4179
486	Other **O.R. Procedures for Multiple Significant Trauma**	RW	4.8793
487	Other Multiple Significant Trauma	RW	2.0057

DRG	Principal Dx/Procedure	Codes	Tips
121 ▽	AMI, initial episode of care *AND* Major Complications *AND* Discharge status, alive	410.0–410.9 (with fifth digit of 1)	■ Describes an acute event, if multiple sites or subsequent sites identified for infarction documented, code all sites. ◆ Non-Q wave codes to subendocardial (410.7x)
484	Craniotomy for multiple significant trauma		■ Craniotomy and principal diagnosis of trauma and at least two injuries (assigned either as principal or secondary) that are defined as significant trauma from different body site categories located under DRG 487
486	Other O.R. procedures for multiple significant trauma		■ Principal diagnosis of trauma and at least two injuries (assigned either as principal or secondary) that are defined as significant trauma from different body site categories located under DRG 487 *AND* O.R. procedure other than craniotomy or limb reattachment, hip and femur procedures
487	Other multiple significant trauma		■ Principal diagnosis of trauma and at least two injuries (assigned either as principal or secondary) that are defined as significant trauma from different body site categories located under DRG 487

■ Coding Tip   ● Documentation Tip   ◆ Encoder Tip   ▽ Targeted DRG

Other Circulatory System Diagnoses without CC

RW 0.5787   **DRG 145**

Potential DRGs

121	Circulatory Disorders with AMI and **Major Complications**, Discharged Alive	RW	1.6169
122	Circulatory Disorders with AMI and **without Major Complications**, Discharged Alive	RW	1.0679
144	Other Circulatory System Diagnoses with CC	RW	1.2260
484	Craniotomy for **Multiple Significant Trauma**	RW	5.4179
486	Other **O.R. Procedures for Multiple Significant Trauma**	RW	4.8793
487	Other Multiple Significant Trauma	RW	2.0057

DRG	Principal Dx/Procedure	Codes	Tips
121 ▽	AMI, initial episode of care *AND* Major Complications *AND* Discharge status, alive	410.0–410.9 (with fifth digit of 1)	■ Describes an acute event, if multiple sites or subsequent sites identified for infarction documented, code all sites. ◆ Non-Q wave codes to subendocardial (410.7x)
122 ▽	AMI, initial episode of care	410.0–410.9 (with fifth digit of 1)	■ *410 Code all sites of MI documented in the medical record.
144	CC condition	See CC section.	
484	Craniotomy for multiple significant trauma		■ Craniotomy and principal diagnosis of trauma and at least two injuries (assigned either as principal or secondary) that are defined as significant trauma from different body site categories located under DRG 487
486	Other O.R. procedures for multiple significant trauma		■ Principal diagnosis of trauma and at least two injuries (assigned either as principal or secondary) that are defined as significant trauma from different body site categories located under DRG 487 *AND* O.R. procedure other than craniotomy or limb reattachment, hip and femur procedures
487	Other multiple significant trauma		■ Principal diagnosis of trauma and at least two injuries (assigned either as principal or secondary) that are defined as significant trauma from different body site categories located under DRG 487

Circulatory System, MDC 5

DRG 478 Other Vascular Procedures with CC RW 2.3743

Potential DRGs

104	Cardiac Valve and Other Major Cardiothoracic Procedures with Cardiac Catheterization	RW	7.9351
105	Cardiac Valve and Other Major Cardiothoracic Procedures without Cardiac Catheterization	RW	5.7088
106	Coronary Bypass with PTCA	RW	7.2936
107	Coronary Bypass with Cardiac Catheterization	RW	5.3751
108	Other Cardiothoracic Procedures	RW	5.3656
109	Coronary Bypass without PTCA or Cardiac Catheterization	RW	3.9401
110	Major Cardiovascular Procedures with CC	RW	4.0492
515	Cardiac Defibrillator Implant without Cardiac Catheterization	RW	5.3366
535	Cardiac Defibrillator Implant with Cardiac Catheterization with Acute Myocardial Infarction/Heart Failure/Shock	RW	8.1560
536	Cardiac Defibrillator Implant with Cardiac Catheterization without Acute Myocardial Infarction/Heart Failure/Shock	RW	6.2775

DRG	Principal Dx/Procedure	Codes	Tips
104	Cardiac valve procedures AND Cardiac catheterization	*35.1, *35.2 37.21, 37.22, 37.23	■ If surgery performed on annulus only, do not use this code, use 35.33.
105	Cardiac valve procedures	*35.1, *35.2	■ If surgery performed on annulus only, do not use this code, use 35.33.
106	Coronary bypass AND PTCA	*36.1, 36.01, 36.02, 36.05	◆ If balloon inflated, code procedure as completed; if balloon could not be inflated, code cardiac catheterization; if balloon tip guided only to extracoronary artery, code arterial catheterization.
107	Coronary bypass AND Cardiac catheterization Angiocardiography	*36.1 37.21–37.23 88.52–88.58	■ Arteriography by Sones, Judkins, or Ricketts and Abrams techniques, direct selective arteriography
108	Resection of vessel with replacement	38.44-38.45	■ Resection abdominal aorta and resection thoracic vessels
109	Coronary bypass	*36.1	
110	Major cardiovascular procedure (e.g., valvotomy, resection of aorta or occlusion procedures)	*35.0, 38.64	
515	Implantation or replacement of automatic cardioverter/defibrillator, total system (AICD) Implantation of automatic cardioverter/ defibrillator lead(s) only Implantation of automatic cardioverter/ defibrillator pulse generator only Replacement of automatic cardioverter/ defibrillator lead(s) only Replacement of automatic cardioverter/ defibrillator pulse generator only	37.94 37.95 37.96 37.97 37.98	■ Implantation of defibrillator with leads; formation of pocket; obtaining defibrillator threshold measurements

DRG	Principal Dx/Procedure	Codes	Tips
535	Implantation or replacement of automatic cardioverter/defibrillator, total system (AICD)	37.94	■ Implantation of defibrillator with leads; formation of pocket; obtaining defibrillator threshold measurements
	Implantation of automatic cardioverter/defibrillator lead(s) only	37.95	
	Implantation of automatic cardioverter/defibrillator pulse generator only	37.96	
	Replacement of automatic cardioverter/defibrillator lead(s) only	37.97	
	Replacement of automatic cardioverter/defibrillator pulse generator only	37.98	
	Cardiac catheterization	37.21, 37.22, 37.23	■ The passage of catheter in heart chambers does not constitute a diagnostic cardiac catheterization. Procedure includes invasive recording of intracardiac and intravascular pressures, tracings, blood sampling, and cardiac output.
	Cardiac electrophysiology study	37.26	■ EPS, programmed electrical stimulation, ICD, implantable stimulation and pacing/recording studies excluding bundle of HIS recording (37.29)
	Angiocardiography	88.52–88.58	■ Arteriography by Sones, Judkins, or Ricketts and Abrams techniques, direct selective arteriography
	AMI, initial episode of care	410.0-410.9 (with fifth digit of 1)	■ Describes an acute event, if multiple sites or subsequent sites identified for infarction documented, code all sites. ◆ Non-Q wave codes to subendocardial (410.7x)
	CHF	*428	◆ PE commonly seen as part of CHFdisease process; when evaluated and treated report as additional diagnosis ■ End-stage congestive heart failure, compensated heart failure, decompensated heart failure, heart failure NOS
	Shock	785.50, 785.51	
536	Implantation or replacement of automatic cardioverter/defibrillator, total system (AICD)	37.94	■ Implantation of defibrillator with leads; formation of pocket; obtaining defibrillator threshold measurements
	Implantation of automatic cardioverter/defibrillator lead(s) only	37.95	
	Implantation of automatic cardioverter/defibrillator pulse generator only	37.96	
	Replacement of automatic cardioverter/defibrillator lead(s) only	37.97	
	Replacement of automatic cardioverter/defibrillator pulse generator only	37.98	
	Cardiac catheterization	37.21, 37.22, 37.23	■ The passage of catheter in heart chambers does not constitute a diagnostic cardiac catheterization. Procedure includes invasive recording of intracardiac and intravascular pressures, tracings, blood sampling, and cardiac output.
	Cardiac electrophysiology study	37.26	■ EPS, programmed electrical stimulation, ICD, implantable stimulation and pacing/recording studies excluding bundle of HIS recording (37.29)

■ Coding Tip   ● Documentation Tip   ◆ Encoder Tip   ▽ Targeted DRG

Circulatory System, MDC 5

DRG 478 (continued)

DRG	Principal Dx/Procedure	Codes	Tips
536 cont.	Angiocardiography	88.52–88.58	■ Arteriography by Sones, Judkins, or Ricketts and Abrams techniques, direct selective arteriography

DRG 479 Other Vascular Procedures without CC RW 1.4300

Potential DRGs

104	**Cardiac Valve Procedures** and other **Major Cardiothoracic Procedures** with **Cardiac Catheterization**	RW	7.9351
105	**Cardiac Valve Procedures** and other **Major Cardiothoracic Procedures** without Cardiac Catheterization	RW	5.7088
106	**Coronary Bypass with PTCA**	RW	7.2936
107	**Coronary Bypass with Cardiac Catheterization**	RW	5.3751
108	**Other Cardiothoracic Procedures**	RW	5.3656
109	Coronary Bypass **without PTCA or Cardiac Catheterization**	RW	3.9401
110	**Major Cardiovascular Procedures with CC**	RW	4.0492
478	Other Vascular Procedures **with CC**	RW	2.3743
515	**Cardiac Defibrillator Implant** without Cardiac Catheterization	RW	5.3366
535	**Cardiac Defibrillator Implant with Cardiac Catheterization** with Acute Myocardial Infarction/Heart Failure/Shock	RW	8.1560
536	**Cardiac Defibrillator Implant with Cardiac Catheterization** without Acute Myocardial Infarction/Heart Failure/Shock	RW	6.2775

DRG	Principal Dx/Procedure	Codes	Tips
104	Cardiac valve procedures **AND** Cardiac catheterization	*35.1, *35.2 37.21, 37.22, 37.23	■ If surgery performed on annulus only, do not use this code, use 35.33.
105	Cardiac valve procedures	*35.1, *35.2	■ If surgery performed on annulus only, do not use this code, use 35.33.
106	Coronary bypass **AND** PTCA	36.01, 36.02, 36.05	◆ If balloon inflated, code procedure as completed; if balloon could not be inflated, code cardiac catheterization; if balloon tip guided only to extracoronary artery, code arterial catheterization.
107	Coronary bypass **AND** Cardiac catheterization Angiocardiography	*36.1 37.21–37.23 88.52–88.58	■ Arteriography by Sones, Judkins, or Ricketts and Abrams techniques, direct selective arteriography
108	Resection of vessel with replacement	38.44–38.45	■ Resection abdominal aorta and resection thoracic vessels
109	Coronary bypass	*36.1	
110	Major cardiovascular procedure (e.g., valvotomy, resection of aorta or occlusion procedures)	*35.0, 38.64 See CC section.	
478	CC condition	See CC section.	

DRG	Principal Dx/Procedure	Codes	Tips
515	Implantation or replacement of automatic cardioverter/defibrillator, total system (AICD)	37.94	■ Implantation of defibrillator with leads; formation of pocket; obtaining defibrillator threshold measurements
	Implantation of automatic cardioverter/ defibrillator lead(s) only	37.95	
	Implantation of automatic cardioverter/ defibrillator pulse generator only	37.96	
	Replacement of automatic cardioverter/ defibrillator lead(s) only	37.97	
	Replacement of automatic cardioverter/ defibrillator pulse generator only	37.98	
535	Implantation or replacement of automatic cardioverter/defibrillator, total system (AICD)	37.94	■ Implantation of defibrillator with leads; formation of pocket; obtaining defibrillator threshold measurements
	Implantation of automatic cardioverter/ defibrillator lead(s) only	37.95	
	Implantation of automatic cardioverter/ defibrillator pulse generator only	37.96	
	Replacement of automatic cardioverter/ defibrillator lead(s) only	37.97	
	Replacement of automatic cardioverter/ defibrillator pulse generator only	37.98	
	Cardiac catheterization	37.21, 37.22, 37.23	■ The passage of catheter in heart chambers does not constitute a diagnostic cardiac catheterization. Procedure includes invasive recording of intracardiac and intravascular pressures, tracings, blood sampling, and cardiac output.
	Cardiac electrophysiology study	37.26	■ EPS, programmed electrical stimulation, ICD, implantable stimulation and pacing/recording studies excluding bundle of HIS recording (37.29)
	Angiocardiography	88.52–88.58	■ Arteriography by Sones, Judkins, or Ricketts and Abrams techniques, direct selective arteriography
	AMI, initial episode of care	410.0-410.9 (with fifth digit of 1)	■ Describes an acute event, if multiple sites or subsequent sites identified for infarction documented, code all sites. ◆ Non-Q wave codes to subendocardial (410.7x)
	CHF	*428	◆ PE commonly seen as part of CHF disease process; when evaluated and treated report as additional diagnosis ■ End-stage congestive heart failure, compensated heart failure, decompensated heart failure, heart failure NOS
	Shock	785.50, 785.51	

■ Coding Tip   ● Documentation Tip   ◆ Encoder Tip   ▽ Targeted DRG

DRG 479 (continued)

DRG	Principal Dx/Procedure	Codes	Tips
536	Implantation or replacement of automatic cardioverter/defibrillator, total system (AICD)	37.94	■ Implantation of defibrillator with leads; formation of pocket; obtaining defibrillator threshold measurements
	Implantation of automatic cardioverter/ defibrillator lead(s) only	37.95	
	Implantation of automatic cardioverter/ defibrillator pulse generator only	37.96	
	Replacement of automatic cardioverter/ defibrillator lead(s) only	37.97	
	Replacement of automatic cardioverter/ defibrillator pulse generator only	37.98	
	Cardiac catheterization	37.21, 37.22, 37.23	■ The passage of catheter in heart chambers does not constitute a diagnostic cardiac catheterization. Procedure includes invasive recording of intracardiac and intravascular pressures, tracings, blood sampling, and cardiac output.
	Cardiac electrophysiology study	37.26	■ EPS, programmed electrical stimulation, ICD, implantable stimulation and pacing/recording studies excluding bundle of HIS recording (37.29)
	Angiocardiography	88.52–88.58	■ Arteriography by Sones, Judkins, or Ricketts and Abrams techniques, direct selective arteriography

DRG 515 Cardiac Defibrillator Implant without Cardiac Catheterization

RW 5.3366

Potential DRGs

104	Cardiac Valve and Other Major Cardiothoracic Procedures with Cardiac Catheterization	RW	7.9351
105	Cardiac Valve and Other Major Cardiothoracic Procedures without Cardiac Catheterization	RW	5.7088
106	Coronary Bypass with PTCA	RW	7.2936
107	Coronary Bypass with Cardiac Catheterization	RW	5.3751
108	Other Cardiothoracic Procedures	RW	5.3656
535	Cardiac Defibrillator Implant with Cardiac Catheterization with Acute Myocardial Infarction/Heart Failure/Shock	RW	8.1560
536	Cardiac Defibrillator Implant with Cardiac Catheterization without Acute Myocardial Infarction/Heart Failure/Shock	RW	6.2775

DRG	Principal Dx/Procedure	Codes	Tips
104	Cardiac valve procedures	*35.1, *35.2	■ If surgery performed on annulus only, do not use this code, use 35.33.
105	Cardiac valve procedures	*35.1, *35.2	■ If surgery performed on annulus only, do not use this code, use 35.33.
106	Percutaneous valvuloplasty Percutaneous coronary angioplasty	35.96, 36.01, 35.02, 36.05	■ Indirect heart revascularization, NOS ■ Balloon angioplasty of coronary artery w/infusion of thrombolytic agent
107	Coronary bypass *AND* Cardiac catheterization Angiocardiography	*36.1 37.21–37.23 88.52–88.58	■ Arteriography by Sones, Judkins, or Ricketts and Abrams techniques, direct selective arteriography

DRG	Principal Dx/Procedure	Codes	Tips
108	Open chest coronary artery angioplasty	36.03	■ Endarterectomy w/patch graft; thromboendarterectom y with patch graft ◆ May be performed on same vessels during a CABG or on vessels not bypassed during a CABG. Only code separately when performed on separate vessels, considered integral to CABG at the same vessel
535	Implantation or replacement of automatic cardioverter/defibrillator, total system (AICD)	37.94	■ Implantation of defibrillator with leads; formation of pocket; obtaining defibrillator threshold measurements
	Implantation of automatic cardioverter/defibrillator lead(s) only	37.95	
	Implantation of automatic cardioverter/defibrillator pulse generator only	37.96	
	Replacement of automatic cardioverter/defibrillator lead(s) only	37.97	
	Replacement of automatic cardioverter/defibrillator pulse generator only	37.98	
	Cardiac catheterization	37.21, 37.22, 37.23	■ The passage of catheter in heart chambers does not constitute a diagnostic cardiac catheterization. Procedure includes invasive recording of intracardiac and intravascular pressures, tracings, blood sampling, and cardiac output.
	Cardiac electrophysiology study	37.26	■ EPS, programmed electrical stimulation, ICD, implantable stimulation and pacing/recording studies excluding bundle of HIS recording (37.29)
	Angiocardiography	88.52–88.58	■ Arteriography by Sones, Judkins, or Ricketts and Abrams techniques, direct selective arteriography
	AMI, initial episode of care	410.0-410.9 (with fifth digit of 1)	■ Describes an acute event, if multiple sites or subsequent sites identified for infarction documented, code all sites. ◆ Non-Q wave codes to subendocardial (410.7x)
	CHF	*428	◆ PE commonly seen as part of CHFdisease process; when evaluated and treated report as additional diagnosis ■ End-stage congestive heart failure, compensated heart failure, decompensated heart failure, heart failure NOS
	Shock	785.50, 785.51	

DRG 515   (continued)

DRG	Principal Dx/Procedure	Codes	Tips
536	Implantation or replacement of automatic cardioverter/defibrillator, total system (AICD)	37.94	■ Implantation of defibrillator with leads; formation of pocket; obtaining defibrillator threshold measurements
	Implantation of automatic cardioverter/defibrillator lead(s) only	37.95	
	Implantation of automatic cardioverter/defibrillator pulse generator only	37.96	
	Replacement of automatic cardioverter/defibrillator lead(s) only	37.97	
	Replacement of automatic cardioverter/defibrillator pulse generator only	37.98	
	Cardiac catheterization	37.21, 37.22, 37.23	■ The passage of catheter in heart chambers does not constitute a diagnostic cardiac catheterization. Procedure includes invasive recording of intracardiac and intravascular pressures, tracings, blood sampling, and cardiac output.
	Cardiac electrophysiology study	37.26	■ EPS, programmed electrical stimulation, ICD, implantable stimulation and pacing/recording studies excluding bundle of HIS recording (37.29)
	Angiocardiography	88.52–88.58	■ Arteriography by Sones, Judkins, or Ricketts and Abrams techniques, direct selective arteriography

Percutaneous Cardiovascular Procedures with AMI
RW 2.6911 **DRG 516**

Potential DRGs

104	Cardiac Valve and Other Major Cardiothoracic Procedures with Cardiac Catheterization	RW	7.9351
105	Cardiac Valve and Other Major Cardiothoracic Procedures without Cardiac Catheterization	RW	5.7088
106	Coronary Bypass with PTCA	RW	7.2936
107	Coronary Bypass with Cardiac Cathe terization	RW	5.3751
108	Other Cardiothoracic Procedures	RW	5.3656
109	Coronary Bypass without PTCA or Cardiac Catheterization	RW	3.9401
110	Major Cardiovascular Procedures with CC	RW	4.0492
115	Permanent Cardiac Pacemaker Implant with AMI, Heart Failure or Shock, or AICD Lead or Generator Procedure	RW	3.5465
515	Cardiac Defibrillator Implant without Cardiac Catheterization	RW	5.3366
526	Percutaneous Cardiovascular Procedure with Drug-Eluting Stent with AMI	RW	2.9891
535	Cardiac Defibrillator Implant with Cardiac Catheterization with Acute Myocardial Infarction/Heart Failure/Shock	RW	8.1560
536	Cardiac Defibrillator Implant with Cardiac Catheterization without Acute Myocardial Infarction/Heart Failure/Shock	RW	6.2775

DRG	Principal Dx/Procedure	Codes	Tips
104	Open valvuloplasty NOS **AND Cardiac catheterization**	35.10, 37.21–37.23	■ The passage of catheter in heart chambers does not constitute a diagnostic cardiac catheterization. Procedure includes invasive recording of intracardiac and intravascular pressures, tracings, blood sampling, and cardiac output.
	Cardiac electrophysiology study	37.26	■ EPS, programmed electrical stimulation, ICD, implantable stimulation and pacing/recording studies excluding bundle of HIS recording (37.29)
	Angiocardiography	88.52–88.58	■ Arteriography by Sones, Judkins, or Ricketts and Abrams techniques, direct selective arteriography
105	Open valvuloplasty NOS	35.10	
106	Coronary bypass	*36.1	
107	Coronary bypass **AND** Cardiac catheterization Angiocardiography	*36.1 37.21–37.23 88.52–88.58	■ Arteriography by Sones, Judkins, or Ricketts and Abrams techniques, direct selective arteriography
108	Open chest coronary artery angioplasty **OR**	36.03	■ Coronary endarterectomy w/patch graft ◆ May be performed on same vessels during a CABG or on vessels not bypassed during a CABG. Only code separately when performed on separate vessels, considered integral to CABG at the same vessel
	Other revascularization of heart (e.g., by arterial implant)	36.2	■ Indirect heart revascularization, NOS
109	Coronary bypass	*36.1	

DRG 516 (continued)

DRG	Principal Dx/Procedure	Codes	Tips
110	Major cardiovascular procedure (e.g., implant, pulsation balloon) *AND* CC condition	37.61, 37.64 See CC section.	◆ Balloon pulsation device inserted for mechanical circulation assistance. Not to be confused with a heart assist system (37.62–37.66) ■ Be sure to review the operative report for code 37.64 Removal of heart assist system. Code 37.64 has recently been moved to DRGs 110 & 111.
115	Hypertensive heart disease with heart failure Hypertensive heart & renal disease with heart failure AMI, initial episode of care Congestive heart failure, unspecified Heart failure NOS Shock, cardiogenic or unspecified *AND* AICD lead or generator procedure	402.01, 402.11, 402.91 404.11, 404.13, 404.91 410.0–410.9 (with fifth digit of 1) 428.0 428.9 785.50, 785.51 37.70–37.76, 37.80–37.87	■ Due to hypertension, hypertensive heart disease, cardiomegaly, cardiopathy, heart failure ■ Cardiorenal disease, cardiovascular renal disease ■ CHF, decompensated ◆ ALTE for newborns; near miss SIDS
515	Cardiac defibrillator implant	37.94–37.98	■ Implantation of defibrillator with leads
526	With insertion of drug-eluting coronary artery stent	36.07	■ Pending FDA approval of drug-eluting stents (code 36.07), DRG 526 is effective for discharges occurring on or after April 1, 2003, and will only be valid for six months during FY 2003 from April through September 2003.
535	Implantation or replacement of automatic cardioverter/defibrillator, total system (AICD) Implantation of automatic cardioverter/defibrillator lead(s) only Implantation of automatic cardioverter/defibrillator pulse generator only Replacement of automatic cardioverter/defibrillator lead(s) only Replacement of automatic cardioverter/defibrillator pulse generator only Cardiac catheterization Cardiac electrophysiology study Angiocardiography	37.94 37.95 37.96 37.97 37.98 37.21, 37.22, 37.23 37.26 88.52–88.58	■ Implantation of defibrillator with leads; formation of pocket; obtaining defibrillator threshold measurements ■ The passage of catheter in heart chambers does not constitute a diagnostic cardiac catheterization. Procedure includes invasive recording of intracardiac and intravascular pressures, tracings, blood sampling, and cardiac output. ■ EPS, programmed electrical stimulation, ICD, implantable stimulation and pacing/recording studies excluding bundle of HIS recording (37.29) ■ Arteriography by Sones, Judkins, or Ricketts and Abrams techniques, direct selective arteriography

DRG	Principal Dx/Procedure	Codes	Tips
535 cont.	AMI, initial episode of care	410.0-410.9 (with fifth digit of 1)	■ Describes an acute event, if multiple sites or subsequent sites identified for infarction documented, code all sites. ◆ Non-Q wave codes to subendocardial (410.7x)
	CHF	*428	◆ PE commonly seen as part of CHF disease process; when evaluated and treated report as additional diagnosis ■ End-stage congestive heart failure, compensated heart failure, decompensated heart failure, heart failure NOS
	Shock	785.50, 785.51	
536	Implantation or replacement of automatic cardioverter/defibrillator, total system (AICD)	37.94	■ Implantation of defibrillator with leads; formation of pocket; obtaining defibrillator threshold measurements
	Implantation of automatic cardioverter/defibrillator lead(s) only	37.95	
	Implantation of automatic cardioverter/defibrillator pulse generator only	37.96	
	Replacement of automatic cardioverter/defibrillator lead(s) only	37.97	
	Replacement of automatic cardioverter/defibrillator pulse generator only	37.98	
	Cardiac catheterization	37.21, 37.22, 37.23	■ The passage of catheter in heart chambers does not constitute a diagnostic cardiac catheterization. Procedure includes invasive recording of intracardiac and intravascular pressures, tracings, blood sampling, and cardiac output.
	Cardiac electrophysiology study	37.26	■ EPS, programmed electrical stimulation, ICD, implantable stimulation and pacing/recording studies excluding bundle of HIS recording (37.29)
	Angiocardiography	88.52–88.58	■ Arteriography by Sones, Judkins, or Ricketts and Abrams techniques, direct selective arteriography

DRG 517 Percutaneous Cardiovascular Procedures RW 2.1598 without AMI with Non-drug Eluting Stent

Potential DRGs

104	**Cardiac Valve** and **Other Major Cardiothoracic Procedures with Cardiac Catheterization**	RW	7.9351
105	**Cardiac Valve** and **Other Major Cardiothoracic Procedures** without Cardiac Catheterization	RW	5.7088
106	**Coronary Bypass with PTCA**	RW	7.2936
107	**Coronary Bypass with Cardiac Catheterization**	RW	5.3751
108	**Other Cardiothoracic Procedures**	RW	5.3656
109	**Coronary Bypass** without PTCA or Cardiac Catheterization	RW	3.9401
110	Major Cardiovascular Procedures with CC	RW	4.0492
111	**Major Cardiovascular Procedures** without CC	RW	2.4797
115	**Permanent Cardiac Pacemaker Implant** with AMI, Heart Failure or Shock, or AICD Lead or Generator Procedure	RW	3.5465
116	**Other Cardiac Pacemaker Implantation**	RW	2.3590
515	**Cardiac Defibrillator Implant** without Cardiac Catheterization	RW	5.3366
516	**Percutaneous Cardiovascular Procedure with AMI**	RW	2.6911
527	Percutaneous Cardiovascular Procedure with Drug-Eluting Stent W/O AMI	RW	2.4483
535	**Cardiac Defibrillator Implant with Cardiac Catheterization** with Acute Myocardial Infarction/Heart Failure/Shock	RW	8.1560
536	**Cardiac Defibrillator Implant with Cardiac Catheterization** without Acute Myocardial Infarction/Heart Failure/Shock	RW	6.2775

DRG	Principal Dx/Procedure	Codes	Tips
104	Open valvuloplasty NOS *AND* Cardiac catheterization	35.10 37.21–37.23	■ The passage of catheter in heart chambers does not constitute a diagnostic cardiac catheterization. Procedure includes invasive recording of intracardiac and intravascular pressures, tracings, blood sampling, and cardiac output.
	Cardiac electrophysiology study	37.26	■ EPS, programmed electrical stimulation, ICD, implantable stimulation and pacing/recording studies excluding bundle of HIS recording (37.29)
	Angiocardiography	88.52–88.58	■ Arteriography by Sones, Judkins, or Ricketts and Abrams techniques, direct selective arteriography
105	Open valvuloplasty NOS	35.10	
106	Coronary bypass	*36.1	
107	Coronary bypass *AND* Cardiac catheterization Angiocardiography	*36.1 37.21–37.23 88.52–88.58	■ Arteriography by Sones, Judkins, or Ricketts and Abrams techniques, direct selective arteriography
108	Open chest coronary artery angioplasty *OR*	36.03	■ Coronary endarterectomy w/patch graft ◆ May be performed on same vessels during a CABG or on vessels not bypassed during a CABG. Only code separately when performed on separate vessels, considered integral to CABG at the same vessel
	Other revascularization of heart (e.g., by arterial implant)	36.2	■ Indirect heart revascularization, NOS
109	Coronary bypass	*36.1	

(continued) DRG 517

DRG	Principal Dx/Procedure	Codes	Tips
110	Major cardiovascular procedure (e.g., implant, pulsation balloon) *AND* CC condition	37.61, 37.64 See CC section.	◆ Balloon pulsation device inserted for mechanical circulation assistance. Not to be confused with a heart assist system (37.62–37.66) ■ Be sure to review the operative report for code 37.64 Removal of heart assist system. Code 37.64 has recently been moved to DRGs 110 & 111.
111	Major cardiovascular procedure (e.g., implant, pulsation balloon)	37.61, 37.64	◆ Balloon pulsation device inserted for mechanical circulation assistance. Not to be confused with a heart assist system (37.62–37.66) ■ Be sure to review the operative report for code 37.64 Removal of heart assist system. Code 37.64 has recently been moved to DRGs 110 & 111.
115	Hypertensive heart disease with heart failure Hypertensive heart & renal disease with heart failure AMI, initial episode of care Congestive heart failure, unspecified Heart failure NOS Shock, cardiogenic or unspecified *AND* AICD lead or generator procedure	402.01, 402.11, 402.91 404.11, 404.13, 404.91 410.0–410.9 (with fifth digit of 1) 428.0 428.9 785.50–785.51 37.70–37.76, 37.80–37.87	■ Due to hypertension, hypertensive heart disease, cardiomegaly, cardiopathy, heart failure ■ Cardiorenal disease, cardiovascular renal disease ■ CHF, decompensated ◆ ALTE for newborns; near miss SIDS
116	Permanent cardiac pacemaker implant (original insertion)	37.80–37.87, 37.95–37.98	
515	Cardiac defibrillator implant	37.94–37.98	■ Implantation of defibrillator with leads
516	AMI, initial episode of care *AND* PTCA	410.0–410.9 (with fifth digit of 1) 36.01, 36.02, 36.05, 36.09	■ PTCA with infusion of thrombolytic agent, coronary atherectomy; PTCA, NOS; balloon angioplasty of coronary vessel
527	With insertion of drug-eluting coronary artery stent	36.07	■ Pending FDA approval of drug-eluting stents (code 36.07), DRG 527 is effective for discharges occurring on or after April 1, 2003, and will only be valid for six months during FY 2003 from April through September 2003.
535	Implantation or replacement of automatic cardioverter/defibrillator, total system (AICD) Implantation of automatic cardioverter/defibrillator lead(s) only Implantation of automatic cardioverter/defibrillator pulse generator only Replacement of automatic cardioverter/defibrillator lead(s) only Replacement of automatic cardioverter/defibrillator pulse generator only	37.94 37.95 37.96 37.97 37.98	■ Implantation of defibrillator with leads; formation of pocket; obtaining defibrillator threshold measurements

■ Coding Tip   ● Documentation Tip   ◆ Encoder Tip   ▽ Targeted DRG

DRG 517 (continued)

DRG	Principal Dx/Procedure	Codes	Tips
535 cont.	Cardiac catheterization	37.21, 37.22, 37.23	■ The passage of catheter in heart chambers does not constitute a diagnostic cardiac catheterization. Procedure includes invasive recording of intracardiac and intravascular pressures, tracings, blood sampling, and cardiac output.
	Cardiac electrophysiology study	37.26	■ EPS, programmed electrical stimulation, ICD, implantable stimulation and pacing/recording studies excluding bundle of HIS recording (37.29)
	Angiocardiography	88.52–88.58	■ Arteriography by Sones, Judkins, or Ricketts and Abrams techniques, direct selective arteriography
	AMI, initial episode of care	410.0-410.9 (with fifth digit of 1)	■ Describes an acute event, if multiple sites or subsequent sites identified for infarction documented, code all sites. ◆ Non-Q wave codes to subendocardial (410.7x)
	CHF	*428	◆ PE commonly seen as part of CHF disease process; when evaluated and treated report as additional diagnosis ■ End-stage congestive heart failure, compensated heart failure, decompensated heart failure, heart failure NOS
	Shock	785.50, 785.51	
536	Implantation or replacement of automatic cardioverter/defibrillator, total system (AICD)	37.94	■ Implantation of defibrillator with leads; formation of pocket; obtaining defibrillator threshold measurements
	Implantation of automatic cardioverter/defibrillator lead(s) only	37.95	
	Implantation of automatic cardioverter/defibrillator pulse generator only	37.96	
	Replacement of automatic cardioverter/defibrillator lead(s) only	37.97	
	Replacement of automatic cardioverter/defibrillator pulse generator only	37.98	
	Cardiac catheterization	37.21, 37.22, 37.23	■ The passage of catheter in heart chambers does not constitute a diagnostic cardiac catheterization. Procedure includes invasive recording of intracardiac and intravascular pressures, tracings, blood sampling, and cardiac output.
	Cardiac electrophysiology study	37.26	■ EPS, programmed electrical stimulation, ICD, implantable stimulation and pacing/recording studies excluding bundle of HIS recording (37.29)
	Angiocardiography	88.52–88.58	■ Arteriography by Sones, Judkins, or Ricketts and Abrams techniques, direct selective arteriography

---

■ Coding Tip   ● Documentation Tip   ◆ Encoder Tip   ▽ Targeted DRG

Percutaneous Cardiovascular Procedures without AMI, without Coronary Artery Stent Implant

RW 1.7494 **DRG 518**

Potential DRGs

104	Cardiac Valve and Other Major Cardiothoracic Procedures with Cardiac Catheterization	RW	7.9351
105	Cardiac Valve and Other Major Cardiothoracic Procedures without Cardiac Catheterization	RW	5.7088
106	Coronary Bypass with PTCA	RW	7.2936
107	Coronary Bypass with Cardiac Catheterization	RW	5.3751
108	Other Cardiothoracic Procedures	RW	5.3656
109	Coronary Bypass without PTCA or Cardiac Catheterization	RW	3.9401
110	Major Cardiovascular Procedures with CC	RW	4.0492
111	Major Cardiovascular Procedures without CC	RW	2.4797
115	Permanent Cardiac Pacemaker Implant with AMI, Heart Failure or Shock, or AICD Lead or Generator Procedure	RW	3.5465
116	Other Cardiac Pacemaker Implantation	RW	2.3590
515	Cardiac Defibrillator Implant without Cardiac Catheterization	RW	5.3366
516	Percutaneous Cardiovascular Procedure with AMI	RW	2.6911
517	Percutaneous Cardiovascular Procedure with Non-Drug Eluting Stent; without AMI	RW	2.1598
535	Cardiac Defibrillator Implant with Cardiac Catheterization with Acute Myocardial Infarction/Heart Failure/Shock	RW	8.1560
536	Cardiac Defibrillator Implant with Cardiac Catheterization without Acute Myocardial Infarction/Heart Failure/Shock	RW	6.2775

DRG	Principal Dx/Procedure	Codes	Tips
104	Open valvuloplasty NOS *AND* Cardiac catheterization	35.10 37.21–37.23	■ The passage of catheter in heart chambers does not constitute a diagnostic cardiac catheterization. Procedure includes invasive recording of intracardiac and intravascular pressures, tracings, blood sampling, and cardiac output.
	Cardiac electrophysiology study	37.26	■ EPS, programmed electrical stimulation, ICD, implantable stimulation and pacing/recording studies excluding bundle of HIS recording (37.29)
	Angiocardiography	88.52–88.58	■ Arteriography by Sones, Judkins, or Ricketts and Abrams techniques, direct selective arteriography
105	Open valvuloplasty NOS	35.10	
106	Coronary bypass	*36.1	
107	Coronary bypass *AND* Cardiac catheterization Angiocardiography	*36.1 37.21–37.23 88.52–88.58	■ Arteriography by Sones, Judkins, or Ricketts and Abrams techniques, direct selective arteriography
108	Open chest coronary artery angioplasty *OR*	36.03	■ Coronary endarterectomy w/patch graft ◆ May be performed on same vessels during a CABG or on vessels not bypassed during a CABG. Only code separately when performed on separate vessels, considered integral to CABG at the same vessel
	Other revascularization of heart (e.g., by arterial implant)	36.2	■ Indirect heart revascularization, NOS

■ Coding Tip   ● Documentation Tip   ◆ Encoder Tip   ▧ Targeted DRG

Circulatory System, MDC 5

DRG 518 (continued)

DRG	Principal Dx/Procedure	Codes	Tips
109	Coronary bypass	*36.1	
110	Major cardiovascular procedure (e.g., implant, pulsation balloon) *AND* CC condition	37.61, 37.64 See CC section.	◆ Balloon pulsation device inserted for mechanical circulation assistance. Not to be confused with a heart assist system (37.62–37.66). ■ Be sure to review the operative report for code 37.64 Removal of heart assist system. Code 37.64 has recently been moved to DRGs 110 & 111.
111	Major cardiovascular procedure (e.g., implant, pulsation balloon)	37.61, 37.64	◆ Balloon pulsation device inserted for mechanical circulation assistance. Not to be confused with a heart assist system (37.62–37.66). ■ Be sure to review the operative report for code 37.64 Removal of heart assist system. Code 37.64 has recently been moved to DRGs 110 & 111.
115	Hypertensive heart disease with heart failure Hypertensive heart & renal disease with heart failure AMI, initial episode of care Congestive heart failure, unspecified Heart failure NOS Shock, cardiogenic or unspecified *AND* AICD lead or generator procedure	402.01, 402.11, 402.91 404.11, 404.13, 404.91 410.0–410.9 (with fifth digit of 1) 428.0 428.9 785.50–785.51 37.70–37.76, 37.80–37.87	■ Due to hypertension, hypertensive heart disease, cardiomegaly, cardiopathy, heart failure ■ Cardiorenal disease, cardiovascular renal disease ■ CHF, decompensated ◆ ALTE for newborns; near miss SIDS
116	Permanent cardiac pacemaker implant (original insertion)	37.80–37.87, 37.95–37.98	
515	Cardiac defibrillator implant	37.94–37.98	■ Implantation of defibrillator with leads
516	AMI, initial episode of care *AND* PTCA	410.0–410.9 (with fifth digit of 1) 36.01, 36.02, 36.05, 36.09	■ PTCA with infusion of thrombolytic agent, coronary atherectomy; PTCA, NOS; balloon angioplasty of coronary vessel
517	PTCA insertion of coronary artery stent(s), non-drug eluting stent	36.01, 36.02, 36.05, 36.09 36.06	■ PTCA with infusion of thrombolytic agent, coronary atherectomy; PTCA, NOS; balloon angioplasty of coronary vessel
535	Implantation or replacement of automatic cardioverter/defibrillator, total system (AICD) Implantation of automatic cardioverter/ defibrillator lead(s) only Implantation of automatic cardioverter/ defibrillator pulse generator only Replacement of automatic cardioverter/ defibrillator lead(s) only Replacement of automatic cardioverter/ defibrillator pulse generator only	37.94 37.95 37.96 37.97 37.98	■ Implantation of defibrillator with leads; formation of pocket; obtaining defibrillator threshold measurements

---

■ Coding Tip   ● Documentation Tip   ◆ Encoder Tip   ▼ Targeted DRG

DRG	Principal Dx/Procedure	Codes	Tips
535 cont.	Cardiac catheterization	37.21, 37.22, 37.23	■ The passage of catheter in heart chambers does not constitute a diagnostic cardiac catheterization. Procedure includes invasive recording of intracardiac and intravascular pressures, tracings, blood sampling, and cardiac output.
	Cardiac electrophysiology study	37.26	■ EPS, programmed electrical stimulation, ICD, implantable stimulation and pacing/recording studies excluding bundle of HIS recording (37.29)
	Angiocardiography	88.52–88.58	■ Arteriography by Sones, Judkins, or Ricketts and Abrams techniques, direct selective arteriography
	AMI, initial episode of care	410.0-410.9 (with fifth digit of 1)	■ Describes an acute event, if multiple sites or subsequent sites identified for infarction documented, code all sites. ◆ Non-Q wave codes to subendocardial (410.7x)
	CHF	*428	◆ PE commonly seen as part of CHFdisease process; when evaluated and treated report as additional diagnosis ■ End-stage congestive heart failure, compensated heart failure, decompensated heart failure, heart failure NOS
	Shock	785.50, 785.51	
536	Implantation or replacement of automatic cardioverter/defibrillator, total system (AICD)	37.94	■ Implantation of defibrillator with leads; formation of pocket; obtaining defibrillator threshold measurements
	Implantation of automatic cardioverter/defibrillator lead(s) only	37.95	
	Implantation of automatic cardioverter/defibrillator pulse generator only	37.96	
	Replacement of automatic cardioverter/defibrillator lead(s) only	37.97	
	Replacement of automatic cardioverter/defibrillator pulse generator only	37.98	
	Cardiac catheterization	37.21, 37.22, 37.23	■ The passage of catheter in heart chambers does not constitute a diagnostic cardiac catheterization. Procedure includes invasive recording of intracardiac and intravascular pressures, tracings, blood sampling, and cardiac output.
	Cardiac electrophysiology study	37.26	■ EPS, programmed electrical stimulation, ICD, implantable stimulation and pacing/recording studies excluding bundle of HIS recording (37.29)
	Angiocardiography	88.52–88.58	■ Arteriography by Sones, Judkins, or Ricketts and Abrams techniques, direct selective arteriography

■ Coding Tip　　● Documentation Tip　　◆ Encoder Tip　　▽ Targeted DRG

DRG 536 Cardiac Defibrillator Implant with Cardiac RW 6.2775 Catheterization without Acute Myocardial Infarction/Heart Failure/Shock

Potential DRGs

104	**Cardiac Valve** and **Other Major Cardiothoracic Procedures** with Cardiac Catheterization	RW	7.9351
106	**Coronary Bypass with PTCA**	RW	7.2936

DRG	Principal Dx/Procedure	Codes	Tips
104	Cardiac valve procedure *AND* Cardiac catheterization	*35.1, *35.2 37.21, 37.22, 37.23	◆ Annuloplasty is included in the valvuloplasty operation
106	Percutaneous valvuloplasty Percutaneous coronary angioplasty	35.96, 36.01, 35.02, 36.05	■ Indirect heart revascularization, NOS ■ Balloon angioplasty of coronary artery w/infusion of thrombolytic agent

Digestive System, MDC 6

Rectal Resection with CC   RW 2.7376   **DRG 146**

Potential DRGs

148 Major Small & Large Bowel Procedures with CC   RW   3.4025

DRG	Principal Dx/Procedure	Codes	Tips
148	Intestinal resection Colostomy *AND* CC condition	45.8 46.10 See CC section.	■ Post-op ileus: Ileus can be an expected event after abdominal surgery and is not a complication unless it is prolonged (usually over six days). It may mean status-post the procedure—not that this is necessarily a complication. Query the physician. ■ Post-op ileus-key terms: adynamic, inhibitory, neurogenic, paralytic

Rectal Resection without CC   RW 1.5375   **DRG 147**

Potential DRGs

146 Rectal Resection with CC   RW   2.7376
148 Major Small & Large Bowel Procedures with CC   RW   3.4025

DRG	Principal Dx/Procedure	Codes	Tips
146	CC condition	See CC section.	■ Post-op ileus: Ileus can be an expected event after abdominal surgery and is not a complication unless it is prolonged (usually over six days). It may mean status-post the procedure—not that this is necessarily a complication. Query the physician. ■ Post-op ileus-key terms: adynamic, inhibitory, neurogenic, paralytic
148	Intestinal resection Colostomy *AND* CC condition	45.8 46.10 See CC section.	■ Post-op ileus: Ileus can be an expected event after abdominal surgery and is not a complication unless it is prolonged (usually over six days). It may mean status-post the procedure—not that this is necessarily a complication. Query the physician. ■ Post-op ileus-key terms: adynamic, inhibitory, neurogenic, paralytic

Digestive System, MDC 6

DRG 148   Major Small & Large Bowel Procedures with CC   RW 3.4025

Potential DRGs

154   Stomach, Esophageal & Duodenal Procedures Age > 17 with CC   RW   4.0212

DRG	Principal Dx/Procedure	Codes	Tips
154	Cricopharyngeal myotomy Intra-abdominal venous shunt Esophagomyotomy *AND* CC condition	29.31 39.1 42.7 See CC section.	◆ Key terms: Mesocaval, portacaval ■ Post-op ileus: Ileus can be an expected event after abdominal surgery and is not a complication unless it is prolonged (usually over six days). It may mean status-post the procedure—not that this is necessarily a complication. Query the physician. ■ Post-op ileus-key terms: adynamic, inhibitory, neurogenic, paralytic

DRG 149   Major Small & Large Bowel Procedures without CC   RW 1.4590

Potential DRGs

148   Major Small & Large Bowel Procedures **with CC**   RW   3.4025
154   Stomach, Esophageal & Duodenal Procedures Age > 17 **with CC**   RW   4.0212

DRG	Principal Dx/Procedure	Codes	Tips
148	Intestinal resection Colostomy *AND* CC condition	45.8 46.10 See CC section.	■ Post-op ileus: Ileus can be an expected event after abdominal surgery and is not a complication unless it is prolonged (usually over six days). It may mean status-post the procedure—not that this is necessarily a complication. Query the physician. ■ Post-op ileus-key terms: adynamic, inhibitory, neurogenic, paralytic
154	Esophagomyotomy *AND* CC condition	42.7 See CC section.	■ Post-op ileus: Ileus can be an expected event after abdominal surgery and is not a complication unless it is prolonged (usually over six days). It may mean status-post the procedure—not that this is necessarily a complication. Query the physician. ■ Post-op ileus-key terms: adynamic, inhibitory, neurogenic, paralytic

DRG 150   Peritoneal Adhesiolysis with CC

No Potential DRGs

Peritoneal Adhesiolysis without CC   RW 1.3061   **DRG 151**

Potential DRGs
150   Peritoneal Adhesiolysis with CC   RW   2.8711

DRG	Principal Dx/Procedure	Codes	Tips
150	Lysis of peritoneal adhesions *AND* CC condition	*54.5 See CC section.	● Adhesiolysis must be determined by physician as significant. ■ Post-op ileus: Ileus can be an expected event after abdominal surgery and is not a complication unless it is prolonged (usually over six days). It may mean status-post the procedure—not that this is necessarily a complication. Query the physician. ■ Post-op ileus-key terms: adynamic, inhibitory, neurogenic, paralytic

Minor Small & Large Bowel Procedures with CC   RW 1.9134   **DRG 152**

Potential DRGs
148   Major Small & Large Bowel Procedures with CC   RW   3.4025

DRG	Principal Dx/Procedure	Codes	Tips
148	Intestinal resection Colostomy Proctopexy *AND* CC condition	45.8 46.10 48.76 See CC section.	◆ Key terms: Delorme repair, puborectalis sling operation ■ Post-op ileus: Ileus can be an expected event after abdominal surgery and is not a complication unless it is prolonged (usually over six days). It may mean status-post the procedure—not that this is necessarily a complication. Query the physician. ■ Post-op ileus-key terms: adynamic, inhibitory, neurogenic, paralytic

Minor Small & Large Bowel Procedures without CC   RW 1.1310   **DRG 153**

Potential DRGs
149   Major Small & Large Bowel Procedures without CC   RW   1.4590
152   Minor Small & Large Bowel Procedures with CC   RW   1.9134

DRG	Principal Dx/Procedure	Codes	Tips
149	Intestinal resection Colostomy Proctopexy	45.8 46.10 48.76	◆ Key terms: Delorme repair, puborectalis sling operation
152	*AND* CC condition	See CC section.	■ Post-op ileus: Ileus can be an expected event after abdominal surgery and is not a complication unless it is prolonged (usually over six days). It may mean status-post the procedure—not that this is necessarily a complication. Query the physician. ■ Post-op ileus-key terms: adynamic, inhibitory, neurogenic, paralytic

■ Coding Tip   ● Documentation Tip   ◆ Encoder Tip   ▽ Targeted DRG

Digestive System, MDC 6

DRG 154 Stomach, Esophageal and Duodenal Procedures Age > 17 with CC

No Potential DRGs

DRG 155 Stomach, Esophageal & Duodenal Procedures, Age > 17 without CC
RW 1.3043

Potential DRGs
148	Major Small & Large Bowel Procedures with CC	RW	3.4025
149	Major Small & Large Bowel Procedures without CC	RW	1.4590
154	Stomach, Esophageal & Duodenal Procedures, Age > 17 with CC	RW	4.0212

DRG	Principal Dx/Procedure	Codes	Tips
148	Intestinal resection Colostomy Proctopexy *AND* CC condition	45.8 46.10 48.76 See CC section.	◆ Key terms: Delorme repair, puborectalis sling operation ■ Post-op ileus: Ileus can be an expected event after abdominal surgery and is not a complication unless it is prolonged (usually over six days). It may mean status-post the procedure—not that this is necessarily a complication. Query the physician. ■ Post-op ileus-key terms: adynamic, inhibitory, neurogenic, paralytic
149	Intestinal resection Colostomy Proctopexy	45.8 46.10 48.76	◆ Key terms: Delorme repair, puborectalis sling operation
154	*AND* CC condition	See CC section.	■ Post-op ileus: Ileus can be an expected event after abdominal surgery and is not a complication unless it is prolonged (usually over six days). It may mean status-post the procedure—not that this is necessarily a complication. Query the physician. ■ Post-op ileus-key terms: adynamic, inhibitory, neurogenic, paralytic

DRG 156 Stomach, Esophageal & Duodenal Procedures, Age 0-17
RW 0.8489

Potential DRGs
148	Major Small & Large Bowel Procedures with CC	RW	3.4025
149	Major Small & Large Bowel Procedures without CC	RW	1.4590
154	Stomach, Esophageal & Duodenal Procedures, Age > 17 with CC	RW	4.0212
155	Stomach, Esophageal & Duodenal Procedures, Age > 17 without CC	RW	1.3043

DRG	Principal Dx/Procedure	Codes	Tips
148	Colostomy Intestinal resection Proctopexy NEC	46.10 45.8 48.76	◆ Key terms: Delorme repair, puborectalis sling operation

(continued)   DRG 156

DRG	Principal Dx/Procedure	Codes	Tips
	AND CC condition	See CC section.	■ Post-op ileus: Ileus can be an expected event after abdominal surgery and is not a complication unless it is prolonged (usually over six days). It may mean status-post the procedure—not that this is necessarily a complication. Query the physician. ■ Post-op ileus-key terms: adynamic, inhibitory, neurogenic, paralytic
149	Intestinal resection Colostomy Proctopexy NEC	45.8 46.10 48.76	◆ Key terms: Delorme repair, puborectalis sling operation
154	Patient's age > 17 *AND* CC condition	See CC section.	■ Post-op ileus: Ileus can be an expected event after abdominal surgery and is not a complication unless it is prolonged (usually over six days). It may mean status-post the procedure—not that this is necessarily a complication. Query the physician. ■ Post-op ileus-key terms: adynamic, inhibitory, neurogenic, paralytic
155	Patient's age >17		

Anal & Stomal Procedures with CC   RW 1.3152   DRG 157

Potential DRGs

148	Major Small & Large Bowel Procedures with CC	RW 3.4025
150	**Peritoneal Adhesiolysis** with CC	RW 2.8711

DRG	Principal Dx/Procedure	Codes	Tips
148	Small or large bowel resection Colostomy *AND* CC condition	*45.6, *45.7 *46.10 See CC section.	■ Post-op ileus: Ileus can be an expected event after abdominal surgery and is not a complication unless it is prolonged (usually over six days). It may mean status-post the procedure—not that this is necessarily a complication. Query the physician. ■ Post-op ileus-key terms: adynamic, inhibitory, neurogenic, paralytic
150	Lysis of peritoneal adhesions *AND* CC condition	*54.5 See CC section.	● Adhesiolysis must be determined by physician as significant. ■ Post-op ileus: Ileus can be an expected event after abdominal surgery and is not a complication unless it is prolonged (usually over six days). It may mean status-post the procedure—not that this is necessarily a complication. Query the physician. ■ Post-op ileus-key terms: adynamic, inhibitory, neurogenic, paralytic

---

■ Coding Tip   ● Documentation Tip   ◆ Encoder Tip   ▽ Targeted DRG

Digestive System, MDC 6

DRG 158   Anal & Stomal Procedures without CC   RW 0.6517

Potential DRGs

150	Peritoneal Adhesiolysis **with CC**	RW	2.8711
151	**Peritoneal Adhesiolysis** without CC	RW	1.3061
157	Anal & Stomal Procedures **with CC**	RW	1.3152

DRG	Principal Dx/Procedure	Codes	Tips
150	Lysis of peritoneal adhesions *AND* CC condition	*54.5 See CC section.	● Adhesiolysis must be determined by physician as significant. ■ Post-op ileus: Ileus can be an expected event after abdominal surgery and is not a complication unless it is prolonged (usually over six days). It may mean status-post the procedure—not that this is necessarily a complication. Query the physician. ■ Post-op ileus-key terms: adynamic, inhibitory, neurogenic, paralytic
151	Lysis of peritoneal adhesions	*54.5	● Adhesiolysis must be determined by physician as significant.
157	CC condition	See CC section.	■ Post-op ileus: Ileus can be an expected event after abdominal surgery and is not a complication unless it is prolonged (usually over six days). It may mean status-post the procedure—not that this is necessarily a complication. Query the physician. ■ Post-op ileus-key terms: adynamic, inhibitory, neurogenic, paralytic

DRG 159   Hernia Procedures Except Inguinal &   RW 1.3744
            Femoral, Age > 17 with CC

Potential DRGs

150	**Peritoneal Adhesiolysis** with CC	RW	2.8711

DRG	Principal Dx/Procedure	Codes	Tips
150	Lysis of peritoneal adhesions *AND* CC condition	*54.5 See CC section.	● Adhesiolysis must be determined by physician as significant. Adhesiolysis must be documented as major focus of attention to warrant use of code. ■ Post-op ileus: Ileus can be an expected event after abdominal surgery and is not a complication unless it is prolonged (usually over six days). It may mean status-post the procedure—not that this is necessarily a complication. Query the physician. ■ Post-op ileus-key terms: adynamic, inhibitory, neurogenic, paralytic

---

■ Coding Tip   ● Documentation Tip   ◆ Encoder Tip   ᵛᵉᵍ Targeted DRG

Hernia Procedures Except Inguinal & Femoral, Age > 17 without CC

RW 0.8219 **DRG 160**

Potential DRGs

150	Peritoneal Adhesiolysis with CC	RW	2.8711
151	Peritoneal Adhesiolysis without CC	RW	1.3061
159	Hernia Procedures Except Inguinal & Femoral, Age > 17 **with CC**	RW	1.3744
161	**Inguinal & Femoral Hernia Procedures**, Age > 17 **with CC**	RW	1.1676

DRG	Principal Dx/Procedure	Codes	Tips
150	Lysis of peritoneal adhesions *AND* CC condition	*54.5 See CC section.	● Adhesiolysis must be determined by physician as significant. ■ Post-op ileus: Ileus can be an expected event after abdominal surgery and is not a complication unless it is prolonged (usually over six days). It may mean status-post the procedure—not that this is necessarily a complication. Query the physician. ■ Post-op ileus-key terms: adynamic, inhibitory, neurogenic, paralytic
151	Lysis of peritoneal adhesions	*54.5	● Adhesiolysis must be determined by physician as significant.
159	CC condition	See CC section.	■ Post-op ileus: Ileus can be an expected event after abdominal surgery and is not a complication unless it is prolonged (usually over six days). It may mean status-post the procedure—not that this is necessarily a complication. Query the physician. ■ Post-op ileus-key terms: adynamic, inhibitory, neurogenic, paralytic
161	Repair of inguinal or femoral hernia *AND* CC condition	*53.0–53.3 See CC section.	■ Post-op ileus: Ileus can be an expected event after abdominal surgery and is not a complication unless it is prolonged (usually over six days). It may mean status-post the procedure—not that this is necessarily a complication. Query the physician. ■ Post-op ileus-key terms: adynamic, inhibitory, neurogenic, paralytic

Inguinal & Femoral Hernia Procedures, Age > 17 with CC

RW 1.1676 **DRG 161**

Potential DRGs

150	**Peritoneal Adhesiolysis** with CC	RW	2.8711

DRG	Principal Dx/Procedure	Codes	Tips
150	Lysis of peritoneal adhesions *AND* CC condition	*54.5 See CC section.	● Adhesiolysis must be determined by physician as significant. ■ Post-op ileus: Ileus can be an expected event after abdominal surgery and is not a complication unless it is prolonged (usually over six days). It may mean status-post the procedure—not that this is necessarily a complication. Query the physician. ■ Post-op ileus-key terms: adynamic, inhibitory, neurogenic, paralytic

■ Coding Tip   ● Documentation Tip   ◆ Encoder Tip   ▽ Targeted DRG

Digestive System, MDC 6

DRG 162 Inguinal & Femoral Hernia Procedures, Age > 17 without CC

RW 0.6446

Potential DRGs

150	Peritoneal Adhesiolysis with CC	RW 2.8711
151	Peritoneal Adhesiolysis without CC	RW 1.3061
161	Inguinal & Femoral Hernia Procedures, Age > 17 **with CC**	RW 1.1676
163	Hernia Procedures, **Age 0–17**	RW 0.6965

DRG	Principal Dx/Procedure	Codes	Tips
150	Lysis of peritoneal adhesions *AND* CC condition	*54.5 See CC section.	● Adhesiolysis must be determined by physician as significant. Adhesiolysis must be documented as major focus of attention to warrant use of code. ■ Post-op ileus: Ileus can be an expected event after abdominal surgery and is not a complication unless it is prolonged (usually over six days). It may mean status-post the procedure—not that this is necessarily a complication. Query the physician. ■ Post-op ileus-key terms: adynamic, inhibitory, neurogenic, paralytic
151	Lysis of peritoneal adhesions	*54.5	
161	CC condition	See CC section.	■ Post-op ileus: Ileus can be an expected event after abdominal surgery and is not a complication unless it is prolonged (usually over six days). It may mean status-post the procedure—not that this is necessarily a complication. Query the physician. ■ Post-op ileus-key terms: adynamic, inhibitory, neurogenic, paralytic
163	Patient's age 0–17		

DRG 163 Hernia Procedures, Age 0–17

RW 0.6965

Potential DRGs

150	Peritoneal Adhesiolysis with CC	RW 2.8711
151	Peritoneal Adhesiolysis without CC	RW 1.3061
159	Hernia Procedures Except Inguinal & Femoral, **Age > 17 with CC**	RW 1.3744
161	Inguinal & Femoral Hernia Procedures, Age > 17 **with CC**	RW 1.1676

DRG	Principal Dx/Procedure	Codes	Tips
150	Lysis of peritoneal adhesions *AND* CC condition	*54.5 See CC section.	● Adhesiolysis must be determined by physician as significant. ■ Post-op ileus: Ileus can be an expected event after abdominal surgery and is not a complication unless it is prolonged (usually over six days). It may mean status-post the procedure—not that this is necessarily a complication. Query the physician. ■ Post-op ileus-key terms: adynamic, inhibitory, neurogenic, paralytic
151	Lysis of peritoneal adhesions	*54.5	● Adhesiolysis must be determined by physician as significant.
159	Patient's age > 17		

■ Coding Tip　　● Documentation Tip　　◆ Encoder Tip　　🖑 Targeted DRG

(continued) **DRG 163**

DRG	Principal Dx/Procedure	Codes	Tips
161	Patient's age > 17 *AND* CC condition	See CC section.	■ Post-op ileus: Ileus can be an expected event after abdominal surgery and is not a complication unless it is prolonged (usually over six days). It may mean status-post the procedure—not that this is necessarily a complication. Query the physician. ■ Post-op ileus-key terms: adynamic, inhibitory, neurogenic, paralytic

Appendectomy with Complicated Principal Diagnosis with CC — RW 2.3306 **DRG 164**

Potential DRGs

150	Peritoneal Adhesiolysis with CC	RW 2.8711

DRG	Principal Dx/Procedure	Codes	Tips
150	Lysis of peritoneal adhesions *AND* CC condition	*54.5 See CC section.	● Adhesiolysis must be determined by physician as significant. ■ Post-op ileus: Ileus can be an expected event after abdominal surgery and is not a complication unless it is prolonged (usually over six days). It may mean status-post the procedure—not that this is necessarily a complication. Query the physician. ■ Post-op ileus-key terms: adynamic, inhibitory, neurogenic, paralytic

Appendectomy with Complicated Principal Diagnosis without CC — RW 1.2302 **DRG 165**

Potential DRGs

150	**Peritoneal Adhesiolysis with CC**	RW 2.8711
164	Appendectomy with Complicated Principal Diagnosis **with CC**	RW 2.3306

DRG	Principal Dx/Procedure	Codes	Tips
150	Lysis of peritoneal adhesions *AND* CC condition	*54.5 See CC section.	● Adhesiolysis must be determined by physician as significant. ■ Post-op ileus: Ileus can be an expected event after abdominal surgery and is not a complication unless it is prolonged (usually over six days). It may mean status-post the procedure—not that this is necessarily a complication. Query the physician. ■ Post-op ileus-key terms: adynamic, inhibitory, neurogenic, paralytic
164	CC condition	See CC section.	■ Post-op ileus: Ileus can be an expected event after abdominal surgery and is not a complication unless it is prolonged (usually over six days). It may mean status-post the procedure—not that this is necessarily a complication. Query the physician. ■ Post-op ileus-key terms: adynamic, inhibitory, neurogenic, paralytic

---

■ Coding Tip   ● Documentation Tip   ◆ Encoder Tip   ⱽᴱᴸ Targeted DRG

Digestive System, MDC 6

DRG 166 Appendectomy without Complicated Principal Diagnosis with CC RW 1.4317

Potential DRGs

150	Peritoneal Adhesiolysis with CC	RW	2.8711
164	Appendectomy with Complicated Principal Diagnosis with CC	RW	2.3306

DRG	Principal Dx/Procedure	Codes	Tips
150	Lysis of peritoneal adhesions *AND* CC condition	*54.5 See CC section.	● Adhesiolysis must be determined by physician as significant. ■ Post-op ileus: Ileus can be an expected event after abdominal surgery and is not a complication unless it is prolonged (usually over six days). It may mean status-post the procedure—not that this is necessarily a complication. Query the physician. ■ Post-op ileus-key terms: adynamic, inhibitory, neurogenic, paralytic
164	Malignant neoplasm appendix Acute appendicitis with peritonitis Abscess of appendix	153.5 540.0 540.1	◆ Key terms: fulminating, gangrenous, obstructive ■ Ruptured appendix with abscess

DRG 167 Appendectomy without Complicated Principal Diagnosis without CC RW 0.8889

Potential DRGs

150	Peritoneal Adhesiolysis with CC	RW	2.8711
151	Peritoneal Adhesiolysis without CC	RW	1.3061
164	Appendectomy with Complicated Principal Diagnosis with CC	RW	2.3306
165	Appendectomy with Complicated Principal Diagnosis without CC	RW	1.2302
166	Appendectomy without Complicated Principal Diagnosis with CC	RW	1.4317

DRG	Principal Dx/Procedure	Codes	Tips
150	Lysis of peritoneal adhesions *AND* CC condition	*54.5 See CC section.	● Adhesiolysis must be determined by physician as significant. ■ Post-op ileus: Ileus can be an expected event after abdominal surgery and is not a complication unless it is prolonged (usually over six days). It may mean status-post the procedure—not that this is necessarily a complication. Query the physician. ■ Post-op ileus-key terms: adynamic, inhibitory, neurogenic, paralytic
151	Peritoneal adhesiolysisis without CC	*54.5	● Adhesiolysis must be determined by physician as significant
164	Malignant neoplasm appendix Acute appendicitis with peritonitis Abscess of appendix *AND* CC condition	153.5 540.0 540.1 See CC section.	◆ Key terms: fulminating, gangrenous, obstructive ■ Ruptured appendix with abscess ■ Post-op ileus: Ileus can be an expected event after abdominal surgery and is not a complication unless it is prolonged (usually over six days). It may mean status-post the procedure—not that this is necessarily a complication. Query the physician. ■ Post-op ileus-key terms: adynamic, inhibitory, neurogenic, paralytic

(continued) **DRG 167**

DRG	Principal Dx/Procedure	Codes	Tips
165	Malignant neoplasm appendix	153.5	
	Acute appendicitis with peritonitis	540.0	◆ Key terms: fulminating, gangrenous, obstructive
	Abscess of appendix	540.1	■ Ruptured appendix with abscess
166	Appendicitis NOS	540.9	◆ Key terms: fulminating, gangrenous,
	AND CC condition	See CC section.	obstructive ■ Post-op ileus: Ileus can be an expected event after abdominal surgery and is not a complication unless it is prolonged (usually over six days). It may mean status-post the procedure—not that this is necessarily a complication. Query the physician. ■ Post-op ileus-key terms: adynamic, inhibitory, neurogenic, paralytic

Other Digestive System Operating Room Procedures with CC **DRG 170**

No Potential DRGs

Other Digestive System O.R. Procedures without CC   RW 1.1912   **DRG 171**

Potential DRGs

150	Peritoneal Adhesiolysis with CC	RW	2.8711
151	Peritoneal Adhesiolysis without CC	RW	1.3061
170	Other Digestive System O.R. Procedures with CC	RW	2.8245

DRG	Principal Dx/Procedure	Codes	Tips
150	Lysis of peritoneal adhesions	*54.5	● Adhesiolysis must be determined by physician as significant.
	AND CC condition	See CC section.	■ Post-op ileus: ileus can be an expected event after abdominal surgery and is not a complication unless it is prolonged (usually over six days). It may mean status-post the procedure—not that this is necessarily a complication. Query the physician. ■ Post-op ileus-key terms: adynamic, inhibitory, neurogenic, paralytic
151	Lysis of peritoneal adhesions	*54.5	● Adhesiolysis must be determined by physician as significant.
170	CC condition	See CC section.	■ Post-op ileus: ileus can be an expected event after abdominal surgery and is not a complication unless it is prolonged (usually over six days). It may mean status-post the procedure—not that this is necessarily a complication. Query the physician. ■ Post-op ileus-key terms: adynamic, inhibitory, neurogenic, paralytic

---

■ Coding Tip	● Documentation Tip	◆ Encoder Tip	▽ Targeted DRG

Digestive System, MDC 6

DRG 172 Digestive Malignancy with CC RW 1.3670

Potential DRGs

150	**Peritoneal Adhesiolysis** with CC	RW	2.8711
154	**Stomach, Esophageal & Duodenal Procedures**, Age >17 with CC	RW	4.0212
170	Other Digestive System O.R. **Procedures** with CC	RW	2.8245

DRG	Principal Dx/Procedure	Codes	Tips
150	Lysis of peritoneal adhesions *AND* CC condition	*54.5 See CC section.	● Adhesiolysis must be determined by physician as significant. ■ Post-op ileus: ileus can be an expected event after abdominal surgery and is not a complication unless it is prolonged (usually over six days). It may mean status-post the procedure—not that this is necessarily a complication. Query the physician. ■ Post-op ileus-key terms: adynamic, inhibitory, neurogenic, paralytic
154	Gastrectomy *AND* CC condition	*43.9 See CC section.	■ Post-op ileus: ileus can be an expected event after abdominal surgery and is not a complication unless it is prolonged (usually over six days). It may mean status-post the procedure—not that this is necessarily a complication. Query the physician. ■ Post-op ileus-key terms: adynamic, inhibitory, neurogenic, paralytic
170	Lymph structure biopsy Open liver biopsy Other destruction of lesion of liver Exploratory lap Peritoneal biopsy	*40.1 50.12 50.29 54.11 54.23	■ Wedge biopsy ◆ Key terms: Bx: mesentery, omentum, peritoneal implant

DRG 173 Digestive Malignancy without CC RW 0.7528

Potential DRGs

150	**Peritoneal Adhesiolysis with CC**	RW	2.8711
154	**Stomach, Esophageal & Duodenal Procedures**, Age >17 with CC	RW	4.0212
170	Other Digestive System O.R. **Procedures with CC**	RW	2.8245
172	Digestive Malignancy **with CC**	RW	1.3670

DRG	Principal Dx/Procedure	Codes	Tips
150	Lysis of peritoneal adhesions *AND* CC condition	*54.5 See CC section.	● Adhesiolysis must be determined by physician as significant. ■ Post-op ileus: ileus can be an expected event after abdominal surgery and is not a complication unless it is prolonged (usually over six days). It may mean status-post the procedure—not that this is necessarily a complication. Query the physician. ■ Post-op ileus-key terms: adynamic, inhibitory, neurogenic, paralytic

(continued) **DRG 173**

DRG	Principal Dx/Procedure	Codes	Tips
154	Gastrectomy *AND* CC condition	*43.9 See CC section.	■ Post-op ileus: ileus can be an expected event after abdominal surgery and is not a complication unless it is prolonged (usually over six days). It may mean status-post the procedure—not that this is necessarily a complication. Query the physician. ■ Post-op ileus-key terms: adynamic, inhibitory, neurogenic, paralytic
170	Biopsy of lymphatic structure Open liver biopsy Other destruction of lesion of liver Exploratory laparotomy Biopsy of peritoneum *AND* CC condition	*40.1 50.12 50.29 54.11 54.23 See CC section.	■ Wedge biopsy ◆ Key terms: Bx: Mesentery, omentum, peritoneal implant ■ Post-op ileus: ileus can be an expected event after abdominal surgery and is not a complication unless it is prolonged (usually over six days). It may mean status-post the procedure—not that this is necessarily a complication. Query the physician. ■ Post-op ileus-key terms: adynamic, inhibitory, neurogenic, paralytic
172	CC condition	See CC section.	

Gastrointestinal Hemorrhage with CC   RW 1.0025 ▽**DRG 174**

Potential DRGs

DRG	Description		RW	Value
154	**Stomach, Esophageal & Duodenal Procedures**, Age > 17 with CC		RW	4.0212
172	**Digestive Malignancy** with CC		RW	1.3670
176	**Complicated Peptic Ulcer**		RW	1.0998

DRG	Principal Dx/Procedure	Codes	Tips
154	Stomach, esophageal, or duodenal procedure *AND* CC condition	42.10, 44.00, 45.31 See CC section.	■ Post-op ileus: ileus can be an expected event after abdominal surgery and is not a complication unless it is prolonged (usually over six days). It may mean status-post the procedure—not that this is necessarily a complication. Query the physician. ■ Post-op ileus-key terms: adynamic, inhibitory, neurogenic, paralytic
172	Digestive malignancy: esophagus stomach small intestine colon secondary malignancy of other digestive organs and spleen	*150 *151 *152 *153 197.8	
176	Duodenal ulcer with perforation or obstruction Gastric ulcer with perforation or obstruction Peptic ulcer with perforation or obstruction	531.31 532.31 533.71	

■ Coding Tip   ● Documentation Tip   ◆ Encoder Tip   ▽ Targeted DRG

Digestive System, MDC 6

DRG 175   Gastrointestinal Hemorrhage without CC   RW 0.5587

Potential DRGs

155	Stomach, Esophageal & Duodenal Procedures, Age > 17 without CC	RW	1.3043
172	Digestive Malignancy with CC	RW	1.3670
173	Digestive Malignancy without CC	RW	0.7528
174	Gastrointestinal Hemorrhage with CC	RW	1.0025
176	Complicated Peptic Ulcer	RW	1.0998

DRG	Principal Dx/Procedure	Codes	Tips
155	Stomach, esophageal, or duodenal procedure	42.01, 43.0, 45.31	

172	Digestive malignancy:
	   esophagus
	   stomach
	   small intestine
	   colon
	   secondary malignancy of other
	      digestive organs and spleen
	AND CC condition
		*150
		*151
		*152
		*153
		197.8
		
		See CC section.	

173	Digestive malignancy:
	   esophagus
	   stomach
	   small intestine
	   colon
	   secondary malignancy of other
	      digestive organs and spleen
	CC condition
		*150
		*151
		*152
		*153
		197.8, 174 2
		
		See CC section.	

174 ▽	Gastric, duodenal, or peptic ulcer: with hemorrhage	*531.0, *532.0, *533.0	◆ Manifestations: hematemesis, melena, occult, hematochezia ◆ Bleeding may be intermittent; code based on physician documenting bleeding ulcer even though endoscopy may not show active bleeding.
176	Duodenal ulcer with perforation or obstruction Gastric ulcer with perforation or obstruction Peptic ulcer with perforation or obstruction	531.31 532.31 533.71	

DRG 176   Complicated Peptic Ulcer   RW 1.0998

Potential DRGs

154	Stomach, Esophageal & Duodenal Procedures, Age > 17 with CC	RW	4.0212
155	Stomach, Esophageal & Duodenal Procedures, Age > 17 without CC	RW	1.3043

DRG	Principal Dx/Procedure	Codes	Tips
154	Esophageal, stomach, or duodenal procedure *AND* CC condition	*42.5, 43.5, 45.32 See CC section.	● Lesion destroyed through electrocoagulation ■ Post-op ileus: ileus can be an expected event after abdominal surgery and is not a complication unless it is prolonged (usually over six days). It may mean status-post the procedure—not that this is necessarily a complication. Query the physician. ■ Post-op ileus-key terms: adynamic, inhibitory, neurogenic, paralytic
155	Esophageal, stomach, or duodenal procedure	*42.5, 43.5, 45.32	● Lesion destroyed through electrocoagulation

Uncomplicated Peptic Ulcer with CC   RW 0.9259 **DRG 177**

Potential DRGs

154	Stomach, Esophageal & Duodenal Procedures, Age > 17 with CC	RW	4.0212
174	Gastrointestinal Hemorrhage with CC	RW	1.0025
176	Complicated Peptic Ulcer	RW	1.0998

DRG	Principal Dx/Procedure	Codes	Tips
154	Esophageal, stomach, or duodenal procedure *AND* CC condition	*42.5, 43.5, 45.32 See CC section.	● Lesion destroyed through electrocoagulation ■ Post-op ileus: ileus can be an expected event after abdominal surgery and is not a complication unless it is prolonged (usually over six days). It may mean status-post the procedure—not that this is necessarily a complication. Query the physician. ■ Post-op ileus-key terms: adynamic, inhibitory, neurogenic, paralytic
174 ▽	Gastric, duodenal, or peptic ulcer: with hemorrhage	*531.0, *532.0, *533.0	◆ Manifestations: hematemesis, melena, occult, hematochezia ◆ Bleeding may be intermittent; code based on physician documenting bleeding ulcer even though endoscopy may not show active bleeding.
176	Gastric, duodenal, or peptic ulcer: with perforation or obstruction	*531.2, *532.2, *533.2	

Uncomplicated Peptic Ulcer without CC   RW 0.6940 **DRG 178**

Potential DRGs

154	Stomach, Esophageal & Duodenal Procedures, Age > 17 with CC	RW	4.0212
155	Stomach, Esophageal & Duodenal Procedures, Age > 17 without CC	RW	1.3043
174	Gastrointestinal Hemorrhage with CC	RW	1.0025
176	Complicated Peptic Ulcer	RW	1.0998
177	Uncomplicated Peptic Ulcer with CC	RW	0.9259

DRG	Principal Dx/Procedure	Codes	Tips
154	Esophageal, stomach, or duodenal procedure *AND* CC condition	*42.5, 43.5, 45.32 See CC section.	● Lesion destroyed through electrocoagulation ■ Post-op ileus: ileus can be an expected event after abdominal surgery and is not a complication unless it is prolonged (usually over six days). It may mean status-post the procedure—not that this is necessarily a complication. Query the physician. ■ Post-op ileus-key terms: adynamic, inhibitory, neurogenic, paralytic
155	Esophageal, stomach, or duodenal procedure	42.5, 43.5, 45.32	● Lesion destroyed through electrocoagulation
174 ▽	Gastric, duodenal, or peptic ulcer: with hemorrhage *AND* CC condition	*531.0, *532.0, *533.0 See CC section.	◆ Manifestations: hematemesis, melena, occult, hematochezia ◆ Bleeding may be intermittent; code based on physician documenting bleeding ulcer even though endoscopy may not show active bleeding.
176	Gastric, duodenal, or peptic ulcer: with perforation or obstruction	*531.2, *532.2, *533.2	
177	CC condition	See CC section	

■ Coding Tip   ● Documentation Tip   ◆ Encoder Tip   ▽ Targeted DRG

Digestive System, MDC 6

DRG 179   Inflammatory Bowel Disease   RW 1.0885

Potential DRGs
150   Peritoneal Adhesiolysis with CC   RW   2.8711

DRG	Principal Dx/Procedure	Codes	Tips
150	Lysis of peritoneal adhesions AND CC condition	*54.5 See CC section.	■ Post-op ileus: ileus can be an expected event after abdominal surgery and is not a complication unless it is prolonged (usually over six days). It may mean status-post the procedure—not that this is necessarily a complication. Query the physician. ◆ Post-op ileus-key terms: adynamic, inhibitory, neurogenic, paralytic

DRG 180▽   Gastrointestinal Obstruction with CC   RW 0.9642

Potential DRGs
188   Other Digestive System Diagnoses, Age > 17 with CC   RW   1.1088

DRG	Principal Dx/Procedure	Codes	Tips
188 ▽	Hernia AND CC condition	*550, *553 See CC section	

DRG 181   Gastrointestinal Obstruction without CC   RW 0.5376

Potential DRGs
180   Gastrointestinal Obstruction with CC   RW   0.9642
188   Other Digestive System Diagnoses, Age > 17 with CC   RW   1.1088

DRG	Principal Dx/Procedure	Codes	Tips
180	CC condition	See CC section.	
188	Hernia AND CC condition	*550, *553 See CC section.	

DRG 182▽   Esophagitis, Gastroenteritis &   RW 0.8223
Miscellaneous Digestive Disorders, Age > 17 with CC

Potential DRGs
174   **Gastrointestinal Hemorrhage** with CC   RW   1.0025
176   **Complicated Peptic Ulcer**   RW   1.0998
179   **Inflammatory Bowel Disease**   RW   1.0885
180   **Gastrointestinal Obstruction** with CC   RW   0.9642
188   **Other Digestive System Diagnoses**, Age > 17 with CC   RW   1.1088
296   **Nutritional & Miscellaneous Metabolic Disorders**, Age > 17 with CC   RW   0.8639

DRG	Principal Dx/Procedure	Codes	Tips
174 ▽	Erosive gastritis with hemorrhage	535.41	◆ Manifestations: hematemesis, melena, occult, hematochezia ◆ Bleeding may be intermittent; code based on physician documenting bleeding ulcer even though endoscopy may not show active bleeding.
176	Gastric, duodenal, or peptic ulcer: with perforation or obstruction	*531.2, *532.2, *533.2	
179	Regional enteritis	*555	◆ Key terms: Crohns disease, granulomatous enteritis

---

(continued) ▽DRG 182

DRG	Principal Dx/Procedure	Codes	Tips
180	Abdominal pain due to small bowel obstruction	*560	
188 ▽	Radiation gastroenteritis Toxic gastroenteritis	558.1 558.2	
296 ▽	Dehydration	276.5	■ IV hydration should be ordered for correct coding. If patient admitted with gastroenteritis and dehydration, w/IV hydration ordered which necessitated the admission, 276.5 is the principal Dx.

Esophagitis, Gastroenteritis & Miscellaneous Digestive Disorders, Age > 17 without CC

RW 0.5759 **DRG 183**

Potential DRGs

174	Gastrointestinal Hemorrhage with CC	RW	1.0025
176	Complicated Peptic Ulcer	RW	1.0998
179	Inflammatory Bowel Disease	RW	1.0885
180	Gastrointestinal Obstruction with CC	RW	0.9642
182	Esophagitis, Gastroenteritis & Miscellaneous Digestive Disorders, Age > 17 with CC	RW	0.8223
188	Other Digestive System Diagnoses, Age > 17 with CC	RW	1.1088
296	Nutritional & Miscellaneous Metabolic Disorders, Age > 17 with CC	RW	0.8639

DRG	Principal Dx/Procedure	Codes	Tips
174 ▽	Erosive gastritis with hemorrhage *AND* CC condition	535.41 See CC section.	◆ Manifestations: hematemesis, melena, occult, hematochezia ◆ Bleeding may be intermittent; code based on physician documenting bleeding ulcer even though endoscopy may not show active bleeding.
176	Gastric, duodenal, or peptic ulcer: with perforation or obstruction	*531.2, *532.2, *533.2	
179	Regional enteritis	*555	◆ Key terms: Crohns disease, granulomatous enteritis
180 ▽	Abdominal pain due to small bowel obstruction *AND* CC condition	*560 See CC section.	◆ Key terms: Paralytic ileus, volvulus, intessusception
182 ▽	CC condition	See CC section.	
188 ▽	Radiation gastroenteritis Toxic gastroenteritis *AND* CC condition	558.1, 558.2 See CC section.	
296 ▽	Dehydration *AND* CC condition	276.5 See CC section.	■ IV hydration should be ordered for correct coding. If patient admitted with gastroenteritis and dehydration, w/IV hydration ordered that necessitated the admission, 276.5 is the principal Dx.

■ Coding Tip   ● Documentation Tip   ◆ Encoder Tip   ▽ Targeted DRG

Digestive System, MDC 6

DRG 184 Esophagitis, Gastroenteritis & Miscellaneous Digestive Disorders, Age 0-17

RW 0.4813

Potential DRGs

174	Gastrointestinal Hemorrhage with CC	RW	1.0025
176	Complicated Peptic Ulcer	RW	1.0998
179	Inflammatory Bowel Disease	RW	1.0885
180	Gastrointestinal Obstruction with CC	RW	0.9642
182	Esophagitis, Gastroenteritis & Miscellaneous Digestive Disorders, **Age > 17** with CC	RW	0.7986
188	Other Digestive System Diagnoses, Age > 17 with CC	RW	1.1088
296	Nutritional & Miscellaneous Metabolic Disorders, Age > 17 with CC	RW	0.8639

DRG	Principal Dx/Procedure	Codes	Tips
174 ▽	Erosive gastritis with hemorrhage *AND* CC condition	535.41 See CC section.	◆ Manifestations: hematemesis, melena, occult, hematochezia ◆ Bleeding may be intermittent; code based on physician documenting bleeding ulcer even though endoscopy may not show active bleeding.
176	Gastric, duodenal, or peptic ulcer: with perforation or obstruction	*531.2, *532.2, *533.2	
179	Regional enteritis	*555	◆ Key terms: Crohns disease, granulomatous enteritis
180 ▽	Abdominal pain due to small bowel obstruction *AND* CC condition	*560 See CC section.	◆ Key terms: Paralytic ileus, volvulus, intessusception
182 ▽	Patient's age > 17 *AND* CC condition	See CC section.	
188 ▽	Radiation gastroenteritis Toxic gastroenteritis *AND* CC condition	558.1, 558.2 See CC section.	
296 ▽	Dehydration *AND* CC condition	276.5 See CC section.	■ IV hydration should be ordered for correct coding. If patient admitted with gastroenteritis and dehydration, w/IV hydration ordered that necessitated the admission, 276.5 is the principal Dx.

DRG 188▽ Other Digestive System Diagnoses, Age > 17 with CC

RW 1.1088

Potential DRGs

172	**Digestive Malignancy** with CC	RW	1.3670
484	**Craniotomy** for Multiple Significant Trauma	RW	5.4179
486	**Other O.R. Procedures for Multiple Significant Trauma**	RW	4.8793
487	Other Multiple Significant Trauma	RW	2.0057

DRG	Principal Dx/Procedure	Codes	Tips
172	Digestive malignancy: esophagus stomach small intestine colon secondary malignancy of other digestive organs and spleen	*150 *151 *152 *153 197.8	

■ Coding Tip ● Documentation Tip ◆ Encoder Tip ▽ Targeted DRG

©2003 Ingenix, Inc.

(continued) **DRG 188**

DRG	Principal Dx/Procedure	Codes	Tips
484	Craniotomy for multiple significant trauma		■ Craniotomy and principal diagnosis of trauma and at least two injuries (assigned either as principal or secondary) that are defined as significant trauma from different body site categories located under DRG 487
486	Other O.R. procedures for multiple significant traum		■ Principal diagnosis of trauma and at least two injuries (assigned either as principal or secondary) that are defined as significant trauma from different body site categories located under DRG 487 *AND* O.R. procedure other than craniotomy or limb reattachment, hip and femur procedures
487	Other multiple significant trauma		■ Principal diagnosis of trauma and at least two injuries (assigned either as principal or secondary) that are defined as significant trauma from different body site categories located under DRG 487

Other Digestive System Diagnoses, Age > 17 without CC

RW 0.5987 **DRG 189**

Potential DRGs

172	**Digestive Malignancy** with CC	RW	1.3670
188	Other Digestive System Diagnoses, Age > 17 **with CC**	RW	1.1088
190	Other Digestive System Diagnoses, **Age 0–17**	RW	0.8104
484	**Craniotomy** for Multiple Significant Trauma	RW	5.4179
486	**Other O.R. Procedures for Multiple Significant Trauma**	RW	4.8793
487	Other Multiple Significant Trauma	RW	2.0057

DRG	Principal Dx/Procedure	Codes	Tips
172	Digestive malignancy: esophagus stomach small intestine colon secondary malignancy of other digestive organs and spleen	*150 *151 *152 *153 197.8	
188 ▽	Hernia	*550, *553	
190	Patient's age 0–17		
484	Craniotomy for multiple significant trauma		■ Craniotomy and principal diagnosis of trauma and at least two injuries (assigned either as principal or secondary) that are defined as significant trauma from different body site categories located under DRG 487
486	Other O.R. procedures for multiple significant traum		■ Principal diagnosis of trauma and at least two injuries (assigned either as principal or secondary) that are defined as significant trauma from different body site categories located under DRG 487 *AND* O.R. procedure other than craniotomy or limb reattachment, hip, and femur procedures

■ Coding Tip   ● Documentation Tip   ◆ Encoder Tip   ▽ Targeted DRG

Digestive System, MDC 6

DRG 189 (continued)

DRG	Principal Dx/Procedure	Codes	Tips
487	Other multiple significant trauma		■ Principal diagnosis of trauma and at least two injuries (assigned either as principal or secondary) that are defined as significant trauma from different body site categories located under DRG 487

DRG 190 Other Digestive System Diagnoses, RW 0.8104
Age 0–17

Potential DRGs

172	**Digestive Malignancy** with CC	RW	1.3670
188	Other Digestive System Diagnoses, Age > 17 **with CC**	RW	1.1088
484	**Craniotomy** for Multiple Significant Trauma	RW	5.4179
486	**Other O.R. Procedures for Multiple Significant Trauma**	RW	4.8793
487	Other Multiple Significant Trauma	RW	2.0057

DRG	Principal Dx/Procedure	Codes	Tips
172	Digestive malignancy: esophagus stomach small intestine colon secondary malignancy of other digestive organs and spleen	*150 *151 *152 *153 197.8	
188 ⦿	Patient's age > 17 *AND* CC condition	See CC section.	
484	Craniotomy for multiple significant trauma		■ Craniotomy and principal diagnosis of trauma and at least two injuries (assigned either as principal or secondary) that are defined as significant trauma from different body site categories located under DRG 487
486	Other O.R. procedures for multiple significant traum		■ Principal diagnosis of trauma and at least two injuries (assigned either as principal or secondary) that are defined as significant trauma from different body site categories located under DRG 487 *AND* O.R. procedure other than craniotomy or limb reattachment, hip, and femur procedures
487	Other multiple significant trauma		■ Principal diagnosis of trauma and at least two injuries (assigned either as principal or secondary) that are defined as significant trauma from different body site categories located under DRG 487

■ Coding Tip   ● Documentation Tip   ◆ Encoder Tip   ⦿ Targeted DRG

Hepatobiliary System & Pancreas, MDC 7

Pancreas, Liver, & Shunt Procedures with CC   DRG 191
No Potential DRGs

Pancreas, Liver & Shunt Procedures without CC   RW 1.8025   DRG 192

Potential DRGs

191	Pancreas, Liver & Shunt Procedures with CC		RW 4.2787

DRG	Principal Dx/Procedure	Codes	Tips
191	CC condition	See CC section.	■ Post-op ileus

Biliary Tract Procedure Except Only Cholecystectomy with or without Common Duct Exploration with CC   DRG 193
No Potential DRGs

Biliary Tract Procedures without CC Except Only Cholecystectomy with or without CDE   RW 1.6030   DRG 194

Potential DRGs

193	Biliary Tract Procedures with CC Except Only Cholecystectomy with or without CDE	RW 3.4211

DRG	Principal Dx/Procedure	Codes	Tips
193	CC condition	See CC section.	■ Post-op ileus

Cholecystectomy with CDE with CC   RW 3.0613   DRG 195

Potential DRGs

193	Biliary Tract Procedures with CC Except Only Cholecystectomy with or without CDE	RW 3.4211

DRG	Principal Dx/Procedure	Codes	Tips
193	Another biliary tract procedure *AND* CC condition .	51.3 See CC section.	■ Anastomosis of gallbladder or bile duct ■ Post-op ileus

Cholecystectomy with CDE without CC   RW 1.6117   DRG 196

Potential DRGs

193	Biliary Tract Procedures with CC Except Only Cholecystectomy with or without CDE	RW 3.4211
195	Cholecystectomy with CDE with CC	RW 3.0613

DRG	Principal Dx/Procedure	Codes	Tips
193	Another biliary tract procedure *AND* CC condition	 See CC section.	■ Anastomosis of gallbladder or bile duct ■ Post-op ileus
195	CC condition	See CC section.	■ Post-op ileus

■ Coding Tip   ● Documentation Tip   ◆ Encoder Tip   � Targeted DRG

         243

DRG 197 Cholecystectomy Except by Laparoscope without CDE with CC   RW 2.5547

Potential DRGs

193	Biliary Tract Procedures with CC Except Only Cholecystectomy with or without CDE	RW 3.4211
195	Cholecystectomy **with CDE** with CC	RW 3.0613

DRG	Principal Dx/Procedure	Codes	Tips
193	Another biliary tract procedure	*51.3	■ Anastomosis of gallbladder or bileduct
195	Common bile duct exploration	51.51	■ Limited to exploration of common duct
	AND CC condition	See CC section.	■ Post-op ileus

DRG 198 Cholecystectomy Except by Laparoscope without CDE without CC   RW 1.1831

Potential DRGs

193	Biliary Tract Procedure with CC Except Only Cholecystectomy with or without CDE	RW 3.4211
194	Biliary Tract Procedure without CC Except Only Cholecystectomy with or without CDE	RW 1.6030
195	Cholecystectomy **with CDE with CC**	RW 3.0613
196	Cholecystectomy **with CDE** without CC	RW 1.6117
197	Cholecystectomy Except by Laparoscope without CDE **with CC**	RW 2.5547
493	**Laparoscopic** Cholecystectomy without CDE **with CC**	RW 1.8302

DRG	Principal Dx/Procedure	Codes	Tips
193	Another biliary tract procedure	*51.3	■ Anastomosis of gallbladder or bile duct
	CC condition	See CC section.	■ Post-op ileus
194	Another biliary tract procedure	*51.3	■ Anastomosis of gallbladder or bile duct
195	Common bile duct exploration	51.51	■ Limited to exploration of common duct
	AND CC condition	See CC section.	■ Post-op ileus
196	Common bile duct exploration	51.51	■ Limited to exploration of common duct
197	CC condition	See CC section.	■ Post-op ileus
493	Laparoscopic cholecystectomy *AND* CC condition	51.23 See CC section.	● By laser ■ Post-op ileus

DRG 199 Hepatobiliary Diagnostic Procedure For Malignancy   RW 2.3953

Potential DRGs

200	Hepatobiliary Diagnostic Procedure for **Nonmalignancy**	RW 3.0415

DRG	Principal Dx/Procedure	Codes	Tips
200	Nonmalignancy *AND* Laparoscopy	572.3 54.21	◆ Portal hypertension

DRG 200 Hepatobiliary Diagnostic Procedure for Nonmalignancy

No Potential DRGs

■ Coding Tip   ● Documentation Tip   ◆ Encoder Tip   ▽ Targeted DRG

Other Hepatobiliary or Pancreas O.R. Procedures　**DRG 201**
Non Potential DRGs

Cirrhosis & Alcoholic Hepatitis　RW 1.3120　**DRG 202**

Potential DRGs

191	Pancreas, Liver & **Shunt Procedures** with CC	RW	4.2787
200	Hepatobiliary Diagnostic Procedure for **Nonmalignancy**	RW	3.0415
201	Other Hepatobiliary or Pancreas O.R. Procedures	RW	3.6841

DRG	Principal Dx/Procedure	Codes	Tips
191	Intra-abdominal shunt Creation of a peritoneovascular shunt *AND* CC condition	39.1 54.94 See CC section.	◆ Mesocaval, portocaval, TIPS (peritoneovenous)
200	Non malignancy Laparoscopy	572.3 54.21	◆ Portal hypertension
201	Ligation of esophageal varix	42.91	

Malignancy of Hepatobiliary System or Pancreas　RW 1.3482　**DRG 203**

Potential DRGs

199	Hepatobiliary **Diagnostic Procedure** for Malignancy	RW	2.3953

DRG	Principal Dx/Procedure	Codes	Tips
199	Hepatobiliary diagnostic procedure	50.12	

Disorders of Pancreas Except Malignancy　RW 1.1675　**DRG 204**

Potential DRGs

203	**Malignancy** of Hepatobiliary System or Pancreas	RW	1.3482
484	**Craniotomy for Multiple Significant Trauma**	RW	5.4179
486	**Other O.R. Procedures for Multiple Significant Trauma**	RW	4.8793
487	**Other Multiple Significant Trauma**	RW	2.0057

DRG	Principal Dx/Procedure	Codes	Tips
203	Malignancy: Neck of pancreas	157.8	
484	Craniotomy for multiple significant trauma		■ Craniotomy and principal diagnosis of trauma and at least two injuries (assigned either as principal or secondary) that are defined as significant trauma from different body site categories located under DRG 487
486	Other O.R. procedures for multiple significant trauma		■ Principal diagnosis of trauma and at least two injuries (assigned either as principal or secondary) that are defined as significant trauma from different body site categories located under DRG 487 *AND* O.R. procedure other than craniotomy or limb reattachment, hip and femur procedures
487	Other multiple significant trauma		■ Principal diagnosis of trauma and at least two injuries (assigned either as principal or secondary) that are defined as significant trauma from different body site categories located under DRG 487

■ Coding Tip　　● Documentation Tip　　◆ Encoder Tip　　▽ Targeted DRG

Hepatobiliary System & Pancreas, MDC 7

DRG 205 Disorders of Liver Except Malignancy, Cirrhosis, & Alcoholic Hepatitis with CC

RW 1.2095

Potential DRGs

202	Cirrhosis and Alcoholic Hepatitis	RW	1.3120
203	Malignancy of Hepatobiliary System or Pancreas	RW	1.3482
484	Craniotomy for Multiple Significant Trauma	RW	5.4179
486	Other O.R. Procedures for Multiple Significant Trauma	RW	4.8793
487	Other Multiple Significant Trauma	RW	2.0057

DRG	Principal Dx/Procedure	Codes	Tips
202	Alcoholic hepatitis Cirrhosis	571.1 571.5	■ Cryptogenic, macro- and micronodular, posthepatic, postnecrotic, portal cirrhosis
203	Malignancy: Neck of pancreas	157.8	
484	Craniotomy for multiple significant trauma		■ Craniotomy and principal diagnosis of trauma and at least two injuries (assigned either as principal or secondary) that are defined as significant trauma from different body site categories located under DRG 487
486	Other O.R. procedures for multiple significant trauma		■ Principal diagnosis of trauma and at least two injuries (assigned either as principal or secondary) that are defined as significant trauma from different body site categories located under DRG 487 *AND* O.R. procedure other than craniotomy or limb reattachment, hip and femur procedures
487	Other multiple significant trauma		■ Principal diagnosis of trauma and at least two injuries (assigned either as principal or secondary) that are defined as significant trauma from different body site categories located under DRG 487

DRG 206 Disorders of Liver Except Malignancy, Cirrhosis, & Alcoholic Hepatitis without CC

RW 0.7071

Potential DRGs

202	Cirrhosis & Alcoholic Hepatitis	RW	1.3120
203	Malignancy of Hepatobiliary System or Pancreas	RW	1.3482
205	Disorders of Liver Except Malignancy, Cirrhosis, & Alcoholic Hepatitis with CC	RW	1.2095
207	Disorders of the Biliary Tract with CC	RW	1.1539
484	Craniotomy for Multiple Significant Trauma	RW	5.4179
486	Other O.R. Procedures for Multiple Significant Trauma	RW	4.8793
487	Other Multiple Significant Trauma	RW	2.0057

DRG	Principal Dx/Procedure	Codes	Tips
202	Alcoholic hepatitis Cirrhosis	571.1 571.5	
203	Malignancy: Neck of pancreas	157.8	
205	CC condition	See CC section.	

(continued) **DRG 206**

DRG	Principal Dx/Procedure	Codes	Tips
207	Disorder of biliary tract, bile ducts *AND* CC condition	576.9 See CC section.	
484	Craniotomy for multiple significant trauma		■ Craniotomy and principal diagnosis of trauma and at least two injuries (assigned either as principal or secondary) that are defined as significant trauma from different body site categories located under DRG 487
486	Other O.R. procedures for multiple significant trauma		■ Principal diagnosis of trauma and at least two injuries (assigned either as principal or secondary) that are defined as significant trauma from different body site categories located under DRG 487 *AND* O.R. procedure other than craniotomy or limb reattachment, hip and femur procedures
487	Other multiple significant trauma		■ Principal diagnosis of trauma and at least two injuries (assigned either as principal or secondary) that are defined as significant trauma from different body site categories located under DRG 487

Disorders of the Biliary Tract with CC   RW 1.1539   **DRG 207**

Potential DRGs
484	Craniotomy for Multiple Significant Trauma	RW 5.4179
486	Other O.R. Procedures for Multiple Significant Trauma	RW 4.8793
487	Other Multiple Significant Trauma	RW 2.0057

DRG	Principal Dx/Procedure	Codes	Tips
484	Craniotomy for multiple significant trauma		■ Craniotomy and principal diagnosis of trauma and at least two injuries (assigned either as principal or secondary) that are defined as significant trauma from different body site categories located under DRG 487
486	Other O.R. procedures for multiple significant trauma		■ Principal diagnosis of trauma and at least two injuries (assigned either as principal or secondary) that are defined as significant trauma from different body site categories located under DRG 487 *AND* O.R. procedure other than craniotomy or limb reattachment, hip and femur procedures
487	Other multiple significant trauma		■ Principal diagnosis of trauma and at least two injuries (assigned either as principal or secondary) that are defined as significant trauma from different body site categories located under DRG 487

■ Coding Tip   ● Documentation Tip   ◆ Encoder Tip   ▼ Targeted DRG

Hepatobiliary System & Pancreas, MDC 7

DRG 208   Disorders of the Biliary Tract without CC   RW 0.6601

Potential DRGs

207	Disorders of the Biliary Tract **with CC**	RW	1.1539
484	**Craniotomy for Multiple Significant Trauma**	RW	5.4179
486	**Other O.R. Procedures for Multiple Significant Trauma**	RW	4.8793
487	**Other Multiple Significant Trauma**	RW	2.0057

DRG	Principal Dx/Procedure	Codes	Tips
207	CC condition	See CC section.	
484	Craniotomy for multiple significant trauma		■ Craniotomy and principal diagnosis of trauma and at least two injuries (assigned either as principal or secondary) that are defined as significant trauma from different body site categories located under DRG 487
486	Other O.R. procedures for multiple significant trauma		■ Principal diagnosis of trauma and at least two injuries (assigned either as principal or secondary) that are defined as significant trauma from different body site categories located under DRG 487 *AND* O.R. procedure other than craniotomy or limb reattachment, hip and femur procedures
487	Other multiple significant trauma		■ Principal diagnosis of trauma and at least two injuries (assigned either as principal or secondary) that are defined as significant trauma from different body site categories located under DRG 487

DRG 493   Laparoscopic Cholecystectomy without CDE with CC   RW 1.8302

Potential DRGs

195	Cholecystectomy **with CDE** with CC	RW	3.0613
197	Cholecystectomy Except by Laparoscope without CDE with CC	RW	2.5547

DRG	Principal Dx/Procedure	Codes	Tips
195	Common bile duct exploration	51.51	■ Limited to exploration of common duct
	AND CC condition	See CC section.	■ Post-op ileus
197	Cholecystectomy (open) *AND* CC condition	51.22 See CC section.	■ Post-op ileus

---

■ Coding Tip	● Documentation Tip	◆ Encoder Tip	▽ Targeted DRG

Laparoscopic Cholecystectomy without CDE without CC
RW 1.0034 **DRG 494**

Potential DRGs

195	Cholecystectomy **with CDE with CC**	RW	3.0613
196	Cholecystectomy **with CDE** without CC	RW	1.6117
197	Cholecystectomy Except by Laparoscope without CDE **with CC**	RW	2.5547
198	Cholecystectomy Except by Laparoscope without CDE without CC	RW	1.1831
493	Laparoscopic Cholecystectomy without CDE **with CC**	RW	1.8302

DRG	Principal Dx/Procedure	Codes	Tips
195	Common bile duct exploration	51.51	■ Limited to exploration of common duct; do not use for incision of cystic duct
	AND CC condition	See CC section.	■ Post-op ileus
196	Common bile duct exploration	51.51	■ Limited to exploration of common duct
197	Cholecystectomy (open) *AND* CC condition	51.22 See CC section.	■ Post-op ileus
198	Cholecystectomy (open)	51.22	
493	CC condition	See CC section.	■ Post-op ileus

Musculoskeletal System, MDC 8

Major Joint & Limb Reattachment Procedures of Lower Extremity
RW 2.0327 **DRG 209**

Potential DRGs

471	**Bilateral or Multiple** Major Joint Procedures of Lower Extremity	RW	3.0576
485	Limb Reattachment, **Hip & Femur** Procedures for **Multiple Significant Trauma**	RW	3.2121

DRG	Principal Dx/Procedure	Codes	Tips
471	Two or more major joint procedures of lower extremity (bilateral if applicable)		
485	Limb reattachment, hip and femur procedures for multiple significant trauma		■ Principal diagnosis of trauma and at least two injuries (assigned either as principal or secondary) that are defined as significant trauma from different body site categories located under DRG 487 *AND* limb reattachment, hip and femur O.R. procedures

*Ensure accurate DRG assignment.
Listed below are the procedure codes found in DRG 209:
  81.51 Total hip replacement
  81.52 Partial hip replacement
  81.53 Revision of hip replacement
  81.54 Total knee replacement
  81.55 Revision of knee replacement
  81.56 Total ankle replacement
  84.26 Foot reattachment
  84.27 Lower leg/ankle reattachment
  84.28 Thigh reattachment

■ Coding Tip   ● Documentation Tip   ◆ Encoder Tip   ▽ Targeted DRG

Musculoskeletal System, MDC 8

DRG 210 Hip & Femur Procedures Except Major Joint, Age > 17 with CC

RW 1.8477

Potential DRGs

485 Limb Reattachment, Hip & Femur Procedures for **Multiple Significant Trauma** RW 3.2121

DRG	Principal Dx/Procedure	Codes	Tips
485	Limb reattachment, hip and femur procedures for multiple significant trauma		■ Principal diagnosis of trauma and at least two injuries (assigned either as principal or secondary) that are defined as significant trauma from different body site categories located under DRG 487 *AND* limb reattachment, hip and femur O.R. procedures

DRG 211 Hip & Femur Procedures Except Major Joint, Age > 17 without CC

RW 1.2544

Potential DRGs

210 Hip & Femur Procedures Except Major Joint, Age > 17 **with CC** RW 1.8477
485 Limb Reattachment, Hip & Femur Procedures for **Multiple Significant Trauma** RW 3.2121

DRG	Principal Dx/Procedure	Codes	Tips
210	Femoral sequestrectomy *AND* CC condition	77.05 See CC section.	
485	Limb reattachment, hip and femur procedures for multiple significant trauma		■ Principal diagnosis of trauma and at least two injuries (assigned either as principal or secondary) that are defined as significant trauma from different body site categories located under DRG 487 *AND* limb reattachment, hip and femur O.R. procedures

DRG 212 Hip & Femur Procedures Except Major Joint, Age 0–17

RW 1.4152

Potential DRGs

210 Hip & Femur Procedures Except Major Joint, **Age > 17 with CC** RW 1.8477
211 Hip & Femur Procedures Except Major Joint, **Age > 17** without CC RW 1.2544
485 Limb Reattachment, Hip & Femur Procedures for **Multiple Significant Trauma** RW 3.2121

DRG	Principal Dx/Procedure	Codes	Tips
210	Femoral sequestrectomy *AND* CC condition	77.05 See CC section.	
211	Patient's age > 17		
485	Limb reattachment, hip and femur procedures for multiple significant trauma		■ Principal diagnosis of trauma and at least two injuries (assigned either as principal or secondary) that are defined as significant trauma from different body site categories located under DRG 487 *AND* limb reattachment, hip and femur O.R. procedures

---

■ Coding Tip   ● Documentation Tip   ◆ Encoder Tip   ▽ Targeted DRG

Amputation for Musculoskeletal System & Connective Tissue Disorders
RW 1.8904 **DRG 213**

Potential DRGs

486   Other O.R. Procedures for **Multiple Significant Trauma**   RW   4.8793

DRG	Principal Dx/Procedure	Codes	Tips
486	Other O.R. procedures for multiple significant trauma		■ Principal diagnosis of trauma and at least two injuries (assigned either as principal or secondary) that are defined as significant trauma from different body site categories located under DRG 487 *AND* O.R. procedure other than craniotomy or limb reattachment, hip and femur procedures

Invalid DRG
DRG 214

No Potential DRGs

Invalid DRG
DRG 215

No Potential DRGs

Biopsies of Musculoskeletal System and Connective Tissue
DRG 216

No Potential DRGs

Wound Debridement and Skin Graft Except Hand, for Musculoskeletal and Connective Tissue Disorders
DRG 217

No Potential DRGs

Lower Extremity & Humerus Procedures Except Hip, Foot, Femur, Age > 17 with CC
RW 1.5750 **DRG 218**

Potential DRGs

486   Other O.R. Procedures for **Multiple Significant Trauma**   RW   4.8793

DRG	Principal Dx/Procedure	Codes	Tips
486	Other O.R. procedures for multiple significant trauma		■ Principal diagnosis of trauma and at least two injuries (assigned either as principal or secondary) that are defined as significant trauma from different body site categories located under DRG 487 *AND* O.R. procedure other than craniotomy or limb reattachment, hip and femur procedures

Musculoskeletal System, MDC 8

DRG 219 Lower Extremity & Humerus Procedures RW 1.0258
Except Hip, Foot, Femur, Age > 17 without CC

Potential DRGs

218	Lower Extremity & Humerus Procedures Except Hip, Foot, Femur, Age > 17 **with CC**	RW	1.5750
486	Other O.R. Procedures for **Multiple Significant Trauma**	RW	4.8793

DRG	Principal Dx/Procedure	Codes	Tips
218	Sequestrectomy, humerus *AND* CC condition	77.02 See CC section.	
486	Other O.R. procedures for multiple significant trauma		■ Principal diagnosis of trauma and at least two injuries (assigned either as principal or secondary) that are defined as significant trauma from different body site categories located under DRG 487 *AND* O.R. procedure other than craniotomy or limb reattachment, hip and femur procedures

DRG 220 Lower Extremity & Humerus Procedures RW 0.5881
Except Hip, Foot, Femur, Age 0–17

Potential DRGs

218	Lower Extremity & Humerus Procedures Except Hip, Foot, Femur, Age > 17 **with CC**	RW	1.5750
219	Lower Extremity & Humerous Procedures Except Hip, Foot, Femur, **Age > 17** without CC	RW	1.0258
486	Other O.R. Procedures for **Multiple Significant Trauma**	RW	4.8793

DRG	Principal Dx/Procedure	Codes	Tips
218	Sequestrectomy, humerus *AND* Age > 17 *AND* CC condition	77.02 See CC section.	
219	Sequestrectomy, humerus *AND* Age > 17	77.02	
486	Other O.R. procedures for multiple significant trauma		■ Principal diagnosis of trauma and at least two injuries (assigned either as principal or secondary) that are defined as significant trauma from different body site categories located under DRG 487 *AND* O.R. procedure other than craniotomy or limb reattachment, hip and femur procedures

DRG 221 Invalid DRG

No Potential DRGs

DRG 222 Invalid DRG

No Potential DRGs

■ Coding Tip   ● Documentation Tip   ◆ Encoder Tip   ▽ Targeted DRG

Major Shoulder/Elbow Procedures, or Other Upper Extremity Procedures with CC

RW 1.0573 **DRG 223**

Potential DRGs

486	Other O.R. Procedures for **Multiple Significant Trauma**	RW	4.8793
491	Major Joint & Limb Reattachment Procedures of the Upper Extremity	RW	1.7139

DRG	Principal Dx/Procedure	Codes	Tips
486	Other O.R. procedures for multiple significant trauma		■ Principal diagnosis of trauma and at least two injuries (assigned either as principal or secondary) that are defined as significant trauma from different body site categories located under DRG 487 *AND* O.R. procedure other than craniotomy or limb reattachment, hip and femur procedures
491	Total shoulder replacement	81.80	■ Includes external and internal fixation and graft of bone or cartilage
	Partial shoulder replacement	81.81	■ Includes external and internal fixation and graft of bone or cartilage
	Total elbow replacement	81.84	■ Includes external and internal fixation and graft of bone or cartilage

Shoulder, Elbow or Forearm Procedures, Except Major Joint Procedure without CC

RW 0.7898 **DRG 224**

Potential DRGs

223	Major Shoulder/Elbow Procedures, or Other Upper Extremity Procedures **with CC**	RW	1.0573
486	Other O.R. Procedures for **Multiple Significant Trauma**	RW	4.8793
491	Major Joint & Limb Reattachment Procedures of the Upper Extremity	RW	1.7139

DRG	Principal Dx/Procedure	Codes	Tips
223	Arthrodesis of shoulder *OR* Arthrodesis of elbow *AND* CC condition	81.23–81.24 See CC section.	■ Includes external and internal fixation and graft of bone or cartilage
486	Other O.R. procedures for multiple significant trauma		■ Principal diagnosis of trauma and at least two injuries (assigned either as principal or secondary) that are defined as significant trauma from different body site categories located under DRG 487 *AND* O.R. procedure other than craniotomy or limb reattachment, hip and femur procedures
491	Total shoulder replacement	81.80	■ Includes external and internal fixation and graft of bone or cartilage
	Partial shoulder replacement	81.81	■ Includes external and internal fixation and graft of bone or cartilage
	Total elbow replacement	81.84	■ Includes external and internal fixation and graft of bone or cartilage

Foot Procedures

RW 1.1704 **DRG 225**

Potential DRGs

213	**Amputation for Musculoskeletal System and Connective Tissue Disorders**	RW	1.8904
217	**Wound Debridement and Skin Graft** Except Hand for Musculoskeletal and Connective Tissue Disorders	RW	3.0020

DRG	Principal Dx/Procedure	Codes	Tips
213	Amputation through midfoot	84.12	■ Transmetatarsal amputation of forefoot, including toes

---

■ Coding Tip   ● Documentation Tip   ◆ Encoder Tip   ▽ Targeted DRG

Musculoskeletal System, MDC 8

DRG 225 (continued)

DRG	Principal Dx/Procedure	Codes	Tips
217	Musculoskeletal and connective tissue disorders WITH Wound debridement	86.22	● Excisional debridement (cutting away) of necrotic, devitalized tissue or slough, may be described as "sharp debridement." Does not include the removal of loose fragments of skin by scissors.
	OR free skin graft	86.60	■ Includes excision of skin for autogenous graft
	OR pedicle graft	86.70	◆ Key term: flap graft

DRG 226 Soft Tissue Procedures with CC   RW 1.5529

Potential DRGs

213	Amputation for Musculoskeletal System and Connective Tissue Disorders	RW	1.8904
217	Wound Debridement and Skin Graft Except Hand for Musculoskeletal and Connective Tissue Disorders	RW	3.0020

DRG	Principal Dx/Procedure	Codes	Tips
213	Amputation through midfoot	84.12	■ Transmetatarsal amputation of forefoot, including toes
217	Musculoskeletal and connective tissue disorders WITH Wound debridement	86.22	● Excisional debridement (cutting away) of necrotic, devitalized tissue or slough, may be described as "sharp debridement." Does not include the removal of loose fragments of skin by scissors.
	OR free skin graft	86.60	■ Includes excision of skin for autogenous graft
	OR pedicle graft	86.70	◆ Key term: flap graft

DRG 227 Soft Tissue Procedures without CC   RW 0.8190

Potential DRGs

226	Soft Tissue Procedures with CC	RW	1.5529

DRG	Principal Dx/Procedure	Codes	Tips
226	Incision of muscle, tendon, fascia, bursa AND CC condition	*83.0 See CC section.	■ Includes aponeuroses, synovial membranes and tendon sheaths

DRG 228 Major Thumb or Joint Procedures, or Other Hand or Wrist Procedures with CC   RW 1.1639

Potential DRGs

486	Other O.R. Procedures for Multiple Significant Trauma	RW	4.8793

DRG	Principal Dx/Procedure	Codes	Tips
486	Other O.R. procedures for multiple significant trauma		■ Principal diagnosis of trauma and at least two injuries (assigned either as principal or secondary) that are defined as significant trauma from different body site categories located under DRG 487 AND O.R. procedure other than craniotomy or limb reattachment, hip and femur procedures

---

■ Coding Tip	● Documentation Tip	◆ Encoder Tip	⩊ Targeted DRG

Hand or Wrist Procedures, Except Major Joint Procedures without CC
RW 0.7064 **DRG 229**

Potential DRGs
228 **Major Thumb or Joint Procedures**, or Other Hand or Wrist Procedures **with CC** RW 1.1639

DRG	Principal Dx/Procedure	Codes	Tips
228	Arthroplasty of carpal joint Arthroplasty of metacarpal joint *AND* CC condition	*81.7 See CC section.	■ Includes external and internal fixation and graft of bone or cartilage

Local Excision & Removal of Internal Fixation Devices of Hip & Femur
DRG 230

No Potential DRGs

Arthroscopy
RW 0.9674 **DRG 232**

Potential DRGs
Any OPEN joint procedure
*Ensure accurate DRG assignment.
  Operating room procedures:

80.20 Arthroscopy NOS
80.21 Shoulder arthroscopy
80.22 Elbow arthroscopy
80.23 Wrist arthroscopy
80.24 Hand & finger arthroscopy
80.25 Hip arthroscopy
80.26 Knee arthroscopy
80.27 Ankle arthroscopy
80.28 Foot & toe arthroscopy
80.29 Arthroscopy NEC

Other Musculoskeletal System & Connective Tissue O.R. Procedures with CC
RW 2.0024 **DRG 233**

Potential DRGs
486 Other O.R. Procedures for **Multiple Significant Trauma**   RW 4.8793

DRG	Principal Dx/Procedure	Codes	Tips
486	Other O.R. procedures for multiple significant trauma		■ Principal diagnosis of trauma and at least two injuries (assigned either as principal or secondary) that are defined as significant trauma from different body site categories located under DRG 487 *AND* O.R. procedure other than craniotomy or limb reattachment, hip and femur procedures

DRG 234 Other Musculoskeletal System & RW 1.1977
Connective Tissue O.R. Procedures without CC

Potential DRGs

233	Other Musculoskeletal System & Connective Tissue O.R. Procedures **with CC**	RW	2.0024
486	Other O.R. Procedures for **Multiple Significant Trauma**	RW	4.8793

DRG	Principal Dx/Procedure	Codes	Tips
233	Repair, pectus deformity *AND* CC condition	34.74 See CC section.	■ Repair of pectus carinatum and excavatum (with implant)
486	Other O.R. procedures for multiple significant trauma		■ Principal diagnosis of trauma and at least two injuries (assigned either as principal or secondary) that are defined as significant trauma from different body site categories located under DRG 487 *AND* O.R. procedure other than craniotomy or limb reattachment, hip and femur procedures

DRG 235 Fractures of Femur RW 0.7580

Potential DRGs

210	**Hip & Femur Procedures** Except Major Joint, Age >17 **with CC**	RW	1.8477
211	**Hip & Femur Procedures** Except Major Joint, Age >17 **without CC**	RW	1.2544
485	**Limb Reattachment, Hip & Femur Procedures for Multiple Significant Trauma**	RW	3.2121
487	Other Multiple Significant Trauma	RW	2.0057

DRG	Principal Dx/Procedure	Codes	Tips
210	Femoral sequestrectomy *AND* CC condtions	77.05 See CC section.	
211	Femoral sequestrectomy	77.05	
485	Limb reattachment, hip and femur procedures for multiple significant trauma		■ Principal diagnosis of trauma and at least two injuries (assigned either as principal or secondary) that are defined as significant trauma from different body site categories located under DRG 487 *AND* limb reattachment, hip and femur O.R. procedures
487	Other multiple significant trauma		■ Principal diagnosis of trauma and at least two injuries (assigned either as principal or secondary) that are defined as significant trauma from different body site categories located under DRG 487

*Ensure accurate DRG assignment.

Listed below are the principal diagnoses found in DRG 235:

821.00 Fracture, femur NOS, closed
821.01 Fracture, femur shaft, closed
821.10 Fracture, femur NOS, open
821.11 Fracture, femur shaft, open
821.20 Fracture, lower end femur NOS, closed
821.21 Fracture, femoral condyle, closed
821.22 Fracture, lower femur epiphysis, closed
821.23 Supracondylar fracture, femur, closed
821.29 Fracture, lower end femur NEC, closed
821.30 Fracture, lower end femur NOS, open
821.31 Fracture, femoral condyle, open
821.32 Fracture, lower femur epiphysis, open
821.33 Supracondylar fracture, femur, open
821.39 Fracture, lower end femur NEC, open

■ Coding Tip   ● Documentation Tip   ◆ Encoder Tip   ▼ Targeted DRG

Fractures of Hip & Pelvis

RW 0.7358 **DRG 236**

Potential DRGs

239	**Pathological Fractures** & Musculoskeletal & Connective Tissue Malignancy	RW 1.0614
485	**Limb Reattachment, Hip & Femur Procedures for Multiple Significant Trauma**	RW 3.2121
487	Other Multiple Significant Trauma	RW 2.0057

DRG	Principal Dx/Procedure	Codes	Tips
239	Pathological fracture	*733.1	■ If pathological fracture is reason for admission, use as principal diagnosis. ● Pathological fracture occurs in a bone weakened by disease and is sometimes produced by minor or slight trauma. Degree of trauma must be determined by physician. ◆ Determine underlying condition, trauma or stress fracture.
485	Limb reattachment, hip and femur procedures for multiple significant trauma		■ Principal diagnosis of trauma and at least two injuries (assigned either as principal or secondary) that are defined as significant trauma from different body site categories located under DRG 487 **AND** limb reattachment, hip and femur O.R. procedures
487	Other multiple significant trauma		■ Principal diagnosis of trauma and at least two injuries (assigned either as principal or secondary) that are defined as significant trauma from different body site categories located under DRG 487

Sprains, Strains & Dislocations of Hip, Pelvis & Thigh

RW 0.5983 **DRG 237**

Potential DRGs

256	Other **Musculoskeletal System & Connective Tissue Diagnoses**	RW 0.8190
485	**Limb Reattachment, Hip & Femur Procedures for Multiple Significant Trauma**	RW 3.2121
487	Other Multiple Significant Trauma	RW 2.0057

DRG	Principal Dx/Procedure	Codes	Tips
256	Pathological dislocation Congenital dislocation	718.25 *754.3	■ Spontaneous dislocation, not recurrent
485	Limb reattachment, hip and femur procedures for multiple significant trauma		■ Principal diagnosis of trauma and at least two injuries (assigned either as principal or secondary) that are defined as significant trauma from different body site categories located under DRG 487 **AND** limb reattachment, hip and femur O.R. procedures
487	Other multiple significant trauma		■ Principal diagnosis of trauma and at least two injuries (assigned either as principal or secondary) that are defined as significant trauma from different body site categories located under DRG 487

■ Coding Tip   ● Documentation Tip   ◆ Encoder Tip   ▽ Targeted DRG

DRG 237 (continued)

*Ensure accurate DRG assignment.
Listed below are the principal diagnoses found in DRG 237:

835.00	Dislocation hip NOS, closed	835.13	Anterior dislocation hip
835.01	Posterior dislocation hip, closed	843.0	Sprain, iliofemoral
835.02	Obturator dislocation hip, closed	843.1	Sprain, ischiocapsular
835.03	Anterior dislocation hip NEC, closed	843.8	Sprain, hip & thigh NEC
835.10	Dislocation hip NOS, open	843.9	Sprain, hip & thigh NOS
835.11	Posterior dislocation hip, open	848.5	Sprain, pelvis
835.12	Obturator dislocation hip, open		

DRG 238 Osteomyelitis   RW 1.3564

Potential DRGs

217   **Wound Debridement & Skin Graft** Except Hand, for Musculoskeletal &   RW   3.0020
       Connective Tissue Disorders

DRG	Principal Dx/Procedure	Codes	Tips
217	Musculoskeletal and connective tissue disorders **WITH** Wound debridement	86.22	● Excisional debridement (cutting away) of necrotic, devitalized tissue or slough, may be described as "sharp debridement." Does not include the removal of loose fragments of skin by scissors.
	OR free skin graft	86.60	■ Includes excision of skin for autogenous graft
	OR pedicle graft	86.70	◆ Key term: flap graft

DRG 239 Pathological Fractures & Musculoskeletal   RW 1.0614
& Connective Tissue Malignancy

Be certain that a procedure has not been missed

DRG 240 Connective Tissue Disorders with CC

No Potential DRGs

DRG 241 Connective Tissue Disorders without CC   RW 0.6358

Potential DRGs

240   Connective Tissue Disorders **with CC**   RW   1.3153

DRG	Principal Dx/Procedure	Codes	Tips
240	Rheumatoid arthritis Systemic rheumatoid arthritis NEC Juvenile rheumatoid arthritis Inflammatory polyarthropathy *AND* CC condition	714.0 714.2 *714.3 714.89 See CC section.	

Septic Arthritis   RW 1.1695 **DRG 242**

Potential DRGs

217   **Wound Debridement & Skin Graft** Except Hand, for Musculoskeletal &   RW   3.0020
      Connective Tissue Disorders

DRG	Principal Dx/Procedure	Codes	Tips
217	Musculoskeletal and connective tissue disorders **WITH** Wound debridement	86.22	● Excisional debridement (cutting away) of necrotic, devitalized tissue or slough, may be described as "sharp debridement." Does not include the removal of loose fragments of skin by scissors.
	OR free skin graft	86.60	■ Includes excision of skin for autogenous graft
	OR pedicle graft	86.70	◆ Key term: flap graft

Medical Back Problems   RW 0.7525 **DRG 243**

Potential DRGs

239   **Pathological Fractures** & Musculoskeletal & Connective Tissue Malignancy   RW   1.0614
486   Other O.R. Procedures for **Multiple Significant Trauma**   RW   4.8793
487   Other Multiple Significant Trauma   RW   2.0057

DRG	Principal Dx/Procedure	Codes	Tips
239	Pathological fracture	*733.1	■ If pathological fracture is reason for admission, use as principal diagnosis. ● Pathological fracture occurs in a bone weakened by disease and is sometimes produced by minor or slight trauma. Degree of trauma must be determined by physician. ◆ Determine underlying condition, trauma or stress fracture.
486	Other O.R. procedures for multiple significant trauma		■ Principal diagnosis of trauma and at least two injuries (assigned either as principal or secondary) that are defined as significant trauma from different body site categories located under DRG 487 **AND** O.R. procedure other than craniotomy or limb reattachment, hip and femur procedures
487	Other multiple significant trauma		■ Principal diagnosis of trauma and at least two injuries (assigned either as principal or secondary) that are defined as significant trauma from different body site categories located under DRG 487

Bone Diseases & Specific Arthropathies   RW 0.7155 **DRG 244**
with CC

Potential DRGs

240   **Connective Tissue Disorders** with CC   RW   1.3153

DRG	Principal Dx/Procedure	Codes	Tips
240	Rheumatoid arthritis Systemic rheumatoid arthritis NEC Juvenile rheumatoid arthritis Inflammatory polyarthropathy *AND* CC condition	714.0 714.2 *714.3 714.89 See CC section.	

■ Coding Tip   ● Documentation Tip   ◆ Encoder Tip   ▽ Targeted DRG

DRG 245 Bone Diseases & Specific Arthropathies without CC   RW 0.4786

Potential DRGs

240	Connective Tissue Disorders with CC	RW	1.3153
241	Connective Tissue Disorders without CC	RW	0.6358
244	Bone Diseases & Specific Arthropathies **with CC**	RW	0.7155

DRG	Principal Dx/Procedure	Codes	Tips
240	Rheumatoid arthritis	714.0	◆ Key terms: atropic polyarthritis, chronic rheumatic arthritis, chronic rheumatic polyarthritis
	Systemic rheumatoid arthritis NEC	714.2	◆ Key term: rheumatoid carditis
	Juvenile rheumatoid arthritis	*714.3	◆ Key term: stills disease
	Inflammatory polyarthropathy	714.89	
	AND CC condition	See CC section.	
241	Rheumatoid arthritis	714.0	◆ Key terms: atropic polyarthritis, chronic rheumatic arthritis, chronic rheumatic polyarthritis
	Systemic rheumatoid arthritis NEC	714.2	◆ Key term: rheumatoid carditis
	Juvenile rheumatoid arthritis	*714.3	◆ Key term: Still's disease
	Inflammatory polyarthropathy	714.89	
244	Specific arthropathies: Gout with other specified manifestations	*274.8	■ Gouty tophi ear, heart, other sites; gouty neuritis
	Osteoarthritis and alllied disorders	*715	■ Bilateral involvement; degenerative, hypertrophic
	AND CC condition	See CC section.	

DRG 246 Nonspecific Arthropathies   RW 0.6063

Potential DRGs

244	Bone Diseases & Specific Arthropathies with CC	RW	0.7155

DRG	Principal Dx/Procedure	Codes	Tips
244	Specific arthropathies: Gout with other specified manifestations	*274.8	■ Gouty tophi of ear, heart, other sites; gouty neuritis
	Osteoarthritis and alllied disorders	*715	■ Bilateral involvement; degenerative, hypertrophic
	AND CC condition	See CC section.	

DRG 247 Signs & Symptoms of Musculoskeletal System & Connective Tissue   RW 0.5724

Potential DRGs

239	Pathological Fractures & Musculoskeletal & Connective Tissue Malignancy	RW	1.0614
241	Connective Tissue Disorders without CC	RW	0.6358
248	Tendinitis, Myositis & Bursitis	RW	0.8585
256	Other Musculoskeletal System & Connective Tissue Diagnoses	RW	0.8190

DRG	Principal Dx/Procedure	Codes	Tips
239	Pathological fracture	*733.1	■ If pathological fracture is reason for admission, use as principal diagnosis. ● Pathological fracture occurs in a bone weakened by disease and is sometimes produced by minor or slight trauma. Degree of trauma must be determined by physician. ◆ Determine underlying condition, trauma or stress fracture.

■ Coding Tip   ● Documentation Tip   ◆ Encoder Tip   🏅 Targeted DRG

(continued) **DRG 247**

DRG	Principal Dx/Procedure	Codes	Tips
241	Rheumatoid arthritis	714.0	◆ Key terms: atropic polyarthritis, chronic rheumatic arthritis, chronic rheumatic polyarthritis
	Systemic rheumatoid arthritis NEC	714.2	◆ Key term: rheumatoid carditis
	Juvenile rheumatoid arthritis	*714.3	◆ Key term: stills disease
	Inflammatory polyarthropathy	714.89	
248	Cause of musculoskeletal difficulty or pain:		
	Adhesive capsulitis of shoulder	726.0	
	Synovitis unspecified	727.00	
	Other bursitis	727.3	
256	Cause of musculoskeletal difficulty or pain:		
	Benign neoplasm bones of skull and face	213.0	■ Meniscus disorder, rupture, tear; old rupture of ligamentous joint NOS
	Articular cartilage disorder	*718. 0	
	Joint contracture	*718. 4	

Tendinitis, Myositis, and Bursitis   **DRG 248**

No Potential DRGs

Aftercare, Musculoskeletal System &   RW 0.6744   **DRG 249**
Connective Tissue

*Ensure accurate DRG assignment.
Principal diagnosis:

905.2	Late effect arm fracture
905.3	Late effect femoral neck fracture
905.4	Late effect leg fracture
905.5	Late effect fracture NEC
905.8	Late effect tendon injury
905.9	Late effect traumatic amputation
996.4	Malfunction internal orthopedic device/graft
996.66	Reaction, internal joint prosthesis
996.67	Reaction, other internal ortho device
996.77	Complication, internal joint prosthesis
996.78	Complication, other internal ortho device
996.90	Complication reattachment extremity NOS
996.91	Complication reattached forearm
996.92	Complication reattached hand
996.93	Complication reattached finger
996.94	Complication reattached arm NEC
996.95	Complication reattached foot
996.96	Complication reattached leg NEC
996.99	Complication reattached part NEC
V52.0	Fitting artificial arm
V52.1	Fitting artificial leg
V53.7	Fitting orthopedic devices
*V54.0	Aftercare, orthopedic, involving removal, fracture plate, other internal fixation device
*V54.1	Aftercare, for healing fracture, traumatic
*V54.2	Aftercare, for healing fracture, pathologic
V54.8	Orthopaedic aftercare NEC
V54.9	Orthopaedic aftercare NOS

Fractures, Sprains, Strains & Dislocations   RW 0.7091   **DRG 250**
of Forearm, Hand, Foot, Age > 17 with CC

Potential DRGs

239	**Pathological Fractures** & Musculoskeletal & Connective Tissue Malignancy	RW	1.0614
486	**Other O.R. Procedures for Multiple Significant Trauma**	RW	4.8793
487	Other **Multiple Significant Trauma**	RW	2.0057

DRG	Principal Dx/Procedure	Codes	Tips
239 ▽	Pathological fracture	*733.1	■ If pathological fracture is reason for admission, use as principal diagnosis. ● Pathological fracture occurs in a bone weakened by disease and is sometimes produced by minor or slight trauma. Degree of trauma must be determined by physician. ◆ Determine underlying condition, trauma or stress fracture.

■ Coding Tip   ● Documentation Tip   ◆ Encoder Tip   ▽ Targeted DRG

DRG 250　(continued)

DRG	Principal Dx/Procedure	Codes	Tips
486	Other O.R. procedures for multiple significant trauma		■ Principal diagnosis of trauma and at least two injuries (assigned either as principal or secondary) that are defined as significant trauma from different body site categories located under DRG 487 *AND* O.R. procedure other than craniotomy or limb reattachment, hip and femur procedures
487	Other multiple significant trauma		■ Principal diagnosis of trauma and at least two injuries (assigned either as principal or secondary) that are defined as significant trauma from different body site categories located under DRG 487

DRG 251　Fractures, Sprains, Strains & Dislocations　RW 0.4578
of Forearm, Hand, Foot, Age > 17 without CC

Potential DRGs

239	**Pathological Fractures** & Musculoskeletal & Connective Tissue Malignancy	RW	1.0614
250	Fractures, Sprains, Strains & Dislocations of Forearm, Hand, Foot, Age > 17 with CC	RW	0.7091
486	**Other O.R. Procedures for Multiple Significant Trauma**	RW	4.8793
487	Other **Multiple Significant Trauma**	RW	2.0057

DRG	Principal Dx/Procedure	Codes	Tips
239 ▽	Pathological fracture	*733.1	■ If pathological fracture is reason for admission, use as principal diagnosis. ● Pathological fracture occurs in a bone weakened by disease and is sometimes produced by minor or slight trauma. Degree of trauma must be determined by physician. ◆ Determine underlying condition, trauma or stress fracture.
250	CC condition	See CC section.	
486	Other O.R. procedures for multiple significant trauma		■ Principal diagnosis of trauma and at least two injuries (assigned either as principal or secondary) that are defined as significant trauma from different body site categories located under DRG 487 *AND* O.R. procedure other than craniotomy or limb reattachment, hip and femur procedures
487	Other multiple significant trauma		■ Principal diagnosis of trauma and at least two injuries (assigned either as principal or secondary) that are defined as significant trauma from different body site categories located under DRG 487

■ Coding Tip　　●　Documentation Tip　　◆　Encoder Tip　　⍟ Targeted DRG

　　　　　　　　　　　　　　　　　　　　　　©2003 Ingenix, Inc.

Fractures, Sprains, Strains & Dislocations of Forearm, Hand, Foot, Age 0–17

RW 0.2553 **DRG 252**

Potential DRGs

239	**Pathological Fractures & Musculoskeletal** & Connective Tissue Malignancy	RW	1.0614
250	Fractures, Sprains, Strains & Dislocations of Forearm, Hand, Foot, Age > 17 **with CC**	RW	0.7091
251	Fractures, Sprains, Strains & Dislocations of Forearm, Hand, Foot, Age > 17 **without CC**	RW	0.4578
486	**Other O.R. Procedures for Multiple Significant Trauma**	RW	4.8793
487	Other **Multiple Significant Trauma**	RW	2.0057

DRG	Principal Dx/Procedure	Codes	Tips
239 ▽YIELD▽	Pathological fracture	*733.1	■ If pathological fracture is reason for admission, use as principal diagnosis. ● Pathological fracture occurs in a bone weakened by disease and is sometimes produced by minor or slight trauma. Degree of trauma must be determined by physician. ◆ Determine underlying condition, trauma or stress fracture.
250	CC condition	See CC section.	
251	Patient's age > 17		
486	Other O.R. procedures for multiple significant trauma		■ Principal diagnosis of trauma and at least two injuries (assigned either as principal or secondary) that are defined as significant trauma from different body site categories located under DRG 487 **AND** O.R. procedure other than craniotomy or limb reattachment, hip and femur procedures
487	Other multiple significant trauma		■ Principal diagnosis of trauma and at least two injuries (assigned either as principal or secondary) that are defined as significant trauma from different body site categories located under DRG 487

Fractures, Sprains, Strains & Dislocations of Upper Arm, Lower Leg Except Foot, Age > 17 with CC

RW 0.7581 **DRG 253**

Potential DRGs

239	**Pathological Fractures** & Musculoskeletal & Connective Tissue Malignancy	RW	1.0614
486	**Other O.R. Procedures for Multiple Significant Trauma**	RW	4.8793
487	Other **Multiple Significant Trauma**	RW	2.0057

DRG	Principal Dx/Procedure	Codes	Tips
239 ▽YIELD▽	Pathological fracture	*733.1	■ If pathological fracture is reason for admission, use as principal diagnosis. ● Pathological fracture occurs in a bone weakened by disease and is sometimes produced by minor or slight trauma. Degree of trauma must be determined by physician. ◆ Determine underlying condition, trauma or stress fracture.

■ Coding Tip   ● Documentation Tip   ◆ Encoder Tip   ▽ Targeted DRG

Musculoskeletal System, MDC 8

DRG 253 (continued)

DRG	Principal Dx/Procedure	Codes	Tips
486	Other O.R. procedures for multiple significant trauma		■ Principal diagnosis of trauma and at least two injuries (assigned either as principal or secondary) that are defined as significant trauma from different body site categories located under DRG 487 *AND* O.R. procedure other than craniotomy or limb reattachment, hip and femur procedures
487	Other multiple significant trauma		■ Principal diagnosis of trauma and at least two injuries (assigned either as principal or secondary) that are defined as significant trauma from different body site categories located under DRG 487

DRG 254 Fractures, Sprains, Strains & Dislocations of Upper Arm, Lower Leg Except Foot, Age > 17 without CC   RW 0.4464

Potential DRGs

239	**Pathological Fractures & Musculoskeletal** & Connective Tissue Malignancy	RW	1.0614
253	Fractures, Sprains, Strains & Dislocations of Upper Arm, Lower Leg Except Foot, Age > 17 **with CC**	RW	0.7581
486	**Other O.R. Procedures for Multiple Significant Trauma**	RW	4.8793
487	Other **Multiple Significant Trauma**	RW	2.0057

DRG	Principal Dx/Procedure	Codes	Tips
239 ▽	Pathological fracture	*733.1	■ If pathological fracture is reason for admission, use as principal diagnosis. ● Pathological fracture occurs in a bone weakened by disease and is sometimes produced by minor or slight trauma. Degree of trauma must be determined by physician. ◆ Determine underlying condition, trauma or stress fracture..
253	CC condition	See CC section.	
486	Other O.R. procedures for multiple significant trauma		■ Principal diagnosis of trauma and at least two injuries (assigned either as principal or secondary) that are defined as significant trauma from different body site categories located under DRG 487 *AND* O.R. procedure other than craniotomy or limb reattachment, hip and femur procedures
487	Other multiple significant trauma		■ Principal diagnosis of trauma and at least two injuries (assigned either as principal or secondary) that are defined as significant trauma from different body site categories located under DRG 487

■ Coding Tip   ● Documentation Tip   ◆ Encoder Tip   ▽ Targeted DRG

Fractures, Sprains, Strains & Dislocations of Upper Arm, Lower Leg Except Foot, Age 0–17

RW 0.2974 **DRG 255**

Potential DRGs

239	**Pathological Fractures & Musculoskeletal** & Connective Tissue Malignancy	RW	1.0614
253	Fractures, Sprains, Strains & Dislocations of Upper Arm, Lower Leg Except Foot, Age > 17 **with CC**	RW	0.7581
486	Other O.R. Procedures for **Multiple Significant Trauma**	RW	4.8793
487	Other **Multiple Significant Trauma**	RW	2.0057

DRG	Principal Dx/Procedure	Codes	Tips
239 ▽	Pathological fracture	*733.1	■ If pathological fracture is reason for admission, use as principal diagnosis. ● Pathological fracture occurs in a bone weakened by disease and is sometimes produced by minor or slight trauma. Degree of trauma must be determined by physician. ◆ Determine underlying condition, trauma or stress fracture..
253	CC condition	See CC section.	
486	Other O.R. procedures for multiple significant trauma		■ Principal diagnosis of trauma and at least two injuries (assigned either as principal or secondary) that are defined as significant trauma from different body site categories located under DRG 487 **AND** O.R. procedure other than craniotomy or limb reattachment, hip and femur procedures
487	Other multiple significant trauma		■ Principal diagnosis of trauma and at least two injuries (assigned either as principal or secondary) that are defined as significant trauma from different body site categories located under DRG 487

Other Musculoskeletal System & Connective Tissue Diagnoses

RW 0.8190 **DRG 256**

Potential DRGs

239	Pathological Fractures & **Musculoskeletal & Connective Tissue Malignancy**	RW	1.0614
486	**Other O.R. Procedures for Multiple Significant Trauma**	RW	4.8793
487	Other **Multiple Significant Trauma**	RW	2.0057

DRG	Principal Dx/Procedure	Codes	Tips
239 ▽	Pathological fracture	*733.1	■ If pathological fracture is reason for admission, use as principal diagnosis. ● Pathological fracture occurs in a bone weakened by disease and is sometimes produced by minor or slight trauma. Degree of trauma must be determined by physician. ◆ Determine underlying condition, trauma or stress fracture..

■ Coding Tip   ● Documentation Tip   ◆ Encoder Tip   ▽ Targeted DRG

Musculoskeletal System, MDC 8

DRG 256 (continued)

DRG	Principal Dx/Procedure	Codes	Tips
486	Other O.R. procedures for multiple significant trauma		■ Principal diagnosis of trauma and at least two injuries (assigned either as principal or secondary) that are defined as significant trauma from different body site categories located under DRG 487 *AND* O.R. procedure other than craniotomy or limb reattachment, hip and femur procedures
487	Other multiple significant trauma		■ Principal diagnosis of trauma and at least two injuries (assigned either as principal or secondary) that are defined as significant trauma from different body site categories located under DRG 487

DRG 471   Bilateral or Multiple Major Joint Procedures of Lower Extremity

No Potential DRGs

DRG 491   Major Joint & Limb Reattachment Procedures of the Upper Extremity   RW 1.7139

Potential DRGs
486   Other O.R. Procedures for **Multiple Significant Trauma**   RW   4.8793

DRG	Principal Dx/Procedure	Codes	Tips
486	Other O.R. procedures for multiple significant trauma		■ Principal diagnosis of trauma and at least two injuries (assigned either as principal or secondary) that are defined as significant trauma from different body site categories located under DRG 487 *AND* O.R. procedure other than craniotomy or limb reattachment, hip and femur procedures

DRG 496   Combined Anterior/Posterior Spinal Fusion   RW 5.6839

*Ensure accurate DRG assignment.
Listed below are the procedure codes used in any combination included in DRG 496.

81.61   Fusion, spinal, 360 degree, single incision approach

OR

One or more of the following procedure codes:
81.02   Other cervical fusion anterior
81.04   Dorsal/dorsolumbar fusion anterior
81.06   Lumbar/lumbosacral fusion anterior
81.32   Refusion, anterior, other cervical
81.34   Refusion, anterior, dorsal/dorsolumbar
81.36   Refusion, anterior, lumbar/lumbosacral

AND

One or more of the following procedure codes:
81.03   Other cervical fusion posterior
81.05   Dorsal/dorsolumbar fusion posterior
81.07   Fusion, lateral, lumbar/lumbosacral
81.08   Lumbar/lumbosacral fusion posterior
81.33   Refusion, posterior, other cervical
81.35   Refusion, posterior, dorsal/dorsolumbar
81.37   Refusion, lateral transverse, lumbar/lumbosacral
81.38   Refusion, posterior, lumbar/lumbosacral

■ Coding Tip   ● Documentation Tip   ◆ Encoder Tip   ▽ Targeted DRG

Spinal Fusion Except Cervical with CC   RW 3.4056 **DRG 497**

Potential DRGs

496   **Combined Anterior/Posterior** Spinal Fusion   RW   5.6839

DRG	Principal Dx/Procedure	Codes	Tips
496	Both anterior and posterior spinal fusion: anterior posterior	 81.06 81.08, 81.61	◆ Includes: 360 degree fusion, combined PLIF, ALIF, TLIF, lumbar, lumbosacral, dorsal, or dorsolumbar technique. ■ Review operative note to identify two operative approaches. ● Two operative notes may be dictated for different incisions/approach.

*Ensure accurate DRG assignment. Listed below are the procedure codes found in DRG 497.

81.00	Spinal fusion NOS	81.31	Refusion, Atlas-axis
81.01	Atlas-axis fusion	81.34	Refusion, anterior, dorsal/dorsolumbar
81.04	Dorsal/dorsolumbar fusion anterior	81.35	Refusion, posterior, dorsal/dorsolumbar
81.05	Dorsal/dorsolumbar fusion posterior	81.36	Refusion, anterior, lumbar/lumbosacral
81.06	Lumbar/lumbosacral fusion anterior	81.37	Refusion, lateral transverse, lumbar/
81.07	Lumbar/lumbosacral fusion lateral		lumbosacral
81.08	Lumbar/lumbosacral fusion posterior	81.38	Refusion, posterior, lumbar/lumbosacral
81.30	Refusion, spinal, NOS	81.39	Refusion, spinal, NEC

Spinal Fusion Except Cervical without CC   RW 2.5319 **DRG 498**

Potential DRGs

496   **Combined Anterior/Posterior Spinal Fusion**   RW   5.6839
497   **Spinal Fusion Except Cervical with CC**   RW   3.4056

DRG	Principal Dx/Procedure	Codes	Tips
496	Both anterior and posterior spinal fusion: anterior posterior	 81.06 81.08, 81.61	◆ Includes: 360 degree fusion, combined PLIF, ALIF, TLIF, lumbar, lumbosacral, dorsal, or dorsolumbar technique ■ Review operative note to identify two operative approaches. ● Two operative notes may be dictated for different incisions/approach.
497	CC condition	See CC section.	◆ Common CCs in spinal surgeries include blood loss anemia and postoperative urinary retention.

*Ensure accurate DRG assignment. Listed below are the procedure codes found in DRG 498.

81.00	Spinal fusion NOS	81.06	Lumbar/lumbosacral fusion anterior
81.04	Dorsal/dorsolumbar fusion anterior	81.07	Lumbar/lumbosacral fusion lateral
81.05	Dorsal/dorsolumbar fusion posterior	81.08	Lumbar/lumbosacral fusion posterior

---

■ Coding Tip   ● Documentation Tip   ◆ Encoder Tip   ⚑ Targeted DRG

Musculoskeletal System, MDC 8

DRG 499   Back & Neck Procedures Except Spinal Fusion with CC   RW 1.4244

Potential DRGs

496	Combined Anterior/Posterior Spinal Fusion	RW	5.6839
497	Spinal Fusion Except Cervical with CC	RW	3.4056

DRG	Principal Dx/Procedure	Codes	Tips

496	Both anterior and posterior spinal fusion:
	  anterior
	  posterior
		
		81.06
		81.08, 81.61
			◆ Includes: 360 degree fusion, combined PLIF, ALIF, TLIF, lumbar, lumbosacral, dorsal, or dorsolumbar technique
			■ Review operative note to identify two operative approaches.
			● Two operative notes may be dictated for different incisions/approach.

497	CC condition	See CC section.	◆ Common CCs in spinal surgeries include blood loss anemia and postoperative urinary retention.

DRG 500   Back & Neck Procedures Except Spinal Fusion without CC   RW 0.9369

Potential DRGs

496	Combined Anterior/Posterior Spinal Fusion	RW	5.6839
497	Spinal Fusion Except Cervical with CC	RW	3.4056
499	Back and Neck Procedures Except Spinal Fusion with CC	RW	1.4244

DRG	Principal Dx/Procedure	Codes	Tips

496	Both anterior and posterior spinal fusion:
	  anterior
	  posterior
		
		81.06
		81.08, 81.61
			◆ Includes: 360 degree fusion, combined PLIF, ALIF, TLIF, lumbar, lumbosacral, dorsal, or dorsolumbar technique
			■ Review operative note to identify two operative approaches.
			● Two operative notes may be dictated for different incisions/approach.

497	CC condition	See CC section.	◆ Common CCs in spinal surgeries include blood loss anemia and postoperative urinary retention.
499	Back and neck procedures except spinal fusion *AND* CC condition	03.02 See CC section.	◆ Common CCs in spinal surgeries include blood loss anemia and postoperative urinary retention.

DRG 501   Knee Procedure with Principal Diagnosis of Infection with CC   RW 2.6393

*Ensure accurate DRG assignment. Listed below are the principal diagnoses found in DRG 501:

711.06 Pyogenic arthritis lower leg
730.06 Acute osteomyelitis lower leg
730.16 Chronic osteomyelitis lower leg
730.26 Unspecified osteomyelitis lower leg
996.66 Infection and inflammatory reaction due to internal joint prosthesis
996.67 Infection and inflammatory reaction due to other internal orthopaedic device

Knee Procedure with Principal Diagnosis of Infection without CC   RW 1.4192   **DRG 502**

Potential DRGs

501   Knee Procedure with Principal Diagnosis of Infection **with CC**   RW   2.6393

DRG	Principal Dx/Procedure	Codes	Tips
501	CC condition	See CC section.	

*Ensure Accurate DRG assignment. Listed below are the principal diagnoses found in DRG 502:

711.06 Pyogenic arthritis lower leg
730.06 Acute osteomyelitis lower leg
730.16 Chronic osteomyelitis lower leg
730.26 Unspecified osteomyelitis lower leg

996.66 Infection and inflammatory reaction due to internal joint prosthesis
996.67 Infection and inflammatory reaction due to other internal orthopaedic device

Knee Procedures without Principal Diagnosis of Infection   RW 1.2233   **DRG 503**

Potential DRGs

501   Knee Procedure with Principal Diagnosis of Infection **with CC**   RW   2.6393
502   Knee Procedure with Principal Diagnosis of Infection without CC   RW   1.4192

DRG	Principal Dx/Procedure	Codes	Tips
501	Pyogenic arthritis lower leg Acute osteomyelitis lower leg Chronic osteomyelitis lower leg Unspecified osteomyelitis lower leg Infection and inflammatory reaction due to internal joint prosthesis Infection and inflammatory reaction due to other internal orthopaedic device *AND* CC condition	711.06 730.06 730.16 730.26 996.66 996.67 See CC section.	◆ Key term: pyarthrosis ■ Necrosis, sequestrum of bone ■ With or without mention of periostitis ◆ Key terms: electrode, pin, rod, screw
502	Pyogenic arthritis lower leg Acute osteomyelitis lower leg Chronic osteomyelitis lower leg Unspecified osteomyelitis lower leg Infection and inflammatory reaction due to internal joint prosthesis Infection and inflammatory reaction due to other internal orthopaedic device	711.06 730.06 730.16 730.26 996.66 996.67	◆ Key term: pyarthrosis ■ Necrosis, sequestrum of bone ■ With or without mention of periostitis ◆ Key term: electrode, pin, rod, screw

Cervical Spinal Fusion with CC   **DRG 519**

No Potential DRGs

Cervical Spinal Fusion without CC   RW 1.5780   **DRG 520**

Potential DRGs

519   Cervical Spinal Fusion **with CC**   RW   2.4266

DRG	Principal Dx/Procedure	Codes	Tips
519	CC condition	See CC section.	◆ Common CCs in spinal surgeries include blood loss anemia and postoperative urinary retention

---

■ Coding Tip   ● Documentation Tip   ◆ Encoder Tip   ▽ Targeted DRG

DRG 537 Local Excision & Removal of Internal Fixation Devices Except Hip and Femur with CC

No Potential DRGs

DRG 538 Local Excision & Removal of Internal Fixation Devices Except Hip and Femur without CC
RW 0.9919

Potential DRGs
537 Local Excision & Removal of Internal Fixation Devices Except Hip and   RW   1.8185
Femur **with CC**

DRG	Principal Dx/Procedure	Codes	Tips
537	CC condition	See CC section.	

Skin, Subcutaneous Tissue & Breast, MDC 9

DRG 257 Total Mastectomy for Malignancy with CC
No Potential DRGs

DRG 258 Total Mastectomy for Malignancy without CC
RW 0.7018

Potential DRGs
257 Total Mastectomy for Malignancy **with CC**   RW   0.8913

DRG	Principal Dx/Procedure	Codes	Tips
257	CC condition	See CC section.	

DRG 259 Subtotal Mastectomy for Malignancy with CC
No Potential DRGs

DRG 260 Subtotal Mastectomy for Malignancy without CC
RW 0.6854

Potential DRGs
258 **Total Mastectomy** for Malignancy without CC   RW   0.7018
259 Subtotal Mastectomy for Malignancy **with CC**   RW   0.9420

DRG	Principal Dx/Procedure	Codes	Tips
258	Total mastectomy	85.31–85.36; 85.41–85.48; 85.7	◆ Key terms: radical (Halsted, Meyer), modifier radical, extended radical (urban), subcutaneous ● May include breast, pectoralis major, minor and regional lymph nodes
259	Subtotal mastectomy AND CC condition	85.23 See CC section.	◆ Key terms: partial, subtotal, segmental

Breast Procedures for Nonmalignancy Except Biopsy and Local Excision
DRG 261

No Potential DRGs

Breast Biopsy & Local Excision for Nonmalignancy
RW 0.9533　**DRG 262**

Potential DRGs

259	Subtotal Mastectomy for Malignancy with CC	RW	0.9420
261	Breast Procedures for Nonmalignancy Except Biopsy & Local Excision	RW	0.8944

DRG	Principal Dx/Procedure	Codes	Tips
259	Subtotal mastectomy *AND* CC condition	85.23 See CC section.	◆ Key terms: partial, subtotal, segmental
261	Breast procedure other than biopsy & local excision: 　Unilateral subcutaneous 　　mammectomy with implant 　Unilateral breast implant 　Removal of breast expander	 85.33 85.53 85.96	

Skin Graft and/or Debridement for Skin Ulcer or Cellulitis with CC
DRG 263

No Potential DRGs

Skin Graft and/or Debridement for Skin Ulcer or Cellulitis without CC
RW 1.0605　**DRG 264**

Potential DRGs

263	Skin Graft &/or Debridement for Skin Ulcer or Cellulitis with CC	RW 2.0556

DRG	Principal Dx/Procedure	Codes	Tips
263	Cellulitis of buttock, Skin ulcer *AND* Excisional debridement *OR* Skin graft, free *AND* CC condition	682.5, 707.x 86.22 86.60 See CC section.	◆ Key terms: abcess, diffuse cellulitis, acute lymphangitis ● May be performed by physician or nonphysician health care provider ● Excisional debridement (cutting away) of necrotic, devitalized tissue or slough, may be described as "sharp debridement." Does not include the removal of loose fragments of skin by scissors.

Skin Graft and/or Debridement Except for Skin Ulcer or Cellulitis with CC
DRG 265

No Potential DRGs

■ Coding Tip　　　● Documentation Tip　　　◆ Encoder Tip　　　▼ Targeted DRG

DRG 266   Skin Graft and/or Debridement Except for   RW 0.8791
Skin Ulcer or Cellulitis without CC

Potential DRGs

265   Skin Graft &/or Debridement Except for Skin Ulcer or Cellulitis **with CC**   RW   1.5984

DRG	Principal Dx/Procedure	Codes	Tips
265	Debridement *OR* Skin graft, free *AND* CC condition	86.22 86.60 See CC section.	● May be performed by physician or nonphysician health care provider ● Excisional debridement (cutting away) of necrotic, devitalized tissue or slough, may be described as "sharp debridement." Does not include the removal of loose fragments of skin by scissors.

DRG 267   Perianal and Pilonidal Procedures

No Potential DRGs

DRG 268   Skin, Subcutaneous Tissue and Breast Plastic
Procedures

No Potential DRGs

DRG 269   Other Skin, Subcutaneous Tissue &   RW 1.7747
Breast Procedures with CC

Potential DRGs

263   Skin Graft &/or Debridement for Skin Ulcer or Cellulitis with CC   RW   2.0556

DRG	Principal Dx/Procedure	Codes	Tips
263	Cellulitis of buttock Skin ulcer *AND* Excisional debridement *OR* Skin graft, free *AND* CC condition	682.5 707.x 86.22 86.60 See CC section.	◆ Key terms: abcess, diffuse cellulitis, acute lymphangitis ● May be performed by physician or nonphysician health care provider ● Excisional debridement (cutting away) of necrotic, devitalized tissue or slough, may be described as "sharp debridement." Does not include the removal of loose fragments of skin by scissors.

Other Skin, Subcutaneous Tissue & Breast Procedures without CC

RW 0.8129 **DRG 270**

Potential DRGs

263	Skin Graft &/or Debridement for Skin Ulcer or Cellulitis with CC	RW	2.0556
264	Skin Graft &/or Debridement for Skin Ulcer or Cellulitis without CC	RW	1.0605
269	Other Skin, Subcutaneous Tissue & Breast Procedures with CC	RW	1.7747

DRG	Principal Dx/Procedure	Codes	Tips
263	Cellulitis of buttock Skin ulcer *AND* Excisional debridement *OR* Skin graft, free *AND* CC condition	682.5 707.x 86.22 86.60 See CC section.	◆ Key terms: abscess, diffuse cellulitis, acute lymphangitis ● May be performed by physician or nonphysician health care provider ● Excisional debridement (cutting away) of necrotic, devitalized tissue or slough, may be described as "sharp debridement." Does not include the removal of loose fragments of skin by scissors.
264	Cellulitis of buttock Skin ulcer *AND* Excisional debridement *OR* Skin graft, free	682.5 707.x 86.22 86.60	◆ Key terms: abscess, diffuse cellulitis, acute lymphangitis ● May be performed by physician or nonphysician health care provider ● Excisional debridement (cutting away) of necrotic, devitalized tissue or slough, may be described as "sharp debridement." Does not include the removal of loose fragments of skin by scissors.
269	Insert vascular access device *AND* CC condition	86.07 See CC section.	◆ Key terms: Port-a-Cath, Perm-a-Cath, Hemo-Cath, subcutaneous port, totally implantable (TIVAD), implanted subcutaneously. ● Insertion is in the central vein and the catheter is anchored to the subcutaneous tissue. No part of the catheter system is brought out through the skin. Indications include: long term access for infusion of chemotherapeutic agents, antibiotics, blood products, total parenteral nutrition, and for hemodialysis

Skin Ulcers

RW 1.0280 **DRG 271**

Potential DRGs

263	Skin Graft &/or Debridement for Skin Ulcer or Cellulitis with CC	RW	2.0556
264	Skin Graft &/or Debridement for Skin Ulcer or Cellulitis without CC	RW	1.0605

DRG	Principal Dx/Procedure	Codes	Tips
263	Cellulitis of buttock Skin ulcer *AND* Excisional debridement *OR* Skin graft, free *AND* CC condition	682.5 707.x 86.22 86.60 See CC section.	◆ Key terms: abscess, diffuse cellulitis, acute lymphangitis ● May be performed by physician or nonphysician health care provider ● Excisional debridement (cutting away) of necrotic, devitalized tissue or slough, may be described as "sharp debridement." Does not include the removal of loose fragments of skin by scissors.

■ Coding Tip	● Documentation Tip	◆ Encoder Tip	℡ Targeted DRG

Skin, Subcutaneous Tissue & Breast, MDC 9

DRG 271   (continued)

DRG	Principal Dx/Procedure	Codes	Tips
264·	Cellulitis of buttock Skin ulcer *AND* Excisional debridement *OR* Skin graft, free	682.5 707.x 86.22 86.60	◆ Key terms: abscess, diffuse cellulitis, acute lymphangitis ● May be performed by physician or nonphysician health care provider ● Excisional debridement (cutting away) of necrotic, devitalized tissue or slough, may be described as "sharp debridement." Does not include the removal of loose fragments of skin by scissors.

DRG 272   Major Skin Disorders with CC
No Potential DRGs

DRG 273   Major Skin Disorders without CC   RW 0.6192
Potential DRGs
272   Major Skin Disorders **with CC**   RW   1.0185

DRG	Principal Dx/Procedure	Codes	Tips
272	Malignant melanoma *AND* CC condition	*172 See CC section.	

DRG 274   Malignant Breast Disorders with CC   RW 1.1574
Potential DRGs
269   Other Skin, Subcutaneous Tissue & Breast Procedures with CC   RW   1.7747

DRG	Principal Dx/Procedure	Codes	Tips
269	Insert vascular access device *AND* CC condition	86.07 See CC section.	◆ Key terms: Port-a-Cath, Perm-a-Cath, Hemo-Cath, subcutaneous port, totally implantable (TIVAD), implanted subcutaneously. ● Insertion is in the central vein and the catheter is anchored to the subcutaneous tissue. No part of the catheter system is brought out through the skin. Indications include: long term access for infusion of chemotherapeutic agents, antibiotics, blood products, total parenteral nutrition, and for hemodialysis

Malignant Breast Disorders without CC   RW 0.5729   **DRG 275**

Potential DRGs

269	Other Skin, Subcutaneous Tissue & Breast Procedures with CC	RW	1.7747
270	Other Skin, Subcutaneous Tissue & Breast Procedures without CC	RW	0.8129
274	Malignant Breast Disorders with CC	RW	1.1574

DRG	Principal Dx/Procedure	Codes	Tips
269	Insert vascular access device *AND* CC condition	86.07 See CC section.	◆ Key terms: Port-a-Cath, Perm-a-Cath, Hemo-Cath, subcutaneous port, totally implantable (TIVAD), implanted subcutaneously. ● Insertion is in the central vein and the catheter is anchored to the subcutaneous tissue.,no part of the catheter system is brought out through the skin. Indications include: long term access for infusion of chemotherapeutic agents, antibiotics, blood products, total parenteral nutrition, and for hemodialysis
270	Insertion of vascular access device	86.07	◆ Key terms: Port-a-Cath, Perm-a-Cath, Hemo-Cath, subcutaneous port, totally implantable (TIVAD), implanted subcutaneously. ● Insertion is in the central vein and the catheter is anchored to the subcutaneous tissue. No part of the catheter system is brought out through the skin. Indications include: long term access for infusion of chemotherapeutic agents, antibiotics, blood products, total parenteral nutrition, and for hemodialysis
274	Breast malignancy *AND* CC condition	*174, *175, 198.81 See CC section.	

Nonmalignant Breast Disorders   RW 0.6471   **DRG 276**

Potential DRGs

274	Malignant Breast Disorders with CC	RW	1.1574

DRG	Principal Dx/Procedure	Codes	Tips
274	Breast malignancy *AND* CC condition	*174, *175, 198.81 See CC section.	

Skin, Subcutaneous Tissue & Breast, MDC 9

DRG 277   Cellulitis, Age > 17 with CC   RW 0.8805
Potential DRGs
263   **Skin Graft &/or Debridement** for Skin Ulcer or Cellulitis **with CC**   RW   2.0556
271   **Skin Ulcers**   RW   1.0280

DRG	Principal Dx/Procedure	Codes	Tips
263	Cellulitis of buttock Skin ulcer *AND* Excisional debridement *OR* Skin graft, free *AND* CC condition	682.5 707.x 86.22 86.60 See CC section.	◆ Key terms: abscess, diffuse cellulitis, acute lymphangitis ● May be performed by physician or nonphysician health care provider ● Excisional debridement (cutting away) of necrotic, devitalized tissue or slough, may be described as "sharp debridement." Does not include the removal of loose fragments of skin by scissors.
271	Ulceration of the leg	707.1x	

DRG 278   Cellulitis, Age > 17 without CC   RW 0.5432
Potential DRGs
263   **Skin Graft &/or Debridement** for Skin Ulcer or Cellulitis **with CC**   RW   2.0556
264   **Skin Graft &/or Debridement** for Skin Ulcer or Cellulitis without CC   RW   1.0605
271   **Skin Ulcers**   RW   1.0280
277   Cellulitis, Age > 17 with CC   RW   0.8805
279   Cellulitis, **Age 0–17**   RW   0.7779

DRG	Principal Dx/Procedure	Codes	Tips
263	Cellulitis of buttock Skin ulcer *AND* Excisional debridement *OR* Skin graft, free *AND* CC condition	682.5 707.x 86.22 86.60 See CC section.	◆ Key terms: abscess, diffuse cellulitis, acute lymphangitis ● May be performed by physician or nonphysician health care provider ● Excisional debridement (cutting away) of necrotic, devitalized tissue or slough, may be described as "sharp debridement." Does not include the removal of loose fragments of skin by scissors.
264	Cellulitis of buttock Skin ulcer *AND* Excisional debridement *OR* Skin graft, free	682.5 707.x 86.22 86.60	◆ Key terms: abscess, diffuse cellulitis, acute lymphangitis ● May be performed by physician or nonphysician health care provider ● Excisional debridement (cutting away) of necrotic, devitalized tissue or slough, may be described as "sharp debridement." Does not include the removal of loose fragments of skin by scissors.
271	Ulceration of the leg	707.1x	
277	Cellulitis *AND* CC condition	*681–*682 See CC section.	◆ Key terms: abscess, diffuse cellulitis, acute lymphangitis
279	Cellulitis *AND* Patient's age 0–17	*681–*682	◆ Key terms: abscess, diffuse cellulitis, acute lymphangitis

Cellulitis, Age 0–17   RW 0.7779   **DRG 279**

Potential DRGs

263	**Skin Graft &/or Debridement** for Skin Ulcer or Cellulitis **with CC**	RW 2.0556
264	**Skin Graft &/or Debridement** for Skin Ulcer or Cellulitis without CC	RW 1.0605
271	**Skin Ulcers**	RW 1.0280
277	Cellulitis, **Age > 17 with CC**	RW 0.8805

DRG	Principal Dx/Procedure	Codes	Tips
263	Cellulitis of buttock Skin ulcer *AND* Excisional debridement *OR* Skin graft, free *AND* CC condition	682.5 707.x 86.22 86.60 See CC section.	◆ Key terms: abscess, diffuse cellulitis, acute lymphangitis ● May be performed by physician or nonphysician health care provider ● Excisional debridement (cutting away) of necrotic, devitalized tissue or slough, may be described as "sharp debridement." Does not include the removal of loose fragments of skin by scissors.
264	Cellulitis of buttock Skin ulcer *AND* Excisional debridement *OR* Skin graft, free	682.5 707.x 86.22 86.60	◆ Key terms: abscess, diffuse cellulitis, acute lymphangitis ● May be performed by physician or nonphysician health care provider ● Excisional debridement (cutting away) of necrotic, devitalized tissue or slough, may be described as "sharp debridement." Does not include the removal of loose fragments of skin by scissors.
271	Ulceration of the leg	707.1x	
277	Cellulitis *AND* CC condition	*681–*682 See CC section.	◆ Key terms: abscess, diffuse cellulitis, acute lymphangitis

Trauma to Skin, Subcutaneous Tissue & Breast, Age > 17 with CC   RW 0.7109   **DRG 280**

Potential DRGs

454	Other Injury, Poisoning & Toxic Effect Diagnoses with CC	RW 0.8153

DRG	Principal Dx/Procedure	Codes	Tips
454	Observation following accident *AND* CC conditions	V71.3, V71.4, V71.6 See CC section.	

Trauma to Skin, Subcutaneous Tissue & Breast, Age > 17 without CC   RW 0.4866   **DRG 281**

Potential DRGs

280	Trauma to Skin, Subcutaneous Tissue & Breast, Age > 17 **with CC**	RW 0.7109
454	**Other Injury, Poisoning & Toxic Effect Diagnoses with CC**	RW 0.8153

DRG	Principal Dx/Procedure	Codes	Tips
280	Contusion *AND* CC condition	*924 See CC section.	
454	Observation following accident *AND* CC conditions	V71.3, V71.4, V71.6 See CC section.	

■ Coding Tip   ● Documentation Tip   ◆ Encoder Tip   Targeted DRG

Skin, Subcutaneous Tissue & Breast, MDC 9

DRG 282 Trauma to the Skin, Subcutaneous Tissue & Breast, Age 0–17

RW 0.2586

Potential DRGs

280	Trauma to Skin, Subcutaneous Tissue & Breast, **Age > 17 with CC**	RW 0.7109
281	Trauma to Skin, Subcutaneous Tissue & Breast, **Age > 17** without CC	RW 0.4866
454	**Other Injury, Poisoning & Toxic Effect Diagnoses with CC**	RW 0.8153
455	**Other Injury, Poisoning & Toxic Effect Diagnoses** without CC	RW 0.4773

DRG	Principal Dx/Procedure	Codes	Tips
280	Contusion *AND* CC condition	*924 See CC section.	
281	Contusion	*924	
454	Observation following accident *AND* CC condition	V71.3, V71.4, V71.6 See CC section.	
455	Observation following accident	V71.3, V71.4, V71.6	

DRG 283 Minor Skin Disorders with CC

RW 0.7322

Potential DRGs

272	**Major Skin Disorders** with CC	RW 1.0185

DRG	Principal Dx/Procedure	Codes	Tips
272	Malignant melanoma *AND* CC condition	*172 See CC section.	

DRG 284 Minor Skin Disorders without CC

RW 0.4215

Potential DRGs

272	**Major Skin Disorders with CC**	RW 1.0185
283	Minor Skin Disorders **with CC**	RW 0.7322

DRG	Principal Dx/Procedure	Codes	Tips
272	Malignant melanoma *AND* CC condition	*172 See CC section.	
283	Lipoma of face *AND* CC condition	214.0 See CC section.	

Endocrine, Nutritional & Metabolic Disorders, MDC 10

Amputation of Lower Limb for Endocrine, Nutritional & Metabolic Disorders   RW 2.0825   **DRG 285**

Potential DRGs
113   Amputation for Circulatory System Disorders Except Upper Limb & Toe   RW   3.0106

DRG	Principal Dx/Procedure	Codes	Tips
113	Diabetes with circulatory disorder *AND* Amputation lower limb NOS	250.7x 84.10	

Adrenal and Pituitary Procedures   **DRG 286**

No Potential DRGs

Skin Grafts and Wound Debridement for Endocrine, Nutritional and Metabolic Disorders   **DRG 287**

No Potential DRGs

Operating Room Procedures for Obesity   RW 2.1498   **DRG 288**

*Ensure accurate DRG assignment. Listed below are the only O.R. procedures found in DRG 288:

44.31   High gastric bypass
44.32   Gastrojejunostomy, percutaneous (endoscopic)
44.39   Other gastroenterostomy
44.5   Revision of gastric anastomosis
44.69   Gastric repair NEC
44.99   Gastric operation NEC

45.90   Intestinal anastomosis NOS
45.91   Small-to-small bowel anastomosis
85.31   Unilateral reduction mammoplasty
85.32   Bilateral reduction mammoplasty
86.83   Size reduction plastic operation
86.89   Skin repair and reconstruction NEC

Parathyroid Procedures   **DRG 289**

No Potential DRGs

Thyroid Procedures   RW 0.8938   **DRG 290**

Potential DRGs
289   **Parathyroid** Procedures   RW   0.9441

DRG	Principal Dx/Procedure	Codes	Tips
289	Parathyroidectomy	*06.8	■ Do not assign code for inadvertent excision of parathyroid glands during a thyroidectomy.

Thyroglossal Procedures   **DRG 291**

No Potential DRGs

■ Coding Tip   ● Documentation Tip   ◆ Encoder Tip   ▽ Targeted DRG

Endocrine, Nutritional & Metabolic Disorders, MDC 10

DRG 292   Other Endocrine, Nutritional & Metabolic   RW 2.7336
O.R. Procedures with CC

Potential DRGs

486   Other O.R. Procedures for Multiple Significant Trauma   RW   4.8793

DRG	Principal Dx/Procedure	Codes	Tips
486	Other O.R. procedures for multiple significant trauma		■ Principal diagnosis of trauma and at least two injuries (assigned either as principal or secondary) that are defined as significant trauma from different body site categories located under DRG 487 *AND* O.R. procedure other than craniotomy or limb reattachment, and hip and femur procedures

DRG 293   Other Endocrine, Nutritional & Metabolic   RW 1.3896
O.R. Procedures without CC

Potential DRGs

120	Other Circulatory System O.R. Procedures	RW	2.3164
292	Other Endocrine, Nutritional & Metabolic O.R. Procedures **with CC**	RW	2.7336
315	**Other Kidney and Urinary Tract O.R. Procedures**	RW	2.0796
442	**Other O.R. Procedures for Injuries with CC**	RW	2.4200
486	Other O.R. Procedures for Multiple Significant Trauma	RW	4.8793

DRG	Principal Dx/Procedure	Codes	Tips
120	Diabetes with peripheral circulatory disorders	250.70, 250.73	
	AND Creation arteriovenostomy for renal dialysis	39.27	◆ Internal formation of AV shunt code 39.27. External vessel-to-vessel shunt (ex, Scribner) code 39.93, arteriovenous fistula
	Revision arteriovenostomy for renal dialysis	39.42	
	Removal of arteriovenostomy for renal dialysis	39.43	
292	Thymus biopsy	07.16	
	AND CC condition	See CC section.	
315	Diabetes with renal manifestations	250.40, 250.43	◆ Internal formation of AV shunt code 39.27. External vessel-to-vessel shunt (ex, Scribner) code 39.93.; Arteriovenous fistula
	AND Creation, arteriovenostomy for renal dialysis	39.27	
	Revision arteriovenostomy for renal dialysis	39.42	◆ Conversion from end-to-end to end-to-side anastomosis
	Removal of arteriovenostomy for renal dialysis	39.43	
442	Principal Dx from MDC 21		◆ Internal formation of AV shunt code 39.27. External vessel-to-vessel shunt (ex, Scribner) code 39.93, arteriovenous fistula
	AND Creation arteriovenostomy for renal dialysis	39.27	
	Revision arteriovenostomy for renal dialysis	39.42	◆ Conversion from end-to-end to end to side anastomosis
	Removal of arteriovenostomy for renal dialysis	39.43	
486	Other O.R. procedures for multiple significant trauma		■ Principal diagnosis of trauma and at least two injuries (assigned either as principal or secondary) that are defined as significant trauma from different body site categories located under DRG 487 *AND* O.R. procedure other than craniotomy or limb reattachment, hip and femur procedures

■ Coding Tip   ● Documentation Tip   ◆ Encoder Tip   ⬥ Targeted DRG

©*2003 Ingenix, Inc.*

Diabetes, Age > 35   RW 0.7800   **DRG 294**

Potential DRGs

130	Peripheral Vascular Disorders with CC	RW	0.9505
287	Skin Graft & Wound Debridement for Endocrine, Nutritional and Met abolic Disorders	RW	1.8899
296	Nutritional & Miscellaneous Metabolic Disorders, Age > 17 with CC	RW	0.8639
331	Other Kidney & Urinary Tract Diagnoses, Age > 17 with CC	RW	1.0618

DRG	Principal Dx/Procedure	Codes	Tips
130 🔻YELD	Diabetic gangrene *AND* CC condition	250.70 250.73 See CC section.	■ Lower extremeity gangrene with no other "cause and effect" relationship, assume that the gangrene is the consequence of a diabetic peripheral vascular circulatory disorder, 250.70, add 785.4 for gangrene.
287	DM with other specified manifestations *AND* Diabetic ulcer *AND* Excisional debridement	250.8x 707.9 86.22	◆ Key terms: chronic, trophic ● May be performed by physician or nonphysician health care provider ● Excisional debridement (cutting away) of necrotic, devitalized tissue or slough, may be described as "sharp debridement." Does not include the removal of loose fragments of skin by scissors.
296 🔻YELD	Dehydration	276.5	■ NIDDM patients are prone to the development of a hyperosmolar state and dehydration. ◆ Key terms: hypovolemia, volume depletion. ■ IV hydration should be ordered for correct coding. If patient admitted with gastroenteritis and dehydration, w/IV hydration ordered which necessitated the admission, 276.5 is the principal Dx.
331	Diabetes with renal manifestations *AND* CC condition	250.40–250.43 See CC section.	

Diabetes, Age 0-35   RW 0.7975   **DRG 295**

Potential DRGs

130	Peripheral Vascular Disorders with CC	RW	0.9505
287	Skin Graft & Wound Debridement for Endocrine, Nutritional & Metabolic Disorders	RW	1.8899
296	Nutritional & Miscellaneous Metabolic Disorders, Age > 17 with CC	RW	0.8639
331	Other Kidney & Urinary Tract Diagnoses, Age > 17 with CC	RW	1.0618

DRG	Principal Dx/Procedure	Codes	Tips
130 🔻YELD	Diabetic gangrene *AND* CC condition	250.70–250.73 See CC section.	■ Lower extremeity gangrene with no other "cause and effect" relationship, assume that the gangrene is the consequence of a diabetic peripheral vascular circulatory disorder, 250.70, add 785.4 for gangrene.

■ Coding Tip   ● Documentation Tip   ◆ Encoder Tip   🔻 Targeted DRG

Endocrine, Nutritional & Metabolic Disorders, MDC 10

DRG 295   (continued)

DRG	Principal Dx/Procedure	Codes	Tips
287	Diabetic ulceration 250.8x *AND* Excisonal debridement	707.9 86.22	● May be performed by physician or nonphysician health care provider performed by physician or nonphysician health care provider. ● Excisional debridement (cutting away) of necrotic, devitalized tissue or slough, may be described as "sharp debridement." Does not include the removal of loose fragments of skin by scissors.
296 ▽	Dehydration	276.5	■ NIDDM patients are prone to the development of a hyperosmolar state and dehydration. ◆ Key terms: hypovolemia, volume depletion. ■ IV hydration should be ordered for correct coding. If patient admitted with gastroenteritis and dehydration, w/IV hydration ordered, which necessitated the admission, 276.5 is the principal Dx. ■ An admission diagnosis of metabolic acidosis in a diabetic, may indicate an additional code diabetic acidosis (250.1) as underlying disease.
331	Diabetes with renal manifestations *AND* CC condition	250.40–250.43 See CC section.	

DRG 296▽ Nutritional & Miscellaneous Metabolic Disorders, Age > 17 with CC   RW 0.8639

Potential DRGs

| 288 | **O.R. Procedures for Obesity** | RW | 2.1498 |
| 320 | **Kidney and Urinary Tract Infections**, Age > 17 with CC | RW | 0.8853 |

DRG	Principal Dx/Procedure	Codes	Tips
288	O.R. procedure performed for obesity	*44.3	◆ Key terms for obesity: exogenous, familial, andogenous, adrenal due to hyperalimentation, morbid, pituitary, thyroid. ◆ Includes Printen and Mason gastric bypasses
320 ▽	Urinary tract infection with coexisting dehydration	599.0, 276.5	● Distinguish between use of term for UTI (localized infection entered the bloodstream) vs. generalized sepsis; only physician can determine sepsis.

Nutritional & Miscellaneous Metabolic Disorders, Age > 17 without CC

RW 0.5085 **DRG 297**

Potential DRGs

288	O.R. Procedures for Obesity	RW	2.1498
296	Nutritional & Miscellaneous Metabolic Disorders, Age > 17 with CC	RW	0.8639
321	Kidney and Urinary Tract Infections, Age > 17 without CC	RW	0.5685

DRG	Principal Dx/Procedure	Codes	Tips
288	O.R. procedure performed for obesity	*44.3	◆ Includes Printen and Mason gastric bypasses
296 ▽	Dehydration AND CC condition	276.5 See CC section.	■ NIDDM patients are prone to the development of a hyperosmolar state and dehydration. ◆ Key terms: hypovolemia, volume depletion. ■ IV hydration should be ordered for correct coding. If patient admitted with gastroenteritis and dehydration, w/IV hydration ordered, which necessitated the admission, 276.5 is the principal Dx. ■ An admission diagnosis of metabolic acidosis in a diabetic, may indicate an additional code, diabetic acidosis (250.1) as underlying disease.
321	Urinary tract infection	599.0	● Distinguish between use of term for UTI (localized infection entered the bloodstream) vs. generalized sepsis; only physician can determine sepsis.

Nutritional & Miscellaneous Metabolic Disorders, Age 0–17

RW 0.4537 **DRG 298**

Potential DRGs

288	O.R. Procedures for Obesity	RW	2.1498
296	Nutritional & Miscellaneous Metabolic Disorders, Age > 17 with CC	RW	0.8639
320	Kidney and Urinary Tract Infections, Age > 17 with CC	RW	0.8853

DRG	Principal Dx/Procedure	Codes	Tips
288	O.R. procedure performed for obesity	*44.3	◆ Includes Printen and Mason gastric bypasses
296 ▽	Dehydration AND CC condition	276.5 See CC section.	■ NIDDM patients are prone to the development of a hyperosmolar state and dehydration. ◆ Key terms: hypovolemia, volume depletion. ■ IV hydration should be ordered for correct coding. If patient admitted with gastroenteritis and dehydration, w/IV hydration ordered, which necessitated the admission, 276.5 is the principal Dx. ■ An admission diagnosis of metabolic acidosis in a diabetic, may indicate an additional code, diabetic acidosis (250.1) as underlying disease.
320	Urinary tract infection AND CC condition	599.0 See CC section.	● Distinguish between use of term for UTI (localized infection entered the bloodstream) vs. generalized sepsis; only physician can determine sepsis.

■ Coding Tip   ● Documentation Tip   ◆ Encoder Tip   ▽ Targeted DRG

DRG 299 Inborn Errors of Metabolism

No Potential DRGs

DRG 300 Endocrine Disorders with CC
RW 1.1001

Potential DRGs

010 Nervous System Neoplasms with CC
RW 1.2448

DRG	Principal Dx/Procedure	Codes	Tips
010	Malignant neoplasm, pineal gland *AND* CC condition	194.4 227.4 See CC section.	◆ Benign neoplasm, pineal gland

DRG 301 Endocrine Disorders without CC
RW 0.6158

Potential DRGs

011	Nervous System Neoplasms without CC	RW 0.8571
300	Endocrine Disorders with CC	RW 1.1001

DRG	Principal Dx/Procedure	Codes	Tips
011	Malignant neoplasm, pineal gland Benign neoplasm pineal gland	194.4 227.4	◆ Benign neoplasm, pineal gland
300	Toxic diffuse goiter *AND* CC condition	*242.0 See CC section.	◆ Key terms: Graves disease, Basedows disease

---

■ Coding Tip   ● Documentation Tip   ◆ Encoder Tip   ▽ Targeted DRG

Kidney and Urinary Tract, MDC 11

Kidney Transplant   DRG 302
No Potential DRGs

Kidney, Ureter and Major Bladder Procedures   DRG 303
for Neoplasm
No Potential DRGs

Kidney, Ureter & Major Bladder   RW 2.3856   DRG 304
Procedures for Non-neoplasm with CC

Potential DRGs

303   Kidney, Ureter & Major Bladder Procedures for Neoplasm   RW   2.3659

DRG	Principal Dx/Procedure	Codes	Tips
303	Open ureteral biopsy AND neoplasm	56.34	

Kidney, Ureter & Major Bladder   RW 1.1854   DRG 305
Procedures for Non-neoplasm without CC

Potential DRGs

303   Kidney, Ureter & Major Bladder Procedures for Neoplasm   RW   2.3659
304   Kidney, Ureter & Major Bladder Procedures for Non-neoplasm with CC   RW   2.3856

DRG	Principal Dx/Procedure	Codes	Tips
303	Open ureteral biopsy AND neoplasm	56.34	
304	Open ureteral biopsy AND CC condition	56.34 See CC section. 997.5, 788.20	◆ Common CC: urinary retention, post-op

Prostatectomy with CC   DRG 306
No Potential DRGs

Prostatectomy without CC   RW 0.6145   DRG 307

Potential DRGs

306   Prostatectomy with CC   RW   1.2257
344   Other Male Reproductive Procedures for Malignancy   RW   1.3306

DRG	Principal Dx/Procedure	Codes	Tips
306	Prostatectomy AND CC condition	*60.2, 60.3, 60.4, 60.5, *60.6, *60.9 See CC section. 997.5, 788.20	◆ Common CC: urinary retention, post-op
344	TURP AND Destruction lesion of bladder transurethral	57.49	

■ Coding Tip   ● Documentation Tip   ◆ Encoder Tip   ⱽᴰ Targeted DRG

Kidney and Urinary Tract, MDC 11

DRG 308   Minor Bladder Procedures with CC   RW 1.5993

Potential DRGs

304   Kidney, Ureter & **Major Bladder Procedures** for Non-neoplasm **with CC**   RW   2.3856

DRG	Principal Dx/Procedure	Codes	Tips
304	Open ureteral biopsy *AND* CC condition	56.34 See CC section. 997.5, 788.20	◆ Common CC: urinary retention, post-op

DRG 309   Minor Bladder Procedures without CC   RW 0.8991

Potential DRGs

304   Kidney, Ureter & **Major Bladder Procedures** for Non-neoplasm **with CC**   RW   2.3856
305   Kidney, Ureter & Major Bladder Procedures for Non-neoplasm **without** CC   RW   1.1854
308   Minor Bladder Procedures **with CC**   RW   1.5993

DRG	Principal Dx/Procedure	Codes	Tips
304	Percutaneous nephrostomy without fragmentation *OR* with fragmentation *AND* CC condition	55.03 55.04 See CC section. 997.5, 788.20	◆ Key terms: nephroscopic nephrostolithotomy, percutaneous pyelostolithotomy ■ Percutaneous nephrostomy with kidney stone disruption, with placement of catheter, with fluoroscopic guidance ◆ Common CC: urinary retention, post-op
305	Percutaneous nephrostomy without fragmentation *OR* with fragmentation	55.03 55.04	◆ Key terms: nephroscopic nephrostolithotomy, percutaneous pyelostolithotomy ■ Percutaneous nephrostomy with kidney stone disruption, with placement of catheter, with fluoroscopic guidance
308	Cystotomy NEC *AND* CC condition	57.19 See CC section. 997.5, 788.20	■ Cystolithotomy ◆ Common CC: urinary retention, post-op

DRG 310   Transurethral Procedures with CC   RW 1.1502

Potential DRGs

306   **Prostatectomy** with CC   RW   1.2257

DRG	Principal Dx/Procedure	Codes	Tips
306	Prostatectomy *AND* CC condition	*60.2, 60.3, 60.4, 60.5, *60.6, *60.9 See CC section. 997.5, 788.20	◆ Common CC: urinary retention, post-op

---

■ Coding Tip   ● Documentation Tip   ◆ Encoder Tip   ▽ Targeted DRG

Transurethral Procedures without CC   RW 0.6258   **DRG 311**

Potential DRGs

306	Prostatectomy with CC	RW	1.2257
310	Transurethral Procedures with CC	RW	1.1502

DRG	Principal Dx/Procedure	Codes	Tips
306	Prostatectomy *AND* CC condition	*60.2, 60.3, 60.4, 60.5, *60.6. *60.9 See CC section. 997.5, 788.20	◆ Common CC: urinary retention, post-op
310	Transurethral procedure *AND* CC condition	997.5, 788.20 See CC section.	◆ Common CC: urinary retention, post-op

Urethral Procedures, Age > 17 with CC   RW 1.0841   **DRG 312**

Potential DRGs

308	Minor Bladder Procedures with CC	RW	1.5993

DRG	Principal Dx/Procedure	Codes	Tips
308	Planned urethral procedure extends to bladder Sphincterotomy *AND* CC condition	57.91 See CC section. 997.5, 788.20	◆ Common CC: urinary retention, post-op

Urethral Procedure, Age > 17 without CC   RW 0.6814   **DRG 313**

Potential DRGs

308	Minor Bladder Procedures with CC	RW	1.5993
309	Minor Bladder Procedures without CC	RW	0.8991
312	Urethral Procedures, Age > 17 with CC	RW	1.0841

DRG	Principal Dx/Procedure	Codes	Tips
308	Planned urethral procedure extends to bladder Sphincterotomy *AND* CC condition	57.91 See CC section. 997.5, 788.20	◆ Common CC: urinary retention, post-op
309	Planned urethral procedure extends to bladder Sphincterotomy	57.91	
312	CC condition	See CC section. 997.5, 788.20	◆ Common CC: urinary retention, post-op

---

■ Coding Tip   ● Documentation Tip   ◆ Encoder Tip   ▼ Targeted DRG

DRG 314   Urethral Procedures, Age 0–17   RW 0.4984

Potential DRGs

308	Minor Bladder Procedures with CC	RW	1.5993
309	Minor Bladder Procedures without CC	RW	0.8991
312	Urethral Procedures, **Age > 17 with CC**	RW	1.0841
313	Urethral Procedures, **Age > 17** without CC	RW	0.6814

DRG	Principal Dx/Procedure	Codes	Tips
308	Planned urethral procedure extends to bladder Sphincterotomy *AND* CC condition	57.91 See CC section. 997.5, 788.20	◆ Common CC: urinary retention, post-op
309	Planned urethral procedure extends to bladder Sphincterotomy	57.91	
312	Patient's age > 17 *AND* CC condition	See CC section. 997.5, 788.20	◆ Common CC: urinary retention, post-op
313	Patient's age > 17		

DRG 315   Other Kidney and Urinary Tract Operating Room Procedures

No Potential DRGs

DRG 316   Renal Failure   RW 1.2987

Potential DRGs

315	Other Kidney & Urinary Tract O.R. Procedures	RW	2.0796

DRG	Principal Dx/Procedure	Codes	Tips
315	Operative procedure in preparation for renal dialysis	39.27	◆ Internal formation of AV shunt code 39.27. External vessel-to-vessel shunt (ex, Scribner) code 39.93.

DRG 317   Admit for Renal Dialysis   RW 0.8503

Potential DRGs

296	Nutritional & Miscellaneous Metabolic Disorders Age >17 with CC	RW	0.8639
315	Other Kidney & Urinary Tract O.R. Procedures	RW	2.0796

DRG	Principal Dx/Procedure	Codes	Tips
296 ▽	Fluid overload *AND* CC condition	276.6 See CC section.	■ Fluid overload is considered a component of CHF and should not be coded separately.
315	Operative procedure in preparation for renal dialysis	39.27	◆ Internal formation of AV shunt code 39.27. External vessel-to-vessel shunt (ex, Scribner) code 39.93.

DRG 318   Kidney & Urinary Tract Neoplasms with CC RW 1.1871

Potential DRGs

303	Kidney, Ureter & Major Bladder Procedures for Neoplasm	RW	2.3659

DRG	Principal Dx/Procedure	Codes	Tips
303	Open ureteral biopsy *AND* Neoplasm	56.34	

■ Coding Tip   ● Documentation Tip   ◆ Encoder Tip   ▽ Targeted DRG

Kidney & Urinary Tract Neoplasms without CC

RW 0.6771 **DRG 319**

Potential DRGs

303	Kidney, Ureter & Major Bladder Procedures for Neoplasm	RW	2.3659
318	Kidney & Urinary Tract Neoplasms **with CC**	RW	1.1871

DRG	Principal Dx/Procedure	Codes	Tips
303	Open ureteral biopsy *AND* Neoplasm	56.34	
318	CC condition	See CC section.	

Kidney & Urinary Tract Infections, Age > 17 with CC

RW 0.8853 ▽**DRG 320**

Potential DRGs

331	Other Kidney & Urinary Tract Diagnoses, Age > 17 with CC	RW	1.0618
416	Septicemia, Age > 17	RW	1.5918

DRG	Principal Dx/Procedure	Codes	Tips
331	Infection due to an indwelling urinary catheter *AND* CC condition	996.64, 599.0 See CC section.	
416 ▽	Septicemia	*038	■ Septicemia with pneumonia; code both. ● If sepsis is documented, it may be coded in absence of positive blood cultures.

Kidney & Urinary Tract Infections, Age > 17 without CC

RW 0.5685 **DRG 321**

Potential DRGs

296	Nutritional & Miscellaneous Metabolic Disorders, Age >17 **with CC**	RW	0.8639
320	Kidney & Urinary Tract Infections, Age > 17 **with CC**	RW	0.8853
331	Other Kidney & Urinary Tract Diagnoses, Age > 17 **with CC**	RW	1.0618
416	Septicemia, Age > 17	RW	1.5918

DRG	Principal Dx/Procedure	Codes	Tips
296 ▽	Dehydration *AND* CC condition	276.5 See CC section.	
320 ▽	Kidney infection Urinary tract infection *AND* CC condition	*590 599.0 See CC section.	
331	Infection due to an indwelling urinary catheter *AND* CC condition	996.64 599.0 See CC section.	
416 ▽	Septicemia	*038	■ Septicemia with pneumonia; code both. ● If sepsis is documented, it may be coded in absence of positive blood cultures.

■ Coding Tip   ● Documentation Tip   ◆ Encoder Tip   ▽ Targeted DRG

DRG 322 Kidney & Urinary Tract Infections, Age 0–17   RW 0.4625

Potential DRGs

320	Kidney & Urinary Tract Infections, **Age > 17 with CC**	RW	0.8853
333	**Other Kidney & Urinary Tract Diagnoses**, Age 0–17	RW	0.9483
416	**Septicemia, Age > 17**	RW	1.5918
417	**Septicemia**, Age 0–17	RW	0.9612

DRG	Principal Dx/Procedure	Codes	Tips
320 ▽	Kidney infection Urinary tract infection *AND* CC condition	*590 599.0 See CC section.	
333	Infection due to an indwelling urinary catheter	996.64, 599.0	
416 ▽	Septicemia *AND* Patient's age > 17	*038	■ Septicemia with pneumonia; code both. ● If sepsis is documented, it may be coded in absence of positive blood cultures.
417	Septicemia	*038	■ Septicemia with pneumonia; code both. ● If sepsis is documented, it may be coded in absence of positive blood cultures.

DRG 323 Urinary Stones with CC &/or Extracorporeal Shock Wave Lithotripsy   RW 0.8088

Potential DRGs

304	**Kidney, Ureter & Major Bladder Procedures for Non-neoplasm with CC**	RW	2.3856
305	**Kidney, Ureter & Major Bladder Procedures for Non-neoplasm** without CC	RW	1.1854

DRG	Principal Dx/Procedure	Codes	Tips
304	Percutaneous nephrostomy without fragmentation *OR* with fragmentation *AND* CC condition	55.03 55.04 See CC section. 997.5, 788.20	◆ Key terms: nephroscopic nephrostolithotomy, percutaneous pyelostolithotomy ■ Percutaneous nephrostomy with kidney stone disruption, with placement of catheter, with fluoroscopic guidance ◆ Common CC: Urinary retention, post-op
305	Percutaneous nephrostomy without fragmentation *OR* with fragmentation	55.03 55.04	◆ Key terms: nephroscopic nephrostolithotomy, percutaneous pyelostolithotomy ■ Percutaneous nephrostomy with kidney stone disruption, with placement of catheter, with fluoroscopic guidance

*Ensure accurate DRG assignment.
Listed below are the only principal diagnoses and procedures found in DRG 323:

274.11 Uric acid nephrolithiasis	594.2 Urethral calculus
591 Hydronephrosis	594.8 Lower urinary calculus NEC
592.0 Calculus of kidney	594.9 Lower urinary calculus NOS
592.1 Calculus of ureter	788.0 Renal colic with CC
592.9 Urinary calculus NOS	*AND*
593.4 Ureteric obstruction NEC	With or Without non-O.R. procedure
593.5 Hydroureter	98.51 Extracorporeal shock wave lithotripsy
594.1 Bladder calculus NEC	[ESWL] of the kidney, ureter &/or bladder

---

■ Coding Tip   ● Documentation Tip   ◆ Encoder Tip   ▽ Targeted DRG

©2003 Ingenix, Inc.

Urinary Stones without CC
RW 0.4797 **DRG 324**

Potential DRGs

304	Kidney, Ureter & Major Bladder Procedures for Non-neoplasm with CC	RW	2.3856
305	**Kidney, Ureter & Major Bladder Procedures for Non-neoplasm** without CC	RW	1.1854
310	**Transurethral Procedures** with CC	RW	1.1502
311	**Transurethral Procedures** without CC	RW	0.6258
323	Urinary Stones **with CC &/or Extracorporeal Shock Wave Lithotripsy**	RW	0.8088

DRG	Principal Dx/Procedure	Codes	Tips
304	Percutaneous nephrostomy without fragmentation	55.03	◆ Key terms: nephroscopic nephrostolithotomy, percutaneous pyelostolithotomy
	OR with fragmentation	55.04	■ Percutaneous nephrostomy with kidney stone disruption, with placement of catheter, with fluoroscopic guidance
	AND CC condition	See CC section. 997.5, 788.20	◆ Common CC: Urinary retention, post-op
305	Percutaneous nephrostomy without fragmentation	55.03	◆ Key terms: nephroscopic nephrostolithotomy, percutaneous pyelostolithotomy
	OR with fragmentation	55.04	■ Percutaneous nephrostomy with kidney stone disruption, with placement of catheter, with fluoroscopic guidance
310	Transurethral removal of urinary stones from ureter and renal pelvis	56.0	
	AND CC condition	See CC section. 997.5, 788.20	◆ Common CC: urinary retention, post-op
311	Transurethral removal of urinary stones from ureter and renal pelvis	56.0	
323	CC condition	See CC section. 997.5, 788.20	◆ Common CC: urinary retention, post-op

Kidney and Urinary Tract Signs and Symptoms, Age >17 with CC
RW 0.6553 **DRG 325**

Potential DRGs

316	**Renal Failure**	RW	1.2987
320	Kidney and Urinary Tract Infections, Age >17 **with CC**	RW	0.8853
331	Other Kidney and Urinary Tract Diagnoses, Age >17 **with CC**	RW	1.0618

DRG	Principal Dx/Procedure	Codes	Tips
316 ▽YIELD	Anuria, oliguria	584.9, 585, 788.5	■ Prenatal/postrenal azotemia (788.9) may be used in reference to acute or chronic renal failure. Further clarify with physician for underlying cause. ■ Anuria, oliguria Deficient secretion of urine, suppression of urinary secretion
	Renal failure	586	■ Uremia, NOS
320 ▽YIELD	Kidney infection	*590	
	Urinary tract infection	599.0	
	AND CC condition	See CC section.	
331	Underlying disease causing the signs & symptoms (e.g., nephrotic syndrome with an unspecified pathological lesion)	581.9	
	AND CC condition	See CC section.	

■ Coding Tip   ● Documentation Tip   ◆ Encoder Tip   ▽YIELD Targeted DRG

Kidney and Urinary Tract, MDC 11

DRG 326   Kidney & Urinary Tract Signs & Symptoms, Age > 17 without CC   RW 0.4206

Potential DRGs

316	**Renal Failure**	RW	1.2987
320	**Kidney and Urinary Tract Infections**, Age > 17 **with CC**	RW	0.8853
321	**Kidney & Urinary Tract Infections**, Age > 17 without CC	RW	0.5685
325	Kidney & Urinary Tract Signs & Symptoms, Age > 17 **with CC**	RW	0.6553
332	**Other Kidney & Urinary Tract Diagnoses**, Age > 17 without CC	RW	0.5982

DRG	Principal Dx/Procedure	Codes	Tips
316 ▽	Anuria, oliguria Renal failure	584.9, 585, 788.5 586	■ Prerenal/postrenal azotemia (788.9) may be used in reference to acute or chronic renal failure. Further clarify with physician for underlying cause. ■ Anuria, oliguria Deficient secretion of urine, suppression of urinary secretion ■ Uremia, NOS
320 ▽	Kidney infection Urinary tract infection *AND* CC condition	*590 599.0 See CC section.	
321	Kidney infection Urinary tract infection	*590 599.0	
325	CC condition	See CC section.	
332	Underlying disease causing the signs & symptoms (e.g., nephrotic syndrome with an unspecified pathological lesion)	581.9	◆ Epstein's tubular, specify lesion

DRG 327   Kidney & Urinary Tract Signs & Symptoms, Age 0–17   RW 0.3727

Potential DRGs

316	**Renal Failure**	RW	1.2987
333	**Other Kidney & Urinary Tract Diagnoses**, Age 0–17	RW	0.9483

DRG	Principal Dx/Procedure	Codes	Tips
316 ▽	Renal failure Anuria, oliguria	584.9, 585, 586 788.5	■ Prerenal/postrenal azotemia (788.9) may be used in reference to acute or chronic renal failure. Further clarify with physician for underlying cause. ■ Uremia, NOS ■ Deficient secretion of urine; suppression of urinary secretion
333	Underlying disease causing the signs & symptoms (e.g., nephrotic syndrome with an unspecified pathological lesion)	581.9	◆ Epstein's tubular, specify lesion

---

Urethral Stricture, Age > 17 with CC RW 0.7613 **DRG 328**

Potential DRGs

320	**Kidney & Urinary Tract Infections**, Age > 17 with CC	RW	0.8853
331	**Other Kidney & Urinary Tract Diagnoses**, Age > 17 with CC	RW	1.0618

DRG	Principal Dx/Procedure	Codes	Tips
320 ▽YIELD	Kidney infection Urinary tract infection *AND* CC condition	*590 599.0 See CC section.	
331	Infection due to an indwelling urinary catheter *AND* CC condition	996.64, 599.0 See CC section.	

Urethral Stricture, Age > 17 without CC RW 0.5296 **DRG 329**

Potential DRGs

320	**Kidney & Urinary Tract Infections**, Age > 17 with CC	RW	0.8853
321	**Kidney & Urinary Tract Infections**, Age > 17 without CC	RW	0.5685
328	Urethral Stricture, Age > 17 **with CC**	RW	0.7613
331	**Other Kidney & Urinary Tract Diagnoses**, Age > 17 **with CC**	RW	1.0618
332	**Other Kidney & Urinary Tract Diagnoses**, Age > 17 without CC	RW	0.5982

DRG	Principal Dx/Procedure	Codes	Tips
320 ▽YIELD	Kidney infection Urinary tract infection *AND* CC condition	*590 599.0 See CC section.	
321	Kidney infection Urinary tract infection	*590 599.0	
328	CC condition	See CC section.	
331	Infection due to an indwelling urinary catheter *AND* CC condition	996.64, 599.0 See CC section.	
332	Urethral stricture due to urinary tract procedure	598.2	

Urethral Stricture, Age 0–17 RW 0.3210 **DRG 330**

Potential DRGs

322	**Kidney & Urinary Tract Infections**, Age 0–17	RW	0.4625
328	Urethral Stricture, **Age > 17 with CC**	RW	0.7613
329	Urethral Stricture, **Age > 17 without CC**	RW	0.5296

DRG	Principal Dx/Procedure	Codes	Tips
322	Kidney infection Urinary tract infection	*590 599.0	
328	Patient's age > 17 *AND* CC condition	598.2 See CC section.	◆ Common CC: post-op urethral stricture
329	Patient's age > 17 *AND* Traumatic urethral stricture	598.1	

DRG 331▽ Other Kidney & Urinary Tract Diagnoses,   RW 1.0618
Age > 17 with CC

Potential DRGs

316	**Renal Failure**	RW	1.2987
484	Craniotomy for **Multiple Significant Trauma**	RW	5.4179
486	**Other O.R. Procedures for Multiple Significant Trauma**	RW	4.8793
487	Other **Multiple Significant Trauma**	RW	2.0057

DRG	Principal Dx/Procedure	Codes	Tips
316 ▽ᵧᵢₑₗ𝒹	Renal failure Anuria, oliguria	584.9, 585, 586 788.5	■ Prenal/postrenal azotemia (788.9) may be used in reference to acute or chronic renal failure. Further clarify with physician for underlying cause. ■ Uremia, NOS ■ Deficient secretion of urine, suppression of urinary secretion
484	Craniotomy for multiple significant trauma		■ Craniotomy and principal diagnosis of trauma and at least two injuries (assigned either as principal or secondary) that are defined as significant trauma from different body site categories located under DRG 487
486	Other O.R. procedures for multiple significant trauma		■ Principal diagnosis of trauma and at least two injuries (assigned either as principal or secondary) that are defined as significant trauma from different body site categories located under DRG 487 *AND* O.R. procedure other than craniotomy or limb reattachment, hip and femur procedures
487	Other multiple significant trauma		■ Principal diagnosis of trauma and at least two injuries (assigned either as principal or secondary) that are defined as significant trauma from different body site categories located under DRG 487

■ Coding Tip   ● Documentation Tip   ◆ Encoder Tip   ▽ Targeted DRG

Other Kidney & Urinary Tract Diagnoses, Age > 17 without CC

RW 0.5982 **DRG 332**

Potential DRGs

316	Renal Failure	RW	1.2987
331	Other Kidney & Urinary Tract Diagnoses, Age > 17 **with CC**	RW	1.0618
333	Other Kidney & Urinary Tract Diagnoses, **Age 0–17**	RW	0.9483
484	Craniotomy for **Multiple Significant Trauma**	RW	5.4179
486	**Other O.R. Procedures for Multiple Significant Trauma**	RW	4.8793
487	**Other Multiple Significant Trauma**	RW	2.0057

DRG	Principal Dx/Procedure	Codes	Tips
316 ▽	Renal failure	584.9, 585, 586	■ Prerenal/postrenal azotemia (788.9) may be used in reference to acute or chronic renal failure. Further clarify with physician for underlying cause.
			■ Uremia, NOS
	Anuria, oliguria	788.5	■ Deficient secretion of urine, suppression of urinary secretion
331	Infection due to an indwelling urinary catheter	996.64, 599.0	
	AND CC condition	See CC section.	
333	Patient's age 0–17 *AND* Infection due to an indwelling urinary catheter	996.64, 599.0	
484	Craniotomy for multiple significant trauma		■ Craniotomy and principal diagnosis of trauma and at least two injuries (assigned either as principal or secondary) that are defined as significant trauma from different body site categories located under DRG 487
486	Other O.R. procedures for multiple significant trauma		■ Principal diagnosis of trauma and at least two injuries (assigned either as principal or secondary) that are defined as significant trauma from different body site categories located under DRG 487 *AND* O.R. procedure other than craniotomy or limb reattachment, hip and femur procedures
487	Other multiple significant trauma		■ Principal diagnosis of trauma and at least two injuries (assigned either as principal or secondary) that are defined as significant trauma from different body site categories located under DRG 487

■ Coding Tip　　● Documentation Tip　　◆ Encoder Tip　　▽ Targeted DRG

DRG 333   Other Kidney & Urinary Tract Diagnoses,   RW 0.9483
Age 0–17

Potential DRGs

316	Renal Failure	RW	1.2987
484	Craniotomy for **Multiple Significant Trauma**	RW	5.4179
486	**Other O.R. Procedures for Multiple Significant Trauma**	RW	4.8793
487	**Other Multiple Significant Trauma**	RW	2.0057

DRG	Principal Dx/Procedure	Codes	Tips
316 ▽	Renal failure Anuria, oliguria	584.9, 585, 586 788.5	■ Prenal/postrenal azotemia (788.9) may be used in reference to acute or chronic renal failure. Further clarify with physician for underlying cause. ■ Uremia, NOS ■ Deficient secretion of urine, suppression of urinary secretion
484	Craniotomy for multiple significant trauma		■ Craniotomy and principal diagnosis of trauma and at least two injuries (assigned either as principal or secondary) that are defined as significant trauma from different body site categories located under DRG 487
486	Other O.R. procedures for multiple significant trauma		■ Principal diagnosis of trauma and at least two injuries (assigned either as principal or secondary) that are defined as significant trauma from different body site categories located under DRG 487 *AND* O.R. procedure other than craniotomy or limb reattachment, hip and femur procedures
487	Other multiple significant trauma		■ Principal diagnosis of trauma and at least two injuries (assigned either as principal or secondary) that are defined as significant trauma from different body site categories located under DRG 487

Male Reproductive System, MDC 12

Major Male Pelvic Procedures with CC   RW 1.4810 **DRG 334**

Potential DRGs

304   Kidney, Ureter & Major Bladder Procedures for Non-neoplasm with CC   RW   2.3856

DRG	Principal Dx/Procedure	Codes	Tips
304	Open renal biopsy *AND* Urinary system postoperative complication	55.24	
	Infection from indwelling urinary catheter	996.64	
	Post-op complication of urinary system	997.5	■ Oliguria, anuria, renal failure specified as due to a procedure

Major Male Pelvic Procedures without CC   RW 1.0835 **DRG 335**

Potential DRGs

304   Kidney, Ureter & Major Bladder Procedures for Non-neoplasm with CC   RW   2.3856
334   Major Male Pelvic Procedures with CC   RW   1.4810

DRG	Principal Dx/Procedure	Codes	Tips
304	Open renal biopsy *AND* Urinary system postoperative complication	55.24	
	Infection from indwelling urinary catheter	996.64	
	Post-op complication of urinary system	997.5	■ Oliguria, anuria, renal failure specified as due to a procedure
334	Partial cystectomy Urinary system postoperative complication infection from indwelling urinary catheter	57.6 996.64	◆ Key terms: excision of bladder dome, trigonectomy, wedge resection
	Post-op complication of urinary system	997.5	■ Oliguria, anuria, renal failure specified as due to a procedure

Transurethral Prostatectomy with CC   RW 0.8595 **DRG 336**

Potential DRGs

306   **Prostatectomy** with CC   RW   1.2257
344   Other Male Reproductive System OR Procedures for Malignancy   RW   1.3306

DRG	Principal Dx/Procedure	Codes	Tips
306	Prostatectomy	*60.2, 60.3, 60.4, 60.5, *60.6, *60.9	◆ Key terms: loop radical (includes prostate, seminal vesicles, and vas ampullae), TULIP-VLAP, TUNA, TUMT. ■ Codes * 60.2, 60.96, 60.97: Principal diagnosis determines DRG assignment from list of codes in MDC 11 versus MDC 12.
	Urinary system postoperative complication	596.0, 598.8	
	Infection from indwelling urinary catheter	996.64	■ If bladder neck obstruction or uretheral stricture is due to some other condition other than BPH assign as principal. When due to BPH, code BPH as principal.
	Post-op complication of urinary system *AND* CC condition	997.5 See CC section.	■ Oliguria, anuria, renal failure specified as due to a procedure

---

■ Coding Tip   ● Documentation Tip   ◆ Encoder Tip   ▽ Targeted DRG

Male Reproductive System, MDC 12

DRG 336   (continued)

DRG	Principal Dx/Procedure	Codes	Tips
344	Destruction malignant lesion of bladder neck	57.49	■ Endoscopic resection of bladder lesion
	AND CC condition	See CC section.	
	Urinary system postoperative complication		
	Infection from indwelling urinary catheter	996.64	
	Post-op complication of urinary system	997.5	■ Oliguria, anuria, renal failure specified as due to a procedure

DRG 337   Transurethral Prostatectomy without CC   RW 0.5869

Potential DRGs

306	**Prostatectomy with CC**	RW	1.2257
307	**Prostatectomy** without CC	RW	0.6145
336	Transurethral Prostatectomy **with CC**	RW	0.8595
344	**Other Male Reproductive System O.R. Procedures for Malignancy**	RW	1.3306

DRG	Principal Dx/Procedure	Codes	Tips
306	Prostatectomy	*60.2, 60.3, 60.4, 60.5, *60.6, *60.9	◆ Key terms: loop radical (includes prostate, seminal vesicles, and vas ampullae), TULIP-VLAP, TUNA, TUMT. ■ Codes * 60.2, 60.96, 60.97: Principal diagnosis determines DRG assignment from list of codes in MDC 11 versus MDC 12.
	Urinary system postoperative complication	596.0, 598.8	
	Infection from indwelling urinary catheter	996.64	■ If bladder neck obstruction or uretheral stricture is due to some other condition other than BPH assign as principal. When due to BPH, code BPH as principal.
	Post-op complication of urinary system	997.5	■ Oliguria, anuria, renal failure specified
	AND CC conditions	See CC section.	as due to a procedure
307	Prostatectomy	*60.2, 60.3, 60.4, 60.5, *60.6, *60.9	◆ Key terms: loop radical (includes prostate, seminal vesicles, and vas ampullae), TULIP-VLAP, TUNA, TUMT. ■ Codes * 60.2, 60.96, 60.97: Principal diagnosis determines DRG assignment from list of codes in MDC 11 versus MDC 12. ■ If bladder neck obstruction or uretheral stricture is due to some other condition other than BPH assign as principal. When due to BPH, code BPH as principal.
336	TURP	*60.2, 60.96, 60.97	■ Codes * 60.2, 60.96, 60.97: Principal diagnosis determines DRG assignment from list of codes in MDC 11 versus MDC 12.
	AND CC condition	See CC section.	
	Urinary system postoperative complication		■ If bladder neck obstruction or uretheral stricture is due to some other condition other than BPH assign as principal. When due to BPH, code BPH as principal.
	Infection from indwelling urinary catheter	996.64	
	Post-op complication of urinary system	997.5	■ Oliguria, anuria, renal failure specified as due to a procedure

(continued)   **DRG 337**

DRG	Principal Dx/Procedure	Codes	Tips
344	Destruction malignant lesion of bladder neck	57.49	■ Endoscopic resection of bladder lesion
	AND CC condition	See CC section.	
	Urinary system postoperative complication		
	Infection from indwelling urinary catheter	996.64	
	Post-op complication of urinary system	997.5	■ Oliguria, anuria, renal failure specified as due to a procedure

Testes Procedures for Malignancy   **DRG 338**
No Potential DRGs

Testes Procedures for Nonmalignancy,   RW 1.1345   **DRG 339**
Age > 17

Potential DRGs
338 Testes Procedures for **Malignancy**   RW 1.2316
344 Other Male Reproductive System O.R. Procedures for **Malignancy**   RW 1.3306

DRG	Principal Dx/Procedure	Codes	Tips
338	Malignant neoplasm of testis	*186	◆ Key term: ectopic, retained
344	Procedure for malignant neoplasm	60.73	◆ Key terms: excision of Mullerian duct cyst, spermatocystectomy
	AND CC condition	See CC section.	
	Urinary system postoperative complication		
	Infection from indwelling urinary catheter	996.64	
	Post-op complication of urinary system	997.5	■ Oliguria, anuria, renal failure specified as due to a procedure

Testes Procedures for Nonmalignancy,   RW 0.2853   **DRG 340**
Age 0–17

Potential DRGs
338 Testes Procedures for **Malignancy**   RW 1.2316
339 Testes Procedures for Nonmalignancy, **Age > 17**   RW 1.1345

DRG	Principal Dx/Procedure	Codes	Tips
338	Malignant neoplasm of testis	*186	◆ Key term: ectopic, retained
339	Patient's age > 17		
	AND Open biopsy testis	62.12	

Penis Procedures   **DRG 341**
No Potential DRGs

Circumcision, Age > 17   **DRG 342**
No Potential DRGs

■ Coding Tip   ● Documentation Tip   ◆ Encoder Tip   ▽ Targeted DRG

Male Reproductive System, MDC 12

DRG 343 Circumcision, Age 0-17   RW 0.1551

Potential DRGs
342   Circumcision, Age > 17   RW   0.7800

DRG	Principal Dx/Procedure	Codes	Tips
342	Patient's age > 17		

DRG 344 Other Male Reproductive O.R. Procedures for Malignancy

No Potential DRGs

DRG 345 Other Male Reproductive System   RW 1.1671
O.R. Procedures Except for Malignancy

Potential DRGs
344   Other Male Reproductive System O.R. Procedures for Malignancy   RW   1.3306

DRG	Principal Dx/Procedure	Codes	Tips
344	Destruction malignant lesion of bladder neck *AND* CC condition Urinary system postoperative complication	57.49 See CC section.	■ Endoscopic resection of bladder lesion
	Infection from indwelling urinary catheter	996.64	
	Post-op complication of urinary system	997.5	■ Oliguria, anuria, renal failure specified as due to a procedure

DRG 346 Malignancy of Male Reproductive System   RW 1.0213
with CC

Potential DRGs
334   Major Male Pelvic Procedures with CC   RW   1.4810
341   Penis Procedures   RW   1.2739
344   Other Male Reproductive System O.R. Procedures for Malignancy   RW   1.3306

DRG	Principal Dx/Procedure	Codes	Tips
334	Partial cystectomy *AND* CC condition Urinary system postoperative complication	57.6 See CC section.	◆ Key terms: excision of bladder dome, trigonectomy, wedge resection
	Infection from indwelling urinary catheter	996.64	
	Post-op complication of urinary system	997.5	■ Oliguria, anuria, renal failure specified as due to a procedure
341	Penis procedures Release of urethral stricture	58.5	◆ Key term: urethrolysis
344	Destruction malignant lesion of bladder neck *AND* CC condition Urinary system postoperative complication	57.49 See CC section.	■ Endoscopic resection of bladder lesion
	Infection from indwelling urinary catheter	996.64	
	Post-op complication of urinary system	997.5	■ Oliguria, anuria, renal failure specified as due to a procedure

---

■ Coding Tip   ● Documentation Tip   ◆ Encoder Tip   ▽ Targeted DRG

Malignancy of Male Reproductive System without CC RW 0.5417 **DRG 347**

Potential DRGs

344	Other Male Reproductive System O.R. Procedures for Malignancy	RW	1.3306
346	Malignancy of Male Reproductive System with CC	RW	1.0213

DRG	Principal Dx/Procedure	Codes	Tips
344	Destruction malignant lesion of bladder neck	57.49	■ Endoscopic resection of bladder lesion
	AND CC condition	See CC section.	
	Urinary system postoperative complication		
	Infection from indwelling urinary catheter	996.64	
	Post-op complication of urinary system	997.5	■ Oliguria, anuria, renal failure specified as due to a procedure
346	Malignant neoplasm of prostate	185	
	AND CC condition	See CC section.	

Benign Prostatic Hypertrophy with CC RW 0.7472 **DRG 348**

*Ensure accurate DRG assignment.
Listed below is the only code found in DRG 348:
*600.0 Hyperplasia of prostate

Benign Prostatic Hypertrophy without CC RW 0.4608 **DRG 349**

Potential DRGs

348	Benign Prostatic Hypertrophy with CC	RW	0.7472

DRG	Principal Dx/Procedure	Codes	Tips
348	CC condition	See CC section.	

Inflammation of the Male Reproductive System RW 0.7370 **DRG 350**

Potential DRGs

336	Transurethral Prostatectomy with CC	RW	0.8595

DRG	Principal Dx/Procedure	Codes	Tips
336	TURP	*60.2	
	AND CC condition	See CC section.	
	Urinary system postoperative complication		
	Infection from indwelling urinary catheter	996.64	
	Post-op complication of urinary system	997.5	■ Oliguria, anuria, renal failure specified as due to a procedure

Sterilization, Male RW 0.2379 **DRG 351**

*Ensure accurate DRG assignment.
Listed below is the only principal diagnosis code found in DRG 351:
   V25.2 Sterilization

■ Coding Tip   ● Documentation Tip   ◆ Encoder Tip   ▽ Targeted DRG

DRG 352   Other Male Reproductive System Diagnoses   RW 0.7097

Potential DRGs

346   Malignancy of Male Reproductive System with CC   RW   1.0213

DRG	Principal Dx/Procedure	Codes	Tips
346	Malignant neoplasm of prostate *AND* CC condition	185 See CC section.	

Female Reproductive System, MDC 13

DRG 353   Pelvic Evisceration, Radical Hysterectomy and Radical Vulvectomy

No Potential DRGs

DRG 354   Uterine, Adnexa Procedures for Non-Ovarian/Adnexal Malignancy with CC   RW 1.4808

Potential DRGs

357   Uterine and Adnexa Procedures for Ovarian or Adnexal Malignancy   RW   2.2737

DRG	Principal Dx/Procedure	Codes	Tips
357	Malignancy of ovary or uterine adnexa *AND* Related procedure	*183, *65	◆ Includes: primary, secondary, and uncertain behavior ● Includes tissue of ovaries and accessory parts: fallopian tube, broad ligament, round ligament

DRG 355   Uterine, Adnexa Procedures for Nonovarian/Adnexal Malignancy without CC   RW 0.8912

Potential DRGs

354   Uterine, Adnexa Procedures for Nonovarian/Adnexal Malignancy with CC   RW   1.4808

DRG	Principal Dx/Procedure	Codes	Tips
354	Malignant neoplasm , uterus, NOS Open uterine biopsy	179 68.13	■ Post-op ileus: ileus can be an expected event after abdominal surgery and is not a complication unless it is prolonged (usually over six days). It may mean status-post the procedure—not that this is necessarily a complication. Query the physician.
	AND CC condition	See CC section. 997.4, 560.1	■ Post-op ileus-key terms: adynamic, inhibitory, neurogenic, paralytic

DRG 356   Female Reproductive System Reconstruction Procedures

No Potential DRGs

DRG 357   Uterine and Adnexal Procedures for Ovarian or Adnexal Malignancy

No Potential DRGs

■ Coding Tip   ● Documentation Tip   ◆ Encoder Tip   ▽ Targeted DRG

Uterine & Adnexa Procedures for Nonmalignancy with CC
RW 1.1807 **DRG 358**

Potential DRGs
357   Uterine & Adnexa Procedures for Ovarian or Adnexal Malignancy   RW   2.2737

DRG	Principal Dx/Procedure	Codes	Tips
357	Malignancy of ovary or adnexa *AND* Related procedure	*183 *65	◆ Includes: primary, secondary, and uncertain behavior ● Includes tissue of ovaries and accessory parts: fallopian tube, broad ligament, round ligament

Uterine & Adnexa Procedures for Nonmalignancy without CC
RW 0.8099 **DRG 359**

Potential DRGs
357   Uterine & Adnexa Procedures for Ovarian or Adnexal Malignancy   RW   2.2737
358   Uterine & Adnexa Procedures for Nonmalignancy with CC   RW   1.1807

DRG	Principal Dx/Procedure	Codes	Tips
357	Malignancy of ovary or adnexa *AND* Related procedure	*183 *65	◆ Includes: primary, secondary, and uncertain behavior ● Includes tissue of ovaries and accessory parts: fallopian tube, broad ligament, round ligament
358	Laparoscopic biopsy of ovary	65.13	■ Post-op ileus: ileus can be an expected event after abdominal surgery and is not a complication unless it is prolonged (usually over six days). It may mean status-post the procedure—not that this is necessarily a complication. Query the physician. ■ Post-op ileus-key terms: adynamic, inhibitory, neurogenic, paralytic
	AND CC condition	See CC section. 997.4, 560.1	

Vagina, Cervix and Vulva Procedures
DRG 360
No Potential DRGs

Laparoscopy and Incisional Tubal Interruption
DRG 361
No Potential DRGs

Endoscopic Tubal Interruption
RW 0.3041 **DRG 362**

Potential DRGs
361   **Laparoscopy & Incisional** Tubal Interruption   RW   1.0793

DRG	Principal Dx/Procedure	Codes	Tips
361	Incisional tubal interruption	66.31, 66.39	■ Includes destruction of solitary fallopian tube

Dilation and Curettage, Conization and Radio-Implant for Malignancy
DRG 363
No Potential DRGs

■ Coding Tip   ● Documentation Tip   ◆ Encoder Tip   ▽ Targeted DRG

Female Reproductive System, MDC 13

DRG 364 Dilation & Curettage & Conization Except for Malignancy   RW 0.9098

Potential DRGs

363   Dilation & Curettage, Conization & Radio-implant for Malignancy   RW   0.9374

DRG	Principal Dx/Procedure	Codes	Tips
363	Malignant neoplasm of uterus, NOS *AND* D&C *OR* Radio-implant	179 69.09 92.27	■ Diagnostic D&C, D&C for removal of blighted ovum

DRG 365 Other Female Reproductive System Operating Room Procedures

No Potential DRGs

DRG 366 Malignancy of Female Reproductive System with CC   RW 1.2826

Potential DRGs

354   Uterine & Adnexa Procedures for Nonovarian/Adnexal Malignancy with CC   RW   1.4808
357   Uterine & Adnexa Procedures for Ovarian or Adnexal Malignancy   RW   2.2737

DRG	Principal Dx/Procedure	Codes	Tips
354	Malignant neoplasm, uterus, NOS Open uterine biopsy	179 68.13	■ Post-op ileus: ileus can be an expected event after abdominal surgery and is not a complication unless it is prolonged (usually over six days). It may mean status-post the procedure—not that this is necessarily a complication. Query the physician.
	AND CC condition	See CC section. 997.4, 560.1	■ Post-op ileus-key terms: adynamic, inhibitory, neurogenic, paralytic
357	Malignancy of ovary or adnexa *AND* Related procedure	*183 *65	◆ Includes: primary, secondary, and uncertain behavior ● Includes tissue of ovaries and accessory parts: fallopian tube, broad ligament, round ligament

DRG 367 Malignancy of Female Reproductive System without CC   RW 0.5588

Potential DRGs

354   Uterine & Adnexa Procedures for Nonovarian/Adnexal Malignancy with CC   RW   1.4808
355   Uterine & Adnexa Procedures for Nonovarian/Adnexal Malignancy without CC   RW   0.8912
357   Uterine & Adnexa Procedures for Ovarian or Adnexal Malignancy   RW   2.2737
366   Malignancy of Female Reproductive System with CC   RW   1.2826

DRG	Principal Dx/Procedure	Codes	Tips
354	Malignant neoplasm, uterus, NOS Open uterine biopsy	179 68.13	■ Post-op ileus: ileus can be an expected event after abdominal surgery and is not a complication unless it is prolonged (usually over six days). It may mean status-post the procedure—not that this is necessarily a complication. Query the physician.
	AND CC condition	See CC section. 997.4, 560.1	■ Post-op ileus-key terms: adynamic, inhibitory, neurogenic, paralytic

---

■ Coding Tip   ● Documentation Tip   ◆ Encoder Tip   ▧ Targeted DRG

(continued) **DRG 367**

DRG	Principal Dx/Procedure	Codes	Tips
355	Malignant neoplasm , uterus, NOS *AND* Open uterine biopsy	179 68.13	
357	Malignancy of ovary or adnexa *AND* Related procedure	*183 *65	◆ Includes: primary, secondary, and uncertain behavior ● Includes tissue of ovaries and accessory parts: fallopian tube, broad ligament, round ligament
366	Malignant neoplasm adnexa *AND* CC condition	183.8 See CC section.	◆ Key terms: tubo-ovarian, utero-ovarian

Infections of the Female Reproductive System **DRG 368**

No Potential DRGs

Menstrual & Other Female Reproductive System Disorders RW 0.6065 **DRG 369**

Potential DRGs
366   Malignancy of Female Reproductive System with CC   RW   1.2826

DRG	Principal Dx/Procedure	Codes	Tips
366	Malignant neoplasm adnexa *AND* CC condition	183.8 See CC section.	◆ Key terms: tubo-ovarian, utero-ovarian

Pregnancy, Childbirth & Puerperium, MDC 14

Cesarean Section with CC **DRG 370**

No Potential DRGs

Cesarean Section without CC RW 0.6317 **DRG 371**

Potential DRGs
370   Cesarean Section with CC   RW   1.0119

DRG	Principal Dx/Procedure	Codes	Tips
370	CC condition	See CC section. 997.4, 560.1	■ Post-op ileus: ileus can be an expected event after abdominal surgery and is not a complication unless it is prolonged (usually over six days). It may mean status-post the procedure—not that this is necessarily a complication. Query the physician. ■ Post-op ileus-key terms: adynamic, inhibitory, neurogenic, paralytic

■ Coding Tip   ● Documentation Tip   ◆ Encoder Tip   ▽ Targeted DRG

DRG 372 Vaginal Delivery with Complicating Diagnoses RW 0.5520

Potential DRGs

374 Vaginal Delivery with Sterilization &/or D&C RW 0.7402

DRG	Principal Dx/Procedure	Codes	Tips
374	D&C NEC Aspiration curettage *OR* Female sterilization procedure	69.09 69.52 66.69	■ Includes: D&C for removal of blighted ovum ♦ Key terms: by cauterization, electrocoagulation, coagulation

DRG 373 Vaginal Delivery without Complicating Diagnoses RW 0.3856

Potential DRGs

372 Vaginal Delivery with Complicating Diagnoses RW 0.5520
374 Vaginal Delivery with Sterilization &/or D&C RW 0.7402
375 Vaginal Delivery with O.R. Procedures Except Sterilization &/or D&C RW 0.5806

DRG	Principal Dx/Procedure	Codes	Tips
372	Placenta previa Hypertension Diabetes Postpartum hemorrhage Anesthesia complications Embolism Infections Mastitis	641.11 642.01 648.01 666.12 668.81 673.01 675.01 675.21	♦ Key terms: incomplete, marginal, partial, total ♦ Key terms: benign, essential, chronic, pre-existing ■ Includes: uterine atony ■ Includes: nipple abscess ■ Includes: lymphangitis of breast
374	D&C NEC Aspiration curettage *OR* Female sterilization procedure	69.09 69.52 69.69	■ Includes: D&C for removal of blighted ovum ♦ Key terms: by cauterization, electrocoagulation, coagulation
375	Selected O.R. procedure except D&C and/or sterilization procedure: cervical biopsy	67.12	■ Includes: punch biopsy

DRG 374 Vaginal delivery with Sterlization and/or Dilation and Curettage

No Potential DRGs

DRG 375 Vaginal Delivery with Operating Room Procedures Except Sterlization and/or Dilation and Curettage

No Potential DRGs

DRG 376 Postpartum & Postabortion Diagnoses without O.R. Procedure RW 0.5693

Potential DRGs

377 Postpartum & Postabortion Diagnoses with O.R. Procedure RW 1.0321

DRG	Principal Dx/Procedure	Codes	Tips
377	Any O.R. procedure		

■ Coding Tip   ● Documentation Tip   ♦ Encoder Tip   ▼ Targeted DRG

Postpartum and Postabortion Diagnoses with Operating Room Procedure
DRG 377

No Potential DRGs

Ectopic Pregnancy
DRG 378

No Potential DRGs

Threatened Abortion
RW 0.3626 **DRG 379**

Potential DRGs
381   Abortion with **Dilation & Curettage, Aspiration Curettage or Hysterotomy**   RW   0.5257

DRG	Principal Dx/Procedure	Codes	Tips
381	Spontaneous or missed abortion **WITH** Dilatation and curettage Aspiration curettage postdelivery Hysterotomy	632 69.01 69.52 74.91	■ Intravaginal misoprostol (Cytotec) placed for induction of labor is an abortifacient used for missed abortions. ■ Includes: Therapeutic abortion by hysterotomy

Abortion without Dilation & Curettage
RW 0.4323 **DRG 380**

Potential DRGs
381   Abortion with Dilation & Curettage, Aspiration Curettage or Hysterotomy   RW   0.5257

DRG	Principal Dx/Procedure	Codes	Tips
381	Spontaneous or missed abortion **WITH** Dilatation and curettage Aspiration curettage postdelivery Hysterotomy	632 69.01 69.52 74.91	■ Intravaginal misoprostol (Cytotec) placed for induction of labor is an abortifacient used for missed abortions. ■ Includes: Therapeutic abortion by hysterotomy

Abortion with Dilation and Curettage, Aspiration Curettage or Hysterotomy
DRG 381

No Potential DRGs

False Labor
RW 0.2190 **DRG 382**

Potential DRGs
379   Threatened Abortion   RW   0.3626

DRG	Principal Dx/Procedure	Codes	Tips
379	Threatened premature labor	644.03	■ Includes: Threatened labor after 22 but prior to 37 weeks gestation

Other Antepartum Diagnoses with Medical Complications
DRG 383

No Potential DRGs

■ Coding Tip   ● Documentation Tip   ◆ Encoder Tip   ⚐ Targeted DRG

DRG 384   Other Antepartum Diagnoses without Medical Complications — RW 0.3485

Potential DRGs

383   Other Antepartum Diagnoses with Medical Complications   RW   0.5123

DRG	Principal Dx/Procedure	Codes	Tips
383	Diabetes Edema Anemia	648.03 646.13 648.23	■ Sequence diabetic complication as principal when admission for regulation of insulin. ■ When more than one complication exists and all are treated, any may be sequenced first.

Newborns & Other Neonates, MDC 15

DRG 385   Neonates, Died, or Transferred to Another Acute Care Facility

No Potential DRGs

DRG 386   Extreme Immaturity or Respiratory Distress Syndrome, Neonate

No Potential DRGs

DRG 387   Prematurity with Major Problems — RW 3.1203

Potential DRGs

386   Extreme Immaturity   RW   4.5687

DRG	Principal Dx/Procedure	Codes	Tips
386	Birthweight less than 1500g and/or gestation less than 28 completed weeks Respiratory distress syndrome	765.05 769	■ Hyaline membrane disease, idiopathic respiratory distress syndrome [IRDS or RDS] of newborn, pulmonary hypofusion syndrome

DRG 388   Prematurity without Major Problems — RW 1.8827

Potential DRGs

386   Extreme Immaturity   RW   4.5687
387   Prematurity with Major Problems   RW   3.1203

DRG	Principal Dx/Procedure	Codes	Tips
386	Birthweight less than 1500g and/or gestation less than 28 completed weeks Respiratory distress syndrome	765.05 769	■ Hyaline membrane disease, idiopathic respiratory distress syndrome [IRDS or RDS] of newborn, pulmonary hypofusion syndrome

---

■ Coding Tip   ● Documentation Tip   ◆ Encoder Tip   ▽ Targeted DRG

(continued)   DRG 388

DRG	Principal Dx/Procedure	Codes	Tips
387	Prematurity *AND* Major problems such as: Postauricular fistula Aneurysm Embolism Cardiac/respiratory arrest Asthma Abscess/cellulitis Asphyxia Anemia Bacteremia	 383.81 414.10 415.19 427.5 493.01 *682 768.5 776.6 790.7	◆ Key terms: mural, ventricular ◆ Key terms: allergic, atopic, childhood, platinum ◆ Key terms: acute abscess, diffuse cellulitis, acute lymphangitis ● Birth asphyxia with neurological involvement; only a physician can ascribe neurological deficits to a low perinatal APGAR

Full Term Neonate with Major Problems   RW 3.2052   DRG 389

Potential DRGs

386	Extreme Immaturity	RW 4.5687

DRG	Principal Dx/Procedure	Codes	Tips
386	Birthweight less than 1500g and/or gestation less than 28 completed weeks Respiratory distress syndrome	765.05 769	■ Hyaline membrane disease, idiopathic respiratory distress syndrome [IRDS or RDS] of newborn, pulmonary hypofusion syndrome

Neonate with Other Significant Problems   RW 1.1344   DRG 390

Potential DRGs

387	Prematurity with Major Problems	RW	3.1203
389	Full Term Neonate with Major Problems	RW	3.2052

DRG	Principal Dx/Procedure	Codes	Tips
387	Prematurity *AND* Major problems such as: Postauricular fistula Aneurysm Embolism Cardiac/respiratory arrest Asthma Abscess/cellulitis Asphyxia Anemia Bacteremia	 383.81 414.10 415.19 427.5 493.01 *682 768.5 776.6 790.7	◆ Key terms: mural, ventricular ◆ Key terms: allergic, atopic, childhood, platinum ◆ Key terms: acute abscess, diffuse cellulitis, acute lymphangitis ● Birth asphyxia with neurological involvement; only a physician can ascribe neurological deficits to a low perinatal APGAR
389	Major problems such as: Postauricular fistula Aneurysm Embolism Cardiac/respiratory arrest Asthma Abscess/cellulitis Asphyxia Anemia Bacteremia	 383.8 1 414.1 0 415.1 9 427.5 493.01 *682 768.5 776.6 790.7	◆ Key terms: mural, ventricular ◆ Key terms: allergic, atopic, childhood, platinum ◆ Key terms: acute abscess, diffuse cellulitis, acute lymphangitis ● Birth asphyxia with neurological involvement; only a physician can ascribe neurological deficits to a low perinatal APGAR

■ Coding Tip   ● Documentation Tip   ◆ Encoder Tip   ▽ Targeted DRG

Newborns & Other Neonates, MDC 15

DRG 391   Normal Newborn   RW 0.1536

Potential DRGs

386	**Extreme Immaturity**	RW	4.5687
387	**Prematurity with Major Problems**	RW	3.1203
388	**Prematurity** without Major Problems	RW	1.8827
389	Full Term Neonate **with Major Problems**	RW	3.2052
390	Neonate **with Other Significant Problems**	RW	1.1344

DRG	Principal Dx/Procedure	Codes	Tips
386	Birthweight less than 1500 and/or gestation less than 28 completed weeks Respiratory distress syndrome	765.05 769	■ Hyaline membrane disease, idiopathic respiratory distress syndrome [IRDS or RDS] of newborn, pulmonary hypofusion syndrome
387	Prematurity *AND* Major problems such as: Postauricular fistula Aneurysm Embolism Cardiac/respiratory arrest Asthma Abscess/cellulitis Asphyxia Anemia Bacteremia	383.81 414.10 415.19 427.5 493.01 *682 768.5 776.6 790.7	◆ Key terms: mural, ventricular ◆ Key terms: allergic, atopic, childhood, platinum ◆ Key terms: acute abscess, diffuse cellulitis, acute lymphangitis ● Birth asphyxia with neurological involvement; only a physician can ascribe neurological deficits to a low perinatal APGAR
388	Prematurity	765.00, 765.06, 765.07, 765.08, *765.1	
389	Major problems such as: Postauricular fistula Aneurysm Embolism Cardiac/respiratory arrest Asthma Abscess/cellulitis Asphyxia Anemia Bacteremia	383.8 1 414.1 0 415.1 9 427.5 493.01 *682 768.5 776.6 790.7	◆ Key terms: mural, ventricular ◆ Key terms: allergic, atopic, childhood, platinum ◆ Key terms: acute abscess, diffuse cellulitis, acute lymphangitis ● Birth asphyxia with neurological involvement; only a physician can ascribe neurological deficits to a low perinatal APGAR
390	Significant problem (those not assigned to DRGs 385–389, 391 or 469)		

Blood & Immunological Disorders, MDC 16

DRG 392   Splenectomy, Age > 17   RW 3.3164

Potential DRGs

486	Other O.R. Procedures for Multiple Significant Trauma	RW	4.8793

DRG	Principal Dx/Procedure	Codes	Tips
486	Other O.R. procedures for multiple significant trauma		■ Principal diagnosis of trauma and at least two injuries (assigned either as principal or secondary) that are defined as significant trauma from different body site categories located under DRG 487 *AND* O.R. procedure other than craniotomy or limb reattachment, hip and femur procedures

Splenectomy, Age 0–17
RW 1.3571 **DRG 393**

Potential DRGs

392	Splenectomy, **Age > 17**	RW 3.3164
486	Other O.R. Procedures for Multiple Significant Trauma	RW 4.8793

DRG	Principal Dx/Procedure	Codes	Tips
392	Patient's age > 17		
486	Other O.R. procedures for multiple significant trauma		■ Principal diagnosis of trauma and at least two injuries (assigned either as principal or secondary) that are defined as significant trauma from different body site categories located under DRG 487 *AND* O.R. procedure other than craniotomy or limb reattachment, hip and femur procedures

Other Operating Room Procedures of the Blood and Blood-forming Organs
DRG 394

No Potential DRGs

Red Blood Cell Disorders, Age > 17
RW 0.8307 **DRG 395**

Potential DRGs

174	Gastrointestinal Hemorrhage with CC	RW 1.0025
296	Nutritional & Miscellaneous Metabolic Disorders, Age > 17 with CC	RW 0.8639
397	Coagulation Disorders	RW 1.2648

DRG	Principal Dx/Procedure	Codes	Tips
174 ▽	Bleeding esophageal varices	456.0	● Varices are common in patients with alcoholic liver disease.
	Gastric ulcer with hemorrhage	*531.0	◆ Manifestations: hematemesis, melena, occult, hematochezia
	Peptic ulcer with hemorrhage	*533.0	◆ Bleeding may be intermittent; code based on physician documenting bleeding ulcer even though endoscopy may not show active bleeding.
	Gastrointestinal hemorrhage *AND* CC condition	*578 See CC section.	◆ Common complications: dehydration, shock, ascites, renal failure, hypotension.
296 ▽	Vitamin A deficiencies Nutritional deficiencies Other metabolic conditions *AND* CC condition	*264 *269 *276 See CC section.	
397	Thrombocytopenia	287.5	■ Pancytopenia includes thrombocytopenia, only then code for pancytopenia (284.8) would be assigned

Red Blood Cell Disorders, Age 0–17
RW 0.6986 **DRG 396**

Potential DRGs

397	Coagulation Disorders	RW 1.2648

DRG	Principal Dx/Procedure	Codes	Tips
397	Thrombocytopenia	287.5	■ Pancytopenia includes thrombocytopenia, only then code for pancytopenia (284.8) would be assigned

---

■ Coding Tip   ● Documentation Tip   ◆ Encoder Tip   ▽ Targeted DRG

Blood & Immunological Disorders, MDC 16

DRG 397 Coagulation Disorders

No Potential DRGs

DRG 398 Reticuloendothelial & Immunity Disorders with CC
RW 1.2360

Potential DRGs

486	Other O.R. Procedures for Multiple Significant Trauma	RW	4.8793
487	Other Multiple Significant Trauma	RW	2.0057
488	HIV with Extensive O.R. Procedure	RW	4.8118
489	**HIV with Major Related Condition**	RW	1.8603

DRG	Principal Dx/Procedure	Codes	Tips
486	Other O.R. procedures for multiple significant trauma		■ Principal diagnosis of trauma and at least two injuries (assigned either as principal or secondary) that are defined as significant trauma from different body site categories located under DRG 487 *AND* O.R. procedure other than craniotomy or limb reattachment, hip and femur procedures
487	Other multiple significant trauma		■ Principal diagnosis of trauma and at least two injuries (assigned either as principal or secondary) that are defined as significant trauma from different body site categories located under DRG 487
488	HIV infection (042) with extensive O.R. procedure (any O.R. procedure not listed in DRG 477)		
489	Major HIV-related diagnosis *WITH* Diagnosis of HIV (042)		

DRG 399 Reticuloendothelial & Immunity Disorders without CC
RW 0.6651

Potential DRGs

398	Reticuloendothelial & Immunity Disorders **with CC**	RW	1.2360
486	**Other O.R. Procedures for Multiple Significant Trauma**	RW	4.8793
487	Other Multiple Significant Trauma	RW	2.0057
488	HIV with Extensive O.R. Procedure	RW	4.8118
489	**HIV with Major Related Condition**	RW	1.8603
490	**HIV with or without Other Related Condition**	RW	1.0512

DRG	Principal Dx/Procedure	Codes	Tips
398	CC condition	See CC section.	
486	Other O.R. procedures for multiple significant trauma		■ Principal diagnosis of trauma and at least two injuries (assigned either as principal or secondary) that are defined as significant trauma from different body site categories located under DRG 487 *AND* O.R. procedure other than craniotomy or limb reattachment, hip and femur procedures
487	Other multiple significant trauma		■ Principal diagnosis of trauma and at least two injuries (assigned either as principal or secondary) that are defined as significant trauma from different body site categories located under DRG 487

■ Coding Tip   ● Documentation Tip   ◆ Encoder Tip   ▽ Targeted DRG

(continued) **DRG 399**

DRG	Principal Dx/Procedure	Codes	Tips
488	HIV infection (042) with extensive O.R. procedure (any O.R. procedure not listed in DRG 477)		
489	Major HIV-related diagnosis **WITH** Diagnosis of HIV (042)		
490	HIV infection (042) with nonmajor HIV-related condition OR HIV infection (042) without HIV-related secondary diagnosis		

Neoplasms, MDC 17

Lymphoma and Nonacute Leukemia with Other O.R. Procedures with CC   **DRG 401**

No Potential DRGs

Lymphoma & Nonacute Leukemia with Other O.R. Procedures without CC   RW 1.1430   **DRG 402**

Potential DRGs
401   Lymphoma & Nonacute Leukemia with Other O.R. Procedures with CC   RW   2.8946

DRG	Principal Dx/Procedure	Codes	Tips
401	Any other O.R. procedure **OR** Radiosurgery **AND** CC condition	*92.3 See CC section.	■ Pancytopenia, 284.8, is not an integral part of myelodysplastic syndrome, assign as additional diagnosis (CC).

Lymphoma & Nonacute Leukemia with CC   RW 1.8197   **DRG 403**

Potential DRGs
473   **Acute Leukemia** without Major O.R. Procedure, Age > 17   RW   3.4885

DRG	Principal Dx/Procedure	Codes	Tips
473	Acute leukemia: Lymphoid Myeloid Monocytic **AND** Patient's age > 17	 *204.0 *205.0 *206.0	◆ Key term: acute lymphoblastic leukemia ◆ Key term: myelogenous, myeloblastic, myelomonocytic Acute promyelocytic leukemia ◆ Acute exacerbation of chronic myelogenous leukemia is included in the code for chronic leukemia.

■ Coding Tip   ● Documentation Tip   ◆ Encoder Tip   ▽ Targeted DRG

Neoplasms, MDC 17

DRG 404 Lymphoma & Nonacute Leukemia without CC   RW 0.8658

Potential DRGs

403	Lymphoma & Nonacute Leukemia **with CC**	RW	1.8197
405	**Acute Leukemia** without Major O.R. Procedure, Age 0–17	RW	1.9241
473	**Acute Leukemia** without Major O.R. Procedure, **Age > 17**	RW	3.4885

DRG	Principal Dx/Procedure	Codes	Tips
403	Hodgkins sarcoma of thorax *AND* CC condition	201.22 See CC section.	■ Pancytopenia, 284.8, is not an integral part of myelodysplastic syndrome, assign as additional diagnosis (CC). ■ Neutropenic enterocolitis can be a complication of chemo in an acute leukemia patient.
405	Acute leukemia: Lymphoid Myeloid Monocytic *AND* Patient's age 0–17	*204.0 *205.0 *206.0	◆ Key terms: acute lymphoblastic leukemia ◆ Key terms: myelogenous, myeloblastic, myelomonocytic ◆ Acute exacerbation of chronic myelogenous leukemia is included in the code for chronic leukemia. Acute promyelocytic leukemia
473	Acute leukemia: Lymphoid Myeloid Monocytic *AND* Patient's age > 17	*204.0 *205.0 *206.0	◆ Key terms: acute lymphoblastic leukemia ◆ Key terms: myelogenous, myeloblastic, myelomonocytic ◆ Acute exacerbation of chronic myelogenous leukemia is included in the code for chronic leukemia ◆ Key term: acute promyelocytic leukemia

DRG 405 Acute Leukemia without Major O.R. Procedure, Age 0–17   RW 1.9241

Potential DRGs

473	Acute Leukemia without Major O.R. Procedure, **Age > 17**	RW	3.4885

DRG	Principal Dx/Procedure	Codes	Tips
473	Acute leukemia: Lymphoid Myeloid Monocytic *AND* Patient's age > 17	*204.0 *205.0 *206.0	◆ Key terms: acute lymphoblastic leukemia ◆ Key terms: myelogenous, myeloblastic, myelomonocytic ◆ Acute exacerbation of chronic myelogenous leukemia is included in the code for chronic leukemia ◆ Key terms: acute promyelocytic leukemia

(continued) DRG 405

*Ensure accurate DRG assignment.
Listed below are the principal diagnoses found in DRG 405:

204.00 Acute lymphoid leukemia without remission
204.01 Acute lymphoid leukemia with remission
205.00 Acute myeloid leukemia without remission
205.01 Acute myeloid leukemia with remission
206.00 Acute monocytic leukemia without remission
206.01 Acute monocytic leukemia with remission
207.00 Acute erythremia without remission
207.01 Acute erythremia with remission
208.00 Acute leukemia NOS without remission
208.01 Acute leukemia NOS with remission

Myeloproliferative Disorders or Poorly Differentiated Neoplasms with Major O.R. Procedures with CC   RW 2.7055 DRG 406

Potential DRGs

170   Other Digestive System O.R. Procedures with CC   RW   2.8245

DRG	Principal Dx/Procedure	Codes	Tips
170	Principal diagnosis from MDC 6 *AND* Control of hemorrhage Total splenectomy Diagnostic procedure liver Diagnostic procedure pancreas Exploratory laparotomy *AND* CC condition (See CC section.)	39.98 41.5 50.19 52.19 54.11 See CC section.	■ Distal esophageal obstruction secondary to neoplasm, 530.3 ■ Exploratory procedure followed by definitive surgery is not coded except for biopsies and incidental appendectomy.

Myeloproliferative Disorders or Poorly Differentiated Neoplasms with Major O.R. Procedures without CC   RW 1.2410 DRG 407

Potential DRGs

406   Myeloproliferative Disorders or Poorly Differentiated Neoplasms with Major O.R.   RW   2.7055
      Procedures with CC

DRG	Principal Dx/Procedure	Codes	Tips
406	CC condition	See CC section.	

Myeloproliferative Disorders or Poorly Differentiated Neoplasms with Other O.R. Procedure   RW 2.1984 DRG 408

Potential DRGs

406   Myeloproliferative Disorders or Poorly Differentiated Neoplasms with   RW   2.7055
      Major O.R. Procedures with CC

DRG	Principal Dx/Procedure	Codes	Tips
406	Major O.R. procedure: Total gastrectomy Cholecystectomy Open biopsy of pancreas Open biopsy of bladder *AND* CC condition	*43.9 *51.12 52.12 57.34 See CC section.	

■ Coding Tip   ● Documentation Tip   ◆ Encoder Tip   ᵂ Targeted DRG

Neoplasms, MDC 17

DRG 409   Radiotherapy

No Potential DRGs

DRG 410   Chemotherapy without Acute Leukemia   RW 1.0833
as Secondary Diagnosis

Potential DRGs

409	Radiotherapy	RW	1.2439
492	Chemotherapy with Acute Leukemia as Secondary Diagnosis	RW	3.8371

DRG	Principal Dx/Procedure	Codes	Tips
409	Radiotherapy concomitant with chemotherapy	V58.0 or V67.1 as principal	■ For patients receiving both chemotherapy and radiation, V58.1 and V58.0, selection of principal diagnosis should be based on documentation in the medical record.
492	Acute leukemia as a secondary Dx: Lymphoid Myeloid Monocytic OR High-dose infusion interleukin-2 (IL-2)	 *204.0 *205.0 *206.0 00.15	◆ Key terms: acute lymphoblastic leukemia ◆ Key terms: myelogenous, myeloblastic, myelomonocytic ◆ Acute exacerbation of chronic myelogenous leukemia is included in the code for chronic leukemia ◆ Key terms: acute promyelocytic leukemia

DRG 411   History of Malignancy without Endoscopy

No Potential DRGs

DRG 412   History of Malignancy with Endoscopy

No Potential DRGs

DRG 413   Other Myeloproliferative Disorders or   RW 1.3224
Poorly Differentiated Neoplasm Diagnosis
with CC

Potential DRGs

408	Myeloproliferative Disorders or Poorly Differentiated Neoplasms with Other O.R. Procedure	RW	2.1984

DRG	Principal Dx/Procedure	Codes	Tips
408	O.R. procedure (except those that group to DRGs 406, 407)		

DRG 414   Other Myeloproliferative Disorders or   RW 0.7370
Poorly Differentiated Neoplasm Diagnosis
without CC

Potential DRGs

408	Myeloproliferative Disorders or Poorly Differentiated Neoplasms with Other O.R. Procedure	RW	2.1984
413	Other Myeloproliferative Disorders or Poorly Differentiated Neoplasm Diagnosis with CC	RW	1.3224

DRG	Principal Dx/Procedure	Codes	Tips
408	O.R. procedure (except those that group to DRGs 406, 407)		

■ Coding Tip   ● Documentation Tip   ◆ Encoder Tip   ▽ Targeted DRG

(continued) **DRG 414**

DRG	Principal Dx/Procedure	Codes	Tips
413	Malignant neoplasm of retroperitoneum *AND* CC condition	158.0 See CC section.	◆ Key terms: periadrenal, perinephric, perirenal

Acute Leukemia without Major O.R. Procedure, Age > 17   RW 3.4885   **DRG 473**

*Ensure accurate DRG assignment. Listed below are the principal diagnoses found in DRG 473:
204.00   Acute lymphoid leukemia without remission
204.01   Acute lymphoid leukemia with remission
205.00   Acute myeloid leukemia without remission
205.01   Acute myeloid leukemia with remission
206.00   Acute monocytic leukemia without remission
206.01   Acute monocytic leukemia with remission
207.00   Acute erythremia without remission
207.01   Acute erythremia with remission
208.00   Acute leukemia NOS without remission
208.01   Acute leukemia NOS with remission

Chemotherapy with Acute Leukemia or With Use of High-Dose Chemotherapy Agent   **DRG 492**

No Potential DRGs

Lymphoma and Leukemia With Major O.R. Procedure with CC   **DRG 539**

No Potential DRGs

Lymphoma and Leukemia With Major O.R. Procedure without CC   RW 1.2891   **DRG 540**

Potential DRGs
539   Lymphoma and Leukemia With Major O.R. Procedure **with CC**   RW   3.3846

DRG	Principal Dx/Procedure	Codes	Tips
539	CC condition	See CC section.	

■ Coding Tip   ● Documentation Tip   ◆ Encoder Tip   ▽ Targeted DRG

Infectious & Parasitic Diseases, MDC 18

DRG 415   Operating Room Procedure for Infectious and Parasitic Diseases

No Potential DRGs

DRG 416▽ Septicemia, Age > 17   RW 1.5918

Potential DRGs

079	**Respiratory Infections & Inflammations**, Age > 17 with CC	RW	1.5974
415	O.R. Procedure for Infectious & Parasitic Diseases	RW	3.6276
475	Respiratory System Diagnosis **with Ventilator Support**	RW	3.6000

DRG	Principal Dx/Procedure	Codes	Tips
079	Cause of pneumonia: *Salmonella* *Klebsiella* *Proteus* *Pseudomonas* *Staphylococcus* Aspiration *AND* CC condition	 003.22 482.0 482.1 482.40 482.83 *507 See CC section.	■ If both aspiration and bacterial pneumonia are documented, code both.
415	Any O.R. procedure		
475 ▽	Continuous mechanical ventilation	96.70–96.79	◆ Key terms: IMV, PEEP, PSV, weaning of intubated patient, endotracheal respiratory assistance, duration includes restarts ■ Mech ventilation used during surgery is not coded unless MD documents unexpected extended period of time following surgery.

DRG 417   Septicemia, Age 0–17   RW 0.9612

Potential DRGs

416	Septicemia, **Age > 17**	RW	1.5918
475	Respiratory System Diagnosis **with Ventilator Support**	RW	3.6000

DRG	Principal Dx/Procedure	Codes	Tips
416 ▽	Patient's age > 17	*038	■ Septicemia with pneumonia; code both. ● If sepsis is documented, it may be coded in absence of positive blood cultures.
475 ▽	Continuous mechanical ventilation	96.70–96.79	◆ Key terms: IMV, PEEP, PSV, weaning of intubated patient, endotracheal respiratory assistance, duration includes restarts ■ Mech ventilation used during surgery is not coded unless MD documents unexpected extended period of time following surgery.

■ Coding Tip   ● Documentation Tip   ◆ Encoder Tip   ▽ Targeted DRG

Postoperative & Post-traumatic Infections   RW 1.0672   **DRG 418**

Potential DRGs
144   Other Circulatory System Diagnoses with CC   RW   1.2260

DRG	Principal Dx/Procedure	Codes	Tips
144	Postoperative infection due to cardiac device, implant or graft *AND* CC condition	996.61 See CC section.	◆ Key terms: infected pacemaker electrode, pulse generator, or pocket

Fever of Unknown Origin, Age > 17 with CC   **DRG 419**

No Potential DRGs

Fever of Unknown Origin, Age > 17 without CC   RW 0.6107   **DRG 420**

Potential DRGs
419   Fever of Unknown Origin, Age >17 with CC   RW   0.8476

DRG	Principal Dx/Procedure	Codes	Tips
419	Fever of unknown origin *AND* CC condition	780.6 See CC section.	

Viral Illness, Age > 17   **DRG 421**

No Potential DRGs

Viral Illness & Fever of Unknown Origin, Age 0–17   RW 0.7248   **DRG 422**

Potential DRGs
419   Fever of Unknown Origin, Age > 17 with CC   RW   0.8476

DRG	Principal Dx/Procedure	Codes	Tips
419	Fever of unknown origin *AND* Patient's age >17 *AND* CC condition	780.6 See CC section.	

Other Infectious and Parasitic Diseases Diagnoses   **DRG 423**

No Potential DRGs

■ Coding Tip   ● Documentation Tip   ◆ Encoder Tip   ▽ Targeted DRG

Mental Diseases & Disorders, MDC 19

DRG 424 Operating Room Procedure with Principal Diagnosis of Mental Illness

No Potential DRGs

DRG 425▽ Acute Adjustment Reaction and Psychosocial Dysfunction   RW 0.6781

Potential DRGs

429	Organic Disturbances & Mental Retardation	RW	0.8291
430	Psychoses	RW	0.6801

DRG	Principal Dx/Procedure	Codes	Tips
429	Senile, presenile, and organic psychotic conditions	*290,*293	
	OR Mental retardation	319	
430 ▽	Simple schizophrenia	*295	
	Affective psychoses	*296	
	Depressive type psychoses	298.0	

DRG 426 Depressive Neuroses   RW 0.5087

Potential DRGs

428	Disorders of Personality & Impulse Control	RW	0.7291
429	Organic Disturbances & Mental Retardation	RW	0.8291
430	Psychoses	RW	0.6801

DRG	Principal Dx/Procedure	Codes	Tips
428	Personality disorders:		■ Dissociative identity disorder
	Multiple personality	300.14	◆ Key terms: fanatic personality
	Paranoid personality	301.0	
	Pathological gambling	312.31	
429	Senile, presenile, and organic psychotic conditions	*290, *293	◆ Key terms: mental deficiency, abnormality
	OR Mental retardation	319	
430 ▽	Simple schizophrenia	*295	
	Affective psychoses	*296	
	Depressive type psychoses	298.0	

DRG 427 Neuroses Except Depressive   RW 0.5012

Potential DRGs

428	Disorders of Personality & Impulse Control	RW	0.7291
429	Organic Disturbances & Mental Retardation	RW	0.8291
430	Psychoses	RW	0.6801
432	Other Mental Disorder Diagnoses	RW	0.6513

DRG	Principal Dx/Procedure	Codes	Tips
428	Personality disorders:		■ Dissociative identity disorder
	Multiple personality	300.14	◆ Key terms: fanatic personality
	Paranoid personality	301.0	
	Pathological gambling	312.31	
429	Senile, presenile, and organic psychotic conditions	*290, *293	
	OR Mental retardation	319	

■ Coding Tip   ● Documentation Tip   ◆ Encoder Tip   ▽ Targeted DRG

(continued) **DRG 427**

DRG	Principal Dx/Procedure	Codes	Tips
430	Simple schizophrenia Affective psychoses Depressive type psychoses	*295 *296 298.0	
432	Other mental disorder: Sleep disorders Bulimia	*307.4 307.51	

Disorders of Personality and Impulse Control **DRG 428**
No Potential DRGs

Organic Disturbances and Mental Retardation **DRG 429**
No Potential DRGs

Psychoses **DRG 430**
No Potential DRGs

Childhood Mental Disorders **DRG 431**
No Potential DRGs

Other Mental Disorder Diagnoses RW 0.6513 **DRG 432**
Potential DRGs
034   Other Disorders of Nervous System with CC   RW   0.9931

DRG	Principal Dx/Procedure	Codes	Tips
034	Insomnia with sleep apnea Hypersomnia *AND* CC condition	780.51 780.53 See CC section.	

Alcohol/Drug Disorders, MDC 20

Alcohol/Drug Abuse or Dependence, Left AMA **DRG 433**
No Potential DRGs for Optimizing Payment

Invalid DRG **DRG 434**
No Potential DRGs for Optimizing Payment

Invalid DRG **DRG 435**
No Potential DRGs for Optimizing Payment

Invalid DRG **DRG 436**
No Potential DRGs for Optimizing Payment

Invalid DRG **DRG 437**
No Potential DRGs for Optimizing Payment

■ Coding Tip   ● Documentation Tip   ◆ Encoder Tip   ▽ Targeted DRG

Alcohol/Drug Disorders, MDC 20

DRG 438 Invalid DRG

No Potential DRGs for Optimizing Payment

DRG 521 Alcohol/Drug Abuse or Dependence with CC
RW 0.7115

Potential DRGs
202   Cirrhosis & Alcoholic Hepatitis   RW   1.3120

DRG	Principal Dx/Procedure	Codes	Tips
202	Alcoholic hepatitis Cirrhosis	571.1 571.2	■ Acute alcoholic liver disease ◆ Key terms: florid, Laennec's

DRG 522 Alcohol/Drug Abuse or Dependence without CC, with Rehabilitation Therapy
RW 0.5226

Potential DRGs
202   Cirrhosis & Alcoholic Hepatitis   RW   1.3120

DRG	Principal Dx/Procedure	Codes	Tips
202	Alcoholic hepatitis Cirrhosis	571.1 571.2	■ Acute alcoholic liver disease ◆ Key terms: florid, Laennec's

DRG 523 Alcohol/Drug Abuse or Dependence without CC, without Rehabilitation Therapy
RW 0.3956

Potential DRGs
202   Cirrhosis & Alcoholic Hepatitis   RW   1.3120
521   Alcohol/Drug Abuse or Dependence **with CC**   RW   0.7115
522   Alcohol/Drug Abuse or Dependence without CC, **with Rehabilitation Therapy**   RW   0.5226

DRG	Principal Dx/Procedure	Codes	Tips
202	Alcoholic hepatitis Cirrhosis	571.1–571.2	■ Acute alcoholic liver disease ◆ Key term: florid, Laennec's
521	Alcohol dependence Drug dependence **AND** CC condition	*303.9, *304 See CC section.	◆ Key terms: chronic alcoholism, dipsomania ■ Drug dependent ■ Drug withdrawal symptoms
522	Alcohol dependence with rehabilitation therapy and detoxification Drug dependence with rehabilitation therapy and detoxification	*303.9, 94.61, 94.63 *304, 94.66	◆ Key terms: chronic alcoholism, dipsomania ■ Drug dependent ■ Drug withdrawal symptoms

Injuries, Poisonings & Toxic Effects of Drugs, MDC 21

Skin Grafts for Injuries   **DRG 439**

No Potential DRGs

Wound Debridement for Injuries   **DRG 440**

No Potential DRGs

Hand Procedures for Injuries   RW 0.9662   **DRG 441**

Potential DRGs

486   Other O.R. Procedures for Multiple Significant Trauma   RW   4.8793

DRG	Principal Dx/Procedure	Codes	Tips
486	Other O.R. procedures for multiple significant trauma		■ Principal diagnosis of trauma and at least two injuries (assigned either as principal or secondary) that are defined as significant trauma from different body site categories located under DRG 487 *AND* O.R. procedure other than craniotomy or limb reattachment, hip and femur procedures

Other O.R. Procedures for Injuries with CC   RW 2.4200   **DRG 442**

Potential DRGs

484   Craniotomy for Multiple Significant Trauma   RW   5.4179
485   Limb Reattachment, Hip & Femur Procedures for Multiple Significant Trauma RW   3.2121
486   Other O.R. Procedures for Multiple Significant Trauma   RW   4.8793

DRG	Principal Dx/Procedure	Codes	Tips
484	Craniotomy for multiple significant trauma		■ Craniotomy and principal diagnosis of trauma and at least two injuries (assigned either as principal or secondary) that are defined as significant trauma from different body site categories located under DRG 487
485	Limb reattachment, hip and femur procedures for multiple significant trauma		■ Principal diagnosis of trauma and at least two injuries (assigned either as principal or secondary) that are defined as significant trauma from different body site categories located under DRG 487 *AND* limb reattachment, hip and femur O.R. procedures
486	Other O.R. procedures for multiple significant trauma		■ Principal diagnosis of trauma and at least two injuries (assigned either as principal or secondary) that are defined as significant trauma from different body site categories located under DRG 487 *AND* O.R. procedure other than craniotomy or limb reattachment, hip and femur procedures

---

■ Coding Tip   ● Documentation Tip   ◆ Encoder Tip   ▽ Targeted DRG

Injuries, Poisonings & Toxic Effects of Drugs, MDC 21

DRG 443 Other O.R. Procedures for Injuries without CC   RW 0.9787

Potential DRGs

442	Other O.R. Procedures for Injuries **with CC**	RW	2.4200
484	**Craniotomy for Multiple Significant Trauma**	RW	5.4179
485	**Limb Reattachment, Hip & Femur Procedures for Multiple Significant Trauma**	RW	3.2121
486	Other O.R. Procedures for **Multiple Significant Trauma**	RW	4.8793

DRG	Principal Dx/Procedure	Codes	Tips
442	Other craniotomy Brain repair *AND* CC condition	01.24 02.92 See CC section.	◆ Key terms: Cranial trephination, exploration, decompression
484	Craniotomy for multiple significant trauma		■ Craniotomy and principal diagnosis of trauma and at least two injuries (assigned either as principal or secondary) that are defined as significant trauma from different body site categories located under DRG 487
485	Limb reattachment, hip and femur procedures for multiple significant trauma		■ Principal diagnosis of trauma and at least two injuries (assigned either as principal or secondary) that are defined as significant trauma from different body site categories located under DRG 487 *AND* limb reattachment, hip and femur O.R. procedures
486	Other O.R. procedures for multiple significant trauma		■ Principal diagnosis of trauma and at least two injuries (assigned either as principal or secondary) that are defined as significant trauma from different body site categories located under DRG 487 *AND* O.R. procedure other than craniotomy or limb reattachment, hip and femur procedures

DRG 444 Traumatic Injury, Age > 17 with CC   RW 0.7475

Potential DRGs

263	**Skin Graft &/or Debridement for Skin Ulcer or Cellulitis** with CC	RW	2.0556
440	**Wound Debridements** for Injuries	RW	1.8878
442	**Other O.R. Procedures for Injuries** with CC	RW	2.4200
484	**Craniotomy for Multiple Significant Trauma**	RW	5.4179
485	**Limb Reattachment, Hip & Femur Procedures for Multiple Significant Trauma**	RW	3.2121
486	**Other O.R. Procedures for Multiple Significant Trauma**	RW	4.8793
487	Other Multiple Significant Trauma	RW	2.0057

DRG	Principal Dx/Procedure	Codes	Tips
263	Cellulitis skin ulcer *AND* Excisional debridement *AND* CC condition	*682 *707 86.22 See CC section.	■ If treatment directed at open wound, code first with cellulitis secondary. If wound does not require treatment or treated earlier, and cellulitis is reason for treatment, assign as principal. ◆ Key terms: acute lymphangitits, diffuse cellulitis, abscess ● May be performed by physician or nonphysician health care provider ● Excisional debridement (cutting away) of necrotic, devitalized tissue or slough, may be described as "sharp debridement." Does not include the removal of loose fragments of skin by scissors.

■ Coding Tip   ● Documentation Tip   ◆ Encoder Tip   ▩ Targeted DRG

DRG	Principal Dx/Procedure	Codes	Tips
440	Excisional debridement	86.22	● May be performed by physician or nonphysician health care provider. ● Excisional debridement (cutting away) of necrotic, devitalized tissue or slough, may be described as "sharp debridement." Does not include the removal of loose fragments of skin by scissors.
442	Operative procedure for injury: Facial bone repair Arthrodesis foot and ankle Above knee amputation ***AND*** CC condition	*76.6 *81.1 84.17 See CC section.	◆ With bone graft, external fixation ◆ Includes conversion BK amputation into AK amputation; reamputation at same site at higher anatomical area.
484	Craniotomy for multiple significant trauma		■ Craniotomy and principal diagnosis of trauma and at least two injuries (assigned either as principal or secondary) that are defined as significant trauma from different body site categories located under DRG 487
485	Limb reattachment, hip and femur procedures for multiple significant trauma		■ Principal diagnosis of trauma and at least two injuries (assigned either as principal or secondary) that are defined as significant trauma from different body site categories located under DRG 487 ***AND*** limb reattachment, hip and femur O.R. procedures
486	Other O.R. procedures for multiple significant trauma		■ Principal diagnosis of trauma and at least two injuries (assigned either as principal or secondary) that are defined as significant trauma from different body site categories located under DRG 487 ***AND*** O.R. procedure other than craniotomy or limb reattachment, hip and femur procedures
487	Other multiple significant trauma		■ Principal diagnosis of trauma and at least two injuries (assigned either as principal or secondary) that are defined as significant trauma from different body site categories located under DRG 487

■ Coding Tip   ● Documentation Tip   ◆ Encoder Tip   ⑂ Targeted DRG

Injuries, Poisonings & Toxic Effects of Drugs, MDC 21

DRG 445   Traumatic Injury, Age > 17 without CC   RW 0.5015

Potential DRGs

264	**Skin Graft &/or Debridement for Skin Ulcer or Cellulitis** without CC	RW	1.0605
440	**Wound Debridements** for Injuries	RW	1.8878
443	**Other O.R. Procedures for Injuries** without CC	RW	0.9787
444	Traumatic Injury, Age > 17**with CC**	RW	0.7475
484	**Craniotomy for Multiple Significant Trauma**	RW	5.4179
485	**Limb Reattachment, Hip & Femur Procedures for Multiple Significant Trauma**	RW	3.2121
486	**Other O.R. Procedures for Multiple Significant Trauma**	RW	4.8793
487	Other Multiple Significant Trauma	RW	2.0057

DRG	Principal Dx/Procedure	Codes	Tips
264	Cellulitis Skin ulcer *AND* Excisional debridement *AND* CC condition	*682 *707 86.22 See CC section.	■ If treatment directed at open wound, code first with cellulitis secondary. If wound does not require treatment or treated earlier, and cellulitis is reason for treatment, assign as principal. Key terms: acute lymphangitits, diffuse cellulitis ● May be performed by physician or nonphysician health care provider. ● Excisional debridement (cutting away) of necrotic, devitalized tissue or slough, may be described as "sharp debridement." Does not include the removal of loose fragments of skin by scissors.
440	Excisional debridement	86.22	● May be performed by physician or nonphysician health care provider. ● Excisional debridement (cutting away) of necrotic, devitalized tissue or slough, may be described as "sharp debridement." Does not include the removal of loose fragments of skin by scissors.
443	Other craniotomy Brain repair	01.24 02.92	◆ Key terms: Cranial trephination, exploration, decompression
444	CC condition	See CC section.	
484	Craniotomy for multiple significant trauma		■ Craniotomy and principal diagnosis of trauma and at least two injuries (assigned either as principal or secondary) that are defined as significant trauma from different body site categories located under DRG 487
485	Limb reattachment, hip and femur procedures for multiple significant trauma		■ Principal diagnosis of trauma and at least two injuries (assigned either as principal or secondary) that are defined as significant trauma from different body site categories located under DRG 487 *AND* limb reattachment, hip and femur O.R. procedures
486	Other O.R. procedures for multiple significant trauma		■ Principal diagnosis of trauma and at least two injuries (assigned either as principal or secondary) that are defined as significant trauma from different body site categories located under DRG 487 *AND* O.R. procedure other than craniotomy or limb reattachment, hip and femur procedures

■ Coding Tip   ● Documentation Tip   ◆ Encoder Tip   ▥ Targeted DRG

    ©2003 Ingenix, Inc.

Injuries, Poisonings & Toxic Effects of Drugs, MDC 21

(continued) **DRG 445**

DRG	Principal Dx/Procedure	Codes	Tips
487	Other multiple significant trauma		■ Principal diagnosis of trauma and at least two injuries (assigned either as principal or secondary) that are defined as significant trauma from different body site categories located under DRG 487

Traumatic Injury, Age 0–17   RW 0.2983   **DRG 446**

Potential DRGs

264	Skin Graft &/or Debridement for Skin Ulcer or Cellulitis without CC	RW	1.0605
440	Wound Debridements for Injuries	RW	1.8878
443	Other O.R. Procedures for Injuries without CC	RW	0.9787
444	Traumatic Injury, Age > 17 with CC	RW	0.7475
484	Craniotomy for Multiple Significant Trauma	RW	5.4179
485	Limb Reattachment, Hip & Femur Procedures for Multiple Significant Trauma	RW	3.2121
486	Other O.R. Procedures for Multiple Significant Trauma	RW	4.8793
487	Other Multiple Significant Trauma	RW	2.0057

DRG	Principal Dx/Procedure	Codes	Tips
264	Cellulitis Skin ulcer *AND* Excisional debridement *AND* CC condition	*682 *707 86.22 See CC section.	■ If treatment directed at open wound, code first with cellulitis secondary. If wound does not require treatment or treated earlier, and cellulitis is reason for treatment, assign as principal. Key terms: acute lymphangitis, diffuse cellulitis ● May be performed by physician or nonphysician health care provider. ● Excisional debridement (cutting away) of necrotic, devitalized tissue or slough, may be described as "sharp debridement." Does not include the removal of loose fragments of skin by scissors.
440	Excisional debridement	86.22	● May be performed by physician or nonphysician health care provider. ● Excisional debridement (cutting away) of necrotic, devitalized tissue or slough, may be described as "sharp debridement." Does not include the removal of loose fragments of skin by scissors.
443	Other craniotomy Brain repair	01.24 02.92	◆ Key terms: cranial trephination, exploration, decompression
444	Patient's age > 17 *AND* CC condition	 See CC section.	
484	Craniotomy for multiple significant trauma		■ Craniotomy and principal diagnosis of trauma and at least two injuries (assigned either as principal or secondary) that are defined as significant trauma from different body site categories located under DRG 487
485	Limb reattachment, hip and femur procedures for multiple significant trauma		■ Principal diagnosis of trauma and at least two injuries (assigned either as principal or secondary) that are defined as significant trauma from different body site categories located under DRG 487 *AND* limb reattachment, hip and femur O.R. procedures

■ Coding Tip   ● Documentation Tip   ◆ Encoder Tip   ▽ Targeted DRG

Injuries, Poisonings & Toxic Effects of Drugs, MDC 21

DRG 446   (continued)

DRG	Principal Dx/Procedure	Codes	Tips
486	Other O.R. procedures for multiple significant trauma		■ Principal diagnosis of trauma and at least two injuries (assigned either as principal or secondary) that are defined as significant trauma from different body site categories located under DRG 487 *AND* O.R. procedure other than craniotomy or limb reattachment, hip and femur procedures
487	Other multiple significant trauma		■ Principal diagnosis of trauma and at least two injuries (assigned either as principal or secondary) that are defined as significant trauma from different body site categories located under DRG 487

DRG 447   Allergic Reactions, Age > 17   RW 0.5238

Potential DRGs
449   **Poisoning & Toxic Effects of Drugs** Age > 17 with CC   RW   0.8352

DRG	Principal Dx/Procedure	Codes	Tips
449	Allergic reaction due to drug *AND* CC condition	995.2 See CC section.	● Medical record should be reviewed to determine sign or symptom of adverse effect. ◆ Key terms: hypersensitivity, idiosyncratic reaction

DRG 448   Allergic Reactions, Age 0–17   RW 0.0981

Potential DRGs
447   **Allergic Reactions, Age > 17**   RW   0.5238
449   **Poisoning & Toxic Effects of Drugs**, Age > 17 with CC   RW   0.8352
450   **Poisoning & Toxic Effects of Drugs**, Age > 17 without CC   RW   0.4246

DRG	Principal Dx/Procedure	Codes	Tips
447	Patient's age > 17		
449	Allergic reaction due to drug *AND* Patient's age > 17 *AND* CC condition	995.2 See CC section.	● Medical record should be reviewed to determine sign or symptom of adverse effect. ◆ Key terms: hypersensitivity, idiosyncratic reaction
450	Allergic reaction due to drug *AND* Patient's age > 17	995.2	● Medical record should be reviewed to determine sign or symptom of adverse effect. ◆ Key terms: hypersensitivity, idiosyncratic reaction

DRG 449   Poisoning & Toxic Effects of Drugs,   RW 0.8352
Age > 17 with CC

Potential DRGs
138   **Cardiac Arrhythmia & Conduction Disorders** with CC   RW   0.8355

DRG	Principal Dx/Procedure	Codes	Tips
138 ▽	Cardiac arrhythmia due to digitalis toxicity *AND* CC condition	*427.8, 972.1, E942.1 See CC section.	■ Review medical record to determine if the toxicity is a poisoning or an adverse effect.

■ Coding Tip   ● Documentation Tip   ◆ Encoder Tip   ▽ Targeted DRG

Poisoning & Toxic Effects of Drugs, Age > 17 without CC

RW 0.4246   **DRG 450**

Potential DRGs

138	Cardiac Arrhythmia & Conduction Disorders with CC	RW	0.8355
139	Cardiac Arrhythmia & Conduction Disorders without CC	RW	0.5160
449	Poisoning & Toxic Effects of Drugs, Age > 17 **with CC**	RW	0.8352

DRG	Principal Dx/Procedure	Codes	Tips
138 ▽	Cardiac arrhythmia due to digitalis toxicity AND CC condition	*427.8, 972.1, E942.1 See CC section.	■ Review medical record to determine if the toxicity is a poisoning or an adverse effect.
139	Cardiac arrhythmia due to digitalis toxicity	*427.8, 972.1, E942.1	■ Review medical record to determine if the toxicity is a poisoning or an adverse effect.
449	Allergic reaction due to drug AND CC condition	995.2 See CC section.	● Medical record should be reviewed to determine sign or symptom of adverse effect. ◆ Key terms: hypersensitivity, idiosyncratic reaction

Poisoning & Toxic Effects of Drugs, Age 0–17

RW 0.2648   **DRG 451**

Potential DRGs

450	Poisoning & Toxic Effects of Drugs, **Age > 17**	RW	0.4246

DRG	Principal Dx/Procedure	Codes	Tips
450	Allergic reaction due to drug AND Patient's age > 17	995.2	● Medical record should be reviewed to determine sign or symptom of adverse effect. ◆ Key terms: hypersensitivity, idiosyncratic reaction

Complications of Treatment with CC

DRG 452

No Potential DRGs

Complications of Treatment without CC

RW 0.5113   **DRG 453**

Potential DRGs

418	Postoperative & Post-traumatic Infections	RW	1.0672
452	Complications of Treatment **with CC**	RW	1.0455

DRG	Principal Dx/Procedure	Codes	Tips
418	Postoperative infection	*998.5	
452	Hemorrhage complicating a procedure Operative laceration	998.11 998.2	■ Hemothorax secondary to a procedure ● Changes in hematocrit occurring 48 hours of the operative event do not necessarily imply hemorrhage, seek physician clarification for abnormal blood loss resulting from a procedure.
	AND CC condition	See CC section.	● Consult physician to determine whether an operative tear is considered an inherent part of the procedure or a complication.

■ Coding Tip	● Documentation Tip	◆ Encoder Tip	▽ Targeted DRG

Injuries, Poisonings & Toxic Effects of Drugs, MDC 21

DRG 454 Other Injury Poisoning and Toxic Effect Diagnoses with CC

No Potential DRGs

DRG 455 Other Injury, Poisoning & Toxic Effect Diagnoses without CC

RW 0.4773

Potential DRGs
454 Other Injury, Poisoning & Toxic Effect Diagnoses **with CC**   RW   0.8153

DRG	Principal Dx/Procedure	Codes	Tips
454	Effects of radiation Hypothermia *AND* CC condition	990 991.6 See CC section.	◆ Key term: radiation sickness

Burns, MDC 22

DRG 456 Invalid DRG
No Potential DRGs

DRG 457 Invalid DRG
No Potential DRGs

DRG 458 Invalid DRG
No Potential DRGs

DRG 459 Invalid DRG
No Potential DRGs

DRG 460 Invalid DRG
No Potential DRGs

DRG 472 Invalid DRG
No Potential DRGs

DRG 504 Extensive Third Degree Burn with Skin Graft
No Potential DRGs

DRG 505 Extensive Third Degree Burn without Skin Graft

RW 2.0006

Potential DRGs
504 Extensive Third Degree Burn **with Skin Graft**   RW   11.6215

DRG	Principal Dx/Procedure	Codes	Tips
504	Third degree burn *AND* Skin graft	85.82–85.84, 86.60–86.63, 86.65–86.69, *86.7, 86.93	◆ Definition: full thickness burn ≥10% of body surface and ≥10% third degree

---

■ Coding Tip   ● Documentation Tip   ◆ Encoder Tip   ▽ Targeted DRG

Full Thickness Burn with Skin Graft of Inhalation Injury with CC or Significant Trauma

RW 4.1070 **DRG 506**

Potential DRGs

504   Extensive Third Degree Burn with Skin Graft   RW   11.6215

DRG	Principal Dx/Procedure	Codes	Tips
504	Third degree burn *AND* Skin graft	85.82–85.84, 86.60–86.63, 86.65–86.69, *86.7, 86.93	◆ Definition: full thickness burn ≥ 10% of body surface and ≥ 10% third degree

Full Thickness Burn with Skin Graft or Inhalation Injury without CC or Significant Trauma

RW 1.8154 **DRG 507**

Potential DRGs

504   Extensive Third Degree Burn with Skin Graft   RW   11.6215
506   Full Thickness Burn with Skin Graft or Inhalation Injury **with CC** or   RW   4.1070
      Significant Trauma

DRG	Principal Dx/Procedure	Codes	Tips
504	Third degree burn *AND* Skin graft	85.82–85.84, 86.60–86.63, 86.65–86.69, *86.7, 86.93	◆ Definition: full thickness burn ≥ 10% of body surface and ≥ 10% third degree
506	Third degree burn *AND* Skin graft *OR* Diagnosis for: Pulmonary insufficiency Acute respiratory failure Burn of lung Inhalation injury *AND* CC condition *OR* Significant trauma diagnosis	85.82–85.84, 86.60–86.63, 86.65–86.69, *86.7, 86.93 518.5, 518.81, 518.84, 947.1 987.9 See CC section.	

Full Thickness Burn without Skin Graft or Inhalation Injury with CC or Significant Trauma

RW 1.3775 **DRG 508**

Potential DRGs

504   Extensive Third Degree Burn with Skin Graft   RW   11.6215
505   Extensive Third Degree Burn without Skin Graft   RW   2.0006
506   Full Thickness Burn **with Skin Graft or Inhalation Injury with CC**   RW   4.1070
      or Significant Trauma

DRG	Principal Dx/Procedure	Codes	Tips
504	Third degree burn *AND* Skin graft	85.82–85.84, 86.60–86.63, 86.65–86.69, *86.7, 86.93	◆ Definition: full thickness burn ≥ 10% of body surface and ≥ 10% third degree
505	Extensive third degree burn		◆ Definition: full thickness burn ≥ 10% of body surface and ≥ 10% third degree

---

DRG 508 (continued)

DRG	Principal Dx/Procedure	Codes	Tips
506	Third degree burn *AND* Skin graft *OR* Diagnosis for: Pulmonary insufficiency Acute respiratory failure Burn of lung Inhalation injury *AND* CC condition *OR* Significant trauma diagnosis	85.82–85.84, 86.60–86.63, 86.65–86.69, *86.7, 86.93 518.5, 518.81, 518.84, 947.1, 987.9 See CC section.	■ Burn categories 941–946, 949 with fourth digit > 2

DRG 509 Full Thickness Burn without Skin Graft or Inhalation Injury without CC or Significant Trauma   RW 0.6426

Potential DRGs

504	Extensive Third Degree Burn with Skin Graft	RW	11.6215
505	Extensive Third Degree Burn without Skin Graft	RW	2.0006
507	Full Thickness Burn with Skin Graft or Inhalation Injury without CC or Significant Trauma	RW	1.8154

DRG	Principal Dx/Procedure	Codes	Tips
504	Third degree burn *AND* Skin graft	85.82–85.84, 86.60–86.63, 86.65–86.69, *86.7, 86.93	◆ Definition: full thickness burn ≥ 10% of body surface and ≥ 10% third degree
505	Extensive third degree burn		◆ Definition: full thickness burn ≥ 10% of body surface and ≥ 10% third degree
507	Third degree burn *AND* Skin graft *OR* Diagnosis for: Pulmonary insufficiency Acute respiratory failure Burn of lung Inhalation injury	 518.5 518.81, 518.84 947.1 987.9	

DRG 510 Nonextensive Burns with CC or Significant Trauma   RW 1.1812

Potential DRGs

504	Extensive Third Degree Burn with Skin Graft	RW	11.6215
505	Extensive Third Degree Burn without Skin Graft	RW	2.0006
506	Full Thickness Burn with Skin Graft or Inhalation Injury with CC or Significant Trauma	RW	4.1070

DRG	Principal Dx/Procedure	Codes	Tips
504	Extensive third degree burn *AND* Skin graft	85.82–85.84, 86.60–86.63, 86.65–86.69, *86.7, 86.93	◆ Definition: full thickness burn ≥ 10% of body surface and ≥ 10% third degree
505	Extensive third degree burn		◆ Definition: full thickness burn ≥ 10% of body surface and ≥ 10% third degree

(continued) **DRG 510**

DRG	Principal Dx/Procedure	Codes	Tips
506	Third degree burn *AND* Skin graft *OR* Diagnosis for: Pulmonary insufficiency Acute respiratory failure Burn of lung Inhalation injury *AND* CC condition *OR* Significant trauma diagnosis	85.82–85.84, 86.60–86.63, 86.65–86.69, *86.7, 86.93 518.5, 518.81, 518.84 947.1 987.9 See CC section.	■ Burn categories 941–946, 949 with fourth digit > 2

Nonextensive Burns without CC or Significant Trauma

RW 0.6753 **DRG 511**

Potential DRGs

504	**Extensive Third Degree Burn with Skin Graft**	RW	11.6215
505	**Extensive Third Degree Burn** without Skin Graft	RW	2.0006
507	**Full Thickness Burn with Skin Graft or Inhalation Injury** without CC or Significant Trauma	RW	1.8154
509	**Full Thickness Burn** without Skin Graft or Inhalation Injury without CC or Significant Trauma	RW	0.6426

DRG	Principal Dx/Procedure	Codes	Tips
504	Extensive third degree burn *AND* Skin graft	85.82–85.84, 86.60–86.63, 86.65–86.69, *86.7, 86.93	◆ Definition: full thickness burn ≥ 10% of body surface and ≥ 10% third degree
505	Extensive third degree burn		◆ Definition: full thickness burn ≥ 10% of body surface and ≥ 10% third degree
507	Third degree burn *AND* Skin graft *OR* Diagnosis for: Pulmonary insufficiency Acute respiratory failure Burn of lung Inhalation injury	85.82–85.84, 86.60–86.63, 86.65–86.69, *86.7, 86.93 518.5, 518.81, 518.84 947.1 987.9	■ Burn categories 941–946, 949 with fourth digit > 2
509	Full thickness third degree burn	*941.3, *941.4, *941.5, *942.3, *942.4, *942.5, *943.3, *943.4, *943.5, *944.3, *944.4, *944.5, *945.3, *945.4, *945.5, 946.3– 946.5, 948.11, 949.3–949.5	

Health Status Factors, MDC 23

DRG 461   Operating Room Procedures with Diagnosis of Other Contact with Health Services

No Potential DRGs

DRG 462   Rehabilitation

No Potential DRGs

DRG 463   Signs & Symptoms with CC   RW 0.6856

Potential DRGs

296   Nutritional & Miscellaneous Metabolic Disorders, Age > 17 with CC   RW   0.8639

DRG	Principal Dx/Procedure	Codes	Tips
296 ▽	Fluid retention	276.6	■ Fluid/volume overload: could be a symptom of CHF, ascites, edema
	Dehydration	276.5	◆ Key terms: hypovolemia, volume depletion ■ IV hydration should be ordered for correct coding. If patient admitted with gastroenteritis and dehydration, w/IV hydration ordered, which necessitated the admission, 276.5 is the principal Dx.
	Abnormal glucose tolerance test *AND* Patient's age > 17 *AND* CC condition	790.2 See CC section.	◆ Codes for nonspecific findings should be assigned only when no definitive diagnosis is documented by the physician.

DRG 464   Signs & Symptoms without CC   RW 0.4982

Potential DRGs

463   Signs & Symptoms with CC   RW   0.6856

DRG	Principal Dx/Procedure	Codes	Tips
463	Chronic fatigue syndrome *AND* CC condition	780.71 See CC section.	■ Do not code signs/symptoms (ex, weakness, headaches, sleep disturbances, muscle pain) considered a component of the syndrome separately.

DRG 465   Aftercare with History of Malignancy as Secondary Diagnosis

No Potential DRGs

DRG 466   Aftercare without History of Malignancy as Secondary Diagnosis

No Potential DRGs

■ Coding Tip   ● Documentation Tip   ◆ Encoder Tip   ▽ Targeted DRG

Other Factors Influencing Health Status   RW 0.5274   **DRG 467**

Potential DRGs

454	Other Injury, Poisoning & Toxic Effect Diagnoses with CC	RW	0.8153
462	Rehabilitation	RW	0.9747

DRG	Principal Dx/Procedure	Codes	Tips
454	Observation following motor vehicle traffic accident *AND* CC condition	V71.4 See CC section.	■ Assigned when no evidence is the suspected condition is found and no treatment is required. Suspected condition is ruled out.
462	Rehabilitation	V57.1–V57.3	◆ Admission for rehab (physical therapy or speech therapy) followed previous injury/illness.

Multiple Significant Trauma, MDC 24

Craniotomy for Multiple Significant Trauma   **DRG 484**

No Potential DRGs

Limb Reattachment, Hip & Femur   RW 3.2121   **DRG 485**
Procedures for Multiple Significant Trauma

Potential DRGs

484	**Craniotomy** for Multiple Significant Trauma	RW	5.4179
486	**Other O.R. Procedures** for Multiple Significant Trauma	RW	4.8793

DRG	Principal Dx/Procedure	Codes	Tips
484	Craniotomy for multiple significant trauma		■ Craniotomy and principal diagnosis of trauma and at least two injuries (assigned either as principal or secondary) that are defined as significant trauma from different body site categories located under DRG 487
486	Other O.R. procedures for multiple significant trauma		■ Principal diagnosis of trauma and at least two injuries (assigned either as principal or secondary) that are defined as significant trauma from different body site categories located under DRG 487 *AND* O.R. procedure other than craniotomy or limb reattachment, hip and femur procedures

Other O.R. Procedures for Multiple   RW 4.8793   **DRG 486**
Significant Trauma

Potential DRGs

484	**Craniotomy** for Multiple Significant Trauma	RW	5.4179

DRG	Principal Dx/Procedure	Codes	Tips
484	Craniotomy for multiple significant trauma		■ Craniotomy and principal diagnosis of trauma and at least two injuries (assigned either as principal or secondary) that are defined as significant trauma from different body site categories located under DRG 487

■ Coding Tip   ● Documentation Tip   ◆ Encoder Tip   ᵂᴱᴳ Targeted DRG

Multiple Significant Trauma, MDC 24

DRG 487   Other Multiple Significant Trauma   RW 2.0057

Potential DRGs

484	Craniotomy for Multiple Significant Trauma	RW	5.4179
485	Limb Reattachment, Hip & Femur Procedures for Multiple Significant Trauma	RW	3.2121
486	Other O.R. Procedures for Multiple Significant Trauma	RW	4.8793

DRG	Principal Dx/Procedure	Codes	Tips
484	Craniotomy for multiple significant trauma		■ Craniotomy and principal diagnosis of trauma and at least two injuries (assigned either as principal or secondary) that are defined as significant trauma from different body site categories located under DRG 487
485	Limb reattachment, hip and femur procedures for multiple significant trauma		■ Principal diagnosis of trauma and at least two injuries (assigned either as principal or secondary) that are defined as significant trauma from different body site categories located under DRG 487 AND limb reattachment, hip and femur O.R. procedures
486	Other O.R. procedures for multiple significant trauma		■ Principal diagnosis of trauma and at least two injuries (assigned either as principal or secondary) that are defined as significant trauma from different body site categories located under DRG 487 AND O.R. procedure other than craniotomy or limb reattachment, hip and femur procedures

HIV Infections, MDC 25

DRG 488   HIV with Extensive Operating Room Procedure

No Potential DRGs

DRG 489   HIV with Major Related Condition   RW 1.8603

Potential DRGs

488	HIV with Extensive O.R. Procedure	RW	4.8118

DRG	Principal Dx/Procedure	Codes	Tips
488	Extensive O.R. procedure: Any operation not listed in DRG 477		

HIV with or without Other Related Condition

RW 1.0512 **DRG 490**

Potential DRGs

488	HIV with **Extensive O.R. Procedure**	RW	4.8118
489	HIV with **Major Related Condition**	RW	1.8603

DRG	Principal Dx/Procedure	Codes	Tips
488	Extensive O.R. procedure: Any operation not listed in DRG 477		
489	Major HIV-related condition: *Salmonella* infection NEC Coccidiosis Candidiasis Primary TB	*003.8 007.2 *112 *010	◆ Key terms: *Isospora belli, Isospora hominis*, isosporiasis

Other DRGS, DRGs Associated with All MDCs and Pre-MDCs

Heart Transplant (Pre-MDC)

DRG 103

No Potential DRGs

Extensive O.R. Procedure Unrelated to Principal Diagnosis

DRG 468

This DRG is not associated with an MDC. No Potential DRGs.

Principal Diagnosis Invalid as Discharge Diagnosis

DRG 469

This DRG is not associated with an MDC. No Potential DRGs.

Ungroupable

DRG 470

This DRG is not associated with an MDC. No Potential DRGs.

Prostatic O.R. Procedure Unrelated to Principal Diagnosis

RW 2.2477 **DRG 476**

This DRG is not associated with an MDC.

*Ensure accurate DRG assignment.
Listed below are the O.R. procedures found in DRG 476:

60.0	Incision of prostate	60.82	Periprostatic excision
60.12	Open biopsy of prostate	60.93	Repair of prostate
60.15	Biopsy of periprostatic tissue	60.94	Control of postoperative hemorrhage of prostate
60.18	Other diagnostic procedures on prostate and periprostatic tissues	60.95	Transurethral balloon dilation of the prostatic urethra
60.21	Transurethral (ultrasound) guided laser-induced prostatectomy (TULIP)	60.96	Destruction, transurethral, microwave thermotherapy, prostate tissue
60.29	Other transurethral prostatectomy	60.97	Destruction, transurethral, other thermotherapy, prostate tissue
60.61	Local excision of lesion of prostate	60.99	Other operations on prostate NEC
60.69	Prostatectomy NEC		
60.81	Periprostatic incision		

■ Coding Tip	● Documentation Tip	◆ Encoder Tip	▽ Targeted DRG

Other DRGS, DRGs Associated with All MDCs and Pre-MDCs

DRG 477   Nonextensive O.R. Procedure Unrelated to Principal Diagnosis
RW 1.8873

This DRG is not associated with an MDC.

Potential DRGs
468   Extensive O.R. Procedure Unrelated to Principal Diagnosis   RW   3.8454

DRG	Principal Dx/Procedure	Codes	Tips
468	Extensive operating room procedure (any O.R. procedure not listed for DRGs 476 & 468)		

DRG 480   Liver Transplant (Pre-MDC)

No Potential DRGs

DRG 481   Bone Marrow Transplant (Pre-MDC)

No Potential DRGs

DRG 482   Tracheostomy for Face, Mouth and Neck Diagnoses (Pre-MDC)
RW 3.4803

Potential DRGs
483   Tracheostomy with **Mech Vent 96+ Hours or Pdx Except Face, Mouth**   RW   16.7762
and Neck Diagnoses

DRG	Principal Dx/Procedure	Codes	Tips
483	Diagnosis except for mouth, larynx or pharynx disorder *AND* Tracheostomy with mechanical ventilation 96+ hours	31.1, 31.21, 31.29, 31.1, 96.72	■ A minitracheostomy is coded as a temporary tracheostomy. ■ Tracheostomy carried out elsewhere prior to admission or in ambulance prior to arrival should not be reported as a current procedure. ● Tracheostomy procedure may be performed either at the bedside and documented in the progress notes or in the operating room and documented in an operative note.

DRG 483   Tracheostomy with Mech Vent 96+ Hours or PDx Except Face, Mouth and Neck Diagnoses (Pre-MDC)

No Potential DRGs

DRG 495   Lung Transplant (Pre-MDC)
RW 8.5551

Potential DRGs
103   Heart Transplant   RW   18.6081

DRG	Principal Dx/Procedure	Codes	Tips
103	Heart-lung transplant	33.6	

■ Coding Tip   ● Documentation Tip   ◆ Encoder Tip   ▽ Targeted DRG

Simultaneous Pancreas/Kidney Transplant (Pre-MDC)   DRG 512

No Potential DRGs

Pancreas Transplant (Pre-MDC)   DRG 513

No Potential DRGs

Complications and Comorbidities (CC) List

The following is a standard list of conditions considered to be complications and comorbidities that when present as a secondary diagnosis may affect DRG assignment. An asterisk (*) indicates a code range is represented.

Code	Code Title
*008.4	Intestinal infection, other specified bacteria
*011	Pulmonary tuberculosis
*012.0	Tuberculous pleurisy
*012.1	Tuberculosis, intrathoracic nodes
*013	Tuberculous meningitis
*014	Tuberculous peritonitis
*016	Tuberculosis, genitourinary system
*017.2	Tuberculosis, peripheral lymph nodes
*017.3	Tuberculosis of eye
*017.4	Tuberculosis of ear
*017.5	Tuberculosis of thyroid gland
*017.6	Tuberculosis of adrenal glands
*017.7	Tuberculosis of spleen
*017.8	Tuberculosis of esophagus
*017.9	Tuberculosis other specified organs
*018	Miliary tuberculosis
031.0	Pulmonary diseases due to other mycobacteria
*036	Meningococcal meningitis
037	Tetanus
*038	Septicemia
040.0	Gas gangrene
042	Human immunodeficiency virus [HIV] disease
046.2	Subacute sclerosing panencephalitis
040.82	Toxic shock syndrome
*052	Varicella
*053.0	Herpes zoster with meningitis
*053.1	Herpes zoster with other nervous system complications
053.79	Herpes zoster, other specified complications
053.8	Unspecified herpes zoster complication
054.3	Herpetic meningoencephalitis
054.5	Herpetic septicemia

Code	Code Title
054.71	Visceral herpes simplex
054.72	Herpes simplex meningitis
054.79	Herpes simplex w/other complications
054.8	Herpes simplex complication w/ unspecified complication
*055	Measles
*056	Rubella
070.2	Viral hepatitis B with hepatic coma
070.3	Viral hepatitis B without mention of hepatic coma
070.4	Viral hepatitis, other specified, with hepatic coma
070.5	Viral hepatitis, other specified, without mention of hepatic coma
070.6	Viral hepatitis, unspecified, with hepatic coma
070.9	Viral hepatitis, unspecified, without mention of hepatic coma
*072	Mumps
079.82	SARS-associated coronavirus
086.0	Chagas' disease with heart involvement
*090.4	Juvenile neurosyphilis
*093	Cardiovascular syphilis
094.0	Tabes dorsalis
094.1	General paresis
094.2	Syphilitic meningitis
094.3	Asymptomatic neurosyphilis
094.81	Syphilitic encephalitis
094.87	Syphilitic ruptured cerebral aneurysm
094.89	Other specified neurosyphilis
094.9	Unspecified neurosyphilis
*098.1	Gonococcal infection (acute) of upper genitourinary tract
112.0	Candidiasis of mouth
112.4	Candidiasis of lung
112.5	Disseminated candidiasis

Code	Code Title	Code	Code Title
112.81	Candidal endocarditis	137.2	Late effects of genitourinary tuberculosis
112.82	Candidal otitis externa		
112.83	Candidal meningitis	138	Late effects of acute poliomyelitis
112.84	Candidiasis of the esophagus	*150	Malignant neoplasm of esophagus
112.85	Candidiasis of the intestine	*151	Malignant neoplasm of stomach
114.0	Primary coccidioidomycosis (pulmonary)	*152	Malignant neoplasm of small intestine
114.2	Coccidioidal meningitis	*153	Malignant neoplasm of colon
114.3	Other forms of progressive coccidioidomycosis	*154	Malignant neoplasm, rectum/rectosig junction/ anus
114.9	Unspecified coccidioidomycosis	*155	Malignant neoplasm of liver & intrahep bile ducts
115.00	Histoplasma capsulatum, w/out mention of manifestation	*156	Malignant neoplasm gallbladder & extrahep bile ducts
115.01	Histoplasma capsulatum meningitis	*157	Malignant neoplasm of pancreas
115.02	Histoplasma capsulatum retinitis	162.2	Malignant neoplasm of main bronchus
115.03	Histoplasma capsulatum pericarditis	162.3	Malignant neoplasm of upper lobe, bronchus, or lung
115.04	Histoplasma capsulatum endocarditis	162.4	Malignant neoplasm of middle lobe, bronchus, or lung
115.05	Histoplasma capsulatum pneumonia	162.5	Malignant neoplasm of lower lobe, bronchus, or lung
*115.1	Infection, Histoplasma duboisii	162.8	Malignant neoplasm of other parts of bronchus or lung
*115.9	Infection, Histoplasmosis, NOS	162.9	Malignant neoplasm of bronchus and lung, unspec site
116.0	Blastomycosis		
116.1	Paracoccidioidomycosis	*163	Malignant neoplasm of pleura
117.3	Aspergillosis	*164	Malignant neoplasm thymus/ heart and mediastinum
117.4	Mycotic mycetomas		
117.5	Cryptococcosis	176.4	Kaposi's sarcoma of lung
117.6	Allescheriosis (Petriellidosis)	176.5	Kaposi's sarcoma of lymph nodes
117.7	Zygomycosis (Phycomycosis or Mucormycosis)	189.0	Malignant neoplasm of kidney, except pelvis
118	Opportunistic mycoses	189.1	Malignant neoplasm of renal pelvis
130.0	Meningoencephalitis due to toxoplasmosis	189.2	Malignant neoplasm of ureter
130.1	Conjunctivitis due to toxoplasmosis	*191	Malignant neoplasm of brain
130.2	Chorioretinitis due to toxoplasmosis	192.0	Malignant neoplasm of cranial nerves
130.3	Myocarditis due to toxoplasmosis	192.1	Malignant neoplasm of cerebral meninges
130.4	Pneumonitis due to toxoplasmosis	192.2	Malignant neoplasm of spinal cord
130.5	Hepatitis due to toxoplasmosis	192.3	Malignant neoplasm of spinal meninges
130.7	Toxoplasmosis of other specified sites	192.8	Malignant neoplasm of other specified sites of nervous system
130.8	Multisystemic disseminated toxoplasmosis		
135	Sarcoidosis	*196	Secondary and unspec malignant neoplasm of lymph nodes
136.3	Pneumocystosis		
137.0	Late effects of respiratory or unspecified tuberculosis		
137.1	Late effects of central nervous system tuberculosis		

Code	Code Title	Code	Code Title
*197	Secondary malignant neoplasm of resp & digestive tracts	276.4	Mixed acid-base balance disorder
*198	Secondary malignant neoplasm other specified sites	276.5	Volume depletion
		276.6	Fluid overload
199.0	Disseminated malignant neoplasm	276.7	Hyperpotassemia
*200	Lymphosarcoma and reticulosarcoma	277.00	Cystic fibrosis without ileus
*201	Hodgkin's disease	277.01	Cystic fibrosis with ileus
*202	Oth malignant neoplasm lymphoid and histiocytic tissue	277.02	Cystic fibrosis with pulmonary manifestations
*203	Multiple myeloma & immunoprolif neoplasms	277.03	Cystic fibrosis with gastrointestinal manifestations
*204	Lymphoid leukemia	277.09	Cystic fibrosis with other manifestations
*205	Myeloid leukemia	279.02	Selective IgM immunodeficiency
*206	Monocytic leukemia	279.03	Other selective immunoglobulin deficiencies
*207	Other specified leukemia		
*208	Leukemia of unspec cell type	279.04	Congenital hypogammaglobulinemia
*242	Thyrotoxicosis with or without goiter	279.05	Immunodeficiency with increased IgM
*250	Diabetes mellitus (except fifth-digit subclassification of 0)	279.06	Common variable immunodeficiency
251.0	Hypoglycemic coma	279.09	Other deficiency of humoral immunity
251.3	Postsurgical hypoinsulinemia	279.1	Deficiency of cell-mediated immunity
252.1	Hypoparathyroidism	279.2	Combined immunity deficiency
253.2	Panhypopituitarism	279.3	Unspecified immunity deficiency
253.5	Diabetes insipidus	279.4	Autoimmune disease, NEC
254.1	Abscess of thymus	279.8	Other specified disorders involving immune mechanism
255.0	Cushing's syndrome		
255.3	Other corticoadrenal overactivity	279.9	Unspecified disorder of immune mechanism
255.4	Corticoadrenal insufficiency		
255.5	Other adrenal hypofunction	280.0	Iron deficiency anemia secondary to blood loss (chronic)
255.6	Medulloadrenal hyperfunction		
*258	Polyglandular dysfunction and related disorders	281.4	Protein-deficiency anemia
		281.8	Anemia assoc w other specified nutritional deficiency
259.2	Carcinoid syndrome		
260	Kwashiorkor	282.41	Thalassemia, sickle-cell, without crisis
261	Nutritional marasmus	282.42	Thalassemia, sickle-cell, with crisis
262	Other severe protein-calorie malnutrition	282.49	Thalassemia, other
*263	Other & unspecified protein-calorie malnutrition	*282.6	Sickle-cell anemia
		*283	Acquired hemolytic anemia
269.0	Deficiency of vitamin K	*284	Aplastic anemia
273.3	Macroglobulinemia	285.0	Sideroblastic anemia
276.0	Hyperosmolality and/or hypernatremia	285.1	Acute posthemorrhagic anemia
		*286	Coagulation defects
267.1	Hyposmolality and/or hyponatremia	*287	Purpura & other hemorhagic conditions
276.2	Acidosis		
276.3	Alkalosis	288.0	Agranulocytosis

Complications & Comorbidities

Code	Code Title	Code	Code Title
288.1	Functional disorders of polymorphonuclear neutrophils	295.31	Paranoid schizophrenia, subchronic condition
289.81	Hypercoagulable state, primary	295.32	Paranoid schizophrenia, chronic condition
289.92	Hypercoagulable state, secondary	295.33	Paranoid schizophrenia, subchr with acute exacerbation
291.0	Alcohol withdrawal delirium		
291.1	Alcohol amnestic syndrome	295.34	Paranoid schizophrenia, chronic w acute exacerbation
291.2	Other alcoholic dementia		
291.3	Alcohol withdrawal hallucinosis	295.40	Acute schizophrenic episode, unspecified condition
291.4	Idiosyncratic alcohol intoxication		
*291.8	Other specified alchoholic psychosis	295.41	Acute schizophrenic episode, subchronic condition
291.9	Unspecified alcoholic psychosis	295.42	Acute schizophrenic episode, chronic condition
*292	Drug psychoses		
293.81	Organic delusional syndrome	295.43	Acute schizophrenic episode, subch w acute exacerbation
293.82	Organic hallucinosis syndrome		
293.83	Organic affective syndrome	295.44	Acute schizophrenic ep chr with acute exacerbation
293.84	Drug depressive syndrome		
295.00	Simple schizophrenia, unspecified condition	295.60	Residual schizophrenia, unspecified condition
295.01	Simple schizophrenia, subchronic condition	295.61	Residual schizophrenia, subchronic condition
295.02	Simple schizophrenia, chronic condition	295.62	Residual schizophrenia, chronic condition
295.03	Simple schizophrenia, subchr w ac exacerbation	295.63	Resid schizophrenia, subchr with acute exacerbation
295.04	Simple schizophrenia, chronic with acute exacerbation	295.64	Resid schizophrenia, chr condition w acute exacerbation
295.10	Disorganized schizophrenia, unspecified condition	295.70	Schizo-affective schizophrenia, unspecified condition
295.11	Disorganized schizophrenia, subchronic condition	295.71	Schizo-affective schizophrenia, subchronic condition
295.12	Disorganized schizophrenia, chronic condition	295.72	Schizo-affective schizophrenia, chronic condition
295.13	Disorg schizophrenia, subchr with acute exacerbation	295.73	Schizo-affective schizophren subchr w acute exacerbation
295.14	Disorg schizophrenia, chronic with acute exacerbation	295.74	Schizo-affective schizophren chr acute exacerbation
295.21	Catatonic schizophrenia, subchronic condition	295.80	Other spec types schizophren unspec condition
295.22	Catatonic schizophrenia, chronic condition	295.81	Other spec types schizophren subchr
295.23	Caton schizophrenia, subchronic w acute exacerbation	295.82	Other specified types of schizophrenia, chronic condition
295.24	Caton schizophrenia, chr with acute exacerbation	295.83	Oth spec types schizophren subchr w acute exacerbation
295.30	Paranoid schizophrenia, unspecified condition	295.84	Oth spec types schizophren chr w acute exacerbation
		295.90	Unspecified schizophrenia, unspecified condition

Code	Code Title	Code	Code Title
295.91	Unspecified schizophrenia, subchronic condition	304.10	Barbitur & similar sedative/hypnotic depen, unspec abuse
295.92	Unspecified schizophrenia, chronic condition	304.11	Barbitur & similar sedative/hypnotic depen, contin abuse
295.93	Unspec schizophren subchr w acute exacerbation	304.12	Barbitur & similar sedative/hypnotic depen, episodic abuse
295.94	Unspec schizophren chr with acute exacerbation	304.20	Cocaine dependence, unspecified
296.04	Manic dis single epi severe, spec w psychotic behavior	304.21	Cocaine dependence, continuous
296.14	Manic dis recurrent epi severe spec w psychotic behavior	304.22	Cocaine dependence, episodic
296.34	Maj depres dis recur epi, severe, spec w psychotic behav	304.40	Amphet & oth psychostimulant dependence, unspecified
296.44	Bipol aff dis manic sev spec w/ psychotic behavior	304.41	Amphet & oth psychostimulant dependence, continuous
296.54	Bipol aff dis depressed, sev spec w psychotic behavior	304.42	Amphet & oth psychostimulant dependence, episodic
296.64	Bipol aff dis mixed, severe, spec w psychotic behavior	304.50	Hallucinogen dependence, unspecified
298.0	Depressive type psychosis	304.51	Hallucinogen dependence, continuous
298.3	Acute paranoid reaction	304.52	Hallucinogen dependence, episodic
298.4	Psychogenic paranoid psychosis	304.60	Drug dependence NEC, unspecified
299.00	Infantile autism, current or active state	304.61	Drug dependence NEC, continuous
299.10	Disintegrative psychosis, current or active state	304.62	Drug dependence NEC, episodic
299.80	Oth spec early childhood psychoses current or active state	304.70	Combin opioid type drug w/ any oth dependence, unspec
299.90	Unspecified childhood psychosis, current or active state	304.71	Combin opioid type drug w any oth depen continuous
303.00	Acute alcoholic intoxication, unspecified drunkenness	304.72	Combin opioid type drug w/ any oth depen episodic
303.01	Acute alcoholic intoxication, continuous drunkenness	304.80	Combin drug depen excl opioid type drug, unspecified
303.02	Acute alcoholic intoxication, episodic drunkenness	304.81	Combin drug depen excl opioid type drug, unspecified
303.90	Oth & unspec alc dep unspec drunkenness	304.82	Combin drug depen excl opioid type drug, episodic
303.91	Oth & unspec alc depen contin drunkenness	304.90	Drug dependence NOS, unspecified
303.92	Oth & unspec alc depen episodic drunkenness	304.91	Drug dependence NOS, continuous
304.00	Opioid type dependence, unspecified abuse	304.92	Drug dependence NOS, episodic
304.01	Opioid type dependence, continuous abuse	305.00	Alcohol abuse, unspecified
304.02	Opioid type dependence, episodic abuse	305.01	Alcohol abuse, continuous
		305.02	Alcohol abuse, episodic
		305.30	Hallucinogenic abuse, unspecified
		305.31	Hallucinogenic abuse, continuous
		305.32	Hallucinogenic abuse, episodic
		305.40	Barbitur & similar sedative or hynotic abuse, unspecified

Complications & Comorbidities

Code	Code Title	Code	Code Title
305.41	Barbitur & similar sedative or hynotic abuse, continuous	345.41	Partial epilep w impair consciousness w intrac epilepsy
305.42	Barbitur & similar sedative or hynotic abuse, episodic	345.51	Partial epilep w/o impair conscious w intractable epilepsy
305.50	Opioid nondependent abuse, unspecified	345.61	Infantile spasms with intractable epilepsy
305.51	Opioid nondependent abuse, continuous	345.71	Epilepsia partialis continua with intractable epilepsy
305.52	Opioid nondependent abuse, episodic	345.81	Other forms of epilepsy with intractable epilepsy
305.60	Cocaine nondependent abuse, unspecified	345.91	Complication, CNS device
305.61	Cocaine nondependent abuse, continuous	348.1	Anoxic brain damage
305.62	Cocaine nondependent abuse	349.1	Nervous system complic. from surgically implanted device
305.70	Amphet/relat sympathomimamine nondependent abuse, unspecified	349.81	Cerebrospinal fluid rhinorrhea
305.71	Amphet/ relat sympathomimetic nondependent abuse contin	349.82	Toxic encephalopathy
		357.0	Acute infective polyneuritis
305.72	Amphet/relat sympathomimetic nondependent abuse, episodic	358.00	Myasthenia gravis, without (acute) exacerbation
305.90	Drug nondependent abuse NEC, unspecified	358.01	Myasthenia gravis, with (acute) exacerbation
305.91	Drug nondependent abuse NEC, continuous	358.1	Myasthenic syndromes in diseases classified elsewhere
305.92	Drug nondependent abuse NEC, episodic	359.0	Congenital hereditary muscular dystrophy
307.1	Anorexia nervosa	359.1	Hereditary progressive muscular dystrophy
*320	Bacterial meningitis	377.00	Unspecified papilledema
*321	Meningitis due to other organisms	377.01	Papilledema associated w increased intracran pressure
*322	Meningitis of unspecified cause	377.02	Papilledema associated with decreased ocular pressure
*324	Intracranial & intraspinal abscess		
325	Phlebitis & thrombophlebitis intracranial venous sinuses	383.01	Subperiosteal abscess of mastoid
331.4	Obstructive hydrocephalus	383.30	Unspecified postmastoidectomy complication
*335	Anterior horn disease	383.81	Postauricular fistula
340	Multiple sclerosis	*394	Mitral valve diseases
343.2	Quadriplegic infantile cerebral palsy	*395	Aortic valve diseases
*344.0	Quadriplegia and quadriparesis	*396	Mitral and aortic valvular diseases
345.01	Generalized nonconvulsive epilepsy w intractable epilepsy	*397	Diseases of other endocardial structures
345.10	Generalized convulsive epilepsy w/o intractable epilepsy	398.0	Rheumatic myocarditis
345.11	Generalized convulsive epilepsy with intractable epilepsy	398.91	Rheumatic heart failure (congestive)
		401.0	Essential hypertension, malignant
345.2	Epileptic petit mal status	*402.0	Hypertensive heart disease
345.3	Epileptic grand mal status	402.11	Benign hypertensive heart disease with CHF

Code	Code Title	Code	Code Title
402.91	Unspecified hypertensive heart disease with heart failure	416.0	Primary pulmonary hypertension
*403.0	Malig hypertensive renal disease	*420	Acute pericarditis
403.11	Benign hypertensive renal disease with renal failure	*421	Acute and subacute endocarditis
403.91	Unspecified hypertensive renal disease with renal failure	*422	Acute myocarditis
*404.0	Hyperten heart & renal disease	423.0	Hemopericardium
404.11	Benign hyperten heart & ren dis w heart failure	423.1	Adhesive pericarditis
404.12	Benign hyperten heart and renal disease with renal failure	423.2	Constrictive pericarditis
404.13	Benign hyperten hrt & ren dis w heart failure & ren failure	*424	Other diseases of endocardium
		*425	Cardiomyopathy
404.91	Unspec hyperten heart and renal disease w heart failure	426.0	Atrioventricular block, complete
404.92	Unspec hyperten heart & renal disease with renal failure	426.12	Mobitz (type) II atrioventricular block
404.93	Unspec hyperten hrt & ren dis w heart failure & renal failure	426.13	Other second degree atrioventricular block
405.01	Secondary renovascular hypertension, malignant	426.53	Other bilateral bundle branch block
		426.54	Trifascicular block
405.09	Other secondary hypertension, malignant	426.6	Other heart block
		426.7	Anomalous atrioventricular excitation
410.01	Acute myocardial infarction, anterolat wall, initial epi care	426.81	Lown-Ganong-Levine syndrome
410.11	Acute myocardial infarction, oth ant wall, initial epi care	426.89	Other specified conduction disorder
		426.9	Conduction disorder NOS
410.21	Acute myocardial infarction, inferolat wall, initial epi care	427.0	Paroxysmal supraventricular tachycardia
410.31	Acute myocardial infarction, inferopost wall, initial epi care	427.1	Paroxysmal ventricular tachycardia
410.41	Acute myocardial infarction, oth inf wall, initial epi care	427.2	Unspecified paroxysmal tachycardia
410.51	Acute myocardial infarction, oth latl wall, initial epi care	*427.3	Atrial fibrillation and flutter
		*427.4	Ventricular fibrillation and flutter
410.61	Acute myocardial infarct, true post wall infarct, initl epi care	427.5	Cardiac arrest
410.71	Acute myocardial infarct, subendo infarct, initial epi care	*428	Heart failure
410.81	Acute myocardial infarct, oth spec sites, initial epi care	428.20	Unspecified systolic heart failure
		428.21	Acute systolic heart failure
410.91	Acute myocardial infarction, unspec site, initial epis care	428.22	Chronic systolic heart failure
		428.23	Acute on chronic systolic heart failure
*411	Other acute and subacute ischemic heart disease	428.30	Unspecified diastolic heart failure
		428.31	Acute diastolic heart failure
*413	Angina pectoris	428.32	Chronic diastolic heart failure
*415	Acute pulmonary heart disease	428.33	Acute on chronic diastolic heart failure
		428.40	Unspecified combined systolic and diastolic heart failure
		428.41	Acute combined systolic and diastolic heart failure
		428.42	Chronic combined systolic and diastolic heart failure
		428.43	Acute on chronic combined systolic and diastolic heart failure

Code	Code Title
429.4	Functional disturbances following cardiac surgery
429.5	Rupture of chordae tendineae
429.6	Rupture of papillary muscle
*429.7	Sequelae myocardial infarction NEC
429.81	Other disorders of papillary muscle
429.82	Hyperkinetic heart disease
430	Subarachnoid hemorrhage
431	Intracerebral hemorrhage
432.0	Nontraumatic extradural hemorrhage
432.1	Subdural hemorrhage
433.01	Occlusion & stenosis basilar artery, w cerebral infarction
433.11	Occlusion & stenosis carotid artery, w cerebral infarction
433.21	Occlusion & stenosis vertebral artery, w cerebral infarction
433.31	Occlu & sten multiple & bilat precerebral artery, w cer infarct
433.81	Occlu & sten oth spec precerebral artery, w cer infarction
433.91	Occlu & sten unspec precerebral artery, w cerebral infarction
434.01	Cerebral thrombosis, with cerebral infarction
434.11	Cerebral embolism, with cerebral infarction
434.91	Unspecified cerebral artery occlusion, w cerebral infarction
436	Acute, but ill-defined, cerebrovascular disease
437.2	Hypertensive encephalopathy
437.4	Cerebral arteritis
437.5	Moyamoya disease
437.6	Nonpyogenic thrombosis of intracranial venous sinus
440.24	Ateroscler native art of extremities w gangrene
*441.0	Dissection of aorta
441.1	Thoracic aneurysm, ruptured
441.3	Abdominal aneurysm, ruptured
441.5	Aortic aneurysm of unspecified site, ruptured
441.6	Thoracoabdominal aneurysm, ruptured
*444	Arterial embolism and thrombosis
445.01	Atheroembolism, upper extremity

Code	Code Title
445.02	Atheroembolism, lower extremity
445.81	Atheroembolism, kidney
445.89	Atheroembolism, other site
446.0	Polyarteritis nodosa
*446.2	Hypersensitivity angiitis
446.3	Lethal midline granuloma
446.4	Wegener's granulomatosis
446.5	Giant cell arteritis
446.6	Thrombotic microangiopathy
446.7	Takayasu's disease
451.0	Phlebitis & thrombophlebitis superfic ves lower extrem
451.11	Phlebitis & thrombophleb femoral vein (deep) (superficial)
451.19	Phlebitis& thrombophleb othr deep ves lower extremities
451.2	Phlebitis & thrombophlebitis lower extremities unspec
451.81	Phlebitis and thrombophlebitis of iliac vein
452	Portal vein thrombosis
*453	Other venous embolism and thrombosis
456.0	Esophageal varices with bleeding
456.20	Esophag varices w bleeding in dis classified elsewhere
459.0	Unspecified hemorrhage
464.11	Acute tracheitis with obstruction
464.21	Acute laryngotracheitis with obstruction
464.31	Acute epiglottitis with obstruction
475	Peritonsillar abscess
478.21	Cellulitis of pharynx or nasopharynx
478.22	Parapharyngeal abscess
478.24	Retropharyngeal abscess
*478.3	Paralysis of vocal cords or larynx
480.3	Pneumonia due to SARS-associated coronavirus
481	Pneumococ pneum (streptococ pneumoniae pneum)
*482	Other bacterial pneumonia
*483	Pneumonia due to other specified organisms
*484	Pneumonia in infect diseases classifed elsewhere
485	Bronchopneumonia, organism unspecified

Code	Code Title
486	Pneumonia, organism unspecified
487.0	Influenza with pneumonia
491.1	Mucopurulent chronic bronchitis
*491.2	Obstructive chronic bronchitis
491.8	Other chronic bronchitis
491.9	Unspecified chronic bronchitis
492.8	Other emphysema
493.01	Extrinsic asthma with status asthmaticus
493.02	Extrinsic asthma, with acute exacerbation
493.11	Intrinsic asthma with status asthmaticus
493.12	Intrinsic asthma, with acute exacerbation
493.20	Chr obstructive asthma w/ o mention status asthmaticus or acute exacerbation or unspecified
493.21	Chronic obstructive asthma with status asthmaticus
493.22	Chronic obstructive asthma, with acute exacerbation
493.91	Unspecified asthma, with status asthmaticus
493.92	Unspecified asthma, with acute exacerbation
494.1	Bronchiectasis, with acute exacerbation
*495	Extrinsic allergic alveolitis
496	Chronic airway obstruction NEC
506.0	Bronchitis & pneumonitis due to fumes and vapors
506.1	Acute pulmonary edema due to fumes and vapors
*507	Pneumonitis due to inhalation of solids or liquids
508.0	Acute pulmonary manifestations due to radiation
508.1	Chr & other pulmonary manifestations due to radiation
510.0	Empyema with fistula
510.9	Empyema without mention of fistula
511.1	Pleurisy w effusion w mention bacterial cause not TB
511.8	Other specified forms of effusion, except tuberculosis
511.9	Unspecified pleural effusion
*512	Pneumothorax

Code	Code Title
*513	Abscess of lung & mediastinum
515	Postinflammatory pulmonary fibrosis
*516	Other alveolar & parietoalveolar pneumonopathy
*517	Lung involvement in conditions classified elsewhere
518.0	Pulmonary collapse
518.1	Interstitial emphysema
518.4	Unspecified acute edema of lung
518.5	Pulmonary insufficiency following trauma and surgery
518.6	Allergic bronchopul aspergillosis
518.81	Respiratory failure
518.82	Other pulmonary insufficiency, NEC
518.83	Chronic respiratory failure
518.84	Acute and chronic respiratory failure
*519.0	Tracheostomy complications
519.2	Mediastinitis
527.3	Abscess of salivary gland
527.4	Fistula of salivary gland
528.3	Cellulitis and abscess of oral soft tissues
530.21	Ulcer, esophagus, with bleeding
530.4	Perforation of esophagus
530.7	Gastroesophageal laceration-hemorrhage syn
530.82	Esophageal hemorrhage
530.84	Tracheoesophageal fistula
*531.0	Acute gastric ulcer w hem
*531.1	Acute gastric ulcer w perf
*531.2	Acute gastric ulcer w hem & perf
531.31	Acu gastric ulcer w/o hem/perf w obstruction
*531.4	Chr or unspec gastric ulcer w hem
*531.5	Chr/ unspec gastric ulcer w perf
*531.6	Chr or unspec gastric ulcer w hem & perf
531.71	Chr gastric ulcer w/o hem perf w obstruction
531.91	Gastric ulcer unspec acute/ chr w/o hem/ perf w obstruct
*532.0	Acute duodenal ulcer w hem
*532.1	Acute duodenal ulcer with perforation
*532.2	Acute duodenal ulcer w hem & perf
532.31	Acute duodenal ulcer w/o hem/ perf with obstruction

Complications & Comorbidities

Code	Code Title	Code	Code Title
*532.4	Chr or unspec duodenal ulcer w hem	535.41	Other specified gastritis with hemorrhage
*532.5	Chr or unspec duodenal ulcer w perf	535.51	Unspecified gastritis & gastroduodenitis with hemorrhage
*532.6	Chr or unspec duodenal ulcer w hem & perf w/o obstruction	535.61	Duodenitis with hemorrhage
532.71	Chr duodenal ulcer w/o hem/perf with obstruction	536.1	Acute dilatation of stomach
532.91	Duoden ulcer unspec acu or chr w/o hem/ perf w obstruct	*536.4	Gastrostomy complications
		537.0	Acquired hypertrophic pyloric stenosis
*533.0	Acu peptic ulcer unspec site w hem	537.3	Other obstruction of duodenum
*533.1	Acu peptic ulcer unspec site w perf w/ o obstruction	537.4	Fistula of stomach or duodenum
*533.2	Acu peptic ulcer unspe site w hem & perf w/o obstruction	537.83	Angiodysplasia of stomach & duodenum w hemorrhage
533.31	Acu peptic ulcer unspec site w hem & perf w obstruction	537.84	Dieulafoy lesion (hemorrhagic) of stomach and duodenum
*533.4	Chr/unspec peptic ulcer unspec site w hem w/o obstruct	*540	Acute appendicitis
*533.5	Chr or unspec peptic ulcer unspec site w perf w/o obstruct	*550.0	Inguinal hernia, with gangrene
*533.6	Chr/unspec peptic ulcer unspec site w hem & perf w/ o obs	*550.1	Inguinal hernia, with obstruction, without mention of gangrene
533.71	Chr peptic ulcer unspec site w/o hemr perf w obstruction	*551	Oth hernia w gangrene , abdominal cavity
533.91	Pep ulcer unspec site unspec acu/chr w/o hem/ perf w obs	*552	Other hernia abdominal cavity with obstruction
*534.0	Acute gastrojejunal ulcer with hemorrhage	557.0	Acute vascular insufficiency of intestine
*534.1	Acu gastrojejunal ulcer w perf	558.1	Gastroenteritis and colitis due to radiation
*534.2	Acute gastrojejunal ulcer w hem & perf	558.2	Toxic gastroenteritis and colitis
534.31	Acu gastrojejunal ulcer w/ o hem/ perf with obstruction	*560	Intestinal obstruction without mention of hernia
*534.4	Chronic/unspec gastrojejunal ulcer w hem w/o obstruction	562.02	Diverticulosis of small intestine with hemorrhage
*534.5	Chronic/unspec gastrojejunal ulcer w perf w/o obstruction	562.03	Divertulitis of small intestine with hemorrhage
*534.6	Chr/unspec gastrojejunal ulcer w hem & perf w/o obstruct	562.12	Diverticulosis of colon with hemorrhage
534.71	Chronic gastrojejunal ulcer w/o hem/ perf w obstruction	562.13	Diverticulitis of colon with hemorrhage
534.91	Gastroje ulcer unspec acu/ chr w/o hem/ perf w obs	566	Abscess of anal and recal regions
535.01	Acute gastritis with hemorrhage	*567	Peritonitis
535.11	Atrophic gastritis with hemorrhage	568.81	Hemoperitoneum (nontraumatic)
535.21	Gastric mucosal hypertrophy with hemorrhage	569.3	Hemorrhage of rectum and anus
		569.5	Abscess of intestine
535.31	Alcoholic gastritis with hemorrhage	*569.6	Complications of colostomy or enterostomy
		569.83	Perforation of intestine

Code	Code Title	Code	Code Title
569.85	Angiodysplasia of intestine with hemorrhage	577.0	Acute pancreatitis
569.86	Dieulafoy lesion (hemorrhagic) of intestine	577.2	Cyst and pseudocyst of pancreas
570	Acute and subacute necrosis of liver	*578	Gastrointestinal hemorrhage
571.2	Alcoholic cirrhosis of liver	579.3	Gastroenteritis and colitis due to radiation
571.49	Other chronic hepatitis	580.0	Acu glomerulonephritis w lesion prolif glomerulonephritis
571.5	Cirrhosis of liver without mention of alcohol	580.4	Acute glomeruloneph w les rapidly progr glomerulonephritis
571.6	Biliary cirrhosis	*580.8	Acute glomerulo w oth spec path les kidney
572.0	Abscess of liver	580.9	Acute glomerulo w unspec path lesion in kidney
572.1	Portal pyemia	*581	Nephrotic syndrome
572.2	Hepatic coma	583.4	Nephr & nephrop not spec acu/chr w rap progr glomerulo
572.4	Hepatorenal syndrome	584.5	Acute renal failure with lesion of tubular necrosis
573.1	Hepatitis in viral diseases classified elsewhere	584.6	Acute renal failure with lesion of renal cortical necrosis
573.2	Hepatitis in other infectious diseases classified elsewhere	584.7	Acu ren failure w les ren medullary (papillary) necrosis
573.3	Unspecified hepatitis	584.8	Acu renal failure w oth spec pathological lesion in kidney
573.4	Hepatic infarction	584.9	Unspecified acute renal failure
*574.0	Calculus gallbladder w acu cholecystitis	585	Chronic renal failure
*574.1	Calculus gallbladder w oth cholecystitis	*590.1	Acu pyelonephritis
574.21	Calculus gallbladder w/o cholecystitis, with obstruction	590.2	Renal and perinephric abscess
*574.3	Calculus bile duct w acu cholecystitis	590.3	Pyeloureteritis cystica
*574.4	Calculus bile duct w oth cholecystitis	*590.8	Unspecified pyelonephritis
*574.5	Calculus bile duct w/o cholecystitis	590.9	Unspecified infection of kidney
*574.6	Calc gallbladder & bile ducts w acu cholecystitis	591	Hydronephrosis
*574.7	Calc gallbladder & bile ducts w oth cholecystitis	592.1	Calculus of ureter
*574.8	Calc gallbl & bile ducts w acu & chr cholecystitis	593.5	Hydroureter
*574.9	Calc gallbladder and bile ducts w/o cholecystitis	595.0	Acute cystitis
575.0	Acute cholecystitis	595.1	Chronic interstitial cystitis
575.12	Acute and chronic cholecystitis	595.2	Other chronic cystitis
575.2	Obstruction of gallbladder	595.4	Cystitis in diseases classified elsewhere
575.3	Hydrops of gallbladder	*595.8	Other specified cystitis
575.4	Perforation of gallbladder	595.9	Unspecified cystitis
575.5	Fistula of gallbladder	596.0	Bladder neck obstruction
576.1	Cholangitis	596.1	Intestinovesical fistula
576.3	Perforation of bile duct	596.2	Vesical fistula, NEC
576.4	Fistula of bile duct	596.4	Atony of bladder
		596.6	Nontraumatic rupture of bladder

Code	Code Title	Code	Code Title
596.7	Hemorrhage into bladder wall	*647.3	TB complicating preg del/ puer
597.0	Urethral abscess	*647.4	Malaria complicating preg del/ puer
598.1	Traumatic urethral stricture	*648.0	Diabetes mellitus complicating preg del/puer
598.2	Postoperative urethral stricture	*648.2	Anemia complicating preg del/ puer
599.0	Urinary tract infection, site not specified	*648.3	Drug depend. complicating preg del/ puer
599.4	Urethral false passage	*648.5	Congen CV disorders complicating preg del/ puer
599.6	Unspecified urinary obstruction		
599.7	Hematuria	*648.6	OthCV dis complicating preg del/ puer
601.0	Acute prostatitis		
601.2	Abscess of prostate	*659.3	Generalized infection during labor
601.3	Prostatocystitis	*665.0	Rupture uterus before lab onset
602.1	Congestion or hemorrhage of prostate	*665.1	Rupture uterus during labor
603.1	Infected hydrocele	666.32	Postpart coag defects w current postpartum complication
604.0	Orchitis, epididymitis & epididymo-orchitis, with abscess	666.34	Postpartum coagulation defects, postpartum complication
611.72	Lump or mass in breast	*668	Complications of anesthesia in delivery
614.0	Acute salpingitis and oophoritis		
614.3	Acute parametritis and pelvic cellulitis	*669.1	Shock in/post lab & del
614.5	Acute/unspecified pelvic peritonitis, female	*669.3	Acute renal failure post labor and delivery
615.0	Acute inflammatory disease of uterus, except cervix	*670	Major puerperal infection
616.3	Abscess of Bartholin's gland	*671.2	Superfic thrombophl comp preg & puer unspec episode
616.4	Other abscess of vulva	*671.3	Deep phlebothrombosis, antepartum, unspec episode
620.7	Hematoma of broad ligament		
*634	Spontaneous abortion	*671.4	Deep phlebothrombosis, postpart unspecified episode
*639	Comp post abortion, ectopic and molar pregnancies	*673	Obst air embolism, unspecified as to episode of care
*640	Hemorrhage in early pregnancy		
*641.0	Placenta previa w/o hem	*674.0	Cerebrovas disorder preg del puer unspec episode care
*641.1	Hem fr placenta previa		
*641.3	Antepar hem ass w coag defects	674.10	Disruption of wound, unspecified as to episode of care
*641.8	Oth antepartum hem		
*641.9	Unspec antepartum hemorrhage	674.12	Disruption cesarean wnd w del w postpartum CC
*642.4	Mild/unspec pre-eclampsia		
*642.5	Severe pre-eclampsia	*674.2	Disruption perineal wound
*642.6	Eclampsia comp preg child/ puer unspec episode of care	*674.5	Cardiomyopathy, peripartum
		675.10	Abscess breast assoc w del, unspec episode of care
*642.7	Pre-eclam/ eclam w prev hyperten comp preg del/ puer	675.11	Abscess breast assoc w del, w or w/o ment antepart cond
*644.0	Threat premature labor		
*644.1	Other threatened labor	675.12	Abscess breast w del, w postpartum complication
*646.6	Infections gu tract in pregnancy		
*646.7	Liver disorders in pregnancy	*680	Carbuncle and furuncle

Code	Code Title
682.0	Cellulitis of face
682.1	Cellulitis of neck
682.2	Cellulitis of trunk
682.3	Cellulitis of arm
682.5	Cellulitis of buttock
682.6	Cellulitis of leg
682.7	Cellulitis of foot
682.8	Cellulitis of site NEC
682.9	Cellulitis, NOS
684	Impetigo
685.0	Pilonidal cyst with abscess
694.4	Pemphigus
694.5	Pemphigoid
695.0	Toxic erythema
696.0	Psoriatic arthropathy
707.0	Decubitus ulcer
*707.1	Ulcer, lower limb, except decubitus
710.0	Systemic lupus erythematosus
710.1	Systemic sclerosis
710.3	Dermatomyositis
710.4	Polymyositis
710.5	Eosinophilia myalgia syndrome
710.8	Other specified diffuse disease of connective tissue
*711.0	Pyogenic arthritis
*711.6	Arthropathy associated with mycoses, site unspecified
714.1	Felty's syndrome
714.2	Oth rheum arthritis with visceral or systemic involvement
*714.3	Polyarticular juv rheumatoid arthritis
*722.8	Postlaminectomy syndrome
723.4	Brachial neuritis or radiculitis NOS
723.5	Torticollis, unspecified
728.0	Infective myositis
728.88	Rhabdomyolysis
*730.0	Acute osteomyelitis
*730.8	Oth inf involving bone in dis class else
*730.9	Unspecified infection of bone
*733.1	Pathologic fracture
*733.8	Malunion of fracture
733.93	Stress fracture of tibia or fibula
733.94	Stress fracture of the metatarsals
733.95	Stress fracture of other bone

Code	Code Title
*741	Spina bifida
745.0	Bulb cordis anom & and anom card sept clos com truncus
*745.1	Complete transposition of great vessels
745.2	Tetralogy of Fallot
745.3	Bulb cordis anom & anom card sep closure com ventricle
745.4	Ventricular septal defect
745.60	Unspecified type congenital endocardial cushion defect
745.69	Other congenital endocardial cushion defect
745.7	Cor biloculare
746.01	Congenital atresia of pulmonary valve
746.02	Congenital stenosis of pulmonary valve
746.1	Congenital tricuspid atresia and stenosis
746.2	Ebstein's anomaly
746.3	Congenital stenosis of aortic valve
746.4	Congenital insufficiency of aortic valve
746.5	Congenital mitral stenosis
746.6	Congenital mitral insufficiency
746.7	Hypoplastic left heart syndrome
746.81	Congenital subaortic stenosis
746.82	Cor triatriatum
746.83	Infundibular pulmonic stenosis
746.84	Congenital obstructive anomalies of heart, NEC
746.86	Congenital heart block
*747.1	Coarctation of aorta
747.22	Aortic atresiaand stenosis of aorta
748.4	Congenital cystic lung
748.5	Congenital agenesis, hypoplasia, and dysplasia of lung
748.61	Congenital bronchiectasis
765.01	Extreme fetal immaturity, less than 500 grams
765.02	Extreme fetal immaturity, 500–749 grams
765.03	Extreme fetal immaturity, 750–999 grams
765.04	Extreme fetal immaturity, 1,000–1,249 grams

Code	Code Title	Code	Code Title
765.05	Extreme fetal immaturity, 1,250–1,499 grams	773.4	Kernicterus isoimmunization of fetus or newborn
765.06	Extreme fetal immaturity, 1,500–1,749 grams	*774.0	Perinatal jaundice from hereditary hemolytic anemias
765.07	Extreme fetal immaturity, 1,750–1,999 grams	774.1	Perinatal jaundice from other excessive hemolysis
765.08	Extreme fetal immaturity, 2,000–2,499 grams	774.2	Neonatal jaundice associated with preterm delivery
767.0	Subdural and cerebral hemorrhage, birth trauma	*774.3	Neonatal jaundice d/t delayed conjugation from other causes
767.11	Injury, scalp, trauma, birth, epicranial subaponeurotic hemorrhage (massive)	774.4	Perinatal jaundice d/t hepatocellular damage
768.5	Severe birth asphyxia	774.5	Perinatal jaundice from other causes
769	Respiratory distress syndrome in newborn	774.7	Kernicterus not d/t isoimmunization
770.0	Congenital pneumonia	775.1	Neonatal diabetes mellitus
770.1	Meconium aspiration syndrome	775.2	Neonatal myasthenia gravis
770.2	Interstitial emphysema and related conditions of newborn	775.3	Neonatal thyrotoxicosis
770.3	Pulmonary hemorrhage of fetus or newborn	775.4	Hypocalcemia and hypomagnesemia of newborn
770.4	Primary atelectasis of newborn	775.5	Other transitory neonatal electrolyte disturbances
770.5	Other and unspecified atelectasis of newborn	775.6	Neonatal hypoglycemia
770.7	Chronic respiratory disease arising in the perinatal period	775.7	Late metabolic acidosis of newborn
770.84	Respiratory failure of newborn	776.0	Hemorrhagic disease of newborn
771.0	Congenital rubella	776.1	Transient neonatal thrombocytopenia
771.1	Congenital cytomegalovirus infection	776.2	Disseminated intravascular coagulation in newborn
771.3	Tetanus neonatorum	776.3	Other transient neonatal disorders of coagulation
771.81	Septicemia [sepsis] of newborn	777.1	Fetal and newborn meconium obstruction
771.83	Bacteremia of newborn	777.2	Intestinal obs due to inspissated milk
*772.1	Intraventricular hemorrhage	777.5	Necrotizing enterocolitis in fetus or newborn
772.2	Fetal and neonatal subarachnoid hemorrhage of newborn	777.6	Perinatal intestinal perforation
772.4	Fetal and neonatal gastrointestinal hemorrhage	778.0	Hydrops fetalis not due to isoimmunization
772.5	Fetal and neonatal adrenal hemorrhage	779.0	Convulsions in newborn
773.0	Hemolyt dis Rh isoimmunization of fetus or newborn	779.1	Other and unspecified cerebral irritability in newborn
773.1	Hemolytic dis abo isoimmunization of fetus or newborn	779.3	Feeding problems in newborn
773.2	Hemolyt dis oth & unspec isoimmun fetus/ newborn	779.4	Drug reactions and intoxications specific to newborn
773.3	Hydrops fetalis due to isoimmunization	779.7	Periventricular leukomalacia
		780.01	Coma
		780.03	Persistent vegetative state
		780.1	Hallucinations

Code	Code Title
780.31	Febrile convulsions
780.39	Other convulsions
781.7	Tetany
785.4	Gangrene
*785.5	Unspecified shock
786.03	Apnea
786.04	Cheyne-Stokes respiration
786.3	Hemoptysis
788.20	Unspecified retention of urine
788.29	Other specified retention of urine
789.5	Ascites
790.7	Bacteremia
791.1	Chyluria
791.3	Myoglobinuria
799.1	Respiratory arrest
799.4	Cachexia
*800	Closed fracture vault skull
*801	Closed fracture base skull
802.1	Fracture nasal bone open
*802.2	Closed fracture mandible
*802.3	Open fracture mandible
802.4	Closed fracture face malar/ maxil/bone
802.5	Open fracture face malar/ maxil/bone
802.6	Closed fracture face orbital floor blow out
802.7	Open fracture, face orbital floor blow out
802.8	Closed fracture, face other facial bone
802.9	Open fracture, face oth facial bone
*803	Other skull fracture
*804	Skull fracture w other bone fracture
*805	Fracture, vertebral column
*806	Fracture, vetebral column w spinal cord injury
807.04	Closed fracture, 4 ribs
807.05	Closed fracture, 5 ribs
807.06	Closed fracture, 6 ribs
807.07	Closed fracture, 7 ribs
807.08	Closed fracture, 8+ ribs
807.09	Closed fracture, mult ribs unsp
*807.1	Open fracture, rib, unspecified
807.2	Closed fracture, sternum
807.3	Open fracture, sternum
807.4	Open fracture, flail chest

Code	Code Title
807.5	Closed fracture, laryn/ trach
807.6	Open fracture, laryn/trach
808.0	Fracture pelvis, acetabulum, closed
808.1	Fracture pelvis, acetabulum, open
808.2	Fracture, pelvis, pubis, closed
808.3	Fracture, pelvis, pubis, open
808.43	Closed fracture w/ disruption pelvis circle
808.49	Closed fracture, pelvis
*808.5	Open fracture, specified part pelvis
808.8	Fracture pelvis, unspecified, closed
808.9	Fracture pelvis unspecified, open
*820	Fracture, neck femur
*821.0	Fracture, shaft or unsp parts femur, closed
*821.1	Open fracture, shaft or unsp part femur shaft
838.19	Open dislocation, foot, other
*839.0	Closed dislocation, cervical vertebra
*839.1	Open dislocation cervical vertebra
*850	Concussion
*851	Cerebral laceration and contusion
*852	Subarachnoid hemorrrhage, no open wound, loc unsp
*853	Other intracranial hemorrhage, post injury
*854	Iintracranial injury, unspecified
*860	Traumatic pneumothorax and hemothorax
861.01	Injury heart, no open wound, contusion
861.02	Injury heart, laceration w/ o penetr chamber
861.03	Injury heart, laceration w/ penetr chamber
*861.1	Injury heart, w/open wound thorax
861.22	Injury lung, no open wound thorax, w laceration
*861.3	Injury, lung w/open wound
862.1	Diaphragm, injury, open
*862.2	Spec intrathoracic organs w/o open wound
*862.3	Oth spec intrathorascic organs w open wound
862.9	Multiple & unspecified intrathor organs w/ open wound

Complications & Comorbidities

Code	Code Title	Code	Code Title
863.1	Injury, stomach, w/open wound into cavity	*875	Open wound, wall
*863.3	Injury, small intestine, w/open wound into cavity	*887	Traumatic amput arm & and
		*896	Traumatic amput foot
*863.5	Injury, colon or rectum, w/open wound into cavity	*897	Traumatic amput leg(s)
		*900	Injury blood vessel, head and neck
*863.9	Injury, GI tract w/open wound into cavity, unsp	901.0	Injury to thoracic aorta
*864	Injury, liver	901.1	Injury to innominate and subclavian arteries
*865	Injury, spleen	901.2	Injury to superior vena cava
*866	Injury, kidney	901.3	Injury to innominate and subclavian veins
*867	Injury, pelvic organs	901.41	Injury to pulmonary artery
*868	Injury, other abdominal organs	901.42	Injury to pulmonary vein
*869	Internal injury,unsp organs	901.83	Injury to multiple blood vessels of thorax
870.3	Penetrating wound, orbit w/ o foreign body	902.20	Injury to celiac and mesenteric arteries, unspecified
870.4	Penetrating wound, orbit w foreign body	902.22	Injury to hepatic artery
870.8	Other spec open wounds ocular adnexa	902.23	Injury to splenic artery
870.9	Unspec open wounds ocular adnexa	902.24	Injury to other specified branches of celiac axis
871.0	Ocular laceration without prolapse of intraocular tissue	902.25	Injury to superior mesenteric artery (trunk)
871.1	Ocular laceration with prolapse or exposure of intraocular tissue	902.26	Injury to primary branches of superior mesenteric artery
871.2	Rupture of eye with partial loss of intraocular tissue	902.27	Injury to inferior mesenteric artery
871.3	Avulsion of eye	902.29	Injury to celiac and mesenteric vessels, other
871.4	Unspecified laceration of eye	*902.3	Injury to portal and splenic veins
871.9	Unspecified open wound of eyeball	*902.4	Injury to renal blood vessels
872.72	Open wound, ear, complicated, ossicles	902.50	Injury to iliac vessel(s), unspecified
872.73	Open wound , ear, complicated, eustachian tube	902.51	Injury to hypogastric artery
		902.52	Injury to hypogastric vein
872.74	Open wound, ear, complicated, cochlea	902.53	Injury to iliac artery
		902.54	Injury to iliac vein
873.33	Open wound, nose, complicated, nasal sinus	902.59	Injury to iliac vessels, other
873.9	Other and unspecified open wound of head, complicated	902.87	Injury to multiple blood vessels of abdomen and pelvis
*874.0	Open wound of larynx and trachea, without mention of complication	904.0	Injury, common femoral, artery
		*925	Crush injury face/scalp and neck
*874.1	Open wound of larynx and trachea, complicated	929.0	Crush injury, multiple site, NEC
		*952	Cord injury, w/o spinal bone injury
874.3	Open wound of thyroid gland, complicated	*953	Injury, nerve root and spinal plexus
		958.0	Air embolism, early comp trauma
874.5	Open wound of pharynx, complicated	958.1	Fat embolism, early comp trauma

Code	Code Title
958.2	Secondary/recur hemorrhage, early comp trauma
958.3	Posttraumatic wound infection, NEC
958.4	Traumatic shock, early comp trauma
958.5	Traumatic anuria, early comp traum
958.7	Traumatic, subcutan emphysema
995.4	Adverse effect, shock d/t anesthesia
995.86	Malignant hyperthermia
995.90	Systemic inflammatory response syndrome, unspecified
995.91	Systemic inflammatory response syndrome due to infectious process without organ dysfunction
995.92	Systemic inflammatory response syndrome due to infectious process with organ dysfunction
995.93	Systemic inflammatory response syndrome due to noninfectious process without organ dysfunction
995.94	Systemic inflammatory response syndrome due to noninfectious process with organ dysfunction
*996.0	Mechanical compl, cardiac dev im/gft
996.1	Mechanical compl, oth vascular dev im/gft
996.2	Mechanical compl, nervous system dev im/gft
996.30	Mechanical compl, GU unsp dev im/gft
996.39	Mechanical compl, GU oth dev
996.4	Mechanical compl, internal ortho dev im/gft
*996.5	Mechanical compl, pros device/impl/graf, oth spec
*996.6	Inf/flam d/t internal prosthetic gft/dev/implant
*996.7	Oth compl internal implt/ gft d/t, unsp dev
*996.8	Complication, transplant organ
*996.9	Complication, reattach extremity
*997.0	Nervous system compl. unsp
997.1	Compl. body system, cardiac
997.2	Compl. body system, periph vascular
997.3	Compl. body system, respiratory
997.4	Compl. body system, digestive system, NEC
997.5	Compl. body system, Urin comp

Code	Code Title
997.62	Complication, amputation stump, infection, chronic
*997.7	Vascular complications of other vessels
997.99	Oth compl other specified body system
998.0	Complication of procedure, postop shock
*998.1	Complication of procedure, hemorrhage
998.2	Complication of procedure, accidental puncture/ laceratoin
998.31	Complication of procedure, disruption internal operation wound
998.32	Complication of procedure, disruption external operation wound
998.4	Complication of procedure, foreign body acc left
*998.5	Infection, postop seroma
998.6	Comp proc pers postop fist
998.7	Complication of proc, acute react foreign body acc left
998.83	Nonhealing surgical wound
998.89	Other complication, specified procedure
998.9	Unsp compl procedure, NEC
999.1	Complicaton medical care, air emb
999.2	Other complicaton medical care, vascular compl
999.3	Other complicaton medical care, infection
999.4	Complicaton medical care, anaph shk d/t serum
999.5	Complicaton medical care, oth serum react
999.6	Complicaton medical care, abo incom react
999.7	Complicaton medical care, rh incom react
999.8	Other complicaton medical care, transfusion reaction
V23.7	Insufficient prenatal care
*V23.8	Other high-risk pregnancy
V23.9	Supervision of high-risk pregnancy, unspecified
V42.0	Kidney transplant status
V42.1	Heart transplant status

Complications & Comorbidities

Code	Code Title
V42.2	Heart valve transplant
V42.6	Lung transplant status
V42.7	Liver transplant status
*V42.8	Other specified organ or tissue replaced by transplant
*V43.2	Status, organ or tissue replaced by other means, heart
V45.1	Renal dialysis status
V46.1	Dependence on ventilator

Most Commonly Missed CC Conditions

Abscess 682.3, 682.5–682.9	**Signs and Symptoms:** Skin or wound infection; may occur more often in people with poor circulation or diabetes mellitus; usually begins at site of injury to skin and quickly intensifies; affected area may be red, hot, and swollen; usual cause is an infection of an operative or traumatic wound, burn, or other lesion **Drug Therapy:** Antibiotics **Laboratory:** Cultures, grain stains, and antibiotic sensitivity tests; blood cultures may be positive **Procedures:** May include punch biopsy, surgical debridement, incision, and drainage; drainage under fluoroscopic, ultrasound, or computed tomography (CT) guidance
Abscess of Bartholin's gland 616.3	**Signs and Symptoms:** Localized pain in region of duct; discomfort when sitting or walking; organisms causing the infection include *Neisseria gonorrhea, Escherichia coli (E. coli), Streptococcus,* and *Trichomonas vaginalis* **Drug Therapy:** Antibiotic therapy **Laboratory:** Blood: Smears/cultures: positive for organism causing infection. Possible increase in white blood cells (WBCs) **Procedures:** Marsupialization of Bartholin's gland cyst; CT scan of pelvis
Acidosis, respiratory/ metabolic/lactic 276.2	**Signs and Symptoms:** Retention of CO_2 and increasing pCO_2; hypoventilation, dyspnea, drowsiness, weakness, malaise, and nausea **Laboratory:** Blood: Arterial blood gases: decreased CO_2 (less than 22); decreased HCO_3 (less than 24); decreased pH (less than 7.35); increased pCO_2 (more than 45); decreased pCO_2 (less than 35); increased blood urea nitrogen (BUN) (over 22); increased potassium (greater than 5.0); decreased potassium (less than 3.5); increased chloride (greater than 105)
Agranulocytosis (Neutropenia) 288.0	**Signs and Symptoms:** Bacterial infection and formation of sores in throat, stomach, or skin; onset is usually acute with fever and chills; ingestion of some drugs can bring on this condition **Drug Therapy:** Treatment of acute infection with appropriate antibiotics **Laboratory:** Blood: WBC markedly decreased, 95% lymphocytes; red blood cells (RBC) and platelets are normal; decreased granulocyte concentration of specific type (i.e., neutropenia, basopenia, eosinopenia) **Culture:** Confirmation of infection **Nurse's Notes:** Protective isolation; frequent monitoring of vital signs

Alcoholism, acute, continuous/ episodic/ unspecified 303.00–303.02	**Signs and Symptoms:** Alcoholism with acute intoxication. Maladaptive behavior, aggressiveness, impaired judgment; characteristic physiologic signs are flushed face, slurred speech, unsteady gait, and incoordination **Continuous:** Daily intake of large amounts or regular heavy drinking on weekends or days off from work **Episodic:** Long periods of sobriety interspersed with binges of heavy drinking lasting weeks or months **Drug Therapy:** B vitamins, antianxiety medications, and Antabuse **Laboratory:** Liver enzymes: Creatine phosphokinase (CPK), lactate dehydrogenase (LDH), serum glutamic oxaloacetic acid (SGOT), serum-glutamic oxaloacetic transminase acid (SGPT), and serum cholesterol may be increased; blood ethanol level may be increased **Nurse's Notes:** Seizure precautions during withdrawal and documentation of withdrawal symptomatology **Procedures:** Detoxification, group, and/or individual therapy **Radiology:** Liver scan and abdominal series; liver biopsy
Alcoholism, chronic, continuous/ episodic/ unspecified 303.90–303.92	**Signs and Symptoms:** Chronic alcohol dependence; symptoms and signs include delirium tremens, acute alcoholic hallucinations, alcoholic hepatitis, or cirrhosis of the liver **Drug Therapy:** B vitamins, antianxiety medications, and Antabuse **Laboratory:** Liver enzymes: CPK, LDH, SGOT, SGPT and serum cholesterol may be increased; blood ethanol level may be increased **Nurse's Notes:** Seizure precautions during withdrawal and documentation of withdrawal symptomatology **Procedures:** Detoxification and group and/or individual therapy **Radiology:** Liver scan and abdominal series; liver biopsy
Alcohol withdrawal syndrome, not elsewhere classified 291.81	**Signs and Symptoms:** Coarse tremor of hands, tongue, and eyelids within several hours of cessation or reduction of alcohol ingestion Development of one or more of the following: nausea or vomiting, fleeting hallucinations (auditory, tactile, or visual), illusions, grand mal seizures, anxiety, insomnia, autonomic hyperactivity, and psychomotor agitation; may cause very noticeable impairment of the sufferer's ability to function at work or in social settings **Drug Therapy:** Benzodiazepines such as Librium for treatment of anxiety; thiamine or large doses of vitamin C and B-complex for fluid imbalances **Laboratory:** Liver enzymes: CPK, LDH, SGOT, SGPT, and serum cholesterol may be increased; blood ethanol level may be increased **Procedures:** Detoxification, group, and/or individual therapy **Radiology:** Liver scan and abdominal series; liver biopsy

Alkalosis, metabolic/ respiratory 276.3	**Signs and Symptoms:** Metabolic alkalosis may show weakness; respirations slow and shallow; uremia; respiratory alkalosis may show drowsiness, giddiness, or paresthesias of the extremities; may be accompanied by a potassium deficiency
	Laboratory: Blood: (metabolic alkalosis): increased bicarbonate, decreased potassium, and increased pH; blood (respiratory alkalosis): Increased bicarbonate excretion, increased pH, and decreased pCO_2
	Radiology: CT scan, abdomen, and head studies
Anemia due to acute blood loss 285.1	**Signs and Symptoms:** Rapid, sudden loss of blood following rupture of an ulcer, trauma, hemophilia, acute leukemia, or excessive blood loss during surgery
	Laboratory: Blood: hemoglobin less than 8 and hematocrit less than 28
	Procedures: Transfusion(s) of blood and blood components; red cell volume, bone marrow scan, upper gastrointestinal studies, colonoscopy, or flexible sigmoidoscopy
Anemia due to chronic blood loss 280.0	**Signs and Symptoms:** Fatigue, anorexia, dyspnea, and irritability; manifestation often is offset by underlying disease; pallor, tenderness of bone, functional heart murmur, tachycardia, and dilatation of heart
	Drug Therapy: Oral iron medication may be administered
	Laboratory: Blood: RBC decreased, hemoglobin less than 8 and hematocrit less than 28
	Procedures: Bone marrow may be normal, hyperplastic, or hypoplastic; red cell volume, bone marrow scan, aspiration or biopsy, upper gastrointestinal studies, colonoscopy, or flexible sigmoidoscopy
Aneurysm of aorta with rupture 441.00–441.03, 441.1, 441.3, 441.5–441.6	**Signs and Symptoms:** Can be immediately fatal; pain is present (constant or paroxysmal) in lower back, groin, and possibly testes; pain is relieved by elevation of knees; numbness and weakness of legs with occasional paralysis; cyanosis, syncope, and shortness of breath
	Drug Therapy: IV and narcotics for pain
	Nurse's Notes: Frequent check of vital signs
	Procedures: Surgical management, whole blood transfusion, and invasive monitoring; transesophageal echocardiography
	Radiology: Chest: calcification of aortic wall; aortography: clinically diagnostic; may show displacement of kidney or ureter; CT thorax and abdominal to scan for confirmation of location

Most Commonly Missed CC Conditions

Angina Pectoris 413.0–413.9	**Signs and Symptoms:** Discomfort in the chest, described as heaviness, pressure, tightness, or squeezing sensation with radiation most usually to the left arm; underlying disease of ischemia causes interruption of coronary blood flow, creating a lack of oxygen supply to the myocardium; attacks may be precipitated by emotion, exertion, cold weather, heavy meals, or tachycardia **Drug Therapy:** May include nitroglycerin, isordil, or procardia **EKG:** Normal at first or during rest; exercise test may show inducing S-T segment depression **Procedures:** Coronary angiography: evidence of significant obstruction of major coronary artery; myocardial perfusion scans; echocardiography; thallium stress test
Anorexia nervosa 307.1	**Signs and Symptoms:** Intense fear of obesity resulting in excessive dieting; high level of activity and alertness, associated endocrinologic and physiologic changes, and distortion in body image **Drug Therapy:** Includes medications for correction of nutritional and metabolic deficiencies and psychotherapeutic drugs **EKG:** Ventricular arrhythmias due to hypokalemia **Laboratory:** Blood: may show evidence of anemia (hemoglobin less than 8, hematocrit less than 28) **Nurse's Notes:** Intake and output, daily weights, and supplemental feedings **Procedures:** Psychotherapy and nutritional counseling
Arrest, cardiac 427.5	**Signs and Symptoms:** Sudden unexpected cessation of cardiac action and absence of heart sounds and/or blood pressure; cardiopulmonary resuscitation performed **Drug Therapy:** May include isoproterenol, atropine, sodium bicarbonate, epinephrine, and calcium gluconate **EKG:** Changes prior to arrest may show bradycardia, tachycardia, or other arrhythmias, fibrillation, or asystole **Physician's/Nurse's Notes:** Resuscitative efforts recorded in notes or "code" sheet **Procedures:** May include intubation and artificial ventilation
Ascites 789.5	**Signs and Symptoms:** Serous fluid effusion and accumulation within the peritoneal cavity **Laboratory:** Blood: possible increase in WBC; albumin/globulin ratio possibly reversed **Nurse's Notes:** Daily weights, intake and output, and daily abdominal measurements **Procedures:** CT scan of abdomen, liver and spleen, abdominal ultrasound; paracentesis, liver biopsy, and insertion of LeVeen Shunt

Atelectasis 518.0	**Signs and Symptoms:** Known as lung collapse; symptomatologies vary with amount of parenchyma involved; dyspnea, cough, and possibly orthopnea **Nurse's Notes:** Deep breathing and coughing; postural drainage (often done by physical therapist) **Procedures:** Bronchoscopy, spirometry, and nebulizer treatments **Radiology:** Chest x-ray: clinically diagnostic; CT scan of thorax
Bacteremia 790.7	**Signs and Symptoms:** Bacteria in the blood; elevated temperature and chills and joint pains **Drug Therapy:** Antibiotics depending on organism sensitivity **Laboratory:** Blood culture: positive **Procedures:** IV hydration; chest films, CT scan of abdomen
Boils 680.0–680.9	**Signs and Symptoms:** Skin and subcutaneous tissue infection most commonly found in hairy areas of the body that are subject to heavy perspiration or irritation; also known as furuncles or carbuncles; symptoms include localized pain and redness **Drug Therapy:** Topical antibiotics **Laboratory:** Culture: positive for *Staphylococcus* or *Streptococcus* organisms **Nurse's Notes:** Warm compresses **Procedures:** Topical application of moist heat; surgical incision and drainage may be indicated
Bronchiectasis with acute exacerbation 494.1	**Signs and Symptoms:** Irreversible dilation of bronchi, usually resulting from chronic infection; may be congenital or acquired; production of foul-smelling sputum in large amounts **Drug Therapy:** May include antibiotics for infection and bronchodilators **Laboratory:** Sputum culture: to rule out bacteria or fungi (Aspergillus) **Nurse's Notes:** Documentation of postural drainage **Procedures:** Bronchoscopy to determine location and extent of disease and pulmonary function studies **Radiology:** Chest x-ray: to rule out tuberculosis and determine fluid level

Bronchitis, chronic 491.1–491.9	**Signs and Symptoms:** Long-standing bronchial infection with mucous and pus secretions in the bronchial tree; persistent cough with usually mucoid tenacious sputum or purulent during infection; progressive breathlessness or wheezing; physical examination may document hyperinflation with decreased breath sounds and bronchi that can be cleared with coughing
	Drug Therapy: May include bronchodilators or antibacterial agents during acute infections and diuretics for edema
	EKG: May show cor pulmonale
	Laboratory: Arterial blood gases: decreased pO_2, increased or normal pCO_2; spirometry before and after bronchodilators
	Nurse's Notes: Postural drainage
	Procedures: O_2 therapy and nebulizer treatments
	Radiology: Chest x-ray: hyperinflation with increased bronchovascular markings in acute exacerbations
Bronchitis, obstructive, chronic 491.20–491.21	**Signs and Symptoms:** Bronchitis combined with airway obstruction or emphysema; advanced disease may be associated with cyanosis with carbon dioxide retention progressing into cor pulmonale
	Drug Therapy: May include both bronchodilators or antibacterial agents, and diuretics for edema
	Laboratory: Throat culture: may be positive for organism causing infection; spirometry before and after bronchodilators, arterial blood gases, thoracic gas volume
	Nurse's Notes: Postural drainage
	Procedures: O_2 therapy and nebulizer treatments
	Radiology: Chest x-ray: clinically diagnostic for obstructive, chronic bronchitis; CT scan of thorax and lung perfusion scan
Cachexia 799.4	**Signs and Symptoms:** Malnutrition and general ill health marked by emaciation and weakness; usually found in patients with cancer and anorexia nervosa
	Drug Therapy: Vitamin supplements
	Laboratory: Blood chemistry may show nutritional and vitamin deficiencies
	Nurse's Notes: Daily weights, intake and output, and supplemental feedings
	Procedures: Total parenteral nutrition; flexible sigmoidoscopy

Cardiomyopathy 425.0–425.9	**Signs and Symptoms:** Usually demonstrated in elderly patients with loss of consciousness, palpitations, and/or dyspnea; palpitations may be evident by bouncing or rapid pulse and skipped heartbeats **Drug Therapy:** May include digoxin, pronestyl, diuretics, and vasodilators **EKG:** May show atrial enlargement, sinus tachycardia, premature ventricular contractions, atrial fibrillation, or ventricular hypertrophy **Nurse's Notes:** Intake and output, daily weights, frequent vital signs, documentation of complete bed rest, and oxygen therapy **Procedures:** Cardiac catheterization, echocardiogram, echocardiography, and possible heart transplant; pacemaker analysis if implanted **Radiology:** Chest x-ray may show cardiac hypertrophy and pleural effusion; MRI of chest
Cellulitis 682.0–682.3, 682.5–682.9	**Signs and Symptoms:** Skin or wound infection; may occur more often in people with poor circulation or diabetes mellitus; usually begins at site of injury to skin and quickly intensifies; affected area may be red, hot, and swollen **Drug Therapy:** Antibiotics **Laboratory:** Cultures, grain stains, and antibiotic sensitivity tests; blood cultures may be positive **Procedures:** May include punch biopsy or surgical debridement; bone scan for presence of osteomyelitis
Cholangitis 576.1	**Signs and Symptoms:** Pain and discomfort in the right upper quadrant of the abdomen, gradually prolonged; anorexia, nausea with possible vomiting, chills, pruritus, and moderate fever (100.4°F to 102.2°F, 38°C to 39°C) **Laboratory:** Blood: increased WBCs and increased eosinophils **Procedures:** Possible liver biopsy for bile stasis or periportal fibrosis; IV fluids **Radiology:** X-ray: operative cholangiography may show marked narrowing of the choledochal lumen and the extent of involvement of the ducts and radicles; percutaneous transhepatic biliary drainage **Surgery:** To remove gallbladder and stones
Convulsions 780.31–780.39	**Signs and Symptoms:** Sudden, violent, involuntary contraction of a group of muscles that may be episodic or paroxysmal, as in a seizure disorder or following a head trauma **Drug Therapy:** May include neurontin, clonazepam, dilantin, tegretol, phenobarbital, or other anticonvulsant drugs **EEG:** Abnormal; may indicate seizure disorder **Radiology:** CT of head, brain scan, or MRI of brain

Cor pulmonale, acute 415.0	**Signs and Symptoms:** Progressive dyspnea, substernal discomfort or pain, persistent cough, wheezing, fatigue, and edema; documentation of infection; most commonly results from chronic obstructive pulmonary disease (COPD); pulmonary hypertension results within hours of onset
	Drug Therapy: May include bronchodilators (e.g., alupent, brethine, aminophylline, bronkosol, epinephrine or theophylline and diuretics, vasodilators, digoxin, antibiotics)
	EKG: Cardiac arrhythmias such as premature atrial and ventricular contractions
	Laboratory: Arterial blood gasmay show poor air exchange (pO_2 75100); hypoxemia indicated by low O_2 saturation (O_2 less than 80); hematocrit often more than 50%; spirometry
	Nurse's Notes: Intake and output, daily weights, fluid restriction, and low-salt diet
	Procedures: Echocardiography or cardiac angiography demonstrating right ventricular hypertrophy
	Respiratory Therapy: May include intermittent positive pressure breathing (IPPB) treatment, use of O_2 (in low concentrations for patients with COPD) and/or use of bronchodilators; pulmonary function studies
Cystitis, acute 595.0	**Signs and Symptoms:** An inflammation of the urinary bladder and ureter characterized by urgency, pain, hematuria, and frequency of urination caused by calculus, bacterial infections, or tumor.
	Drug Therapy: May include Cipro, Septra or Bactrim, and Pyridium
	Laboratory: Urinalysis: evidence of WBCs and RBCs in urine; urine culturepositive; *E. coli* is the most common organism causing cystitis.
Cystitis, chronic 595.1-595.2	**Signs and Symptoms:** Prolonged urinary tract infections with long-standing complications of urethral stricture, leukoplakia, or urinary retention
	Drug Therapy: May include Cipro, Septra, and Bactrim
	Laboratory: Urinalysis: evidence of WBC and RBC urine culture: may be positive for organism causing infection (most common is *E. coli*)
Dehydration 276.5	**Signs and Symptoms:** Excessive loss of water from the body tissue with a disturbance of the electrolytes, such as sodium, chloride, and potassium; also called volume depletion syndrome; physical signs and symptoms include loss of skin turgor, dry mucous membranes, thirst, lethargy, lowered tension of the eyeballs, pinched faces, a rapid resting pulse, and hypotension in the recumbent position
	Drug Therapy: Oral replenishment of fluids or intravenous administration of fluids; in severe dehydration, rapid infusion of blood plasma is indicated; in less severe conditions, saline may be infused
	Laboratory: Blood chemistry may show electrolyte disturbance (i.e., low potassium [less than 3.5 mEq/L])
	Nurse's Notes: Monitoring intake and output

Disease, Addison's 255.4	**Signs and Symptoms:** Features of crisis include anorexia, headache, weakness, dizziness, nausea, vomiting, apprehension, diarrhea, abdominal pain and syncope; chronic Addison's disease may show symptoms resembling hypoglycemia (i.e., hunger, sweating, irritability, nervousness and depression) **Drug Therapy:** Glucocorticoid and mineralocorticoid replacement **Laboratory:** Blood: sodium and glucose decreased; potassium level increased; azotemia present; plasma cortisol levels decreased; 24-hour urine for 17 ketosteroids and 17 hydroxycorticosteroids to establish baseline urine steroids **Nurse's Notes:** Record of intake and output, weight, and vital signs
Disease, hypertensive heart and renal, malignant 404.00	**Signs and Symptoms:** History of renal disease, headache, fatigue, and irritability; evidence of renal failure; elevated blood pressure (systolic greater than 160 and diastolic greater than 100); malignant hypertension diastolic pressure above 140 mm Hg, or lower diastolic pressure described as rising and irregular, or accompanied by focal neurological deficits **Drug Therapy:** Parenteral antihypertensive therapy, with a rapid acting agent such as the vasodilator Nitrostat **EKG:** Possible tachycardia **Laboratory:** BUN level greater than 20 and creatinine above 2.5 **Nurse's Notes:** Frequent monitoring of vital signs, intake and output, and low-sodium diet **Procedures:** Possible kidney transplant and dialysis, arteriogram, bicycle stress testing, and echocardiography **Radiology:** Renal scan and urography
Disease, hypertensive heart, benign, with heart failure 402.11	**Signs and Symptoms:** Elevated blood pressure (systolic greater than 160 and diastolic greater than 100); symptoms may include headache, fatigue, irritability, dyspnea, and cardiac arrhythmia **Drug Therapy:** May include hydrochlorothiazide, aldoril, altrace, lopressor, or lasix **EKG:** Tachycardia, bradycardia, or PVCs **Nurse's Notes:** Frequent monitoring of vital signs, intake and output, and oxygen therapy **Procedures:** Ophthalmoscopy: retinopathy, spirometry, arteriogram, bicycle stress testing, echocardiography, and Swan-Ganz catheterization **Radiology:** Chest x-ray: may indicate cardiac enlargement

Disease, hypertensive heart, malignant, with heart failure 402.01	**Signs and Symptoms:** Atherosclerosis, history of uncontrolled blood pressure and history of oliguria with varying degrees of renal insufficiency; onset of elevated blood pressure is usually sudden in nature; malignant hypertension diastolic pressure above 140 mm Hg, or lower diastolic pressure described as rising and irregular, or accompanied by focal neurological deficits
	Drug Therapy: Parenteral antihypertensive therapy, with a rapid acting agent such as the vasodilator Nitrostat; may include hydrochlorothiazide, aldoril, altrace, lopressor, or lasix
	Laboratory: BUN greater than 20 and creatinine greater than 2.5
	Nurse's Notes: Frequent monitoring of vital signs with evidence of rapidly accelerated high blood pressure (diastolic greater than 100, systolic greater than 140) and sodium-restricted diet
	Procedures: Ophthalmoscopy: retinopathy, arteriogram, bicycle stress testing, echocardiography, and swan-ganz catheterization
	Radiology: Chest x-ray: heart failure
Disease, hypertensive heart, unspecified, with heart failure 402.91	**Signs and Symptoms:** Atherosclerosis, obesity, ischemic heart disease, headaches, features of myocardial infarction and paroxysmal nocturnal dyspnea
	Drug Therapy: May include hydrochlorothiazide, aldoril, altrace, lopressor, or lasix
	Nurse's Notes: Frequent monitoring of vital signs with evidence of high blood pressure (diastolic greater than 100, systolic greater than 140)
	Procedures: Ophthalmoscopy: retinopathy and papilledema, arteriogram, bicycle stress testing, echocardiography, and swan-ganz catheterization
	Radiology: Chest x-ray: heart failure and cardiac enlargement
Disease, pulmonary, obstructive, chronic (COPD) 496	**Signs and Symptoms:** Irreversible and progressive condition characterized by diminished inspiratory and expiratory capacity of the lungs; exacerbation's of progressive worsening or deterioration with increased shortness of breath, weakness, wheezing, activity intolerance, retained airway secretion due to mild dehydration, or ineffective cough; expiratory slowing despite prolonged and intensive therapy
	Drug Therapy: May include bronchodilators or antibiotics in acute infections; Biaxin, Ceftin
	Laboratory: Arterial blood gases: pO_2 is usually lower than normal and pCO_2 is usually higher than normal
	Procedures: Pulmonary function test show slowing of forced expiration volume (FEV), which is disproportionate to any reduction in forced volume capacity (FVC); a ratio of FEV/FVC of less than 60%; intensification of bronchodilator therapy, liquification, evacuation of secretions, and controlled oxygen supplementation, and cardiopulmonary exercise testing
	Radiology: Chest x-ray: emphysema predominating and increased lung size

Effusion, pleural 511.9	**Signs and Symptoms:** Collection of fluid in the pleura; includes transudates, exudates, empyema, hemothorax, and chylous effusion; a few milliliters of pleural fluid is normal (less than 25 ml); dry cough, signs of congestion, tachycardia, dyspnea, and possible pleuritic pain **Drug Therapy:** May include a diuretic agent such as Lasix or digoxin **Procedures:** Thoracentesis, pleural biopsy, lung perfusion scan **Radiology:** Chest x-ray: usually diagnostic of this condition; ultrasound of chest wall
Emphysema 492.8	**Signs and Symptoms:** Manifestations modified by influences of associated pulmonary disease, condition, exertional dyspnea, cough, wheezing, and weakness **Drug Therapy:** May include bronchodilators (e.g., atrovent, albuterol, aminophylline) **Laboratory:** Arterial blood gases: evidence of CO_2 retention **Radiology:** Chest x-ray: radiolucency of lung during full expiration; possible accentuation of hilar marking **Respiratory Therapy:** Pulmonary functionvital capacity reduced; low-flow oxygen therapy
Endometritis **(acute)** 615.0	**Signs and Symptoms:** Features of salpingitis and vaginal discharge **Drug Therapy:** May include appropriate antibiotics and possibly vaginal creams **Laboratory:** Blood: increased WBC; vaginal smear: positive; culture of vaginal discharge: positive
Failure, heart, **congestive (CHF),** **unspecified** 428.0	**Signs and Symptoms:** Dyspnea is present with orthopnea and paroxysmal nocturnal dyspnea present in more advanced failure; other symptoms include peripheral edema, irritability, weakness, and neck (jugular) vein distention; cyanosis is present on occasion; heart rate is irregular; moist rales are present in bases of lungs with productive cough; confusion is usually present **Drug Therapy:** May include digoxin, diuretics and vasodilators, examples, altrace, aldoril, vasotec, zestril **EKG:** Tachycardia and atrial enlargement **Laboratory:** Possible increase in plasma volume above 5% of body weight **Nurse's Notes:** Frequent monitoring of vital signs, intake and output, antiembolism hose, low-sodium diet, oxygen therapy, daily weights, fluid restriction, and rotating tourniquets **Procedures:** Echocardiography, cardiac blood pool imaging, pulmonary artery monitoring, and cardiac catheterization **Radiology:** Chest x-ray: may show cardiac hypertrophy, pleural effusion or pulmonary venous congestion; S3 chest sound and pulmonary edema or pulmonary vascular congestion on chest x-ray

Fibrillation, atrial 427.31	**Signs and Symptoms:** Occurs as a result of other conditions, such as congestive heart failure and sepsis, or after bypass or valve replacement surgery; symptoms include palpitations, dyspnea, dizziness, fainting, and apprehension **Drug Therapy:** May include the ongoing use of digoxin, diuretics, and quinidine; calan, cardizem, coumadin **EKG:** Atrial rate over 400/minute with a variable ventricular rate; absence of P waves **Procedures:** Cardioversion and echocardiography
Fibrillation, ventricular 427.41	**Signs and Symptoms:** A life-threatening cardiac emergency; absence of effective cardiac action resulting in loss of pulse, respirations, and blood pressure; seizures and death can occur **Drug Therapy:** Lidocaine, procainamide, calan, cardizem, and digitalis **EKG:** Bizarre (QRS) complexes; ventricular rhythm chaotic and rapid **Nurse's Notes:** CPR and oxygen therapy **Procedures:** Cardiopulmonary resuscitation and defibrillation
Failure, renal, chronic/acute 584.5–585	**Signs and Symptoms:** Lethargy, fatigue, anorexia, nausea, dyspnea, weakness, thirst, oliguria, bradycardia or tachycardia and hematuria **EKG:** Arrhythmias of all types due to electrolyte imbalance **Laboratory:** Urinalysis: low specific gravity, high specific gravity if due to prerenal or postrenal factors, RBC, protein, traces of glucose, casts, epithelial cells; Blood: increase in WBCs during infection; increase of BUN and creatinine **Nurse's Notes:** Daily weights and intake and output; often with acute failure urine output is less than 500 ml per day **Procedures:** Dialysis; renal scan, ultrasound of kidney, kidney biopsy
Failure, respiratory 518.81, 518.83– 518.84	**Signs and Symptoms:** Inability of the pulmonary and cardiac systems to maintain an adequate exchange of carbon dioxide and oxygen in the lungs; acute respiratory failure (ARF) is a life-threatening emergency; symptoms include increase in sputum production, cough, and shortness of breath **Laboratory:** Arterial blood gases: increased pCO_2 (greater than 50) and decreased pO_2 (less than 50), pH less than 7.35 could be an indication **Procedures:** O_2 therapy and artificial ventilation **Radiology:** Chest x-ray: may show congestion caused by an infectious process or an obstructive process such as emphysema or chronic obstructive pulmonary disease
Fistula of bladder 596.2	**Signs and Symptoms:** Urinary incontinence, dysuria and vaginal irritation **Drug Therapy:** May include antibiotic therapy **Procedures:** Cystoscopy; surgery to repair fistula

Flutter, atrial 427.32	**Signs and Symptoms:** Palpitation, weakness, dizziness, syncope, anxiety and feeling of impending death **Drug Therapy:** May include digoxin, quinidine, propranolol, calan, cardizem, digitalis **EKG:** P waves in regular rhythm (250–350 per minute) and PR interval prolonged, varying with degree of AV block **Nurse's Notes:** Documentation of rapid, regular atrial rate between 220 and 360 per minute **Procedures:** Cardioversion, atrial pacemaker, and vagal stimulation
Fracture, pathological 733.10–733.19	**Signs and Symptoms:** Fracture resulting in weakened bone tissue (e.g., osteoporosis, neoplasms, and osteomalacia.); pain, swelling, discoloration, and tenderness at fracture site **Procedures:** Surgery to reduce and immobilize fracture; traction and wound care may be necessary **Radiology:** Skeletal x-ray: diagnostic of pathological fracture; CT scan and MRI; bone scan
Hematemesis 578.0	**Signs and Symptoms:** Vomiting of blood or "coffee ground material" **Drug Therapy:** May include vasopressin **Laboratory:** Stool may show blood in specimen; may show decreased hemoglobin and hematocrit **Nurse's Notes:** Frequent monitoring of vital signs and intake and output **Procedures:** IV therapy for volume replacement and endoscopy **Radiology:** X-rays may include uppergastrointestinal to determine source of hemorrhage, arteriography, and nuclear scans
Hematuria 599.7	**Signs and Symptoms:** Blood in the urine **Drug Therapy:** May include agents for treatment of underlying cause (e.g., urinary tract infection) (Cipro, Septra, or Bactrim) **Laboratory:** Urinalysis: red blood cells in urine specimen, indicating hemorrhage or infectious process; Blood: elevated erythrocyte sedimentation rate (ESR) **Radiology:** CT of pelvis, cystourethrogram, retrograde pyelogram
Hemorrhage, gastrointestinal 578.9	**Signs and Symptoms:** May be evident by vomiting of blood or signs of blood in stool (black and tarry) **Laboratory:** Stool may show blood in specimen; may show decreased hemoglobin and hematrocrit **Nurse's Notes:** Frequent monitoring of vital signs and intake and output **Procedures:** Endoscopy and colonoscopy **Radiology:** X-rays may include upper and lower gastrointestinal tract studies to determine source of bleeding

Hydrocele, infected 603.1	**Signs and Symptoms:** Inflammation, infection of the spermatic cord or testis **Laboratory:** Culture: fluid fibrinous, purulent or hemorrhagic, depending on underlying disease **Radiology:** Testicular scan or ultrasound
Hydronephrosis 591	**Signs and Symptoms:** Colicky, dull, aching flank pain; hematuria in about 10% of patients and urinary tract infections are common with symptoms of pyuria, fever, and discomfort **Drug Therapy:** Treatment for urinary tract infection symptoms with antibiotics **Procedures:** Cystoscopy with contrast to visualize anatomic deformity **Radiology:** Renal scan; ultrasound of kidney, pelvis, or guided nephrostomy drainage needed for severe obstruction, infection, or stones; retrograde pyelogram
Hyponatremia 276.1	**Signs and Symptoms:** Less than normal amount of sodium in the blood, caused by inadequate excretion of water or by excessive water in the circulating bloodstream due to vomiting, diarrhea, cirrhosis or drugs such as diuretics; symptoms include muscle cramps, lethargy, nausea, and seizures **Laboratory:** Blood chemistry: low sodium **Nurse's Notes:** Intake and output
Ileus, paralytic (adynamic) 560.1	**Signs and Symptoms:** Vomiting, cramps, pain, abdominal distention, absent bowel sounds, and obstipation; causes include peritoneal irritation and most cases of adynamic are postoperative **Procedures:** Nasogastric tube to remove intestinal contents; Miller-Abbott tube to decompress the intestine **Nurse's Notes:** Monitoring of pulse, blood pressure, and urine flow; parenteral fluids **Radiology:** Plain abdominal x-ray will show distended gas-filled loops in the small intestine

Infarction, myocardial, acute, initial episode 410.91	**Signs and Symptoms:** Deep severe substernal pain with radiation to back, jaw, or left arm; pain may be mild or even unrecognized in some patients; unresponsive to nitroglycerin; may be preceded by angina pectoris; signs of left heart failure may be predominant; arrhythmias and apprehension may often accompany the acute myocardial infarction
	Drug Therapy: May include use of morphine IM or intravenous to relieve pain; antiarrhythmic medication may also be administered, such as lidocaine, calan, quinidine
	EKG: Evidence of acute ischemia and infarction pattern
	Laboratory: Cardiac enzymes: increased CPK, SGOT, LDH, CK-MB, and/or LD-1 fractions
	Nurse's Notes: Intake and output and cardiopulmonary resuscitation in the event of cardiac arrest
	Procedures: Coronary angiography and O_2 therapy; thallium stress testing, myocardial perfusion scan
Infection of urinary tract 599.0	**Signs and Symptoms:** Dysuria or burning pain on urination, frequency of urination and sometimes retention of urine; fever, chills, general malaise, and hematuria.
	Drug Therapy: Appropriate antibiotic
	Laboratory: Urinalysis: WBC, RBC, and bacteria; urine culture positive for organism causing infection showing greater than 100,000 colonies of a single organism; urinalysis showing greater than 5 WBCs per high power field
	Radiology: Cystourethrogram, retrograde pyelogram, renal scan, or ultrasound of kidneys
Ischemia, coronary, acute and subacute 411.0–411.89	**Signs and Symptoms:** Arteriosclerotic heart disease, elevated cholesterol, disease of aortic valve, thoracic pain, anemia, dizziness, syncope, and dyspnea
	Drug Therapy: May include nitroglycerin, lidocaine, pronestyl, digoxin, quinidine, and potassium supplement administered intravenously
	EKG: Documentation may indicate subacute ischemia
	Laboratory: Potassium: may show a decrease in level indicating cardiac damage; enzymes slightly elevated cholesterol level greater than 250; anemia (hemoglobin less than 8 and hematocrit less than 28)
	Nurse's Notes: May document cardiac monitoring or CCU services
	Procedures: Stress EKG and cardiac catheterization, echocardiogram, myocardial perfusion studies, and gated blood pool imaging
	Radiology: Chest x-ray may show cardiac enlargement and increased hilar markings

Malnutrition (protein calorie) 262.0–263.9	**Signs and Symptoms:** Weakness, emaciation, loss of subcutaneous fat and multiple vitamin deficiencies; increased likelihood of infections and other disease processes; can result in electrolyte imbalances
	Drug Therapy: May include hydration and vitamin supplements; other supplements may include potassium
	Laboratory: Blood: may be indicative of iron deficiency anemia, low vitamin levels, and low protein levels
	Nurse's Notes: Intake and output and dietary supplements
	Procedures: Total parenteral nutrition (TPN)
	Radiology: X-ray: decreased mineralization of bone
Melena 578.1	**Signs and Symptoms:** Black, tarry stools with digested blood
	Laboratory: Stool may show blood in specimen; may show decreased hemoglobin and hematrocrit
	Nurse's Notes: Frequent monitoring of vital signs and intake and output
	Procedures: Sigmoidoscopy and colonoscopy
	Radiology: X-ray may include upper and/or lower gastrointestinal tract to determine source of hemorrhage, and may include barium enema, angiogram, and nuclear scans.
Myocarditis, acute 422.90	**Signs and Symptoms:** Inflammation of the myocardium caused by viral, bacterial, or fungal infection; precordial or substernal discomfort with severe dyspnea and later, abdominal discomfort in the right upper quadrant; rapidly progressive clinical course can be complicated by congestive heart failure
	Drug Therapy: May include antiarrhythmic drugs to control arrhythmias, antibiotics for underlying infection, and anti-inflammatory drugs
	EKG: Tachycardia, intraventricular, or bundle branch abnormalities
	Laboratory: CPK, SGOT, and LDH may be elevated; viral antibody titers, WBCs, and erythrocyte sedimentation rates are also elevated
	Nurse's Notes: Oxygen therapy, frequent vital signs, and documentation of bed rest
	Procedures: Endomyocardial biopsy and echocardiogram
	Radiology: Chest x-ray: cardiac enlargement
Myositis, infective 728.0	**Signs and Symptoms:** Pain in muscles, possible fever and chills with muscle swelling
	Laboratory: Blood: CBCs, WBCs, ESR and eosinophils elevated
	Radiology: Arteriography may show displacement of arteries and abnormal vascular patterns
Neuritis or radiculitis, brachial 723.4	**Signs and Symptoms:** Weakness of neck, inside forearm, and shoulder; this can sometimes occur after an injection of tetanus or diphtheria antitoxins
	Radiology: X-ray, cervical and shoulder; possible bone scan

Obstruction, urinary 599.6	**Signs and Symptoms:** Unable to urinate and feeling of not emptying; pain, hematuria, and changes in urinary output **Drug Therapy:** May include agents such as cipro, bactrim, or septra and analgesics for pain **Procedures:** Cystoscopy may be performed to diagnose obstruction or as a means to remove the obstruction **Radiology:** X-ray: may be diagnostic of obstruction; plain abdominal films would be followed by an intravenous pyelogram
Orchitis with abscess 604.0	**Signs and Symptoms:** Inflammation and infection of testes; area may be reddened and tender **Drug Therapy:** Antibiotic therapy and diethylstilbestrol for mumps or orchitis **Laboratory:** Blood: WBCs may be elevated; culture: positive **Nurse's Notes:** Bed rest and ice pack to scrotum
Pancreatitis (acute) 577.0	**Signs and Symptoms:** Damage to the biliary tract by alcohol, infectious disease, trauma, or certain drugs; jaundice will occur in patients with common bile duct obstruction; continuous pain in the epigastric area and sometimes referred to the back; abdomen is distended and tender; fever is present **Drug Therapy:** May include large doses of antibiotics and drugs to control pain **Laboratory:** Blood: WBCs are elevated as well as amylase, leucine aminopeptidase, bilirubin, and lipase **Procedures:** Intravenous hydration and nasogastric tube for suction **Radiology:** X-ray: stomach and duodenum are displaced, and calcification of pancreas is evident; CT scan to identify presence and extent of pancreatitis
Pericarditis, acute, unspecified 420.90	**Signs and Symptoms:** Onset is usually abrupt and often preceded by sharp precordial or substernal pain, radiating to the neck; precordial pain can be distinguished from ischemic coronary pain because it usually is not aggravated by thoracic motion; fever, chills, and weakness are common; pericardial friction rub is heard as a scratchy or leathery sound **Drug Therapy:** Intravenous antibiotics, corticosteroids, and anti-inflammatory drugs such as aspirin **EKG:** Tachycardia, S-T segment elevation, and atrial arrhythmias **Laboratory:** WBC count 15,000–20,000, SGOT increased (above 40 units), and PPD skin test is positive if caused by tuberculosis; positive gram stain and positive culture **Nurse's Notes:** Documentation of complete bed rest, frequent monitoring of vital signs and oxygen therapy **Procedures:** Pericardiocentesis fluid may be hemorrhagic or straw-colored; echocardiogram if pericardial effusion is present **Radiology:** Chest x-ray: usually serial for the purpose of ruling out cause of pleuritic chest pain; may show slight cardiac hypertrophy

Most Commonly Missed
CC Conditions

Peritonitis 567.0–567.9	**Signs and Symptoms:** Inflammation of the peritoneum caused by acute irritating substances or bacteria entering the abdominal cavity by perforation of an organ in the gastrointestinal tract, the reproductive tract or a penetrating wound; abdominal pain with nausea and vomiting, and chills **Drug Therapy:** IV antibiotics such as doxycycline, cefoxitin, clindamycin, and gentamicin **Laboratory:** Blood: elevated WBCs; positive gram strain and positive culture **Nurse's Notes:** Documentation of abdominal distention, ascites and possibly elevated temperature **Radiology:** Abdominal x-ray, ileus
Phlebitis and thrombophlebitis of femoral vein 451.11	**Signs and Symptoms:** Inflammation of a vein generally followed by a clot; affected area may be hot and tender to touch; other symptoms include swelling of the extremity, pain, and cyanosis **Drug Therapy:** May include heparin given intravenously or subcutaneously followed by a course of oral anticoagulants **Laboratory:** Increase in platelet and leucocyte count; frequent prothrombin time monitoring **Radiology:** X-ray: may be diagnostic of the affected area; Arteriography may be diagnostic of location of thrombus
Phlebitis and thrombophlebitis of superficial vessels, lower extremities 451.0	**Signs and Symptoms:** Inflammation of vein generally followed by a clot; may be hot and tender to touch **Drug Therapy:** May include administration of anticoagulant agent such as heparin **Radiology:** X-ray: may be diagnostic of the affected area; arteriography may be diagnostic of the location of the clot
Phlebitis, following infusion, perfusion, or tranfusion 999.2	**Signs and Symptoms:** Inflammation of a vein and can occur following infusion, perfusion, or transfusion; the area may be red, hot, swollen, and tender to the touch **Drug Therapy:** Need for antibiotics or anticoagulants such as heparin to avoid clot formation **Nurse's Notes:** Attention to the site; change or relocation of the IV may be necessary **Radiology:** Extremity venogram, lung perfusion scan

Pneumonia, organism unspecified 486	**Signs and Symptoms:** Lung infection may be due to a number of organisms that may cause the infection; symptoms include cough, fever, chills, and sometimes general aching
	Drug Therapy: Appropriate antibiotic therapy is usually given according to organism
	Laboratory: Blood: Elevated WBCs; culture (sputum) is positive for *Haemophilus influenzae, Klebsiella, Pseudomonas, Staphylococcus, Streptococcus*, or other specified bacteria
	Nurse's Notes: Oxygen therapy and analgesics for chest pain
	Procedures: May include bronchoscopy
	Radiology: Chest x-ray may show infiltrates
Pneumothorax 512.8	**Signs and Symptoms:** Collapse of the lung caused by the collection of air in the pleural space; usually sudden in onset; pain in chest on involved side, radiating to neck; cough and rapid onset of severe dyspnea; cyanosis and asymmetrical chest wall movement also present
	Procedures: Oxygen therapy
	Radiology: X-ray: outline of collapsed lung; mediastinal shift to opposite side
	Respiratory Therapy: Pulmonary functionvital capacity decreased
	Surgery: Chest tube placement
Prostatitis, acute 601.0	**Signs and Symptoms:** Inflammation of the prostate gland caused by infection; dysuria, frequency, urgency, burning, and painful urination
	Drug Therapy: May include appropriate antibiotic
	Laboratory: Urinalysis: evidence of WBC, RBC, and bacteria; urine culture may identify organism causing infection
	Nurse's Notes: Force fluids and sitz baths
	Procedures: Possible suprapubic cystostomy; ultrasound of prostate
Retention, urinary, unspecified 788.20	**Signs and Symptoms:** Acquired obstruction or a congenital defect; patient is unable to urinate or completely empty bladder; may also be due to a neurological disorder, such as multiple sclerosis, or trauma, such as a spinal cord injury
	Drug Therapy: May include bactrim or septra
	Nurse's Notes: Documentation of residual urine volume and intake and output; also bladder training
	Procedures: Cystoscopy may be performed to determine reason for obstruction; cystometrogram to measure pressure and capacity of bladder
	Radiology: IVP may be performed for diagnostic purposes.
Seizure, petit mal, with intractable epilepsy 345.01	**Signs and Symptoms:** Momentary loss of memory with twitching face and upper extremities; may be characterized by momentary staring into space; also known as "absence seizure"
	Drug Therapy: May include dilantin or phenobarbital, neurontin, clonazepam
	EEG: Diagnostic

Septicemia 038.9	**Signs and Symptoms:** Chills, skin eruptions, fever, nausea, leukocytosis, vomiting, diarrhea, and prostration **Drug Therapy:** Antibiotics **Laboratory:** Blood cultures; serial white blood cell counts, between 15,000 and 30,000 with a left shift; platelet count decreased; BUN and creatinine are increased; common contaminant is *Staphylococcus epidermidis*
Shock, cardiogenic 785.51	**Signs and Symptoms:** A life-threatening emergency requiring intensive stabilizing measures; most often occurs as the result of a myocardial infarction, end-stage cardiomyopathy, or possibly a malfunction of the mitral valve; rapidly developing mental confusion with weakness, cyanosis, oliguria, tachycardia, and gallop rhythm; systolic pressure drops to 50; skin is cool and moist **Drug Therapy:** May include morphine to control chest pain, dopamine, norepinephrine, and nitroprusside **EKG:** Ventricular fibrillation may be present **Laboratory:** May show serum acidosis; BUN and creatinine are elevated, as are CPK, LDH, SGOT, and SGPT; arterial blood gases demonstrate acidosis and hypoxia **Nurse's Notes:** May indicate a weak rapid pulse, cardiac monitoring, and intake and output **Procedures:** Pulmonary artery pressure monitoring and pulmonary capillary wedge pressure; may also include intra-aortic balloon pump **Radiology:** Chest x-ray may show pulmonary edema
Shock, septic 785.59	**Signs and Symptoms:** May include septic shock due to management of underlying disease; hypotension and fever may be present except in chronically ill or elderly patients; onset of abrupt chills, nausea, vomiting, and diarrhea; documentation of extreme exhaustion (prostration) **Drug Therapy:** Dopamine for renal perfusion, IV antibiotics **EKG:** May demonstrate conduction defect and/or ventricular fibrillation **Laboratory:** Blood: May show acidosis or elevated BUN and creatinine, leukocytosis, or neutropenia **Procedures:** Invasive monitoring with a pulmonary artery catheter **Radiology:** Chest x-ray: may show pulmonary edema

Status, renal dialysis V45.1	**Signs and Symptoms:** Presence of arteriovenous shunt or arteriovenous fistula for hemodialysis, or peritoneal catheter (Tenckoff) for continuous ambulatory peritoneal dialysis; diagnosis of chronic renal disease, such as chronic renal failure, diabetic nephropathy, nephrosclerosis, or status postnephrectomy is indicative of renal dialysis; complications of vascular access include thrombosis, infection, and hemorrhage **Drug Therapy:** Multivitamin supplements (B-complex, folic acid, vitamin C); ferrous sulfate 500–900 mg/day; an anabolic steroid; and oral phosphate to maintain serum phosphate within normal levels; Epoetin alfa is the principal treatment for anemia **Laboratory:** Urinalysis: maintain RBC volume in the range of 33%, protein; blood increase in WBCs for infection; increase of BUN and creatinine **Nurse's Notes:** Daily fluid intake is limited to 500–1000 mL plus measured urinary output; assessment includes weight gain, blood pressure, nutrition balances, and psychosocial and community resources **Procedures:** Hemodialysis access examination by duplex scan to assess arterial inflow and venous outflow
Tachycardia, paroxysmal, supraventricular 427.0	**Signs and Symptoms:** Abrupt onset and termination of palpitations; often asymptomatic although patient may be aware of a rapid heartbeat some patients complain of throbbing vessels of the throat, dyspnea, sweating, dizziness, syncope, weakness, and polyuria **Drug Therapy:** May include propranolol, quinidine, or calan **EKG:** Premature atrial beats, abnormally shaped P waves; regular rhythm at 150–220 beats per minute **Procedures:** May include intracardiac electrophysiologic studies and vagal stimulation; may also see reduced vital capacity and increased cardiac output and circulation time
Tachycardia, paroxysmal, unspecified 427.2	**Signs and Symptoms:** Fluttering sensation in the chest, weakness, faintness, and nausea **Drug Therapy:** May include quinidine, procainamide, calan **EKG:** Uninterrupted series of beats
Tachycardia, paroxysmal, ventricular 427.1	**Signs and Symptoms:** Associated with ischemic heart disease, especially myocardial infarction; precordial pain; sudden onset usually preceded by premature ventricular beats; pulse rate of 150–210 per minute **Drug Therapy:** May include quinidine, procainamide, and calan **EKG:** Wide QRS complexes **Nurse's Notes:** Cardiopulmonary resuscitation **Procedures:** Cardioversion

Most Commonly Missed CC Conditions

Ulcer, decubitus 707.0	**Signs and Symptoms:** Also known as a bedsore or pressure sore; occurs most frequently in debilitated patients who are bed- or wheelchair-confined; is a result of loss of circulation to a susceptible body area, such as a bony prominence. **Drug Therapy:** May include topical antibiotic ointments **Nurse's Notes:** May show special mattresses used for treatment and prevention of spread of ulcer, dressing changes, and treatment of decubitus **Procedures:** Fourth stage ulcers may be debrided; whirlpool debridements in physical therapy may be required
Varices, esophageal, bleeding 456.0	**Signs and Symptoms:** Hematemesis can sometimes be an indication of an esophageal bleed **Drug Therapy:** Peripheral venous or central arterial vasopressin **Procedures:** Esophagoscopy, diagnostic; barium swallow, diagnostic; balloon tamponade **Surgery:** Endoscopic sclerosis of bleeding varices

CC Principal Diagnosis Exclusion List

008.41 CC Excl: 001.1, 002.0, 002.9, 003.0, 004.9, 005.0-005.2, 006.0-006.2, 006.9, 007.1-007.9, 008.00-008.49, 008.5, 008.61-008.69, 008.8, 009.0, 014.80-014.86, 112.85, 129, 487.8, 536.3, 536.8, 555.0-555.9, 556.0-556.9, 557.0-557.9, 558.2, 558.3, 558.9, 564.1, 775.0-775.9, 777.5, 777.8

008.42 CC Excl: see Code 008.41

008.43 CC Excl: see Code 008.41

008.44 CC Excl: see Code 008.41

008.45 CC Excl: see Code 008.41

008.46 CC Excl: see Code 008.41

008.47 CC Excl: see Code 008.41

008.49 CC Excl: see Code 008.41

011.0x CC Excl: 011.00-011.96, 012.00-012.86, 017.90-017.96, 018.00-018.96, 031.0, 031.2, 031.8-031.9, 041.81-041.89, 041.9, 137.0, 139.8, 480.0-487.1, 494.0-494.1, 495.0-495.9, 496, 500-505, 506.0-506.9, 507.0-507.8, 508.0-508.9, 517.1, 518.89

011.1x CC Excl: see Code 011.0

011.2x CC Excl: see Code 011.0

011.3x CC Excl: see Code 011.0

011.4x CC Excl: see Code 011.0

011.5x CC Excl: see Code 011.0

011.6x CC Excl: **For codes 011.60-011.65:** see Code 011.0; CC Excl: **For code 011.66:** 011.66, 139.8, 480.0-487.1, 494.0-494.1, 495.0-495.9, 496, 500-505, 506.0-506.9, 507.0-507.8, 508.0-508.9, 517.1, 518.89

011.7x CC Excl: see Code 011.0

011.8x CC Excl: see Code 011.0

011.9x CC Excl: see Code 011.0

012.0x CC Excl: see Code 011.0

012.1x CC Excl: see Code 011.0

013.0x CC Excl: 003.21, 013.00-013.16, 013.40-013.56, 013.80-013.96, 017.90-017.96, 031.2, 031.8-031.9, 036.0, 041.81-041.89, 041.9, 047.0-047.9, 049.0-049.1, 053.0, 054.72, 072.1, 090.42, 091.81, 094.2, 098.89, 100.81, 112.83, 114.2, 115.01, 115.11, 115.91, 130.0, 137.1, 139.8, 320.0-320.9, 321.0-321.8, 322.0-322.9, 349.89, 349.9, 357.0

013.1x CC Excl: see Code 013.0

013.2x CC Excl: 013.20-013.36, 013.60-013.96, 017.90-017.96, 031.2, 031.8-031.9, 041.81-041.89, 041.9, 137.1, 139.8

013.3x CC Excl: see Code 013.2

013.4x CC Excl: 013.00-013.16, 013.40-013.56, 013.80-013.96, 017.90-017.96, 031.2, 031.8-031.9, 041.81-041.89, 041.9, 137.1, 139.8

013.5x CC Excl: see Code 013.4

013.6x CC Excl: 013.20-013.36, 013.60-013.96, 017.90-017.96, 031.2, 031.8-031.9, 041.81-041.89, 041.9, 137.1, 139.8

013.8x CC Excl: 013.80-013.96, 017.90-017.96, 031.2, 031.8-031.9, 041.81-041.89, 041.9, 137.1, 139.8

013.9x CC Excl: see Code 013.8

014.0x CC Excl: 014.00-014.86, 017.90-017.96, 031.2, 031.8-031.9, 041.81-041.89, 041.9, 139.8

014.8x CC Excl: **For code 014.80:** see Code 014.0,CC Excl: **For code 014.81:** 014.81, 139.8,CC Excl: **For code 014.82:** 014.00-014.86, 017.90-017.96, 031.2, 031.8-031.9, 041.81-041.89, 041.9, 139.8,CC Excl: **For code** 014.83-014.86: see Code 014.82

016.0x CC Excl: 016.00-016.36, 016.90-016.96, 017.90-017.96, 031.2, 031.8-031.9, 041.81-041.89, 041.9, 137.2, 139.8

016.1x CC Excl: see Code 016.0

016.2x CC Excl: see Code 016.0

016.3x CC Excl: see Code 016.0

016.4x CC Excl: 016.40-016.56, 016.90-016.96, 017.90-017.96, 031.2, 031.8-031.9, 041.81-041.89, 041.9, 137.2, 139.8

016.5x CC Excl: see Code 016.4

016.6x CC Excl: 016.60-016.96, 017.90-017.96, 031.2, 031.8-031.9, 041.81-041.89, 041.9, 137.2, 139.8

016.7x CC Excl: see Code 016.6

016.9x CC Excl: 016.90-016.96, 017.90-017.96, 031.2, 031.8-031.9, 041.81-041.89, 041.9, 137.2, 139.8

017.2x CC Excl: 017.20-017.26, 017.90-017.96, 031.2, 031.8-031.9, 041.81-041.89, 041.9, 139.8

017.3x CC Excl: 017.30-017.36, 017.90-017.96, 031.2, 031.8-031.9, 041.81-041.89, 041.9, 139.8

017.4x CC Excl: 017.40-017.46, 017.90-017.96, 031.2, 031.8-031.9, 041.81-041.89, 041.9, 139.8

017.5x CC Excl: 017.50-017.56, 017.90-017.96, 031.2, 031.8-031.9, 041.81-041.89, 041.9, 139.8

017.6x CC Excl: 017.60-017.66, 017.90-017.96, 031.2, 031.8-031.9, 041.81-041.89, 041.9, 139.8

017.7x CC Excl: 017.70-017.76, 017.90-017.96, 031.2, 031.8-031.9, 041.81-041.89, 041.9, 139.8

017.8x CC Excl: 017.80-017.96, 031.2, 031.8-031.9, 041.81-041.89, 041.9, 139.8

017.9x CC Excl: 017.90-017.96, 031.2, 031.8-031.9, 041.81-041.89, 041.9, 139.8

018.0x CC Excl: 017.90-017.96, 018.00-018.96, 031.2, 031.8-031.9, 041.81-041.89, 041.9, 139.8

018.8x CC Excl: see Code 018.0

018.9x CC Excl: see Code 018.0

031.0 CC Excl: 011.00-011.96, 012.00-012.86, 017.90-017.96, 031.0, 031.2, 031.9, 041.81-041.89, 041.9, 137.0, 139.8, 480.0-480.9, 481, 482.0-482.9, 483.0, 483.1, 483.8, 484.1-484.8, 485-486, 487.0-487.1, 494.0-494.1, 495.0-495.9, 496, 500-505, 506.0-506.9, 507.0-507.8, 508.0-508.9, 517.1, 518.89

036.0 CC Excl: 003.21, 013.00-013.16, 036.0, 036.89, 036.9, 041.81-041.89, 041.9, 047.0-047.9, 049.0-049.1, 053.0, 054.72, 072.1, 090.42, 091.81, 094.2, 098.89, 100.81, 112.83, 114.2, 115.01, 115.11, 115.91, 130.0, 139.8, 320.0-320.9, 321.0-321.8, 322.0-322.9, 349.89, 349.9, 357.0

036.1 CC Excl: 036.1, 036.89, 036.9, 041.81-041.89, 041.9, 139.8

036.2 CC Excl: 003.1, 020.2, 036.2, 036.89, 036.9, 038.0, 038.10-038.11, 038.19, 038.2-038.9, 041.81-041.89, 041.9, 054.5, 139.8, 995.90-995.94

036.3 CC Excl: 036.3, 036.89, 036.9, 041.81-041.89, 041.9, 139.8

036.40 CC Excl: 036.40, 036.89, 036.9, 041.81-041.89, 041.9, 139.8

036.41 CC Excl: 036.41, 036.89, 036.9, 041.81-041.89, 041.9, 139.8

036.42 CC Excl: 036.42, 036.89, 036.9, 041.81-041.89, 041.9, 139.8

036.43 CC Excl: 036.43, 041.81-041.89, 041.9, 139.8

036.81 CC Excl: 036.81, 036.89, 036.9, 041.81-041.89, 041.9, 139.8

036.82 CC Excl: 036.82, 036.89, 036.9, 041.81-041.89, 041.9, 139.8

036.89 CC Excl: 036.89, 036.9, 041.81-041.89, 041.9, 139.8

036.9 CC Excl: see Code 036.89

037 CC Excl: 037, 139.8

038.0 CC Excl: 003.1, 020.2, 036.2, 038.0-038.9, 040.82, 040.89, 041.00-041.05, 041.09-041.11, 041.19, 041.2-041.7, 041.81-041.86, 041.89, 041.9, 054.5, 139.8, 995.90-995.94, V09.0-V09.91

038.10 CC Excl: see Code 038.0

038.11 CC Excl: see Code 038.0

038.19 CC Excl: see Code 038.0

038.2 CC Excl: see Code 038.0

038.3 CC Excl: see Code 038.0

038.40 CC Excl: see Code 038.0

038.41 CC Excl: see Code 038.0

038.42 CC Excl: see Code 038.0

038.43 CC Excl: see Code 038.0

038.44 CC Excl: see Code 038.0

038.49 CC Excl: see Code 038.0

038.8 CC Excl: see Code 038.0

038.9 CC Excl: see Code 038.0

040.0 CC Excl: 040.0, 139.8

040.82 CC Excl: 040.82, 780.91-780.94, 780.99, 785.50-785.52, 785.59, 785.9, 799.81-799.89

042 CC Excl: 042, 139.8

046.2 CC Excl: 046.2, 139.8

052.0 CC Excl: 051.9, 052.0, 052.7-052.9, 078.88-078.89, 079.81, 079.88-079.89, 079.98-079.99, 139.8

052.1 CC Excl: 051.9, 052.1, 052.7-052.9, 078.88-078.89, 079.81, 079.88-079.89, 079.98-079.99, 139.8

052.7 CC Excl: 051.9, 052.7-052.9, 078.88-078.89, 079.81, 079.88-079.89, 079.98-079.99, 139.8

052.8 CC Excl: see Code 052.7

052.9 CC Excl: see Code 052.7

053.0 CC Excl: 003.21, 013.00-013.16, 036.0, 047.0-047.9, 049.0-049.1, 053.0-053.19, 053.79, 053.8-053.9, 054.72, 054.79, 054.8-054.9, 072.1, 078.88-078.89, 079.81, 079.88-079.89, 079.98-079.99, 090.42, 091.81, 094.2, 098.89, 100.81, 112.83, 114.2, 115.01, 115.11, 115.91, 130.0, 139.8, 320.0-320.9, 321.0-321.8, 322.0-322.9, 349.89, 349.9, 357.0

053.10 CC Excl: 053.0-053.19, 053.79, 053.8-053.9, 054.72, 054.79, 054.8-054.9, 078.88-078.89, 079.81, 079.88-079.89, 079.98-079.99, 139.8

053.11   CC Excl: see Code 053.10
053.12   CC Excl: see Code 053.10
053.13   CC Excl: see Code 053.10
053.19   CC Excl: see Code 053.10
053.79   CC Excl: 053.0-053.9, 054.0-054.71,
         054.73, 054.79, 054.8-054.9, 078.88-
         078.89, 079.81, 079.88-079.89, 079.98-
         079.99, 139.8
053.8   CC Excl: see Code 053.79
054.3   CC Excl: 054.3, 054.79, 054.8-054.9,
         139.8
054.5   CC Excl: 003.1, 020.2, 036.2, 038.0,
         038.10-038.11, 038.19, 038.2-038.9,
         054.5, 054.79, 054.8-054.9, 139.8,
         995.90-995.94
054.71   CC Excl: 054.71, 054.72, 054.79, 054.8-
         054.9, 139.8
054.72   CC Excl: 003.21, 013.00-013.16, 036.0,
         047.0-047.9, 049.0-049.1, 053.0,
         054.72, 054.79, 054.8-054.9, 072.1,
         090.42, 091.81, 094.2, 098.89, 100.81,
         112.83, 114.2, 115.01, 115.11, 115.91,
         130.0, 139.8, 320.0-320.9, 321.0-321.8,
         322.0-322.9, 349.89, 349.9, 357.0
054.79   CC Excl: 054.79, 054.8-054.9, 078.88-
         078.89, 079.81, 079.88-079.89, 079.98-
         079.99, 139.8
054.8   CC Excl: see Code 054.79
055.0   CC Excl: 055.0, 055.79, 055.8-055.9,
         078.88-078.89, 079.81, 079.88-079.89,
         079.98-079.99, 139.8
055.1   CC Excl: 055.1, 055.79, 055.8-055.9,
         078.88-078.89, 079.81, 079.88-079.89,
         079.98-079.99, 139.8
055.2   CC Excl: 055.2, 055.79, 055.8-055.9,
         078.88-078.89, 079.81, 079.88-079.89,
         079.98-079.99, 139.8
055.71   CC Excl: 055.71, 055.79, 055.8-055.9,
         078.88-078.89, 079.81, 079.88-079.89,
         079.98-079.99, 139.8
055.79   CC Excl: 055.79, 055.8-055.9, 078.88-
         078.89, 079.81, 079.88-079.89, 079.98-
         079.99, 139.8
055.8   CC Excl: 055.79, 055.8-055.9, 056.09,
         078.88-078.89, 079.81, 079.88-079.89,
         079.98-079.99, 139.8
056.00   CC Excl: 056.00-056.09, 056.79, 056.8-
         056.9, 078.88-078.89, 079.81, 079.88-
         079.89, 079.98-079.99, 139.8
056.01   CC Excl: see Code 056.00
056.09   CC Excl: see Code 056.00
056.71   CC Excl: 056.71-056.9, 078.88-078.89,
         079.81, 079.88-079.89, 079.98-079.99,
         139.8
056.79   CC Excl: see Code 056.00

056.8   CC Excl: 056., 056.01, 056.79, 056.8-
         056.9, 078.88-078.89, 079.81, 079.88-
         079.89, 079.98-079.99, 139.8
070.2   CC Excl: 070.0-070.9, 078.88-078.89,
         079.81, 079.88-079.89, 079.98-079.99,
         139.8
070.3   CC Excl: 070.0-070.9, 078.88-078.89,
         079.81, 079.88-079.89, 079.98-079.99,
         139.8
070.41   CC Excl: 070.0-070.9, 078.88-078.89,
         079.81, 079.88-079.89, 079.98-079.99,
         139.8
070.42   CC Excl: see Code 070.41
070.43   CC Excl: see Code 070.41
070.44   CC Excl: see Code 070.41
070.49   CC Excl: see Code 070.41
070.51   CC Excl: 070.0-070.9, 078.88-078.89,
         079.81, 079.88-079.89, 079.98-079.99,
         139.8
070.52   CC Excl: see Code 070.51
070.53   CC Excl: see Code 070.51
070.54   CC Excl: see Code 070.51
070.59   CC Excl: see Code 070.51
070.6   CC Excl: see Code 070.51
070.9   CC Excl: see Code 070.51
072.0   CC Excl: 072.0, 072.79, 072.8-072.9,
         078.88-078.89, 079.81, 079.88-079.89,
         079.98-079.99, 139.8
072.1   CC Excl: 003.21, 013.00-013.16, 036.0,
         047.0-047.9, 049.0-049.1, 053.0,
         054.72, 072.1, 072.79, 072.8-072.9,
         078.88-078.89, 079.81, 079.98-079.99,
         090.42, 091.81, 094.2, 098.89, 100.81,
         112.83, 114.2, 115.01, 115.11, 115.91,
         130.0, 139.8, 320.0-320.9, 321.0-321.8,
         322.0-322.9, 349.89, 349.9, 357.0
072.2   CC Excl: 072.2, 072.79, 072.8-072.9,
         078.88-078.89, 079.81, 079.88-079.89,
         079.98-079.99, 139.8
072.3   CC Excl: 072.3, 072.79, 072.8-072.9,
         078.88-078.89, 079.81, 079.88-079.89,
         079.98-079.99, 139.8
072.71   CC Excl: 072.71, 072.79, 072.8-072.9,
         078.88-078.89, 079.81, 079.88-079.89,
         079.98-079.99, 139.8
072.72   CC Excl: 072.72, 072.79, 072.8-072.9,
         078.88-078.89, 079.81, 079.88-079.89,
         079.98-079.99, 139.8
072.79   CC Excl: 072.79, 072.8-072.9, 078.88-
         078.89, 079.81, 079.88-079.89, 079.98-
         079.99, 139.8
072.8   CC Excl: 072.79, 072.8-072.9, 078.88-
         078.89, 079.81, 079.88-079.89, 079.98-
         079.99

CC Exclusion List

079.82 CC Excl: 011.00-012.16, 012.80-012.86, 017.90-017.96, 021.2, 0310, 03.91, 079.82-079.89, 115.05, 115.15, 115.95, 122.1, 130.4, 136.3, 480.0-480.2, 480.8-487.1, 494.0-508.9, 517.1, 517.8, 518.89, 519.8-519.9

086.0 CC Excl: 086.0, 139.8

090.40 CC Excl: 090.0-090.9, 091.0-091.9, 092.0, 092.9, 093.0-093.9, 094.0-094.9, 095.0-095.9, 096, 097.0-097.9, 099.40-099.59, 099.8, 099.9, 139.8

090.41 CC Excl: see Code 090.40

090.42 CC Excl: 003.21, 013.00-013.16, 036.0, 047.0-047.9, 049.0-049.1, 053.0, 054.72, 072.1, 090.0-090.9, 091.0-091.9, 092.0, 092.9, 093.0-093.9, 094.0-094.9, 095.0-095.9, 096, 097.0-097.9, 098.89, 099.40-099.59, 099.8, 099.9, 100.81, 112.83, 114.2, 115.01, 115.11, 115.91, 130.0, 139.8, 320.0-320.9, 321.0-321.8, 322.0-322.9, 349.89, 349.9, 357.0

090.49 CC Excl: see Code 090.40

093.0 CC Excl: see Code 090.40

093.1 CC Excl: see Code 090.40

093.20 CC Excl: see Code 090.40

093.21 CC Excl: see Code 090.40

093.22 CC Excl: see Code 090.40

093.23 CC Excl: see Code 090.40

093.24 CC Excl: see Code 090.40

093.81 CC Excl: see Code 090.40

093.82 CC Excl: see Code 090.40

093.89 CC Excl: see Code 090.40

093.9 CC Excl: see Code 090.40

094.0 CC Excl: see Code 090.40

094.1 CC Excl: see Code 090.40

094.2 CC Excl: 003.21, 013.00-013.16, 036.0, 047.0-047.9, 049.0-049.1, 053.0, 054.72, 072.1, 090.0-090.9, 091.0-091.9, 092.0, 092.9, 093.0-093.9, 094.0-094.9, 095.0-095.9, 096, 097.0-097.9, 098.89, 099.40-099.59, 099.8, 099.9, 100.81, 112.83, 114.2, 115.01, 115.11, 115.91, 130.0, 139.8, 320.0-320.9, 321.0-321.8, 322.0-322.9, 349.89, 349.9, 357.0

094.3 CC Excl: see Code 090.40

094.81 CC Excl: see Code 090.40

094.87 CC Excl: see Code 090.40

094.89 CC Excl: see Code 090.40

094.9 CC Excl: see Code 090.40

098.0 CC Excl: 098.0-098.39, 098.89, 099.40-099.59, 099.8, 099.9, 139.8

098.10 CC Excl: see Code 098.0

098.11 CC Excl: see Code 098.0

098.12 CC Excl: see Code 098.0

098.13 CC Excl: see Code 098.0

098.14 CC Excl: see Code 098.0

098.15 CC Excl: see Code 098.0

098.16 CC Excl: see Code 098.0

098.17 CC Excl: see Code 098.0

098.19 CC Excl: see Code 098.0

112.0 CC Excl: 112.0-112.9, 117.9, 139.8

112.4 CC Excl: see Code 112.0

112.5 CC Excl: see Code 112.0

112.81 CC Excl: see Code 112.0

112.82 CC Excl: see Code 112.0

112.83 CC Excl: 003.21, 013.00-013.16, 036.0, 047.0-047.9, 049.0-049.1, 053.0, 054.72, 072.1, 090.42, 091.81, 094.2, 098.89, 100.81, 112.0-112.9, 114.2, 115.01, 115.11, 115.91, 117.9, 130.0, 139.8, 320.0-320.9, 321.0-321.8, 322.0-322.9, 349.89, 349.9, 357.0

112.84 CC Excl: see Code 112.0

112.85 CC Excl: see Code 112.0

114.0 CC Excl: 114.0, 114.3, 114.4-114.5, 114.9, 117.9, 139.8

114.2 CC Excl: 003.21, 013.00-013.16, 036.0, 047.0-047.9, 049.0-049.1, 053.0, 054.72, 072.1, 090.42, 091.81, 094.2, 098.89, 100.81, 112.83, 114.2-114.9, 115.01, 115.11, 115.91, 117.9, 130.0, 139.8, 320.0-320.9, 321.0-321.8, 322.0-322.9, 349.89, 349.9, 357.0

114.3 CC Excl: 114.3, 114.9, 117.9, 139.8

114.9 CC Excl: see Code 114.3

115.0x CC Excl: **For code 115.00:** 115.00, 115.09, 115.90, 115.99, 117.9, 139.8; CC Excl: **For code 115.01:** 003.21, 013.00-013.16, 036.0, 047.0-047.9, 049.0-049.1, 053.0, 054.72, 072.1, 090.42, 091.81, 094.2, 098.89, 100.81, 112.83, 114.2, 115.00-115.01, 115.09, 115.11, 115.90-115.91, 115.99, 117.9, 130.0, 139.8, 320.0-320.9, 321.0-321.8, 322.0-322.9, 349.89, 349.9, 357.0; CC Excl: **For code 115.02:** 115.00, 115.02, 115.09, 115.90, 115.92, 115.99, 117.9, 139.8; CC Excl: **For code 115.03:** 115.00, 115.03, 115.09, 115.90, 115.93, 115.99, 117.9, 139.8; CC Excl: **For code 115.04:** 115.00, 115.04, 115.09, 115.90, 115.94, 115.99, 117.9, 139.8; CC Excl: **For code 115.05:** 115.00, 115.05, 115.09, 115.90, 115.95, 115.99, 117.9, 139.8, 480.0-480.9, 481, 482.0-482.7, 482.81-482.84, 482.89, 482.9, 483.0, 483.1, 483.8, 484.1-484.8, 485-486, 487.0-487.1, 494.0-494.1, 495.0-495.9, 496, 500-505, 506.0-506.9, 507.0-507.8, 508.0-508.9, 517.1, 518.89

115.1x CC Excl: **For code 115.10**: 115.10,
115.19, 115.90, 115.99, 117.9, 139.8;
CC Excl: **For code 115.11**: 003.21,
013.00-013.16, 036.0, 047.0-047.9,
049.0-049.1, 053.0, 054.72, 072.1,
090.42, 091.81, 094.2, 098.89, 100.81,
112.83, 114.2, 115.01, 115.10-115.11,
115.19, 115.90-115.91, 115.99, 117.9,
130.0, 139.8, 320.0-320.9, 321.0-321.8,
322.0-322.9, 349.89, 349.9, 357.0; CC
Excl: **For code 115.12**: 115.10, 115.12,
115.19, 115.90, 115.92, 115.99, 117.9,
139.8; CC Excl: **For code 115.13**:
115.10, 115.13, 115.19, 115.90, 115.93,
115.99, 117.9, 139.8; CC Excl: **For code
115.14**: 115.10, 115.14, 115.19, 115.90,
115.94, 115.99, 117.9, 139.8; CC Excl:
For code 115.15: 115.05, 115.10,
115.15, 115.19, 115.90, 115.95, 115.99,
117.9, 139.8, 480.0-480.9, 481, 482.0-
482.7, 482.81-482.83, 482.89, 482.9,
483.0, 483.1, 483.8, 484.1-484.8, 485-
486,487.0-487.1, 494.0-494.1, 495.0-
495.9, 496, 500-505, 506.0-506.9,
507.0-507.8, 508.0-508.9, 517.1,
518.89;CC Excl: **For code 115.19**:
115.10, 115.19, 115.90, 115.99, 117.9,
139.8

115.9x CC Excl: **For code 115.90**: 115.90,
115.99, 117.9, 139.8; CC Excl: **For code
115.91**: 003.21, 013.00-013.16, 036.0,
047.0-047.9, 049.0-049.1, 053.0,
054.72, 072.1, 090.42, 091.81, 094.2,
098.89, 100.81, 112.83, 114.2, 115.01,
115.11, 115.91, 115.99, 117.9, 130.0,
139.8, 320.0-320.9, 321.0-321.8, 322.0-
322.9, 349.89, 349.9, 357.0; CC Excl:
For code 115.92: 115.92, 115.99, 117.9,
139.8; CC Excl: **For code 115.93**:
115.93, 115.99, 117.9, 139.8; CC Excl:
For code 115.94: 115.94, 115.99, 117.9,
139.8; CC Excl: **For code 115.95**:
115.05, 115.15, 115.95, 115.99, 117.9,
139.8;CC Excl: **For code 115.99**: 115.99,
117.9, 139.8

116.0 CC Excl: 116.0, 117.9, 139.8
116.1 CC Excl: 116.1, 117.9, 139.8
117.3 CC Excl: 117.3, 117.9, 139.8
117.4 CC Excl: 117.4, 117.9, 139.8
117.5 CC Excl: 117.5, 117.9, 139.8
117.6 CC Excl: 117.6, 117.9, 139.8
117.7 CC Excl: 117.7, 117.9, 139.8
118 CC Excl: 117.9, 118, 139.8
130.0 CC Excl: 130.0, 130.7-130.9, 139.8
130.1 CC Excl: 130.1, 130.7-130.9, 139.8
130.2 CC Excl: 130.2, 130.7-130.9, 139.8
130.3 CC Excl: 130.3, 130.7-130.9, 139.8

130.4 CC Excl: 130.4, 130.7-130.9, 139.8,
480.0-480.9, 481, 482.0-482.7, 482.81-
482.83, 482.89, 482.9, 483.0, 483.1,
483.8, 484.1-484.8, 485-486, 487.0-
487.1, 494.0-494.1, 495.0-495.9, 496,
500-505, 506.0-506.9, 507.0-507.8,
508.0-508.9, 517.1, 518.89
130.5 CC Excl: 130.5-130.9, 139.8
130.7 CC Excl: 130.7-130.9, 139.8
130.8 CC Excl: see Code 130.7
135 CC Excl: 135, 139.8
136.3 CC Excl: 136.3, 139.8, 480.0-480.9,
481, 482.0-482.7, 482.81-482.83,
482.89, 482.9, 483.0, 483.1, 483.8,
484.1-484.8, 485-486, 487.0-487.1,
494.0-494.1, 495.0-495.9, 496, 500-
505, 506.0-506.9, 507.0-507.8, 508.0-
508.9, 517.1, 518.89
137.0 CC Excl: 137.0, 139.8
137.1 CC Excl: 137.1, 139.8
137.2 CC Excl: 137.2, 139.8
138 CC Excl: 138, 139.8
150.0 CC Excl: 150.0-150.9, 159.0, 159.8-
159.9, 176.3, 195.8, 199.0-199.1, 239.0,
239.8-239.9
150.1 CC Excl: see Code 150.0
150.2 CC Excl: see Code 150.0
150.3 CC Excl: see Code 150.0
150.4 CC Excl: see Code 150.0
150.5 CC Excl: see Code 150.0
150.8 CC Excl: see Code 150.0
150.9 CC Excl: see Code 150.0
151.0 CC Excl: 151.0-151.9, 159.0, 159.8-
159.9, 176.3, 195.8, 199.0-199.1, 239.0,
239.8-239.9
151.1 CC Excl: see Code 151.0
151.2 CC Excl: see Code 151.0
151.3 CC Excl: see Code 151.0
151.4 CC Excl: see Code 151.0
151.5 CC Excl: see Code 151.0
151.6 CC Excl: see Code 151.0
151.8 CC Excl: see Code 151.0
151.9 CC Excl: see Code 151.0
152.0 CC Excl: 152.0, 152.8-152.9, 159.0,
159.8-159.9, 176.3, 195.8, 199.0-199.1,
239.0, 239.8-239.9
152.1 CC Excl: 152.1, 152.8-152.9, 159.0,
159.8-159.9, 176.3, 195.8, 199.0-199.1,
239.0, 239.8-239.9
152.2 CC Excl: 152.2, 152.8-152.9, 159.0,
159.8-159.9, 176.3, 195.8, 199.0-199.1,
239.0, 239.8-239.9
152.3 CC Excl: 152.3-152.9, 159.0, 159.8-
159.9, 176.3, 195.8, 199.0-199.1, 239.0,
239.8-239.9

CC Exclusion List

152.8 CC Excl: 152.8-152.9, 159.0, 159.8-
159.9, 176.3, 195.8, 199.0-199.1, 239.0,
239.8-239.9

152.9 CC Excl: see Code 152.8

153.0 CC Excl: 153.0, 153.8-153.9, 159.0,
159.8-159.9, 176.3, 195.8, 199.0-199.1,
239.0, 239.8-239.9

153.1 CC Excl: 153.1, 153.8-153.9, 159.0,
159.8-159.9, 176.3, 195.8, 199.0-199.1,
239.0, 239.8-239.9

153.2 CC Excl: 153.2, 153.8-153.9, 159.0,
159.8-159.9, 176.3, 195.8, 199.0-199.1,
239.0, 239.8-239.9

153.3 CC Excl: 153.3, 153.8-153.9, 159.0,
159.8-159.9, 176.3, 195.8, 199.0-199.1,
239.0, 239.8-239.9

153.4 CC Excl: 153.4, 153.8-153.9, 159.0,
159.8-159.9, 176.3, 195.8, 199.0-199.1,
239.0, 239.8-239.9

153.5 CC Excl: 153.5, 153.8-153.9, 159.0,
159.8-159.9, 176.3, 195.8, 199.0-199.1,
239.0, 239.8-239.9

153.6 CC Excl: 153.6, 153.8-153.9, 159.0,
159.8-159.9, 176.3, 195.8, 199.0-199.1,
239.0, 239.8-239.9

153.7 CC Excl: 153.7-153.9, 159.0, 159.8-
159.9, 176.3, 195.8, 199.0-199.1, 239.0,
239.8-239.9

153.8 CC Excl: 153.8-153.9, 159.0, 159.8-
159.9, 176.3, 195.8, 199.0-199.1, 239.0,
239.8-239.9

153.9 CC Excl: see Code 153.8

154.0 CC Excl: 154.0, 154.8, 159.0, 159.8-
159.9, 176.3, 195.8, 199.0-199.1, 239.0,
239.8-239.9

154.1 CC Excl: 154.1, 154.8, 159.0, 159.8-
159.9, 176.3, 195.8, 199.0-199.1, 239.0,
239.8-239.9

154.2 CC Excl: 154.2-154.8, 159.0, 159.8-
159.9, 176.3, 195.8, 199.0-199.1, 239.0,
239.8-239.9

154.3 CC Excl: see Code 154.2

154.8 CC Excl: 154.8, 159.0, 159.8-159.9,
176.3, 195.8, 199.0-199.1, 239.0,
239.8-239.9

155.0 CC Excl: 155.0-155.2, 159.0, 159.8-
159.9, 176.3, 195.8, 199.0-199.1, 239.0,
239.8-239.9

155.1 CC Excl: see Code 155.0

155.2 CC Excl: see Code 155.0

156.0 CC Excl: 156.0, 156.8-156.9, 159.0,
159.8-159.9, 176.3, 195.8, 199.0-199.1,
239.0, 239.8-239.9

156.1 CC Excl: 156.1, 156.8-156.9, 159.0,
159.8-159.9, 176.3, 195.8, 199.0-199.1,
239.0, 239.8-239.9

156.2 CC Excl: 156.2-156.9, 159.0, 159.8-
159.9, 176.3, 195.8, 199.0-199.1,

156.8 CC Excl: 156.8-156.9, 159.0, 159.8-
159.9, 176.3, 195.8, 199.0-199.1, 239.0,
239.8-239.9

156.9 CC Excl: see Code 156.8

157.0 CC Excl: 157.0-157.9, 159.0, 159.8-
159.9, 176.3, 195.8, 199.0-199.1, 239.0,
239.8-239.9

157.1 CC Excl: see Code 157.0

157.2 CC Excl: see Code 157.0

157.3 CC Excl: see Code 157.0

157.4 CC Excl: see Code 157.0

157.8 CC Excl: see Code 157.0

157.9 CC Excl: see Code 157.0

162.2 CC Excl: 162.2, 162.8-162.9, 165.8-
165.9, 176.4, 195.8, 199.0-199.1, 239.1,
239.8-239.9

162.3 CC Excl: 162.3, 162.8-162.9, 165.8-
165.9, 176.4, 195.8, 199.0-199.1, 239.1,
239.8-239.9

162.4 CC Excl: 162.4, 162.8-162.9, 165.8-
165.9, 176.4, 195.8, 199.0-199.1, 239.1,
239.8-239.9

162.5 CC Excl: 162.5-162.9, 165.8-165.9,
176.4, 195.8, 199.0-199.1, 239.1,
239.8-239.9

162.8 CC Excl: 162.8-162.9, 165.8-165.9,
176.4, 195.8, 199.0-199.1, 239.1,
239.8-239.9

162.9 CC Excl: see Code 162.8

163.0 CC Excl: 163.0-163.9, 165.8-165.9,
195.8, 199.0-199.1, 239.1, 239.8-239.9

163.1 CC Excl: see Code 163.0

163.8 CC Excl: see Code 163.0

163.9 CC Excl: see Code 163.0

164.0 CC Excl: 164.0

164.1 CC Excl: 164.1

164.2 CC Excl: 164.2-164.9, 165.8-165.9,
195.8, 199.0-199.1, 239.1, 239.8-239.9

164.3 CC Excl: see Code 164.2

164.8 CC Excl: see Code 164.2

164.9 CC Excl: see Code 164.2

176.4 CC Excl: 162.8-162.9, 165.8-165.9,
176.4, 195.8, 199.0-199.1, 239.1,
239.8-239.9

176.5 CC Excl: 176.5, 195.8, 196.0-196.9,
199.0-199.1, 239.8-239.9

189.0 CC Excl: 189.0-189.1, 189.8-189.9,
195.8, 199.0-199.1, 239.5, 239.8-239.9

189.1 CC Excl: see Code 189.0

189.2 CC Excl: 189.2, 189.8-189.9, 195.8,
199.0-199.1, 239.5, 239.8-239.9

191.0 CC Excl: 191.0-191.9, 192.0-192.1,
192.8-192.9, 195.8, 199.0-199.1, 239.6-
239.9

191.1 CC Excl: see Code 191.0
191.2 CC Excl: see Code 191.0
191.3 CC Excl: see Code 191.0
191.4 CC Excl: see Code 191.0
191.5 CC Excl: see Code 191.0
191.6 CC Excl: see Code 191.0
191.7 CC Excl: see Code 191.0
191.8 CC Excl: see Code 191.0
191.9 CC Excl: see Code 191.0
192.0 CC Excl: 192.0, 192.8-192.9, 195.8, 199.0-199.1, 239.6-239.9
192.1 CC Excl: 192.1, 192.8-192.9, 195.8, 199.0-199.1, 239.6-239.9
192.2 CC Excl: 192.2, 192.8-192.9, 195.8, 199.0-199.1, 239.6-239.9
192.3 CC Excl: 192.3-192.9, 195.8, 199.0-199.1, 239.6-239.9
192.8 CC Excl: 191.0-191.9, 192.0-192.9, 195.8, 199.0-199.1, 239.6-239.9
196.0 CC Excl: 176.5, 195.8, 196.0-196.9, 199.0-199.1, 239.8-239.9
196.1 CC Excl: see Code 196.0
196.2 CC Excl: see Code 196.0
196.3 CC Excl: see Code 196.0
196.5 CC Excl: see Code 196.0
196.6 CC Excl: see Code 196.0
196.8 CC Excl: see Code 196.0
196.9 CC Excl: see Code 196.0
197.0 CC Excl: 195.8, 197.0, 197.3, 198.89, 199.0-199.1, 239.8-239.9
197.1 CC Excl: 195.8, 197.1, 197.3, 198.89, 199.0-199.1, 239.8-239.9
197.2 CC Excl: 195.8, 197.2-197.3, 198.89, 199.0-199.1, 239.8-239.9
197.3 CC Excl: 195.8, 197.0-197.3, 198.89, 199.0-199.1, 239.8-239.9
197.4 CC Excl: 195.8, 197.4, 197.8, 198.89, 199.0-199.1, 239.8-239.9
197.5 CC Excl: 195.8, 197.5, 197.8, 198.89, 199.0-199.1, 239.8-239.9
197.6 CC Excl: 195.8, 197.6, 197.8, 198.89, 199.0-199.1, 239.8-239.9
197.7 CC Excl: 195.8, 197.7-197.8, 198.89, 199.0-199.1, 239.8-239.9
197.8 CC Excl: 195.8, 197.4-197.8, 198.89, 199.0-199.1, 239.8-239.9
198.0 CC Excl: 195.8, 198.0-198.1, 198.89, 199.0-199.1, 239.8-239.9
198.1 CC Excl: see Code 198.0
198.2 CC Excl: 195.8, 198.2, 198.89, 199.0-199.1, 239.8-239.9
198.3 CC Excl: 195.8, 198.3, 198.89, 199.0-199.1, 239.8-239.9
198.4 CC Excl: 195.8, 198.4, 198.89, 199.0-199.1, 239.8-239.9

198.5 CC Excl: 195.8, 198.5, 198.89, 199.0-199.1, 239.8-239.9
198.6 CC Excl: 195.8, 198.6, 198.89, 199.0-199.1, 239.8-239.9
198.7 CC Excl: 195.8, 198.7, 198.89, 199.0-199.1, 239.8-239.9
198.81 CC Excl: 195.8, 198.81, 198.89, 199.0-199.1, 239.8-239.9
198.82 CC Excl: 195.8, 198.82, 198.89, 199.0-199.1, 239.8-239.9
198.89 CC Excl: 195.8, 198.89, 199.0-199.1, 239.8-239.9
199.0 CC Excl: see Code 198.89
200.0x CC Excl: For code 200.00: 200.00-200.08, 239.8-239.9: For code 200.01: 200.00, 200.01, 200.08, 239.8-239.9; For code 200.02: 200.00, 200.02, 200.08, 239.8-239.9; For code 200.03: 200.00, 200.03, 200.08, 239.8-239.9; For code 200.04: 200.00, 200.04, 200.08, 239.8-239.9; For code 200.05: 200.00, 200.05, 200.08, 239.8-239.9; For code 200.06: 200.00, 200.06, 200.08, 239.8-239.9; For code 200.07: 200.00, 200.07-200.08, 239.8-239.9; For code 200.08: 200.00-200.08, 239.8-239.9
200.1x CC Excl: For code 200.10: 200.10-200.18, 239.8-239.9; For code 200.11: 200.10, 200.11, 200.18, 239.8-239.9; For code 200.12: 200.10, 200.12, 200.18, 239.8-239.9; For code 200.13: 200.10, 200.13, 200.18, 239.8-239.9; For code 200.14: 200.10, 200.14, 200.18, 239.8-239.9; For code 200.15: 200.10, 200.15, 200.18, 239.8-239.9; For code 200.16: 200.10, 200.16, 200.18, 239.8-239.9; For code 200.17: 200.10, 200.17-200.18, 239.8-239.9; For code 200.18: 200.10-200.18, 239.8-239.9
200.2x CC Excl: For code 200.20: 200.20-200.28, 239.8-239.9; For code 200.21: 200.20, 200.21, 200.28, 239.8-239.9; For code 200.22: 200.20, 200.22, 200.28, 239.8-239.9; For code 200.23: 200.20, 200.23, 200.28, 239.8-239.9; For code 200.24: 200.20, 200.24, 200.28, 239.8-239.9; For code 200.25: 200.20, 200.25, 200.28, 239.8-239.9; For code 200.26: 200.20, 200.26, 200.28, 239.8-239.9; For code 200.27: 200.20, 200.27-200.28, 239.8-239.9; For code 200.28: 200.20-200.28, 239.8-239.9

CC Exclusion List

200.8x CC Excl: **For code 200.80:** 200.80-200.88, 239.8-239.9; **For code 200.81:** 200.80, 200.81, 200.88, 239.8-239.9; **For code 200.82:** 200.80, 200.82, 200.88, 239.8-239.9; **For code 200.83:** 200.80, 200.83, 200.88, 239.8-239.9; **For code 200.84:** 200.80, 200.84, 200.88, 239.8-239.9; **For code 200.85:** 200.80, 200.85, 200.88, 239.8-239.9; **For code 200.86:** 200.80, 200.86, 200.88, 239.8-239.9; **For code 200.87:** 200.80, 200.87-200.88, 239.8-239.9; **For code 200.88:** 200.80-200.88, 239.8-239.9

201.0x CC Excl: **For code 201.00:** 201.00-201.08, 201.90, 239.8-239.9; **For code 201.01:** 201.00, 201.01, 201.08, 201.90-201.91, 239.8-239.9; **For code 201.02:** 201.00, 201.02, 201.08, 201.90, 201.92, 239.8-239.9; **For code 201.03:** 201.00, 201.03, 201.08, 201.90, 201.93, 239.8-239.9; **For code 201.04:** 201.00, 201.04, 201.08, 201.90, 201.94, 239.8-239.9; **For code 201.05:** 201.00, 201.05, 201.08, 201.90, 201.95, 239.8-239.9; **For code 201.06:** 201.00, 201.06, 201.08, 201.90, 201.96, 239.8-239.9; **For code 201.07:** 201.00, 201.07-201.08, 201.90, 201.97, 239.8-239.9; **For code 201.08:** 201.00-201.08, 201.90, 201.98, 239.8-239.9

201.1x CC Excl: **For code 201.10:** 201.10-201.18, 201.90, 201.98, 239.8-239.9; **For code 201.11:** 201.10, 201.11, 201.18, 201.90-201.91, 201.98, 239.8-239.9; **For code 201.12:** 201.10, 201.12, 201.18, 201.90, 201.92, 201.98, 239.8-239.9; **For code 201.13:** 201.10, 201.13, 201.18, 201.90, 201.93, 201.98, 239.8-239.9; **For code 201.14:** 201.10, 201.14, 201.18, 201.90, 201.94, 201.98, 239.8-239.9; **For code 201.15:** 201.10, 201.15, 201.18, 201.90, 201.95, 201.98, 239.8-239.9; **For code 201.16:** 201.10, 201.16, 201.18, 201.90, 201.96, 201.98, 239.8-239.9; **For code 201.17:** 201.10, 201.17-201.18, 201.90, 201.97-201.98, 239.8-239.9; **For code 201.18:** 201.10-201.18, 201.90, 201.98, 239.8-239.9

201.2x CC Excl: **For code 201.20:** 201.20-201.28, 201.90, 201.98, 239.8-239.9; **For code 201.21:** 201.20, 201.21, 201.28, 201.90-201.91, 201.98, 239.8-239.9; **For code 201.22:** 201.20, 201.22, 201.28, 201.90, 201.92, 201.98, 239.8-239.9; **For code 201.23:** 201.20, 201.23, 201.28, 201.90, 201.93, 201.98, 239.8-239.9; **For code 201.24:** 201.20, 201.24, 201.28, 201.90, 201.94, 201.98, 239.8-239.9; **For code 201.25:** 201.20, 201.25, 201.28, 201.90, 201.95, 201.98, 239.8-239.9; **For code 201.26:** 201.20, 201.26, 201.28, 201.90, 201.96, 201.98, 239.8-239.9; **For code 201.27:** 201.20, 201.27-201.28, 201.90, 201.97-201.98, 239.8-239.9; **For code 201.28:** 201.20-201.28, 201.90, 201.98, 239.8-239.9

201.4x CC Excl: **For code 201.40:** 201.40-201.48, 201.90, 201.98, 239.8-239.9; **For code 201.41:** 201.40, 201.41, 201.48, 201.90-201.91, 201.98, 239.8-239.9; **For code 201.42:** 201.40, 201.42, 201.48, 201.90, 201.92, 201.98, 239.8-239.9; **For code 201.43:** 201.40, 201.43, 201.48, 201.90, 201.93, 201.98, 239.8-239.9; **For code 201.44:** 201.40, 201.44, 201.48, 201.90, 201.94, 201.98, 239.8-239.9; **For code 201.45:** 201.40, 201.45, 201.48, 201.90, 201.95, 201.98, 239.8-239.9; **For code 201.46:** 201.40, 201.46, 201.48, 201.90, 201.96, 201.98, 239.8-239.9; **For code 201.47:** 201.40, 201.47-201.48, 201.90, 201.97-201.98, 239.8-239.9; **For code 201.48:** 201.40-201.48, 201.90, 201.98, 239.8-239.9

201.5x CC Excl: **For code 201.50:** 201.50-201.58, 201.90, 201.98, 239.8-239.9; **For code 201.51:** 201.50, 201.51, 201.58, 201.90-201.91, 201.98, 239.8-239.9; **For code 201.52:** 201.50, 201.52, 201.58, 201.90, 201.92, 201.98, 239.8-239.9; **For code 201.53:** 201.50, 201.53, 201.58, 201.90, 201.93, 201.98, 239.8-239.9; **For code 201.54:** 201.50, 201.54, 201.58, 201.90, 201.94, 201.98, 239.8-239.9; **For code 201.55:** 201.50, 201.55, 201.58, 201.90, 201.95, 201.98, 239.8-239.9; **For code 201.56:** 201.50, 201.56, 201.58, 201.90, 201.96, 201.98, 239.8-239.9; **For code 201.57:** 201.50, 201.57-201.58, 201.90, 201.97-201.98, 239.8-239.9; **For code 201.58:** 201.50-201.58, 201.90, 201.98, 239.8-239.9

201.6x   CC Excl: **For code 201.60:** 201.60-201.68, 201.90, 201.98, 239.8-239.9; **For code 201.61:** 201.60, 201.61, 201.68, 201.90-201.91, 201.98, 239.8-239.9; **For code 201.62:** 201.60, 201.62, 201.68, 201.90, 201.92, 201.98, 239.8-239.9; **For code 201.63:** 201.60, 201.63, 201.68, 201.90, 201.93, 201.98, 239.8-239.9; **For code 201.64:** 201.60, 201.64, 201.68, 201.90, 201.94, 201.98, 239.8-239.9; **For code 201.65:** 201.60, 201.65, 201.68, 201.90, 201.95, 201.98, 239.8-239.9; **For code 201.66:** 201.60, 201.66, 201.68, 201.90, 201.96, 201.98, 239.8-239.9; **For code 201.67:** 201.60, 201.67-201.68, 201.90, 201.97-201.98, 239.8-239.9; **For code 201.68:** 201.60-201.68, 201.90, 201.98, 239.8-239.9

201.7x   CC Excl: **For code 201.70:** 201.70-201.78, 201.90, 201.98, 239.8-239.9; **For code 201.71:** 201.70, 201.71, 201.78, 201.91, 201.98, 239.8-239.9; **For code 201.72:** 201.70, 201.72, 201.78, 201.92, 201.98, 239.8-239.9; **For code 201.73:** 201.70, 201.73, 201.78, 201.93, 201.98, 239.8-239.9; **For code 201.74:** 201.70, 201.74, 201.78, 201.94, 201.98, 239.8-239.9; **For code 201.75:** 201.70, 201.75, 201.78, 201.95, 201.98, 239.8-239.9;**For code 201.76:** 201.70, 201.76, 201.78, 201.96, 201.98, 239.8-239.9;**For code 201.77:** 201.70, 201.77-201.78, 201.97-201.98, 239.8-239.9;**For code 201.78:** 201.70-201.78, 201.98, 239.8-239.9

201.9x   CC Excl: **For code 201.90:** 201.90-201.98, 239.8-239.9; **For code 201.91:** 201.90, 201.91, 201.98, 239.8-239.9; **For code 201.92:** 201.90, 201.92, 201.98, 239.8-239.9; **For code 201.93:** 201.90, 201.93, 201.98, 239.8-239.9; **For code 201.94:** 201.90, 201.94, 201.98, 239.8-239.9; **For code 201.95:** 201.90, 201.95, 201.98, 239.8-239.9; **For code 201.96:** 201.90, 201.96, 201.98, 239.8-239.9; **For code 201.97:** 201.90, 201.97-201.98, 239.8-239.9; **For code 201.98:** 201.90-201.98, 239.8-239.9

202.0x   CC Excl: **For code 202.00:** 202.00-202.08, 202.80, 202.90, 239.8-239.9; **For code 202.01:** 202.00, 202.01, 202.08, 202.81, 202.91, 239.8-239.9; **For code 202.02:** 202.00, 202.02, 202.08, 202.82, 202.92, 239.8-239.9;**For code 202.03:** 202.00, 202.03, 202.08, 202.83, 202.93, 239.8-239.9;**For code 202.04:** 202.00, 202.04, 202.08, 202.84, 202.94, 239.8-239.9;**For code 202.05:** 202.00, 202.05, 202.08, 202.85, 202.95, 239.8-239.9;**For code 202.06:** 202.00, 202.06, 202.08, 202.86, 202.96, 239.8-239.9;**For code 202.07:** 202.00, 202.07-202.08, 202.87, 202.97, 239.8-239.9;**For code 202.08:** 202.00-202.08, 202.88, 202.98, 239.8-239.9

202.1x   CC Excl: **For code 202.10:** 202.10-202.18, 202.80, 202.90, 239.8-239.9;**For code 202.11:** 202.10, 202.11, 202.18, 202.81, 202.91, 239.8-239.9;**For code 202.12:** 202.10, 202.12, 202.18, 202.82, 202.92, 239.8-239.9;**For code 202.13:** 202.10, 202.13, 202.18, 202.83, 202.93, 239.8-239.9;**For code 202.14:** 202.10, 202.14, 202.18, 202.84, 202.94, 239.8-239.9;**For code 202.15:** 202.10, 202.15, 202.18, 202.85, 202.95, 239.8-239.9;**For code 202.16:** 202.10, 202.16, 202.18, 202.86, 202.96, 239.8-239.9;**For code 202.17:** 202.10, 202.17-202.18, 202.87, 202.97, 239.8-239.9;**For code 202.18:** 202.10-202.18, 202.88, 202.98, 239.8-239.9

202.2x   CC Excl: **For code 202.20:** 202.20-202.28, 202.80, 202.90, 239.8-239.9; **For code 202.21:** 202.20, 202.21, 202.28, 202.81, 202.91, 239.8-239.9; **For code 202.22:** 202.20, 202.22, 202.28, 202.82, 202.92, 239.8-239.9;**For code 202.23:** 202.20, 202.23, 202.28, 202.83, 202.93, 239.8-239.9;**For code 202.24:** 202.20, 202.24, 202.28, 202.84, 202.94, 239.8-239.9;**For code 202.25:** 202.20, 202.25, 202.28, 202.85, 202.95, 239.8-239.9;**For code 202.26:** 202.20, 202.26, 202.28, 202.86, 202.96, 239.8-239.9;**For code 202.27:** 202.20, 202.27-202.28, 202.87, 202.97, 239.8-239.9;**For code 202.28:** 202.20-202.28, 202.88, 202.98, 239.8-239.9

CC Exclusion List

202.3x CC Excl: **For code 202.30:** 202.30-
202.38, 202.80, 202.90, 239.8-239.9;
For code 202.31: 202.30, 202.31,
202.38, 202.81, 202.91, 239.8-239.9;
For code 202.32: 202.30, 202.32,
202.38, 202.82, 202.92, 239.8-
239.9;**For code 202.33:** 202.30, 202.33,
202.38, 202.83, 202.93, 239.8-
239.9;**For code 202.34:** 202.30, 202.34,
202.38, 202.84, 202.94, 239.8-
239.9;**For code 202.35:** 202.30, 202.35,
202.38, 202.85, 202.95, 239.8-
239.9;**For code 202.36:** 202.30, 202.36,
202.38, 202.86, 202.96, 239.8-
239.9;**For code 202.37:** 202.30, 202.37-
202.38, 202.87, 202.97, 239.8-
239.9;**For code 202.38:** 202.30-202.38,
202.88, 202.98, 239.8-239.9

202.4x CC Excl: **For code 202.40:** 202.40-
202.48, 202.80, 202.90, 239.8-239.9;
For code 202.41: 202.40, 202.41,
202.48, 202.81, 202.91, 239.8-
239.9;**For code 202.42:** 202.40, 202.42,
202.48, 202.82, 202.92, 239.8-
239.9;**For code 202.43:** 202.40, 202.43,
202.48, 202.83, 202.93, 239.8-
239.9;**For code 202.44:** 202.40, 202.44,
202.48, 202.84, 202.94, 239.8-
239.9;**For code 202.45:** 202.40, 202.45,
202.48, 202.85, 202.95, 239.8-
239.9;**For code 202.46:** 202.40, 202.46,
202.48, 202.86, 202.96, 239.8-
239.9;**For code 202.47:** 202.40, 202.47-
202.48, 202.87, 202.97, 239.8-
239.9;**For code 202.48:** 202.40-202.48,
202.88, 202.98, 239.8-239.9

202.5x CC Excl: **For code 202.50:** 202.50-
202.58, 202.80, 202.90, 239.8-
239.9;**For code 202.51:** 202.50, 202.51,
202.58, 202.81, 202.91, 239.8-
239.9;**For code 202.52:** 202.50, 202.52,
202.58, 202.82, 202.92, 239.8-
239.9;**For code 202.53:** 202.50, 202.53,
202.58, 202.83, 202.93, 239.8-
239.9;**For code 202.54:** 202.50, 202.54,
202.58, 202.84, 202.94, 239.8-
239.9;**For code 202.55:** 202.50, 202.55,
202.58, 202.85, 202.95, 239.8-
239.9;**For code 202.56:** 202.50, 202.56,
202.58, 202.86, 202.96, 239.8-
239.9;**For code 202.57:** 202.50, 202.57-
202.58, 202.87, 202.97, 239.8-
239.9;**For code 202.58:** 202.50-202.58,
202.88, 202.98, 239.8-239.9

202.6x CC Excl: **For code 202.60:** 202.60-
202.68, 202.80, 202.90, 239.8-239.9;
For code 202.61: 202.60, 202.61,
202.68, 202.81, 202.91, 239.8-
239.9;**For code 202.62:** 202.60, 202.62,
202.68, 202.82, 202.92, 239.8-
239.9;**For code 202.63:** 202.60, 202.63,
202.68, 202.83, 202.93, 239.8-
239.9;**For code 202.64:** 202.60, 202.64,
202.68, 202.84, 202.94, 239.8-
239.9;**For code 202.65:** 202.60, 202.65,
202.68, 202.85, 202.95, 239.8-
239.9;**For code 202.66:** 202.60, 202.66,
202.68, 202.86, 202.96, 239.8-
239.9;**For code 202.67:** 202.60, 202.67-
202.68, 202.87, 202.97, 239.8-
239.9;**For code 202.68:** 202.60-202.68,
202.88, 202.98, 239.8-239.9

202.8x **For code 202.81:** 202.80, 202.81,
202.88, 202.91, 239.8-239.9; **For code
202.82:** 202.80, 202.82, 202.88, 202.92,
239.8-239.9; **For code 202.83:** 202.80,
202.83, 202.88, 202.93, 239.8-239.9;
For code 202.84: 202.80, 202.84,
202.88, 202.94, 239.8-239.9; **For code
202.85:** 202.80, 202.85, 202.88, 202.95,
239.8-239.9; **For code 202.86:** 202.80,
202.86, 202.88, 202.96, 239.8-239.9;
For code 202.87: 202.80, 202.87-
202.88, 202.97, 239.8-239.9; **For code
202.88:** 202.80-202.88, 202.98, 239.8-
239.9

202.9x CC Excl: **For code 202.90:** 202.90-
202.98, 239.8-239.9; **For code 202.91:**
202.90, 202.91, 202.98, 239.8-239.9;
For code 202.92: 202.90, 202.92,
202.98, 239.8-239.9; **For code 202.93:**
202.90, 202.93, 202.98, 239.8-239.9;
For code 202.94: 202.90, 202.94,
202.98, 239.8-239.9; **For code 202.95:**
202.90, 202.95, 202.98, 239.8-239.9;
For code 202.96: 202.90, 202.96,
202.98, 239.8-239.9; **For code 202.97:**
202.90, 202.97-202.98, 239.8-239.9;
For code 202.98: 202.90-202.98, 239.8-
239.9

203.0x CC Excl: 203.00-203.81, 204.00-204.91,
205.00-205.91, 206.00-206.91, 207.00-
207.81, 208.00-208.91, 239.8-239.9

203.1x CC Excl: see Code 203.0
203.8x CC Excl: see Code 203.0
204.0x CC Excl: see Code 203.0
204.1x CC Excl: see Code 203.0
204.2x CC Excl: see Code 203.0
204.8x CC Excl: see Code 203.0
204.9x CC Excl: see Code 203.0

205.0x CC Excl: see Code 203.0
205.1x CC Excl: see Code 203.0
205.2x CC Excl: see Code 203.0
205.3x CC Excl: see Code 203.0
205.8x CC Excl: see Code 203.0
205.9x CC Excl: see Code 203.0
206.0x CC Excl: see Code 203.0
206.1x CC Excl: see Code 203.0
206.2x CC Excl: see Code 203.0
206.8x CC Excl: see Code 203.0
206.9x CC Excl: see Code 203.0
207.0x CC Excl: see Code 203.0
207.1x CC Excl: see Code 203.0
207.2x CC Excl: see Code 203.0
207.8x CC Excl: see Code 203.0
208.0x CC Excl: see Code 203.0
208.1x CC Excl: see Code 203.0
208.2x CC Excl: see Code 203.0
208.8x CC Excl: see Code 203.0
208.9x CC Excl: see Code 203.0
242.0x CC Excl: 017.50-017.56, 017.90-017.96,
        240.0, 240.9, 241.0-241.9, 242.00-
        242.91, 243, 244.0-244.9, 245.0-245.9,
        246.0-246.9, 259.8-259.9
242.1x CC Excl: see Code 242.0
242.2x CC Excl: see Code 242.0
242.3x CC Excl: see Code 242.0
242.4x CC Excl: see Code 242.0
242.8x CC Excl: see Code 242.0
242.9x CC Excl: see Code 242.0
250.0   CC Excl: For codes 250.01-250.03:
        250.00-250.93, 251.0-251.3, 259.8-
        259.9
250.1   CC Excl: For codes 250.11-250.13:
        250.00-250.93, 251.0-251.3, 259.8-
        259.9
250.2   CC Excl: For codes 250.21-250.23:
        250.00-250.93, 251.0-251.3, 259.8-
        259.9
250.3   CC Excl: For codes 250.31-250.33:
        250.00-250.93, 251.0-251.3, 259.8-
        259.9
250.4   CC Excl: For codes 250.41-250.43:
        250.00-250.93, 251.0-251.3, 259.8-
        259.9
250.5   CC Excl: For codes 250.51-250.3:
        250.00-250.93, 251.0-251.3, 259.8-
        259.9
250.6   CC Excl: For codes 250.61-250.63:
        250.00-250.93, 251.0-251.3, 259.8-
        259.9
250.7   CC Excl: For codes 250.71-250.73:
        250.00-250.93, 251.0-251.3, 259.8-
        259.9

250.8   CC Excl: For codes 250.81-250.83:
        250.00-250.93, 251.0-251.3, 259.8-
        259.9
250.9   CC Excl: For codes 250.91-250.93:
        250.00-250.93, 251.0-251.3, 259.8-
        259.9
251.0   CC Excl: 250.00-250.93, 251.0-251.3,
        259.8-259.9
251.3   CC Excl: see Code 251.0
252.1   CC Excl: 252.0-252.9, 259.8-259.9
253.2   CC Excl: 253.0-253.9, 259.8-259.9
253.5   CC Excl: 253.1-253.2, 253.4-253.9,
        259.8-259.9
254.1   CC Excl: 254.0-254.1, 254.8-254.9,
        259.8-259.9
255.0   CC Excl: 255.0-255.2, 259.8-259.9
255.3   CC Excl: 017.60-017.66, 017.90-017.96,
        255.3-255.9, 259.8-259.9
255.4   CC Excl: see Code 255.3
255.5   CC Excl: see Code 255.3
255.6   CC Excl: see Code 255.3
258.0   CC Excl: 240.0, 240.9, 241.0-241.9,
        242.00-242.91, 243, 244.0-244.9,
        245.0-245.9, 246.0-246.9, 250.00-
        250.93, 251.0-251.9, 252.0-252.9,
        253.0-253.9, 254.0-254.9, 255.0-255.9,
        256.0-256.2, 256.31-256.39, 256.4-
        256.9, 257.0-257.9, 258.0-258.9, 259.0-
        259.9
258.1   CC Excl: see Code 258.0
258.8   CC Excl: see Code 258.0
258.9   CC Excl: see Code 258.0
259.2   CC Excl: 259.2-259.3, 259.8-259.9
260   CC Excl: 260-262, 263.0-263.9
261   CC Excl: see Code 260
262   CC Excl: see Code 260
263.0   CC Excl: see Code 260
263.1   CC Excl: see Code 260
263.2   CC Excl: see Code 260
263.8   CC Excl: see Code 260
263.9   CC Excl: see Code 260
269.0   CC Excl: 269.0
273.3   CC Excl: 273.0-273.9
276.0   CC Excl: 276.0-276.9
276.1   CC Excl: see Code 276.0
276.2   CC Excl: see Code 276.0
276.3   CC Excl: see Code 276.0
276.4   CC Excl: see Code 276.0
276.5   CC Excl: see Code 276.0
276.6   CC Excl: see Code 276.0
276.7   CC Excl: see Code 276.0
276.9   CC Excl: see Code 276.0
277.00 CC Excl: 277.00-277.09
277.01 CC Excl: see Code 277.00
277.02 CC Excl: see Code 277.00

277.03   CC Excl: see Code 277.00
277.09   CC Excl: see Code 277.00
279.02   CC Excl: 279.02-279.9
279.03   CC Excl: see Code 279.02
279.04   CC Excl: see Code 279.02
279.05   CC Excl: see Code 279.02
279.06   CC Excl: see Code 279.02
279.09   CC Excl: see Code 279.02
279.10   CC Excl: see Code 279.02
279.11   CC Excl: see Code 279.02
279.12   CC Excl: see Code 279.02
279.13   CC Excl: see Code 279.02
279.19   CC Excl: see Code 279.02
279.2   CC Excl: see Code 279.02
279.3   CC Excl: see Code 279.02
279.4   CC Excl: see Code 279.02
279.8   CC Excl: see Code 279.02
279.9   CC Excl: see Code 279.02
280.0   CC Excl: 280.0-280.9, 281.0-281.9,
         282.0-282.9, 283.0-283.9, 284.0-284.9,
         285.0-285.9, 289.81-289.9, 517.3
281.4   CC Excl: see Code 280.0
281.8   CC Excl: see Code 280.0
282.41   CC Excl: see Code 280.0
282.42   CC Excl: see Code 280.0
282.49   CC Excl: see Code 280.0
282.60   CC Excl: see Code 280.0
282.61   CC Excl: see Code 280.0
282.62   CC Excl: see Code 280.0
282.63   CC Excl: see Code 280.0
282.64   CC Excl: see Code 280.0
282.68   CC Excl: see Code 280.0
282.69   CC Excl: see Code 280.0
283.0   CC Excl: see Code 280.0
283.10   CC Excl: see Code 280.0
283.11   CC Excl: see Code 280.0
283.19   CC Excl: see Code 280.0
283.2   CC Excl: see Code 280.0
283.9   CC Excl: see Code 280.0
284.0   CC Excl: see Code 280.0
284.8   CC Excl: see Code 280.0
284.9   CC Excl: see Code 280.0
285.0   CC Excl: see Code 280.0
285.1   CC Excl: 280.0-280.9, 281.0-281.9,
         282.0-282.9, 283.0-283.9, 284.0, 284.8,
         285.0-285.9, 289.81-289.9, 517.3,
         958.2
286.0   CC Excl: 286.0-286.9, 287.0-287.9,
         289.81-289.9
286.1   CC Excl: see Code 286.0
286.2   CC Excl: see Code 286.0
286.3   CC Excl: see Code 286.0
286.4   CC Excl: see Code 286.0
286.5   CC Excl: see Code 286.0

286.6   CC Excl: see Code 286.0
286.7   CC Excl: see Code 286.0
286.9   CC Excl: see Code 286.0
287.0   CC Excl: see Code 286.0
287.1   CC Excl: see Code 286.0
287.2   CC Excl: see Code 286.0
287.3   CC Excl: see Code 286.0
287.4   CC Excl: see Code 286.0
287.5   CC Excl: see Code 286.0
287.8   CC Excl: see Code 286.0
287.9   CC Excl: see Code 286.0
288.0   CC Excl: 288.0-288.9, 289.81-289.9
288.1   CC Excl: see Code 288.0
289.81   see Code 288.0
289.82   see Code 288.0
291.0   CC Excl: 291.0-291.9, 292.0-292.9,
         293.0-293.9, 294.0-294.9, 303.00-
         303.93, 304.00-304.91, 305.00-305.03,
         305.20-305.93, 790.3
291.1   CC Excl: see Code 291.0
291.2   CC Excl: see Code 291.0
291.3   CC Excl: see Code 291.0
291.4   CC Excl: see Code 291.0
291.81   CC Excl: 291.0-291.9, 292.0-292.9,
         293.0-293.9, 294.0-294.9, 303.00-
         303.93, 304.00-304.93, 305.00-305.03,
         305.20-305.93, 790.3
291.89   CC Excl: see Code 291.81
291.9   CC Excl: see Code 291.0
292.0   CC Excl: see Code 291.0
292.11   CC Excl: see Code 291.0
292.12   CC Excl: see Code 291.0
292.2   CC Excl: see Code 291.0
292.81   CC Excl: see Code 291.0
292.82   CC Excl: see Code 291.0
292.83   CC Excl: see Code 291.0
292.84   CC Excl: see Code 291.0
292.89   CC Excl: see Code 291.0
292.9   CC Excl: see Code 291.0
293.81   CC Excl: 291.0-291.7, 291.81, 291.89,
         291.9, 292.0-292.9, 293.0-293.9, 294.0-
         294.9, 303.00-303.93, 304.00-304.93,
         305.00-305.03, 305.20-305.93, 790.3
293.82   CC Excl: see Code 293.81
293.83   CC Excl: see Code 293.81
293.84   CC Excl: see Code 293.81
295.0   CC Excl: For codes 295.00-295.04:
         295.00-295.95, 296.00-296.99, 297.0-
         297.9, 298.0-298.9, 299.00-299.91,
         300.00-300.9, 301.0-301.9, 306.0-
         306.9, 307.0-307.9, 308.0-308.9, 309.0-
         309.9, 310.0-310.9, 311, 312.00-312.9,
         313.0-313.9, 314.00-314.9, 315.00-
         315.9, 316-317, 318.0-318.2, 319

295.1	CC Excl: For codes 295.10-295.14: see Code 295.0
295.2	CC Excl: For codes 295.21-295.24: see Code 295.0
295.3	CC Excl: For codes 295.30_295.34: see Code 295.0
295.4	CC Excl: For codes 295.40-295.44: see Code 295.0
295.6	CC Excl: For codes 295.60-295.64: see Code 295.0
295.7	CC Excl: For codes 295.70-295.74: see Code 295.0
295.8	CC Excl: For codes 295.80-295.84: see Code 295.0
295.9	CC Excl: For codes 295.90-295.94: see Code 295.0
296.0	CC Excl: **For code 296.04**: see Code 295.0
296.1	CC Excl: **For code 296.14**: see Code 295.0
296.3	CC Excl: **For code 296.34**: see Code 295.0
296.4	CC Excl: **For code 296.44**: see Code 295.0
296.5	CC Excl: **For code 296.54**: see Code 295.0
296.6	CC Excl: **For code 296.64**: see Code 295.0
298.0	CC Excl: see Code 295.0
298.3	CC Excl: see Code 295.0
298.4	CC Excl: see Code 295.0
299.0	CC Excl: **For code 299.00**: see Code 295.0
299.1	CC Excl: **For code 299.10**: see Code 295.0
299.8	CC Excl: **For code 299.80**: see Code 295.0
299.9	CC Excl: **For code 299.90**: see Code 295.0
303.0	CC Excl: For codes 303.00-303.02: 291.0-291.9, 292.0-292.9, 303.00-303.93, 304.00-304.91, 305.00-305.03, 305.20-305.93, 790.3
303.9	CC Excl: For codes 303.90-303.92: see Code 303.0
304.0	CC Excl: For codes 304.00-304.02: see Code 303.0
304.1	CC Excl: For codes 304.10-304.12: see Code 303.0
304.2	CC Excl: For codes 304.20-304.22: see Code 303.0
304.4	CC Excl: For codes 304.40-304.42: see Code 303.0
304.5	CC Excl: For codes 304.50-304.52: see Code 303.0
304.6	CC Excl: For codes 304.60-304.62: see Code 303.0
304.7	CC Excl: For codes 304.70-304.72: see Code 303.0
304.8	CC Excl: For codes 304.80-304.82: see Code 303.0
304.9	CC Excl: For codes 304.90-304.92: see Code 303.0
305.0	CC Excl: For codes 305.00-305.02: see Code 303.0
305.3	CC Excl: For codes 305.30-305.32: see Code 303.0
305.4	CC Excl: For codes 305.40-305.42: see Code 303.0
305.5	CC Excl: For codes 305.50-305.52: see Code 303.0
305.6	CC Excl: For codes 305.60-305.62: see Code 303.0
305.7	CC Excl: For codes 305.70-305.72: see Code 303.0
305.9	CC Excl: For codes 305.90-305.92: see Code 303.0
307.1	CC Excl: 306.4, 306.8-306.9, 307.1, 307.50-307.59, 309.22
320.0	CC Excl: 003.21, 013.00-013.16, 036.0, 047.0-047.9, 049.0-049.1, 053.0, 054.72, 072.1, 090.42, 091.81, 094.2, 098.89, 100.81, 112.83, 114.2, 115.01, 115.11, 115.91, 130.0, 250.60-250.63, 250.80-250.93, 320.0-320.9, 321.0-321.8, 322.0-322.9, 349.89, 349.9, 357.0
320.1	CC Excl: see Code 320.0
320.2	CC Excl: see Code 320.0
320.3	CC Excl: see Code 320.0
320.7	CC Excl: see Code 320.0
320.81	CC Excl: see Code 320.0
320.82	CC Excl: see Code 320.0
320.89	CC Excl: see Code 320.0
320.9	CC Excl: see Code 320.0
321.0	CC Excl: see Code 320.0
321.1	CC Excl: see Code 320.0
321.2	CC Excl: 003.21, 013.00-013.16, 036.0, 047.0-047.9, 049.0-049.1, 053.0, 054.72, 072.1, 090.42, 091.81, 094.2, 098.89, 100.81, 112.83, 114.2, 115.01, 115.11, 115.91, 130.0, 320.0-320.9, 321.0-321.8, 322.0-322.9, 349.89, 349.9, 357.0

CC Exclusion List

321.3	CC Excl: 003.21, 013.00-013.16, 036.0, 047.0-047.9, 049.0-049.1, 053.0, 054.72, 072.1, 090.42, 091.81, 094.2, 098.89, 100.81, 112.83, 114.2, 115.01, 115.11, 115.91, 130.0, 250.60-250.63, 250.80-250.93, 320.0-320.9, 321.0-321.8, 322.0-322.9, 349.89, 349.9, 357.0
321.4	CC Excl: see Code 321.3
321.8	CC Excl: see Code 321.3
322.0	CC Excl: see Code 321.3
322.1	CC Excl: see Code 321.3
322.2	CC Excl: see Code 321.3
322.9	CC Excl: see Code 321.3
324.0	CC Excl: 006.5, 013.20-013.36, 250.60-250.63, 250.80-250.93, 324.0-324.9, 325, 348.8-348.9
324.1	CC Excl: 006.5, 013.20-013.36, 250.60-250.63, 250.80-250.93, 324.1
324.9	CC Excl: 006.5, 013.20-013.36, 250.60-250.63, 250.80-250.93, 324.0-324.9, 325
325	CC Excl: see Code 324.9
331.4	CC Excl: 250.60-250.63, 250.80-250.93, 331.3-331.7, 331.82-331.89, 331.9, 348.8-348.9, 741.00-741.03, 742.3-742.4, 742.59, 742.8-742.9
335.0	CC Excl: 250.60-250.63, 250.80-250.93, 334.8-334.9, 335.0, 335.10-335.9, 336.0-336.9, 337.0-337.9, 349.89, 349.9
335.10	CC Excl: see Code 335.0
335.11	CC Excl: see Code 335.0
335.19	CC Excl: see Code 335.0
335.20	CC Excl: see Code 335.0
335.21	CC Excl: see Code 335.0
335.22	CC Excl: see Code 335.0
335.23	CC Excl: see Code 335.0
335.24	CC Excl: see Code 335.0
335.29	CC Excl: see Code 335.0
335.8	CC Excl: see Code 335.0
335.9	CC Excl: see Code 335.0
340	CC Excl: 250.60-250.63, 250.80-250.93, 340, 341.8-341.9
343.2	CC Excl: 250.60-250.63, 250.80-250.93, 342.00-342.92, 343.0-343.9, 344.00-344.61, 344.9, 348.8-348.9, 349.89, 349.9, 742.59, 742.8-742.9
344.00	CC Excl: see Code 343.2
344.01	CC Excl: see Code 343.2
344.02	CC Excl: see Code 343.2
344.03	CC Excl: see Code 343.2
344.04	CC Excl: see Code 343.2
344.09	CC Excl: see Code 343.2
345.0	CC Excl: For code 345.01: 250.60-250.63, 345.00-345.91, 348.8-348.9, 349.89, 349.9
345.1	CC Excl: see Code 345.01
345.2	CC Excl: 250.60-250.63, 250.80-250.93, 345.00-345.91, 348.8-348.9, 349.89, 349.9
345.3	CC Excl: see Code 345.2
345.4	CC Excl: For code 345.41: 250.60-250.63, 345.00-345.91, 348.8-348.9, 349.89, 349.9
345.5	CC Excl: For code 345.51: see Code 345.4
345.6	CC Excl: For code 345.61: see Code 345.4
345.7	CC Excl: For code 345.71: see Code 345.4
345.8	CC Excl: For code 345.81: see Code 345.4
345.9	CC Excl: For code 345.91: see Code 345.4
348.1	CC Excl: 250.60-250.63, 250.80-250.93, 348.1-348.2, 349.89, 349.9
349.1	CC Excl: 250.60-250.63, 250.80-250.93, 349.1, 349.89, 349.9
349.81	CC Excl: 250.60-250.63, 250.80-250.93, 349.81, 349.89, 349.9
349.82	CC Excl: 013.60-013.66, 017.90-017.96, 036.1, 049.8-049.9, 052.0, 054.3, 062.0-062.9, 063.0-063.9, 072.2, 090.41, 094.81, 130.0, 250.60-250.63, 250.80-250.93, 323.0-323.9, 348.3, 348.8-348.9, 349.82-349.89, 349.9
357.0	CC Excl: 003.21, 013.00-013.16, 036.0, 036.89, 036.9, 041.81-041.89, 041.9, 047.0-047.9, 049.0-049.1, 053.0, 054.72, 072.1, 090.42, 091.81, 094.2, 098.89, 100.81, 112.83, 114.2, 115.01, 115.11, 115.91, 130.0, 139.8, 320.0-320.9, 321.0-321.8, 322.0-322.9, 349.89, 349.9, 357.0
358.0x	CC Excl: 250.60-250.63, 250.80-250.93, 349.89, 349.9, 358.00-358.1
358.1	CC Excl: see Code 358.0
359.0	CC Excl: 250.60-250.63, 250.80-250.93, 349.89, 349.9, 359.00-359.1
359.1	CC Excl: see Code 359.0
377.00	CC Excl: 017.30-017.36, 017.90-017.96, 036.81, 250.50-250.53, 250.80-250.93, 377.00-377.03, 377.14, 377.24, 379.8, 379.90, 379.99, 743.8-743.9
377.01	CC Excl: see Code 377.00
377.02	CC Excl: see Code 377.00

383.01	CC Excl: 015.60-015.66, 017.40-017.46, 017.90-017.96, 383.00-383.9, 388.71-388.72, 388.8-388.9, 744.00, 744.02, 744.09, 744.29, 744.3
383.30	CC Excl: see Code 383.01
383.81	CC Excl: see Code 383.01
394.0	CC Excl: 390, 391.8-391.9, 394.0-394.9, 396.0-396.9, 397.9, 398.90, 398.99, 424.0, 459.89, 459.9
394.1	CC Excl: see Code 394.0
394.2	CC Excl: see Code 394.0
394.9	CC Excl: see Code 394.0
395.0	CC Excl: 390, 391.8-391.9, 395.0-395.9, 396.0-396.9, 397.9, 398.90, 398.99, 424.1, 459.89, 459.9
395.1	CC Excl: see Code 395.0
395.2	CC Excl: see Code 395.0
395.9	CC Excl: see Code 395.0
396.0	CC Excl: 390, 391.8-391.9, 394.0-394.9, 395.0-395.9, 396.0-396.9, 397.9, 398.90, 398.99, 424.0-424.1, 459.89, 459.9
396.1	CC Excl: see Code 396.0
396.2	CC Excl: see Code 396.0
396.3	CC Excl: see Code 396.0
396.8	CC Excl: see Code 396.0
396.9	CC Excl: see Code 396.0
397.0	CC Excl: 397.0, 398.90, 398.99, 424.2, 459.89, 459.9
397.1	CC Excl: 397.1, 398.90, 398.99, 424.3, 459.89, 459.9
397.9	CC Excl: 390, 391.1, 391.8-391.9, 394.0-394.9, 395.0-395.9, 397.1, 397.9, 398.90, 398.99, 421.0-421.9, 424.0-424.99, 459.89, 459.9
398.0	CC Excl: 390, 391.2-391.9, 398.0, 398.90, 398.99, 422.0, 422.90-422.99, 429.0, 429.71, 429.79, 459.89, 459.9
398.91	CC Excl: 398.90-398.99, 402.01, 402.11, 402.91, 428.0-428.9, 459.89, 459.9
401.0	CC Excl: 401.0-401.9, 402.00-402.91, 403.00-403.91, 404.00-404.93, 405.01-405.99, 459.89, 459.9
402.00	CC Excl: see Code 401.0
402.01	CC Excl: 398.91, 401.0-401.9, 402.00-402.91, 403.00-403.91, 404.00-404.93, 405.01-405.99, 428.0-428.9, 459.89, 459.9
402.11	CC Excl: see Code 402.01
402.91	CC Excl: see Code 402.01
403.0x	CC Excl: 401.0-401.9, 402.00-402.91, 403.00-403.91, 404.00-404.93, 405.01-405.99, 459.89, 459.9
403.1	CC Excl: For code 403.11: see Code 403.0
403.9	CC Excl: For code 403.91: see Code 403.0
404.0x	CC Excl: see Code 403.0
404.1	CC Excl: For codes 404.11-404.13: see Code 403.0
404.9	CC Excl: For codes 404.91-404.93: see Code 403.0
405.01	CC Excl: 401.0-401.9, 402.00-402.91, 403.00-403.91, 404.00-404.93, 405.01-405.99, 459.89, 459.9
405.09	CC Excl: see Code 405.01
410.0	CC Excl: For code 410.01: 410.00-410.92, 459.89, 459.9
410.1	CC Excl: For code 410.11: see Code 410.0
410.2	CC Excl: For code 410.21: see Code 410.0
410.3	CC Excl: For code 410.31: see Code 410.0
410.4	CC Excl: For code 410.41: see Code 410.0
410.5	CC Excl: For code 410.51: see Code 410.0
410.6	CC Excl: For code 410.61: see Code 410.0
410.7	CC Excl: For code 410.71: see Code 410.0
410.8	CC Excl: For code 410.81: see Code 410.0
410.9	CC Excl: For code 410.91: see Code 410.0
411.0	CC Excl: 411.0, 411.81, 411.89, 459.89, 459.9
411.1	CC Excl: 410.00-410.92, 411.1-411.89, 413.0-413.9, 414.8-414.9, 459.89, 459.9
411.81	CC Excl: 410.00-410.92, 411.0-411.89, 413.0-413.9, 414.8-414.9, 459.89, 459.9
411.89	CC Excl: see Code 411.81
413.0	CC Excl: 410.00-410.92, 411.1-411.89, 413.0-413.9, 414.8-414.9, 459.89, 459.9
413.1	CC Excl: see Code 413.0
413.9	CC Excl: see Code 413.0
415.0	CC Excl: 415.0, 416.8-416.9, 459.89, 459.9
415.11	CC Excl: 415.11, 415.19, 459.89, 459.9
415.19	CC Excl: 415.11, 415.19, 459.89, 459.9
416.0	CC Excl: 416.0, 416.8-416.9, 417.8-417.9, 459.89, 459.9
420.0	CC Excl: 391.0, 393, 420.0-420.99, 423.8-423.9, 459.89, 459.9

420.90	CC Excl: see Code 420.0
420.91	CC Excl: see Code 420.0
420.99	CC Excl: see Code 420.0
421.0	CC Excl: 391.1, 397.9, 421.0-421.9, 424.90-424.99, 459.89, 459.9
421.1	CC Excl: see Code 421.0
421.9	CC Excl: see Code 421.0
422.0	CC Excl: 391.2, 398.0, 422.0-422.99, 429.0, 429.71, 429.79, 459.89, 459.9
422.90	CC Excl: see Code 422.0
422.91	CC Excl: see Code 422.0
422.92	CC Excl: see Code 422.0
422.93	CC Excl: see Code 422.0
422.99	CC Excl: see Code 422.0
423.0	CC Excl: 423.0-423.9, 459.89, 459.9
423.1	CC Excl: see Code 423.0
423.2	CC Excl: see Code 423.0
424.0	CC Excl: 394.0-394.9, 396.0-396.9, 424.0, 459.89, 459.9
424.1	CC Excl: 395.0-395.9, 396.0-396.9, 424.1, 459.89, 459.9
424.2	CC Excl: 397.0, 424.2, 459.89, 459.9
424.3	CC Excl: 397.1, 424.3, 459.89, 459.9
424.90	CC Excl: 424.90-424.99, 459.89, 459.9
424.91	CC Excl: see Code 424.90
424.99	CC Excl: see Code 424.90
425.0	CC Excl: 425.0-425.9, 459.89, 459.9
425.1	CC Excl: see Code 425.0
425.2	CC Excl: see Code 425.0
425.3	CC Excl: see Code 425.0
425.4	CC Excl: see Code 425.0
425.5	CC Excl: see Code 425.0
425.7	CC Excl: see Code 425.0
425.8	CC Excl: see Code 425.0
425.9	CC Excl: see Code 425.0
426.0	CC Excl: 426.0-426.9, 427.0-427.5, 427.89, 459.89, 459.9
426.12	CC Excl: see Code 426.0
426.13	CC Excl: see Code 426.0
426.54	CC Excl: see Code 426.0
426.6	CC Excl: see Code 426.0
426.7	CC Excl: see Code 426.0
426.81	CC Excl: see Code 426.0
426.89	CC Excl: see Code 426.0
426.9	CC Excl: see Code 426.0
427.0	CC Excl: see Code 426.0
427.1	CC Excl: see Code 426.0
427.2	CC Excl: see Code 426.0
427.31	CC Excl: see Code 426.0
427.32	CC Excl: see Code 426.0
427.41	CC Excl: see Code 426.0
427.42	CC Excl: see Code 426.0
427.5	CC Excl: 427.0-427.5, 459.89, 459.9

428.0	CC Excl: 398.91, 402.01, 402.11, 402.91, 428.0-428.9, 459.89, 459.9, 518.4
428.1	CC Excl: 398.91, 402.01, 402.11, 402.91, 428.0-428.9, 459.89, 459.9
428.20	CC Excl: See code 428.0
428.21	CC Excl: See code 428.0
428.22	CC Excl: See code 428.0
428.23	CC Excl: See code 428.0
428.30	CC Excl: See code 428.0
428.31	CC Excl: See code 428.0
428.32	CC Excl: See code 428.0
428.33	CC Excl: See code 428.0
428.40	CC Excl: See code 428.0
428.41	CC Excl: See code 428.0
428.42	CC Excl: See code 428.0
428.43	CC Excl: See code 428.0
428.9	CC Excl: see Code 428.1
429.4	CC Excl: 429.4, 429.71, 429.79, 459.89, 459.9
429.5	CC Excl: 429.5, 429.71, 429.79, 459.89, 459.9
429.6	CC Excl: 429.6, 429.71, 429.79, 429.81, 459.89, 459.9
429.71	CC Excl: 422.0-422.99, 429.0, 429.4-429.82, 459.89, 459.9, 745.0-745.9, 746.89, 746.9, 747.83, 747.89, 747.9, 759.7-759.89
429.79	CC Excl: see Code 429.71
429.81	CC Excl: 429.6, 429.71, 429.79, 429.81, 459.89, 459.9
429.82	CC Excl: 429.71, 429.79, 429.82, 459.89, 459.9
430	CC Excl: 430, 431, 432.0-432.9, 459.89, 459.9, 780.01-780.09, 800.00-800.99, 801.00-801.99, 803.00-803.99, 804.00-804.96, 850.0-850.9, 851.00-851.99, 852.00-852.19, 852.21-852.59, 853.00-853.19, 854.00-854.19
431	CC Excl: see Code 430
432.0	CC Excl: see Code 430
432.1	CC Excl: see Code 430
433.0	CC Excl: **For code 433.01:** 250.70-250.93, 433.00-433.91, 435.0, 459.89, 459.9
433.1	CC Excl: **For code 433.11:** 250.70-250.93, 433.00-433.91, 459.89, 459.9
433.2	CC Excl: **For code 433.21:** 250.70-250.93, 433.00-433.91, 435.1, 459.89, 459.9
433.3	CC Excl: **For code 433.31:** see Code 433.11
433.8	CC Excl: **For code 433.81:** see Code 433.01
433.9	CC Excl: **For code 433.91:** see Code 433.01

434.0   CC Excl: **For code 434.01:** 250.70-
        250.93, 434.00-434.91, 436, 459.89,
        459.9

434.1   CC Excl: **For code 434.11:** see Code
        434.01

434.9   CC Excl: **For code 434.91:** see Code
        434.01

436   CC Excl: 250.70-250.93, 430-431,
        432.0-432.9, 434.00-434.91, 436,
        459.89, 459.9, 780.01-780.09, 800.00-
        800.99, 801.00-801.99, 803.00-803.99,
        804.00-804.96, 850.0-850.9, 851.00-
        851.99, 852.00-852.19, 852.21-852.59,
        853.00-853.19, 854.00-854.19

437.2   CC Excl: 250.70-250.93, 437.2, 459.89,
        459.9

437.4   CC Excl: 250.70-250.93, 437.4, 459.89,
        459.9

437.5   CC Excl: 250.70-250.93, 437.5, 459.89,
        459.9

437.6   CC Excl: 250.70-250.93, 437.6, 459.89,
        459.9

440.24 CC Excl: 440.24, 780.91-780.99, 785.4,
        799.81-799.89

441.00 CC Excl: 250.70-250.93, 441.00-441.9,
        459.89, 459.9

441.01 CC Excl: see Code 441.00

441.02 CC Excl: see Code 441.00

441.03 CC Excl: see Code 441.00

441.1   CC Excl: see Code 441.00

441.3   CC Excl: see Code 441.00

441.5   CC Excl: see Code 441.00

441.6   CC Excl: see Code 441.00

444.0   CC Excl: 250.70-250.93, 444.0, 444.89,
        444.9, 459.89, 459.9

444.1   CC Excl: 250.70-250.93, 444.1, 444.89,
        444.9, 459.89, 459.9

444.21 CC Excl: 250.70-250.93, 444.21,
        444.89, 444.9, 459.89, 459.9

444.22 CC Excl: 250.70-250.93, 444.22,
        444.89, 444.9, 459.89, 459.9

444.81 CC Excl: 250.70-250.93, 444.81-444.9,
        459.89, 459.9

444.89 CC Excl: 250.70-250.93, 444.89, 444.9,
        459.89, 459.9

444.9   CC Excl: see Code 444.89

445.01 CC Excl: 250.70-250.73, 250.80-250.83,
        250.90-250.93, 444.89, 444.9, 445.01,
        459.89, 459.9

445.02 CC Excl: 250.70-250.73, 250.80-250.83,
        250.90-250.93, 444.89, 444.9, 445.02,
        459.89, 459.9

445.81 CC Excl: 250.70-250.73, 250.80-250.83,
        250.90-250.93, 444.89, 444.9, 445.81,
        459.89, 459.9

445.89 CC Excl: 250.70-250.73, 250.80-250.83,
        250.90-250.93, 444.89, 444.9, 445.89,
        459.9

446.0   CC Excl: 250.70-250.93, 446.0-446.7,
        459.89, 459.9

446.20 CC Excl: see Code 446.0

446.21 CC Excl: see Code 446.0

446.29 CC Excl: see Code 446.0

446.3   CC Excl: see Code 446.0

446.4   CC Excl: see Code 446.0

446.5   CC Excl: see Code 446.0

446.6   CC Excl: see Code 446.0

446.7   CC Excl: see Code 446.0

451.0   CC Excl: 250.70-250.93, 451.0-451.9,
        459.89, 459.9

451.11 CC Excl: see Code 451.0

451.19 CC Excl: see Code 451.0

451.2   CC Excl: see Code 451.0

451.81 CC Excl: see Code 451.0

452   CC Excl: 250.70-250.93, 452, 453.8-
        453.9, 459.89, 459.9

453.0   CC Excl: 250.70-250.93, 453.0, 453.8-
        453.9, 459.89, 459.9

453.1   CC Excl: 250.70-250.93, 453.1, 453.8-
        453.9, 459.89, 459.9

453.2   CC Excl: 250.70-250.93, 453.2, 453.8-
        453.9, 459.89, 459.9

453.3   CC Excl: 250.70-250.93, 453.3, 453.8-
        453.9, 459.89, 459.9

453.8   CC Excl: 250.70-250.93, 453.8-453.9,
        459.89, 459.9

453.9   CC Excl: see Code 453.8

456.0   CC Excl: 251.5, 456.0, 456.20, 459.89,
        459.9, 530.20-530.21, 530.7, 530.82,
        530.85, 531.00-531.91, 532.00-532.91,
        533.00-533.91, 534.00-534.91, 535.01,
        535.11, 535.21, 535.31, 535.41, 535.51,
        535.61, 537.83, 562.02-562.03, 562.12-
        562.13, 569.3, 569.85, 578.0-578.9

456.20 CC Excl: 456.0, 456.20, 459.89, 459.9,
        530.82

459.0   CC Excl: 459.0, 459.89, 459.9

464.11 CC Excl: 012.20-012.86, 017.90-017.96,
        464.10-464.31, 519.8-519.9

464.21 CC Excl: see Code 464.11

464.31 CC Excl: see Code 464.11

475   CC Excl: 475, 519.8-519.9

478.21 CC Excl: 478.20-478.24, 519.8-519.9

478.22 CC Excl: see Code 478.21

478.24 CC Excl: see Code 478.21

478.30 CC Excl: 478.30-478.34, 478.5, 478.70,
        519.8-519.9

478.31 CC Excl: see Code 478.30

478.32 CC Excl: see Code 478.30

478.33 CC Excl: see Code 478.30

CC Exclusion List

478.34 CC Excl: see Code 478.30

480.3 CC Excl: 011.00-012.16, 012.80-012.86, 017.90-017.96, 021.2, 0310, 03.91, 115.05, 115.15, 115.95, 122.1, 130.4, 136.3, 480.0-487.1, 494.0-508.9, 517.1, 517.8, 518.89, 519.8-519.9

481 CC Excl: 011.00-011.06, 011.10-011.16, 011.20-011.26, 011.30-011.36, 011.40-011.46, 011.50-011.56, 011.60-011.66, 011.70-011.76, 011.80-011.86, 011.90-011.96, 012.00-012.06, 012.10-012.16, 012.80-012.86, 017.90-017.96, 021.2, 031.0, 039.1, 115.05, 115.15, 115.95, 122.1, 130.4, 136.3, 480.0-480.2, 480.8-480.9, 481, 482.0-482.2, 482.30-482.32, 482.39, 482.4, 482.81-482.84, 482.89, 482.9, 483.0-483.1, 483.8, 484.1, 484.3, 484.5-484.8, 485, 486, 487.0-487.1, 494.0-494.1, 495.0-495.9, 496, 500, 501, 502, 503, 504, 505, 506.0-506.4, 506.9, 507.0-507.1, 507.8, 508.0-508.1, 508.8, 508.9, 517.1-517.8, 518.89, 519.8, 519.9, 748.61

482.0 CC Excl: see Code 481
482.1 CC Excl: see Code 481
482.2 CC Excl: see Code 481
482.30 CC Excl: see Code 481
482.31 CC Excl: see Code 481
482.32 CC Excl: see Code 481
482.39 CC Excl: see Code 481
482.40 CC Excl: see Code 481
482.41 CC Excl: see Code 481
482.49 CC Excl: see Code 481
482.81 CC Excl: see Code 481
482.82 CC Excl: see Code 481
482.83 CC Excl: see Code 481
482.84 CC Excl: see Code 481
482.89 CC Excl: see Code 481
482.9 CC Excl: see Code 481
483.0 CC Excl: see Code 481
483.1 CC Excl: see Code 481
483.8 CC Excl: see Code 481
484.1 CC Excl: see Code 481
484.3 CC Excl: see Code 481
484.5 CC Excl: see Code 481
484.6 CC Excl: see Code 481
484.7 CC Excl: see Code 481
484.8 CC Excl: see Code 481
485 CC Excl: see Code 481
486 CC Excl: see Code 481
487.0 CC Excl: see Code 481
491.1 CC Excl: 491.1-491.9, 493.20-493.21
491.20 CC Excl: see Code 491.1
491.21 CC Excl: see Code 491.1
491.8 CC Excl: see Code 491.1

491.9 CC Excl: see Code 491.1
492.8 CC Excl: 492.0, 492.8, 493.20-493.21
493.0 CC Excl: **For code 493.01 and 493.02:** 493.00-493.92, 517.8, 518.89, 519.8-519.9

493.1 CC Excl: **For code 493.11 and 493.12:** see Code 493.0

493.2 CC Excl: **For code 493.20 and 493.21:** 491.1-493.92, 517.8, 518.89, 519.8-519.9; **For code 493.22:** 493.00-493.92, 517.8, 518.89, 519.8-519.9

493.9 CC Excl: **For code 493.91 and 493.92:** 493.00-493.92, 517.8, 518.89, 519.8-519.9

494.1 CC Excl: 017.90-017.96, 487.1, 494.1, 496, 506.1, 506.4, 506.9, 748.61

495.0 CC Excl: 011.00-011.96, 012.00-012.16, 012.80-012.86, 017.90-017.96, 021.2, 031.0, 039.1, 115.05, 115.15, 115.95, 122.1, 130.4, 136.3, 480.0-480.9, 481, 482.0-482.7, 482.81-482.84, 482.89, 482.9, 483.0, 483.1, 483.8, 484.1-484.8, 485-486, 487.0-487.1, 494.0-494.1, 495.0-495.9, 496, 500-505, 506.0-506.9, 507.0-507.8, 508.0-508.9, 517.1, 517.8, 518.89, 519.8-519.9, 748.61

495.1 CC Excl: see Code 495.0
495.2 CC Excl: see Code 495.0
495.3 CC Excl: see Code 495.0
495.4 CC Excl: see Code 495.0
495.5 CC Excl: see Code 495.0
495.6 CC Excl: see Code 495.0
495.7 CC Excl: see Code 495.0
495.8 CC Excl: see Code 495.0
495.9 CC Excl: see Code 495.0
496 CC Excl: 017.90-017.96, 487.1, 494.0-494.1, 496, 506.1, 506.4, 506.9, 748.61

506.0 CC Excl: 011.00-011.96, 012.10-012.16, 012.80-012.86, 017.90-017.96, 021.2, 031.0, 039.1, 115.05, 115.15, 115.95, 122.1, 130.4, 136.3, 480.0-480.9, 481, 482.0-482.7, 482.81-482.84, 482.89, 482.9, 483.0, 483.1, 483.8, 484.1-484.8, 485-486, 487.0-487.1, 494.0-494.1, 495.0-495.9, 496, 500-505, 506.0-506.9, 507.0-507.8, 508.0-508.9, 517.1, 517.8, 518.89, 519.8-519.9, 748.61

506.1 CC Excl: see Code 506.0
507.0 CC Excl: see Code 506.0
507.1 CC Excl: see Code 506.0
507.8 CC Excl: see Code 506.0
508.0 CC Excl: see Code 506.0
508.1 CC Excl: see Code 506.0
510.0 CC Excl: 510.0, 510.9, 517.8, 518.89, 519.8-519.9

510.9   CC Excl: see Code 510.0
511.1   CC Excl: 011.00-011.96, 012.00-012.16, 012.80-012.86, 017.90-017.96, 511.0-511.9, 517.8, 518.89, 519.8-519.9
511.8   CC Excl: see Code 511.1
511.9   CC Excl: see Code 511.1
512.0   CC Excl: 512.0-512.1, 512.8, 517.8, 518.89, 519.8-519.9
512.1   CC Excl: see Code 512.0
512.8   CC Excl: see Code 512.0
513.0   CC Excl: 006.4, 011.00-011.96, 012.00-012.16, 012.80-012.86, 017.90-017.96, 513.0, 519.8-519.9
513.1   CC Excl: 513.1, 519.8-519.9
515   CC Excl: 011.00-011.96, 012.00-012.16, 012.80-012.86, 017.90-017.96, 494.0-494.1, 495.0-495.9, 496, 500-505, 506.0-506.9, 507.0-507.8, 508.0-508.9, 515, 516.0-516.9, 517.2, 517.8, 518.89, 519.8-519.9, 748.61
516.0   CC Excl: see Code 515
516.1   CC Excl: see Code 515
516.2   CC Excl: see Code 515
516.3   CC Excl: see Code 515
516.8   CC Excl: see Code 515
516.9   CC Excl: see Code 515
517.1   CC Excl: 011.00-011.96, 012.00-012.16, 012.80-012.86, 017.90-017.96, 480.0-480.9, 481, 482.0-482.7, 482.81-482.84, 482.89, 482.9, 483.0, 483.1, 483.8, 484.1-484.8, 485-486, 487.0-487.1, 494.0-494.1, 495.0-495.9, 496, 500-505, 506.0-506.9, 507.0-507.8, 508.0-508.9, 515, 516.0-516.9, 517.1-517.8, 518.89, 519.8-519.9, 748.61
517.2   CC Excl: 011.00-011.96, 012.00-012.16, 012.80-012.86, 017.90-017.96, 494.0-494.1, 495.0-495.9, 496, 500-505, 506.0-506.9, 507.0-507.8, 508.0-508.9, 515, 516.0-516.9, 517.2, 517.8, 518.89, 519.8-519.9, 748.61
517.8   CC Excl: see Code 517.2
518.0   CC Excl: 518.0, 519.8-519.9
518.1   CC Excl: 518.1, 519.8-519.9
518.4   CC Excl: 040.82, 398.91, 428.0-428.9, 518.4, 519.8-519.9, 534.11
518.5   CC Excl: 518.5, 519.8-519.9
518.6   CC Excl: 518.6, 519.8-519.9
518.81 CC Excl: 518.81-518.89, 519.8-519.9, 799.1
518.82 CC Excl: see Code 518.81
518.83 CC Excl: see Code 518.81
518.84 CC Excl: see Code 518.81
519.00 CC Excl: 519.0-519.1, 519.8-519.9
519.01 CC Excl: see Code 519.00
519.02 CC Excl: see Code 519.00

519.09 CC Excl: see Code 519.00
519.2   CC Excl: 519.2-519.3, 519.8-519.9
527.3   CC Excl: 527.0-527.9, 537.89, 537.9
527.4   CC Excl: see Code 527.3
528.3   CC Excl: 528.0, 528.3, 529.0, 529.2
530.21 CC Excl: 251.5, 456.0, 530.20-530.21, 530.7, 530.82, 530.85, 531.00-531.91, 532.00-532.91, 534.00-534.91, 535.01, 535.11, 535.21, 535.31, 535.41, 535.51, 535.61, 573.83, 573.89, 562.02-532.03, 562.12-562.13, 569.3, 569.85, 578.0-578.9
530.4   CC Excl: 530.4, 530.7-530.81, 530.83-530.9
530.7   CC Excl: 251.5, 456.0, 530.20-530.21, 530.4, 530.7-530.9, 531.00-531.91, 532.00-532.91, 533.00-533.91, 534.00-534.91, 535.01, 535.11, 535.21, 535.31, 535.41, 535.51, 535.61, 537.83, 562.02-562.03, 562.12-562.13, 569.3, 569.85, 578.0-578.9
530.82 CC Excl: 251.5, 456.0, 456.20, 459.89-459.9, 530.20-530.21, 530.7, 530.82, 530.85, 531.00-531.21, 531.30-531.31, 531.40-531.91, 532.00-532.91, 533.00-533.91, 534.00-534.51, 534.61, 534.70-534.91, 535.01-535.11, 535.21, 535.31, 535.41, 535.51, 535.61, 537.83, 562.02-562.03, 562.12-562.13, 569.3, 569.85, 578.0-578.9
530.84 CC Excl: 530.4, 530.7, 530.81, 530.83-530.9
531.0x CC Excl: 251.5, 456.0, 530.20-530.21, 530.7, 530.82, 530.85, 531.00-531.91, 532.00-532.91, 533.00-533.91, 534.00-534.91, 535.01, 535.11, 535.21, 535.31, 535.41, 535.51, 535.61, 537.83, 537.89, 537.9, 562.02-562.03, 562.12-562.13, 569.3, 569.85, 578.0-578.9
531.1x CC Excl: see Code 531.0
531.2x CC Excl: see Code 531.0
531.3x CC Excl: For code 531.31: see code 531.0
531.4x CC Excl: see Code 531.0
531.5x CC Excl: see Code 531.0
531.6x CC Excl: see Code 531.0
531.7x CC Excl: For code 531.71: see code 531.0
531.9   CC Excl: For code 531.91: see code 531.0
532.0x CC Excl: 251.5, 456.0, 530.20-530.21, 530.7, 530.82, 530.85, 531.00-531.91, 532.00-532.91, 533.00-533.91, 534.00-534.91, 535.01, 535.11, 535.21, 535.31, 535.41, 535.51, 535.61, 537.3, 537.83, 537.89, 537.9, 562.02-562.03, 562.12-562.13, 569.3, 569.85, 578.0-578.9

CC Exclusion List

532.1x CC Excl: see Code 532.0
532.2x CC Excl: see Code 532.0
532.3   CC Excl: **For code 532.31**: see Code 532.0
532.4x CC Excl: see Code 532.0
532.5x CC Excl: see Code 532.0
532.6x CC Excl: see Code 532.0
532.7   CC Excl: **For code 532.71**: see Code 532.0
532.9   CC Excl: **For code 532.91**: see Code 532.0
533.0x CC Excl: see Code 532.0
533.1x CC Excl: see Code 532.0
533.2x CC Excl: see Code 532.0
533.3   CC Excl: **For code 533.31**: see Code 532.0
533.4x CC Excl: see Code 532.0
533.5x CC Excl: see Code 532.0
533.6x CC Excl: see Code 532.0
533.7   CC Excl: **For code 533.71**: see Code 532.0
533.9   CC Excl: **For code 533.91**: see Code 532.0
534.0x CC Excl: 251.5, 456.0, 530.20-530.21, 530.7, 530.82, 530.85, 531.00-531.91, 532.00-532.91, 533.00-533.91, 534.00-534.91, 535.01, 535.11, 535.21, 535.31, 535.41, 535.51, 535.61, 537.83, 537.89, 537.9, 562.02-562.03, 562.12-562.13, 569.3, 569.85, 578.0-578.9
534.1x CC Excl: see Code 534.0
534.2x CC Excl: see Code 534.0
534.3   CC Excl: **For code 534.31**: see Code 534.0
534.4x CC Excl: see Code 534.0
534.5x CC Excl: see Code 534.0
534.6x CC Excl: see Code 534.0
534.7   CC Excl: **For code 534.71**: see Code 534.0
534.9   CC Excl: **For code 534.91**: see Code 534.0
535.0   CC Excl: **For code 535.01**: 251.5, 456.0, 530.20-530.21, 530.7, 530.82, 530.85, 531.00-531.91, 532.00-532.91, 533.00-533.91, 534.00-534.91, 535.01, 535.11, 535.21, 535.31, 535.41, 535.51, 535.61, 537.83, 562.02-562.03, 562.12-562.13, 569.3, 569.85, 578.0-578.9
535.1   CC Excl: **For code 535.11**: see Code 535.01
535.2   CC Excl: **For code 535.21**: see Code 535.01
535.3   CC Excl: **For code 535.31**: see Code 535.01

535.4   CC Excl: **For code 535.41**: see Code 535.01
535.5   CC Excl: **For code 535.51**: see Code 535.01
535.6   CC Excl: **For code 535.61**: see Code 535.01
536.1   CC Excl: 536.1
536.40 CC Excl: 536.40-536.49, 997.4, 997.71, 997.91, 997.99, 998.81, 998.83-998.9
536.41 CC Excl: see Code 536.40
536.42 CC Excl: see Code 536.40
536.49 CC Excl: see Code 536.40
537.0   CC Excl: 536.3, 536.8-536.9, 537.0, 537.3, 750.5, 750.8-750.9, 751.1, 751.5
537.3   CC Excl: 537.3, 750.8-750.9, 751.1, 751.5
537.4   CC Excl: 537.4, 750.8-750.9, 751.5
537.83 CC Excl: 251.5, 456.0, 530.20-530.21, 530.7, 530.82, 530.85, 531.00-531.91, 532.00-532.91, 533.00-533.91, 534.00-534.91, 535.01, 535.11, 535.21, 535.31, 535.41, 535.51, 535.61, 537.83, 562.02-562.03, 562.12-562.13, 569.3, 569.85, 578.0-578.9
537.84 CC Excl: 251.5, 456.0, 530.20-530.21, 530.7, 530.82, 530.85, 531.00-531.01, 531.10-531.11, 531.20-531.21, 531.30-531.31, 531.40-531.41, 531.50-531.51, 531.60-531.61, 531.70-531.71, 531.90-531.91, 532.00-532.01, 532.10-532.11, 532.20-532.21, 532.30-532.31, 532.40-532.41, 532.50-532.51, 532.60-532.61, 532.70-532.71, 532.90-532.91, 533.00-533.01, 533.10-533.11, 533.20-533.21, 533.30-533.31, 533.40-533.41, 533.50-533.51, 533.60-533.61, 533.70-533.71, 533.90-533.91, 534.00-534.01, 534.10-534.11, 534.20-534.21, 534.30-534.31, 534.40-534.41, 534.50-534.51, 534.60-534.61, 534.70-534.71, 534.90-534.91, 535.01, 535.11, 535.21, 535.31, 535.41, 535.51, 535.61, 537.83-537.84, 562.02-562.03, 562.12-562.13, 569.3, 569.85, 578.0-578.1, 578.9
540.0x CC Excl: 537.89, 537.9, 540.0-540.9, 541-542, 543.0, 543.9
540.1x CC Excl: see Code 540.0
540.9   CC Excl: see Code 540.0
550.0   CC Excl: 537.89, 537.9, 550.00-550.93, 552.8-552.9, 553.8-553.9
550.1   CC Excl: see Code 550.0
551.00 CC Excl: 537.89, 537.9, 551.00-551.03, 552.8-552.9, 553.00-553.03, 553.8-553.9
551.01 CC Excl: see Code 551.0
551.02 CC Excl: see Code 551.0

551.03   Excl: see Code 551.0
551.1x   CC Excl: 537.89, 537.9, 551.1-551.29, 552.1-552.29, 552.8-552.9, 553.1-553.29, 553.8-553.9
551.20   CC Excl: see Code 551.1
551.21   CC Excl: see Code 551.1
551.29   CC Excl: see Code 551.1
551.3   CC Excl: 551.3, 552.3, 552.8-552.9, 553.3, 553.8-553.9
551.8   CC Excl: 537.89, 537.9, 550.00-550.93, 551.00-551.9, 552.00-552.9, 553.00-553.9
551.9   CC Excl: see Code 551.8
552.00   CC Excl: 537.89, 537.9, 551.00-551.03, 552.00-552.03, 552.8-552.9, 553.00-553.03, 553.8-553.9
552.01   CC Excl: see Code 552.00
552.02   CC Excl: see Code 552.00
552.03   CC Excl: see Code 552.00
552.1   CC Excl: 551.1-551.29, 552.1-552.29, 552.8-552.9, 553.8-553.9
552.20   CC Excl: see Code 552.1
552.21   CC Excl: see Code 552.1
552.29   CC Excl: see Code 552.1
552.3   CC Excl: 551.3, 552.3-552.9, 553.3-553.9
552.8   CC Excl: 550.00-550.93, 551.00-551.9, 552.00-552.9, 553.00-553.9
552.9   CC Excl: see Code 552.8
557.0   CC Excl: 557.0-557.1
558.1   CC Excl: 558.1
558.2   CC Excl: 558.2
560.0   CC Excl: 560.0-560.9, 569.89, 569.9
560.1   CC Excl: see Code 560.0
560.2   CC Excl: see Code 560.0
560.30   CC Excl: see Code 560.0
560.31   CC Excl: see Code 560.0
560.39   CC Excl: see Code 560.0
560.81   CC Excl: see Code 560.0
560.89   CC Excl: see Code 560.0
560.9   CC Excl: see Code 560.0
562.02   CC Excl: 251.5, 456.0, 530.20-530.21, 530.7, 530.82, 530.85, 531.00-531.91, 532.00-532.91, 533.00-533.91, 534.00-534.91, 535.01, 535.11, 535.21, 535.31, 535.41, 535.51, 535.61, 537.83, 562.02-562.03, 562.12-562.13, 569.3, 569.85, 578.0-578.9
562.03   CC Excl: see Code 562.02
562.12   CC Excl: see Code 562.02
562.13   CC Excl: see Code 562.02
566   CC Excl: 566
567.0   CC Excl: 567.0-567.9, 569.89, 569.9
567.1   CC Excl: see Code 567.0
567.2   CC Excl: see Code 567.0

567.8   CC Excl: see Code 567.0
567.9   CC Excl: see Code 567.0
568.81   CC Excl: 568.81
569.3   CC Excl: 251.5, 456.0, 530.20-530.21, 530.7, 530.82, 530.85, 531.00-531.91, 532.00-532.91, 533.00-533.91, 534.00-534.91, 535.01, 535.11, 535.21, 535.31, 535.41, 535.51, 535.61, 537.83, 562.02-562.03, 562.12-562.13, 569.3, 569.85, 578.0-578.9
569.5   CC Excl: 569.5
569.60   CC Excl: 569.60-569.69
569.61   CC Excl: see code 596.60
569.62   CC Excl: 536.40-536.49, 569.60-569.69, 997.4, 997.71, 997.91, 997.99, 998.81, 998.83-998.9
569.69   CC Excl: see code 596.60
569.83   CC Excl: 569.83
569.85   CC Excl: 251.5, 456.0, 530.20-530.21, 530.7, 530.82, 530.85, 531.00-531.91, 532.00-532.91, 533.00-533.91, 534.00-534.91, 535.01, 535.11, 535.21, 535.31, 535.41, 535.51, 535.61, 537.83, 562.02-562.03, 562.12-562.13, 569.3, 569.85, 578.0-578.9
569.86   CC Excl: 251.5, 465.0, 530.20-530.21, 530.7, 530.82, 530.85, 531.00-531.01, 531.10-531.11, 531.20-531.21, 531.30-531.31, 531.40-531.41, 531.50-531.51, 531.60-531.61, 531.70-531.71, 531.90-531.91, 532.00-532.01, 532.10-532.11, 532.20-532.21, 532.30-532.31, 532.40-532.41, 532.50-532.51, 532.60-532.61, 532.70-532.71, 532.90-532.91, 533.00-533.01, 533.10-533.11, 533.20-533.21, 533.30-533.31, 533.40-533.41, 533.50-533.51, 533.60-533.61, 533.70-533.71, 533.90-533.91, 534.00-534.01, 534.10-534.11, 534.20-534.21, 534.30-534.31, 534.40-534.41, 534.50-534.51, 534.60-534.61, 534.70-534.71, 534.90-534.91, 535.01, 535.11, 535.21, 535.31, 535.41, 535.51, 535.61, 537.83, 537.84, 562.02-562.03, 562.12-562.13, 569.3, 569.85-569.86, 578.0-578.1, 578.9
570   CC Excl: 570, 573.4-573.9
571.2   CC Excl: 571.2, 573.8-573.9
571.49   CC Excl: 571.49, 571.5-571.9, 573.8-573.9
571.5   CC Excl: see Code 571.49
571.6   CC Excl: see Code 571.49
572.0   CC Excl: 006.3, 572.0-572.1, 573.8-573.9
572.1   CC Excl: see Code 572.0
572.2   CC Excl: 572.2, 573.8-573.9
572.4   CC Excl: 572.4, 573.8-573.9

CC Exclusion List

573.1	CC Excl: 573.1-573.3, 573.8-573.9
573.2	CC Excl: see Code 573.1
573.3	CC Excl: see Code 573.1
573.4	CC Excl: 570, 573.4-573.9
574.0x	CC Excl: **For code 574.00:** 574.00-574.21, 574.40, 574.60-574.61, 574.80-574.81, 575.0, 575.10-575.12, 575.9, 576.8-576.9; CC Excl: **For code 574.01:** 574.00-574.21, 574.60-574.61, 574.80-574.81, 575.0, 575.10-575.12, 575.9, 576.8-576.9
574.1x	CC Excl: see Code 574.01
574.2x	CC Excl: **For code 574.21:** see Code 574.01
574.3x	CC Excl: 574.30-574.51, 574.60-574.61, 574.70-574.71, 574.80-574.81, 574.90-574.91, 575.0, 575.10-575.12, 576.8-576.9
574.4x	CC Excl: see Code 574.3
574.5x	CC Excl: see Code 574.3
574.6x	CC Excl: 574.60-574.61, 575.0, 575.10-575.12, 575.9, 576.8-576.9
574.7x	CC Excl: 574.30-574.31, 574.40-574.41, 574.50-574.51, 574.60-574.61, 574.70-574.71, 574.80-574.81, 574.90-574.91, 575.0, 575.10-575.12, 576.8-576.9
574.8x	CC Excl: 574.80-574.81, 575.0, 575.10-575.12, 575.9, 576.8-576.9
574.9x	CC Excl: see Code 574.7
575.0	CC Excl: 574.60-574.61, 574.80-574.81, 575.0, 575.10-575.12, 575.9, 576.8-576.9
575.12	CC Excl: 575.0, 575.10-575.12, 575.9, 576.8-576.9
575.2	CC Excl: 575.2-575.9, 576.8-576.9
575.3	CC Excl: see Code 575.2
575.4	CC Excl: see Code 575.2
575.5	CC Excl: see Code 575.2
576.1	CC Excl: 576.1, 576.8-576.9
576.3	CC Excl: 576.3-576.4, 576.8-576.9
576.4	CC Excl: see Code 576.3
577.0	CC Excl: 577.0-577.1, 577.8-577.9
577.2	CC Excl: 577.2, 577.8-577.9
578.0	CC Excl: 251.5, 456.0, 530.20-530.21, 530.7, 530.82, 530.85, 531.00-531.91, 532.00-532.91, 533.00-533.91, 534.00-534.91, 535.01, 535.11, 535.21, 535.31, 535.41, 535.51, 535.61, 537.83, 562.02-562.03, 562.12-562.13, 569.3, 569.85, 578.0-578.9
578.1	CC Excl: see Code 578.0
578.9	CC Excl: see Code 578.0
579.3	CC Excl: 579.3-579.9

580.0	CC Excl: 016.00-016.06, 016.30-016.36, 016.90-016.96, 017.90-017.96, 098.10, 098.19, 098.30-098.31, 098.89, 112.2, 131.00, 131.8-131.9, 250.40-250.43, 250.80-250.93, 274.10, 274.19, 580.0-580.9, 581.0-581.9, 582.0-582.9, 583.0-583.9, 584.5-584.9, 585-587, 588.0-588.9, 589.0-589.9, 590.00-590.9, 591, 593.0-593.2, 593.89, 593.9, 599.7-599.9
580.4	CC Excl: see Code 580.0
580.81	CC Excl: see Code 580.0
580.89	CC Excl: 016.00-016.06, 016.30-016.36, 016.90-016.96, 017.90-017.96, 098.10, 098.19, 098.30-098.31, 098.89, 112.2, 131.00, 131.8-131.9, 274.10, 274.19, 580.0-580.9, 581.0-581.9, 582.0-582.9, 583.0-583.9, 584.5-584.9, 585-587, 588.0-588.9, 589.0-589.9, 590.00-590.9, 591, 593.0-593.2, 593.89, 593.9, 599.7-599.9
580.9	CC Excl: 016.00-016.06, 016.30-016.36, 016.90-016.96, 017.90-017.96, 098.10, 098.19, 098.30-098.31, 098.89, 112.2, 131.00, 131.8-131.9, 250.40-250.43, 250.80-250.93, 274.10, 274.19, 580.0-580.9, 581.0-581.9, 582.0-582.9, 583.0-583.9, 584.5-584.9, 585-587, 588.0-588.9, 589.0-589.9, 590.00-590.09, 591, 593.0-593.2, 593.89, 593.9, 599.7-599.9
581.0	CC Excl: see Code 580.9
581.1	CC Excl: see Code 580.9
581.2	CC Excl: see Code 580.9
581.3	CC Excl: see Code 580.9
581.81	CC Excl: see Code 580.9
581.89	CC Excl: see Code 580.9
581.9	CC Excl: see Code 580.9
583.4	CC Excl: see Code 580.9
584.5	CC Excl: 250.40-250.43, 250.80-250.93, 274.10, 274.19, 580.0-580.9, 581.0-581.9, 582.0-582.9, 583.0-583.9, 584.5-584.9, 585-587, 588.0-588.9, 589.0-589.9, 590.00-590.9, 591, 593.0-593.2, 593.89, 593.9, 599.7-599.9, 753.0, 753.20-753.23, 753.29, 753.3, 753.9
584.6	CC Excl: see Code 584.5
584.7	CC Excl: see Code 584.5
584.8	CC Excl: 250.40-250.43, 250.80-250.93, 274.10, 274.19, 580.0-580.9, 581.0-581.9, 582.0-582.9, 583.0-583.9, 584.5-584.9, 585-587, 588.0-588.9, 589.0-589.9, 590.00-590.9, 591, 593.0-593.2, 593.89, 593.9, 599.7-599.9

584.9   CC Excl: 250.40-250.43, 250.80-250.93,
         274.10, 274.19, 580.0-580.9, 581.0-
         581.9, 582.0-582.9, 583.0-583.9, 584.5-
         584.9, 585-587, 588.0-588.9, 589.0-
         589.9, 590.00-590.9, 591, 593.0-593.2,
         593.89, 593.9, 599.7-599.9, 753.0,
         753.20-753.23, 753.29, 753.3, 753.9

585   CC Excl: see Code 584.9

590.10   CC Excl: 016.00-016.06, 016.30-016.36,
         016.90-016.96, 017.90-017.96, 098.10,
         098.19, 098.30-098.31, 098.89, 112.2,
         131.00, 131.8-131.9, 250.40-250.43,
         250.80-250.93, 274.10, 274.19, 580.0-
         580.9, 581.0-581.9, 582.0-582.9, 583.0-
         583.9, 584.5-584.9, 585-587, 588.0-
         588.9, 589.0-589.9, 590.00-590.9, 591,
         593.0-593.2, 593.89, 593.9, 599.0,
         599.7-599.9

590.11   CC Excl: see Code 590.10

590.2   CC Excl: see Code 590.10

590.3   CC Excl: 016.00-016.06, 016.30-016.36,
         016.90-016.96, 017.90-017.96, 098.10,
         098.19, 098.30-098.31, 098.89, 112.2,
         131.00, 131.8-131.9, 274.10, 274.19,
         580.0-580.9, 581.0-581.9, 582.0-582.9,
         583.0-583.9, 584.5-584.9, 585-587,
         588.0-588.9, 589.0-589.9, 590.00-
         590.9, 591, 593.0-593.2, 593.89, 593.9,
         599.0, 599.7-599.9

590.80   CC Excl: see Code 590.3

590.81   CC Excl: see Code 590.3

590.9   CC Excl: see Code 590.3

591   CC Excl: see Code 590.3

592.1   CC Excl: 592.0-592.9, 593.3-593.5,
         593.89, 593.9, 594.0-594.9, 599.6-
         599.9

593.5   CC Excl: 593.3-593.5, 593.89, 593.9,
         595.0-595.9, 596.8-596.9, 599.0, 599.6-
         599.9, 753.4-753.5, 753.9

595.0   CC Excl: 016.10-016.16, 016.30-016.36,
         016.90-016.96, 017.90-017.96, 098.0,
         098.11, 098.2, 098.39, 098.89, 112.2,
         131.00, 131.8-131.9, 593.3-593.5,
         593.89, 593.9, 595.0-595.9, 596.8-
         596.9, 599.0, 599.6-599.9

595.1   CC Excl: see Code 595.0

595.2   CC Excl: see Code 595.0

595.4   CC Excl: see Code 595.0

595.81   CC Excl: see Code 595.0

595.82   CC Excl: see Code 595.0

595.89   CC Excl: see Code 595.0

595.9   CC Excl: see Code 595.0

596.0   CC Excl: 185, 188.0-188.9, 189.3-189.9,
         596.0, 596.4, 596.51-596.59, 596.8-
         596.9, 600.00-600.9, 601.0-601.9,
         602.0-602.9

596.1   CC Excl: 098.0, 098.2, 098.39, 098.89,
         596.1-596.2, 596.8-596.9, 599.7-599.9,
         788.1

596.2   CC Excl: see Code 596.1

596.4   CC Excl: 596.4, 596.51-596.59, 596.8-
         596.9, 599.7-599.9, 788.1

596.6   CC Excl: 596.6-596.9, 599.7-599.9,
         788.1

596.7   CC Excl: see Code 596.6

597.0   CC Excl: 098.0, 098.2, 098.39, 098.89,
         099.40-099.49, 112.2, 131.00, 131.02,
         131.8-131.9, 597.0-597.89, 598.00-
         598.01, 598.8-598.9, 599.0, 599.6-
         599.9, 607.1-607.83, 607.85, 607.89,
         607.9, 608.4, 608.81, 608.85, 608.87,
         608.89, 752.61-752.65, 752.69, 752.81-
         752.9, 753.6-753.9, 788.1

598.1   CC Excl: 098.0, 098.2, 098.39, 098.89,
         131.02, 598.1-598.9, 599.6-599.9,
         752.61-752.65, 752.69, 753.6-753.9,
         788.1

598.2   CC Excl: see Code 598.1

599.0   CC Excl: 098.2, 098.39, 098.89, 099.40-
         099.49, 112.2, 131.00, 131.8-131.9,
         590.10-590.9, 591, 593.89, 593.9,
         595.0-595.9, 599.0, 599.6-599.9, 788.1,
         996.64

599.4   CC Excl: 597.0-597.89, 598.00-598.9,
         599.1-599.9, 607.1-607.83, 607.85,
         607.89, 607.9, 608.4, 608.81, 608.85,
         608.87, 608.89, 752.61-752.65, 752.69,
         752.81-752.9, 753.9, 788.1

599.6   CC Excl: 185, 188.0-188.9, 189.2-189.9,
         274.11, 344.61, 592.1, 592.9, 593.3-
         593.5, 593.89, 593.9, 594.0-594.9,
         595.0-595.9, 596.0, 596.51-596.59,
         596.8-596.9, 597.0-597.89, 598.00-
         598.9, 599.0-599.9, 600.00-600.9,
         601.0-601.9, 602.0-602.9, 753.0-753.9,
         788.1

599.7   CC Excl: 592.0-592.9, 593.89, 593.9,
         594.0-594.9, 596.6-596.7, 599.7-599.9

601.0   CC Excl: 098.12, 098.32, 098.89, 112.2,
         131.00, 131.03, 131.8-131.9, 600.00-
         600.9, 601.0-601.9, 602.0-602.9

601.2   CC Excl: see Code 601.0

601.3   CC Excl: see Code 601.0

602.1   CC Excl: see Code 601.0

603.1   CC Excl: 112.1, 131.00, 131.8-131.9,
         603.0-603.9

604.0   CC Excl: 072.0, 098.13-098.14, 098.33-
         098.34, 098.89, 112.2, 131.00, 131.8-
         131.9, 604.0-604.99

611.72   CC Excl: 610.0-610.9, 611.0-611.9

614.0 CC Excl: 016.60-016.96, 017.90-017.96, 098.15-098.17, 098.35-098.37, 098.89, 112.2, 131.00, 131.8-131.9, 614.0-614.9, 615.0-615.9, 616.8-616.9, 625.8-625.9, 629.8-629.9, 752.81-752.9

614.3 CC Excl: see Code 614.0

614.5 CC Excl: see Code 614.0

615.0 CC Excl: 016.60-016.96, 017.90-017.96, 098.15-098.17, 098.35-098.37, 098.89, 112.2, 131.00, 131.8-131.9, 614.0-614.9, 615.0-615.9, 616.0, 616.8-616.9, 621.8-621.9, 625.8-625.9, 629.8-629.9, 752.81-752.9

616.3 CC Excl: 016.70-016.96, 017.90-017.96, 112.1-112.2, 131.00-131.01, 131.8-131.9, 616.10-616.9, 624.3-624.9, 625.8-625.9, 629.8-629.9, 752.81-752.9

616.4 CC Excl: see Code 616.3

620.7 CC Excl: 620.6-620.9, 625.8-625.9, 629.8-629.9, 752.81-752.9

634.0 CC Excl: 634.00-634.92, 635.00-635.92, 636.00-636.92, 637.00-637.92, 638.0-638.9, 640.00-640.93, 641.00-641.23, 646.80-646.93, 648.90-648.94, 650, 669.40-669.44, 669.80-669.94

634.1x CC Excl: see Code 634.0

634.2x CC Excl: see Code 634.0

634.3x CC Excl: see Code 634.0

634.4x CC Excl: see Code 634.0

634.5x CC Excl: see Code 634.0

634.6x CC Excl: see Code 634.0

634.7x CC Excl: see Code 634.0

634.8x CC Excl: see Code 634.0

634.9x CC Excl: see Code 634.0

639.0 CC Excl: 639.0, 639.2-639.9, 640.00-640.93, 641.00-641.23, 646.80-646.93, 648.90-648.94, 650, 669.40-669.44, 669.80-669.94

639.1 CC Excl: 639.1-639.9, 640.00-640.93, 641.00-641.23, 646.80-646.93, 648.90-648.94, 650, 669.40-669.44, 669.80-669.94

639.2 CC Excl: 639.2-639.9, 640.00-640.93, 641.00-641.23, 646.80-646.93, 648.90-648.94, 650, 669.40-669.44, 669.80-669.94

639.3 CC Excl: see Code 639.2

639.4 CC Excl: see Code 639.2

639.5 CC Excl: see Code 639.2

639.6 CC Excl: see Code 639.2

639.8 CC Excl: see Code 639.2

639.9 CC Excl: see Code 639.2

640.0 CC Excl: **For codes 640.00-640.03:** 640.00-640.93, 641.00-641.13, 646.80-646.93, 648.90-648.94, 650, 669.40-669.44, 669.80-669.94

640.8 CC Excl: **For codes 640.80-640.83:** see Code 640.0

640.9 CC Excl: **For codes 640.90-640.93:** see Code 640.0

641.0 CC Excl: **For codes 641.00-641.03:** see Code 640.0

641.1 CC Excl: **For codes 641.10-641.13:** see Code 640.0

641.3 CC Excl: **For codes 641.30-641.33:** 641.30-641.93, 646.80-646.93, 648.90-648.94, 650, 669.40-669.44, 669.80-669.94

641.8 CC Excl: **For codes 641.80-641.83:** see Code 641.3

641.9 CC Excl: **For codes 641.90-641.93:** see Code 641.3

642.4x CC Excl: 642.00-642.94, 646.10-646.14, 646.80-646.93, 648.90-648.94, 650, 669.40-669.44, 669.80-669.94

642.5x CC Excl: see Code 642.4

642.6x CC Excl: see Code 642.4

642.7x CC Excl: see Code 642.4

644.0 CC Excl: **For codes 644.00, 644.03:** 644.00-644.21, 646.80-646.93, 648.90-648.94, 650, 669.40-669.44, 669.80-669.94

644.1 CC Excl: **For codes 644.10, 644.13:** see Code 644.0

646.6x CC Excl: 646.60-646.64, 646.80-646.93, 648.90-648.94, 650, 669.40-669.44, 669.80-669.94

646.7 CC Excl: **For codes 646.70-646.73:** 646.70-646.93, 648.90-648.94, 650, 669.40-669.44, 669.80-669.94

647.3x CC Excl: 646.80-646.93, 647.30-647.34, 648.90-648.94, 650, 669.40-669.44, 669.80-669.94

647.4x CC Excl: 646.80-646.93, 647.30-647.34, 648.90-648.94, 650, 669.40-669.44, 669.80-669.94

648.0x CC Excl: 646.80-646.93, 648.00-648.04, 648.90-648.94, 650, 669.40-669.44, 669.80-669.94

648.2x CC Excl: 646.80-646.93, 648.20-648.24, 648.90-648.94, 650, 669.40-669.44, 669.80-669.94

648.3x CC Excl: 646.80-646.93, 648.30-648.34, 648.90-648.94, 650, 669.40-669.44, 669.80-669.94

648.5x CC Excl: 646.80-646.93, 648.50-648.64, 648.90-648.94, 650, 669.40-669.44, 669.80-669.94

648.6x CC Excl: see Code 648.5

659.3 CC Excl: **For codes 659.30-659.33:**
646.80-646.93, 648.90-648.94, 650,
659.30-659.33, 669.40-669.44, 669.80-
669.94

665.0 CC Excl: **For codes 665.01, 665.03:**
646.80-646.93, 648.90-648.94, 650,
655.70-655.73,665.00-665.11, 665.50-
665.54, 665.80-665.94, 669.40-669.44,
669.80-669.94

665.1 CC Excl: **For codes 665.10, 665.11:** see
Code 665.0

666.3 CC Excl: **For Codes 666.32-666.34:**
646.80-646.93, 648.90-648.94, 650,
666.00-666.34, 669.40-669.44, 669.80-
669.94

668.0x CC Excl: 646.80-646.93, 648.90-648.94,
650, 668.00-668.04, 669.40-669.44,
669.80-669.94

668.1x CC Excl: 646.80-646.93, 648.90-648.94,
650, 668.10-668.14, 669.40-669.44,
669.80-669.94

668.2x CC Excl: 646.80-646.93, 648.90-648.94,
650, 668.20-668.24, 669.40-669.44,
669.80-669.94

668.8x CC Excl: 646.80-646.93, 648.90-648.94,
650, 668.80-668.94, 669.40-669.44,
669.80-669.94

668.9x CC Excl: see Code 668.8

669.1x CC Excl: 646.80-646.93, 648.90-648.94,
650, 669.10-669.14, 669.40-669.44,
669.80-669.94

669.3x CC Excl: 646.80-646.93, 648.90-648.94,
650, 669.30-669.44, 669.80-669.94

670.0 CC Excl: **For codes 670.00, 670.02,
670.04:** 646.80-646.93, 648.90-648.94,
650, 669.40-669.44, 669.80-669.94,
670.00-670.04

671.2x CC Excl: 646.80-646.93, 648.90-648.94,
650, 669.40-669.44, 669.80-669.94,
671.20-671.94

671.3 CC Excl: **For codes 671.30, 671.31,
671.33:** see Code 671.2

671.4 CC Excl: For codes 671.40, 671.42,
671.44: see Code 671.2

673.0x CC Excl: 646.80-646.93, 648.90-648.94,
650, 669.40-669.44, 669.80-669.94,
673.00-673.84

673.1x CC Excl: see Code 673.0
673.2x CC Excl: see Code 673.0
673.3x CC Excl: see Code 673.0
673.8x CC Excl: see Code 673.0

674.0x CC Excl: 646.80-646.93, 648.90-648.94,
650, 669.40-669.44, 669.80-669.94,
674.00-674.04,674.50-674.54

674.1 CC Excl: **For Codes 674.10-674.12:**
646.80-646.93, 648.90-648.94, 650,
669.40-669.44, 669.80-669.94, 674.10,
674.34

674.2 CC Excl: **For Codes 674.20, 674.22,
674.24:** see Code 674.1

674.5x CC Excl: 646.80-646.93, 648.90-648.94,
650, 669.40-669.44, 669.80-669.94,
674.00-674.04, 674.50-674.54

675.1 CC Excl: For codes 675.10-675.12:
646.80-646.93, 648.90-648.94, 650,
669.40-669.44, 669.80-669.94, 675.00-
675.94

680.0 CC Excl: 017.00-017.06, 017.90-017.96,
040.82, 040.89, 041.00-041.89, 041.9,
680.0, 680.8-680.9, 686.00-686.01,
686.09, 686.1-686.9, 705.83, 709.8,
V09.0-V09.91

680.1 CC Excl: 017.00-017.06, 017.90-017.96,
040.82, 040.89, 041.00-041.89, 041.9,
680.1, 680.8-680.9, 686.00-686.01,
686.09, 686.1-686.9, 705.83, 709.8,
V09.0-V09.91

680.2 CC Excl: 017.00-017.06, 017.90-017.96,
040.82, 040.89, 041.00-041.89, 041.9,
680.2, 680.8-680.9, 686.00-686.01,
686.09, 686.1-686.9, 705.83, 709.8,
V09.0-V09.91

680.3 CC Excl: 017.00-017.06, 017.90-017.96,
040.82, 040.89, 041.00-041.89, 041.9,
680.3, 680.8-680.9, 686.00-686.01,
686.09, 686.1-686.9, 705.83, 709.8,
V09.0-V09.91

680.4 CC Excl: 017.00-017.06, 017.90-017.96,
040.82, 040.89, 041.00-041.89, 041.9,
680.4, 680.8-680.9, 686.00-686.01,
686.09, 686.1-686.9, 705.83, 709.8,
V09.0-V09.91

680.5 CC Excl: 017.00-017.06, 017.90-017.96,
040.82, 040.89, 041.00-041.89, 041.9,
680.5, 680.8-680.9, 686.00-686.01,
686.09, 686.1-686.9, 705.83, 709.8,
V09.0-V09.91

680.6 CC Excl: 017.00-017.06, 017.90-017.96,
040.82, 040.89, 041.00-041.89, 041.9,
680.6, 680.8-680.9, 686.00-686.01,
686.09, 686.1-686.9, 705.83, 709.8,
V09.0-V09.91

680.7 CC Excl: 017.00-017.06, 017.90-017.96,
040.82, 040.89, 041.00-041.89, 041.9,
680.7-680.9, 686.00-686.01, 686.09,
686.1-686.9, 705.83, 709.8, V09.0-
V09.91

CC Exclusion List

680.8   CC Excl: 017.00-017.06, 017.90-017.96, 040.82, 040.89, 041.00-041.89, 041.9, 680.8-680.9, 686.00-686.01, 686.09, 686.1-686.9, 705.83, 709.8, V09.0-V09.91

680.9   CC Excl: see Code 680.8

682.0   CC Excl: 017.00-017.06, 017.90-017.96, 040.82, 040.89, 041.00-041.89, 041.9, 682.0, 682.8-682.9, 686.00-686.01, 686.09, 686.1-686.9, 705.83, 709.8, V09.0-V09.91

682.1   CC Excl: 017.00-017.06, 017.90-017.96, 040.82, 040.89, 041.00-041.89, 041.9, 682.1, 682.8-682.9, 686.00-686.01, 686.09, 686.1-686.9, 705.83, 709.8, V09.0-V09.91

682.2   CC Excl: 017.00-017.06, 017.90-017.96, 040.82, 040.89, 041.00-041.89, 041.9, 682.2, 682.8-682.9, 686.00-686.01, 686.09, 686.1-686.9, 705.83, 709.8, V09.0-V09.91

682.3   CC Excl: 017.00-017.06, 017.90-017.96, 040.82, 040.89, 041.00-041.89, 041.9, 682.3, 682.8-682.9, 686.00-686.01, 686.09, 686.1-686.9, 705.83, 709.8, V09.0-V09.91

682.5   CC Excl: 017.00-017.06, 017.90-017.96, 040.82, 040.89, 041.00-041.89, 041.9, 682.5, 682.8-682.9, 686.00-686.01, 686.09, 686.1-686.9, 705.83, 709.8, V09.0-V09.91

682.6   CC Excl: 017.00-017.06, 017.90-017.96, 040.82, 040.89, 041.00-041.89, 041.9, 682.6, 682.8-682.9, 686.00-686.01, 686.09, 686.1-686.9, 705.83, 709.8, V09.0-V09.91

682.7   CC Excl: 017.00-017.06, 017.90-017.96, 040.82, 040.89, 041.00-041.89, 041.9, 682.7-682.9, 686.00-686.01, 686.09, 686.1-686.9, 705.83, 709.8, V09.0-V09.91

682.8   CC Excl: 017.00-017.06, 017.90-017.96, 040.82, 040.89, 041.00-041.89, 041.9, 682.8-682.9, 686.00-686.01, 686.09, 686.1-686.9, 705.83, 709.8, V09.0-V09.91

682.9   CC Excl: see Code 682.8

684   CC Excl: 684, 686.00-686.01, 686.09, 686.1-686.9, 709.8

685.0   CC Excl: 685.0-685.1, 709.8

694.4   CC Excl: 694.4-694.9, 709.8

694.5   CC Excl: see Code 694.4

695.0   CC Excl: 695.0-695.4, 709.8

696.0   CC Excl: 015.80-015.96, 017.90-017.96, 036.82, 056.71, 098.50-098.51, 098.59, 098.89, 696.0, 711.00-711.99, 712.10-712.99, 713.0-713.8, 714.0, 715.00, 715.09-715.10, 715.18, 715.20-715.98, 716.00-716.99, 718.00-718.08, 719.00-719.09, 719.10, 719.18-719.19, 719.20-719.99

707.0   CC Excl: 707.0, 707.8-707.9, 709.8

707.10 CC Excl: 440.23, 707.10-707.19, 707.8-707.9, 709.8

707.11 CC Excl: See code 707.10

707.12 CC Excl: See code 707.10

707.13 CC Excl: See code 707.10

707.14 CC Excl: See code 707.10

707.15 CC Excl: See code 707.10

707.19 CC Excl: See code 707.10

710.0   CC Excl: 710.0

710.1   CC Excl: 710.1

710.3   CC Excl: 710.3

710.4   CC Excl: 710.4

710.5   CC Excl: 292.0-292.9, 293.0-293.9, 710.5

710.8   CC Excl: 710.8

711.0   CC Excl: **For code 711.00:** 015.80-015.96, 017.90-017.96, 036.82, 056.71, 098.50-098.51, 098.59, 098.89, 711.00, 714.0, 715.00, 715.09-715.10, 715.18-715.98, 716.00-716.99, 718.00-718.08, 719.00-719.10, 719.18-719.99 **For code 711.01:** 015.80-015.96, 017.90-017.96, 036.82, 056.71, 098.50-098.51, 098.59, 098.89, 711.00-711.01, 711.08-711.11, 711.18-711.21, 711.28-711.31, 711.38-711.41, 711.48-711.51, 711.58-711.61, 711.68-711.71, 711.78-711.81, 711.88-711.91, 711.98-711.99, 712.10-712.11, 712.18-712.21, 712.28-712.31, 712.38-712.81, 712.88-712.91, 712.98-712.99, 713.0-713.8, 714.0, 715.00, 715.09-715.11, 715.18-715.21, 715.28, 715.91, 715.98, 716.00-716.01, 716.08-716.11, 716.18-716.21, 716.28-716.31, 716.38-716.41, 716.48-716.51, 716.58-716.61, 716.68-716.81, 716.88-716.91, 716.98-716.99, 718.00-718.01, 718.08, 719.00-719.01, 719.08-719.11, 719.18-719.21, 719.28-719.31, 719.38-719.41, 719.48-719.51, 719.58-719.61, 719.68-719.7, 717.80-717.81, 719.88-719.91, 719.98-719.99; **For code 711.02:** 015.80-015.96, 017.90-017.96, 036.82, 056.71, 098.50-098.51, 098.59, 098.89, 711.00, 711.02, 711.08-711.10, 711.12, 711.18-711.20, 711.22, 711.28-711.30, 711.32, 711.38-711.40, 711.42, 711.48-711.50, 711.52, 711.58-711.60, 711.62, 711.68-711.70, 711.72, 711.78-711.80, 711.82, 711.88-711.90, 711.92, 711.98-711.99, 712.10, 712.12, 712.18-712.20, 712.22, 712.28-712.30, 712.32, 712.38-712.80, 712.82, 712.88-712.90, 712.92, 712.98-712.99, 713.0-713.8, 714.0, 715.00, 715.09-715.10, 715.12, 715.18, 715.20, 715.22, 715.28, 715.30, 715.32, 715.38-715.90, 715.92, 715.98, 716.00, 716.02, 716.08-716.10, 716.12, 716.18-716.20, 716.22, 716.28-716.30, 716.32, 716.38-716.40, 716.42, 716.48-716.50, 716.52, 716.58-716.60, 716.62, 716.68, 716.80, 716.82, 716.88-716.90, 716.92, 716.98-716.99, 718.00, 718.02, 718.08, 719.00, 719.02, 719.08-719.10, 719.12, 719.18-719.20, 719.22, 719.28-719.30, 719.32, 719.38-719.40, 719.42, 719.48-719.50, 719.52, 719.58-719.60, 719.62, 719.68-719.7, 719.80, 719.88-719.90, 719.92, 719.98-719.99 **For code 711.03:** 015.80-015.96, 017.90-017.96, 036.82, 056.71, 098.50-

711.0   098.51, 098.59, 098.89, 711.00, 711.03,
cont.   711.08-711.10, 711.13, 711.18-711.20, 711.23, 711.28-711.30, 711.33, 711.38-711.40, 711.43, 711.48-711.50, 711.53, 711.58-711.60, 711.63, 711.68-711.70, 711.73, 711.78-711.80, 711.83, 711.88-711.90, 711.93, 711.98-711.99, 712.10, 712.13, 712.18-712.20, 712.23, 712.28-712.30, 712.33, 712.38-712.80, 712.83, 712.88-712.90, 712.93, 712.98-712.99, 713.0-713.8, 714.0, 715.00, 715.09-715.10, 715.13, 715.18, 715.20, 715.23, 715.28, 715.30, 715.33, 715.38-715.90, 715.93, 715.98, 716.00, 716.03, 716.08-716.10, 716.13, 716.18-716.20, 716.23, 716.28-716.30, 716.33, 716.38-716.40, 716.43, 716.48-716.50, 716.53, 716.58-716.60, 716.63, 716.68, 716.80, 716.83, 716.88-716.90, 716.93, 716.98-716.99, 718.00, 718.03, 718.08, 719.00, 719.03, 719.08-719.10, 719.13, 719.18-719.20, 719.23, 719.28-719.30, 719.33, 719.38-719.40, 719.43, 719.48-719.50, 719.53, 719.58-719.60, 719.63, 719.68-719.7, 719.80, 719.83, 719.88-719.90, 719.93, 719.98-719.99 **For code 711.04:** 015.80-015.96, 017.90-017.96, 036.82, 056.71, 098.50-098.51, 098.59, 098.89, 711.00, 711.04, 711.08-711.10, 711.14, 711.18-711.20, 711.24, 711.28-711.30, 711.34, 711.38-711.40, 711.44, 711.48-711.50, 711.54, 711.58-711.60, 711.64, 711.68-711.70, 711.74, 711.78-711.80, 711.84, 711.88-711.90, 711.94, 711.98-711.99, 712.10, 712.14, 712.18-712.20, 712.24, 712.28-712.30, 712.34, 712.38-712.80, 712.84, 712.88-712.90, 712.94, 712.98-712.99, 713.0-713.8, 714.0, 715.00-715.10, 715.14, 715.18, 715.20, 715.24, 715.28, 715.30, 715.34, 715.38-715.90, 715.94, 715.98, 716.00, 716.04, 716.08-716.10, 716.14, 716.18-716.20, 716.24, 716.28-716.30, 716.34, 716.38-716.40, 716.44, 716.48-716.50, 716.54, 716.58-716.60, 716.64, 716.68, 716.80, 716.84, 716.88-716.90, 716.94, 716.98-716.99, 718.00, 718.04, 718.08, 719.00, 719.04, 719.08-719.10, 719.14, 719.18-719.20, 719.24, 719.28-719.30, 719.34, 719.38-719.40, 719.44, 719.48-719.50, 719.54, 719.58-719.60, 719.64, 719.68-719.7, 719.80, 719.84, 719.88-719.90, 719.94, 719.98-719.99: **For code 711.05:** 015.80-015.96, 017.90-017.96, 036.82, 056.71, 098.50-098.51, 098.59, 098.89, 711.00, 711.05, 711.08-711.10, 711.15, 711.18-711.20, 711.25,

711.0 cont. 711.28-711.30, 711.35, 711.38-711.40, 711.45, 711.48-711.50, 711.55, 711.58-711.60, 711.65, 711.68-711.70, 711.75, 711.78-711.80, 711.85, 711.88-711.90, 711.95, 711.98-711.99, 712.10, 712.15, 712.18-712.20, 712.25, 712.28-712.30, 712.35, 712.38-712.80, 712.85, 712.88-712.90, 712.95, 712.98-712.99, 713.0-713.8, 714.0, 715.00, 715.09-715.10, 715.15, 715.18, 715.20, 715.25, 715.28, 715.30, 715.35, 715.38-715.90, 715.95, 715.98, 716.00, 716.05, 716.08-716.10, 716.15, 716.18-716.20, 716.25, 716.28-716.30, 716.35, 716.38-716.40, 716.45, 716.48-716.50, 716.55, 716.58-716.60, 716.65, 716.68, 716.80, 716.85, 716.88-716.90, 716.95, 716.98-716.99, 718.00, 718.05, 718.08, 719.00, 719.05, 719.08-719.10, 719.15, 719.18-719.20, 719.25, 719.28-719.30, 719.35, 719.38-719.40, 719.45, 719.48-719.50, 719.55, 719.58-719.60, 719.65, 719.68-719.7, 719.80, 719.85-719.88-719.90, 719.95, 719.98-719.99 **For code 711.06:** 015.80-015.96, 017.90-017.96, 036.82, 056.71, 098.50-098.51, 098.59, 098.89, 711.00, 711.06, 711.08-711.10, 711.16, 711.18-711.20, 711.26, 711.28-711.30, 711.36, 711.38-711.40, 711.46, 711.48-711.50, 711.56, 711.58-711.60, 711.66, 711.68-711.70, 711.76, 711.78-711.80, 711.86, 711.88-711.90, 711.96, 711.98-711.99, 712.10, 712.16, 712.18-712.20, 712.26, 712.28-712.30, 712.36, 712.38-712.80, 712.86, 712.88-712.90, 712.96, 712.98-712.99, 713.0-713.8, 714.0, 715.00, 715.09-715.10, 715.16, 715.18, 715.20, 715.26, 715.28, 715.30, 715.36, 715.38-715.90, 715.96, 715.98, 716.00, 716.06, 716.08-716.10, 716.16, 716.18-716.20, 716.26, 716.28-716.30, 716.36, 716.38-716.40, 716.46, 716.48-716.50, 716.56, 716.58-716.60, 716.66, 716.68, 716.80, 716.86, 716.88-716.90, 716.96, 716.98-716.99, 718.00, 718.08, 719.00, 719.06, 719.08-719.10, 719.16, 719.18-719.20, 719.26, 719.28-719.30, 719.36, 719.38-719.40, 719.46, 719.48-719.50, 719.56, 719.58-719.60, 719.66, 719.68-719.7, 719.80, 719.86, 719.88-719.90, 719.96, 719.98-719.99 **For code 711.07:** 015.80-015.96, 017.90-017.96, 036.82, 056.71, 098.50-098.51, 098.59, 098.89, 711.00, 711.07-711.10, 711.17-711.20, 711.27-711.30, 711.37-711.40, 711.47-711.50, 711.57-711.60, 711.67-711.70,

711.0 cont. 711.77-711.80, 711.87-711.90, 711.97-711.99, 712.10, 712.17-712.20, 712.27-712.30, 712.37-712.80, 712.87-712.90, 712.97-712.99, 713.0-713.8, 714.0, 715.00, 715.09-715.10, 715.17-715.18, 715.20, 715.27-715.28, 715.30, 715.37-715.90, 715.97-715.98, 716.00, 716.07-716.10, 716.17-716.20, 716.27-716.30, 716.37-716.40, 716.47-716.50, 716.57-716.60, 716.67-716.68, 716.80, 716.87-716.90, 716.97-716.99, 718.00, 718.07-718.08, 719.00, 719.07-719.10, 719.17-719.20, 719.27-719.30, 719.37-719.40, 719.47-719.50, 719.57-719.60, 719.67-719.7, 719.80, 719.87-719.90, 719.97-719.99 **For code 711.08:** 015.80-015.96, 017.90-017.96, 036.82, 056.71, 098.50-098.51, 098.59, 098.89, 711.00-711.99, 712.10-712.99, 713.0-713.8, 714.0, 715.00, 715.09-715.10, 715.18-715.98, 716.00-716.99, 718.00-718.08, 719.00-719.10, 719.18-719.99 **For code 711.09:** see Code 711.08

711.6 CC Excl: **For code 711.60:** see Code 711.08: **For code 711.61:** 015.80-015.96, 017.90-017.96, 036.82, 056.71, 098.50-098.51, 098.59, 098.89, 711.00-711.01, 711.08-711.11, 711.18-711.21, 711.28-711.31, 711.38-711.41, 711.48-711.51, 711.58-711.61, 711.68-711.71, 711.78-711.81, 711.88-711.91, 711.98-711.99, 712.10-712.11, 712.18-712.21, 712.28-712.31, 712.38-712.81, 712.88-712.91, 712.98-712.99, 713.0-713.8, 714.0, 715.00, 715.09-715.11, 715.18-715.21, 715.28, 715.30-715.31, 715.38-715.91, 715.98, 716.00-716.01, 716.08-716.11, 716.18-716.21, 716.28-716.31, 716.38-716.41, 716.48-716.51, 716.58-716.61, 716.68, 716.80-716.81, 716.88-716.91, 716.98-716.99, 718.00-718.01, 718.08, 719.00-719.01, 719.08-719.11, 719.18-719.21, 719.28-719.31, 719.38-719.41, 719.48-719.51, 719.58-719.61, 719.68-719.7, 719.81, 719.88-719.91, 719.98-719.99: **For code 711.62:** 015.80-015.96, 017.90-017.96, 036.82, 056.71, 098.50-098.51, 098.59, 098.89, 711.00, 711.02, 711.08-711.10, 711.12, 711.18-711.20, 711.22, 711.28-711.30, 711.32, 711.38-711.40, 711.42, 711.48-711.50, 711.52, 711.58-711.60, 711.62, 711.68-711.70, 711.72, 711.78-711.80, 711.82, 711.88-711.90, 711.92, 711.98-711.99, 712.10, 712.12, 712.18-712.20, 712.22, 712.28-712.30, 712.32, 712.38-712.80, 712.82, 712.88-712.90,

711.6
cont.
712.92, 712.98-712.99, 713.0-713.8,
714.0, 715.00, 715.09-715.10, 715.12,
715.18, 715.20, 715.22, 715.28, 715.30,
715.32, 715.38-715.90, 715.92, 715.98,
716.00, 716.02, 716.08-716.10, 716.12,
716.18-716.20, 716.22, 716.28-716.30,
716.32, 716.38-716.40, 716.42, 716.48-
716.50, 716.52, 716.58-716.60, 716.62,
716.68, 716.80, 716.82, 716.88-716.90,
716.92, 716.98-716.99, 718.00, 718.02,
718.08, 719.00, 719.02, 719.08-719.10,
719.12, 719.18-719.20, 719.22, 719.28-
719.30, 719.32, 719.38-719.40, 719.42,
719.48-719.50, 719.52, 719.58-719.60,
719.62, 719.68-719.7, 719.80, 719.82,
719.88-719.90, 719.92, 719.98-719.99:
For code 711.63: 015.80-015.96,
017.90-017.96, 036.82, 056.71, 098.50-
098.51, 098.59, 098.89, 711.00, 711.03,
711.08-711.10, 711.13, 711.18-711.20,
711.23, 711.28-711.30, 711.33, 711.38-
711.40, 711.43, 711.48-711.50, 711.53,
711.58-711.60, 711.63, 711.68-711.70,
711.73, 711.78-711.80, 711.83, 711.88-
711.90, 711.93, 711.98-711.99, 712.10,
712.13, 712.18-712.20, 712.23, 712.28-
712.30, 712.33, 712.38-712.80, 712.83,
712.88-712.90, 712.93, 712.98-712.99,
713.0-713.8, 714.0, 715.00, 715.09-
715.10, 715.13, 715.18, 715.20, 715.23,
715.28, 715.30, 715.33, 715.38-715.90,
715.93, 715.98, 716.00, 716.03, 716.08-
716.10, 716.13, 716.18-716.20, 716.23,
716.28-716.30, 716.33, 716.38-716.40,
716.43, 716.48-716.50, 716.53, 716.58-
716.60, 716.63, 716.68, 716.80, 716.83,
716.88-716.90, 716.93, 716.98-716.99,
718.00, 718.03, 718.08, 719.00, 719.03,
719.08-719.10, 719.13, 719.18-719.20,
719.23, 719.28-719.30, 719.33, 719.38-
719.40, 719.43, 719.48-719.50, 719.53,
719.58-719.60, 719.63, 719.68-719.7,
719.80, 719.83, 719.88-719.90, 719.93,
719.98-719.99 For code 711.64: 015.80-
015.96, 017.90-017.96, 036.82, 056.71,
098.50-098.51, 098.59, 098.89, 711.00,
711.04, 711.08-711.10, 711.14, 711.18-
711.20, 711.24, 711.28-711.30, 711.34,
711.38-711.40, 711.44, 711.48-711.50,
711.5, 711.58-711.60, 711.64, 711.68-
711.70, 711.74, 711.78-711.80, 711.84,
711.88-711.90, 711.94, 711.98-711.99,
712.10, 712.14, 712.18-712.20, 712.24,
712.28-712.30, 712.34, 712.38-712.80,
712.84, 712.88-712.90, 712.94, 712.98-
712.99, 713.0-713.8, 714.0, 715.00-
715.10, 715.14, 715.18,

711.6
cont.
715.20, 715.24, 715.28, 715.30,
715.34, 715.38-715.90, 715.94, 715.98,
716.00, 716.04, 716.08-716.10, 716.14,
716.18-716.20, 716.24, 716.28-716.30,
716.34, 716.38-716.40, 716.44, 716.48-
716.50, 716.54, 716.58-716.60, 716.64,
716.68, 716.80, 716.84, 716.88-716.90,
716.94, 716.98-716.99, 718.00, 718.04,
718.08, 719.00, 719.04, 719.08-719.10,
719.14, 719.18-719.20, 719.24, 719.28-
719.30, 719.34, 719.38-719.40, 719.44,
719.48-719.50, 719.54, 719.58-719.60,
719.64, 719.68-719.7, 719.80, 719.84,
719.88-719.90, 719.94, 719.98-719.99
For code 711.65: 015.80-015.96,
017.90-017.96, 036.82, 056.71, 098.50-
098.51, 098.59, 098.89, 711.00, 711.05,
711.08-711.10, 711.15, 711.18-711.20,
711.25, 711.28-711.30, 711.35, 711.38-
711.40, 711.45, 711.48-711.50, 711.55,
711.58-711.60, 711.65, 711.68-711.70,
711.75, 711.78-711.80, 711.85, 711.88-
711.90, 711.95, 711.98-711.99, 712.10,
712.15, 712.18-712.20, 712.25, 712.28-
712.30, 712.35, 712.38-712.80, 712.85,
712.88-712.90, 712.95, 712.98-712.99,
713.0-713.8, 714.0, 715.00, 715.09-
715.10, 715.15, 715.18, 715.20, 715.25,
715.28, 715.30, 715.35, 715.38-715.90,
715.95, 715.98, 716.00, 716.05, 716.08-
716.10, 716.15, 716.18-716.20, 716.25,
716.28-716.30, 716.35, 716.38-716.40,
716.45, 716.48-716.50, 716.55, 716.58-
716.60, 716.65, 716.68, 716.80, 716.85,
716.88-716.90, 716.95, 716.98-716.99,
718.00, 718.05, 718.08, 719.00, 719.05,
719.08-719.10, 719.15, 719.18-719.20,
719.25, 719.28-719.30, 719.35, 719.38-
719.40, 719.45, 719.48-719.50, 719.55,
719.58-719.60, 719.65, 719.68-719.7,
719.80, 719.85, 719.88-719.90, 719.95,
719.98-719.99; For code 711.66:
015.80-015.96, 017.90-017.96, 036.82,
056.71, 098.50-098.51, 098.59, 098.89,
711.00, 711.06, 711.08-711.10, 711.16,
711.18-711.20, 711.26, 711.28-711.30,
711.36, 711.38-711.40, 711.46, 711.48-
711.50, 711.56, 711.58-711.60, 711.66,
711.68-711.70, 711.76, 711.78-711.80,
711.86, 711.88-711.90, 711.96, 711.98-
711.99, 712.10, 712.16, 712.18-712.20,
712.26, 712.28-712.30, 712.36, 712.38-
712.80, 712.86, 712.88-712.90, 712.96,
712.98-712.99, 713.0-713.8, 714.0,
715.00, 715.09-715.10, 715.16, 715.18,
715.20, 715.26, 715.28, 715.30, 715.36,
715.38-715.90,

711.6
cont. 715.96, 715.98, 716.00, 716.06, 716.08-716.10, 716.16, 716.18-716.20, 716.26, 716.28-716.30, 716.36, 716.38-716.40, 716.46, 716.48-716.50, 716.56, 716.58-716.60, 716.66, 716.68, 716.80, 716.86, 716.88-716.90, 716.96, 716.98-716.99, 718.00, 718.08, 719.00, 719.06, 719.08-719.10, 719.16, 719.18-719.20, 719.26, 719.28-719.30, 719.36, 719.38-719.40, 719.46, 719.48-719.50, 719.56, 719.58-719.60, 719.66, 719.68-719.7, 719.80, 719.86, 719.88-719.90, 719.96, 719.98-719.99 **For code 711.67:** 015.80-015.96, 017.90-017.96, 036.82, 056.71, 098.50-098.51, 098.59, 098.89, 711.00, 711.07-711.10, 711.17-711.20, 711.27-711.30, 711.37-711.40, 711.47-711.50, 711.57-711.60, 711.67-711.70, 711.77-711.80, 711.87-711.90, 711.97-711.99, 712.10, 712.17-712.20, 712.27-712.30, 712.37-712.80, 712.87-712.90, 712.97-712.99, 713.0-713.8, 714.0, 715.00, 715.09-715.10, 715.17-715.18, 715.20, 715.27-715.28, 715.30, 715.37-715.90, 715.97-715.98, 716.00, 716.07-716.10, 716.17-716.20, 716.27-716.30, 716.37-716.40, 716.47-716.50, 716.57-716.60, 716.67-716.80, 716.87-716.90, 716.97-716.99, 718.00, 718.07-718.08, 719.00, 719.07-719.10, 719.17-719.20, 719.27-719.30, 719.37-719.40, 719.47-719.50, 719.57-719.60, 719.67-719.7, 719.80, 719.87-719.90, 719.97-719.99 **For code 711.68:** 015.80-015.96, 017.90-017.96, 036.82, 056.71, 098.50-098.51, 098.59, 098.89, 711.00-711.99, 712.10-712.99, 713.0-713.8, 714.0, 715.00, 715.09-715.10, 715.18-715.98, 716.00-716.99, 718.00-718.08, 719.00-719.10, 719.18-719.99 **For code 711.69:** see Code 711.68

714.1 CC Excl: 036.82, 056.71, 711.00-711.99, 712.10-712.99, 713.0-713.8, 714.0-714.4, 715.00, 715.09-715.10, 715.18-715.98, 716.00-716.99, 718.00-718.08, 719.00-719.10, 719.18-719.7, 719.80-719.99

714.2 CC Excl: see Code 714.1
714.30 CC Excl: see Code 714.1
714.31 CC Excl: see Code 714.1
714.32 CC Excl: see Code 714.1
714.33 CC Excl: see Code 714.1
722.80 CC Excl: 722.51-722.93
722.81 CC Excl: see Code 722.80
722.82 CC Excl: see Code 722.80
722.83 CC Excl: see Code 722.80
723.4 CC Excl: 722.6-722.71, 722.80-722.81, 722.90-722.91, 723.0-723.9

723.5 CC Excl: 053.71, 722.6-722.71, 722.80-722.81, 722.90-722.91, 723.0-723.9

728.0 CC Excl: 728.0, 728.11-728.3, 728.81, 728.86

728.86 CC Excl: 728.0, 728.11-728.19, 728.2, 728.3, 728.82, 728.86

728.88 CC Excl: 728.0, 728.11-728.3, 728.81, 728.86, 728.88

730.0 CC Excl: **For code 730.00:** 015.50-015.56, 015.70-015.76, 015.90-015.96, 017.90-017.96, 730.00-730.39, 730.80-730.99 **For code 730.01:** 015.50-015.56, 015.70-015.76, 015.90-015.96, 017.90-017.96, 730.00, 730.08-730.11, 730.18-730.21, 730.28-730.31, 730.38-730.39, 730.80-730.81, 730.88-730.91, 730.98-730.99 **For code 730.02:** 015.50-015.56, 015.70-015.76, 015.90-015.96, 017.90-017.96, 730.00, 730.08-730.10, 730.12, 730.18-730.20, 730.22, 730.28-730.30, 730.32, 730.38-730.39, 730.80, 730.82, 730.88-730.90, 730.92, 730.98-730.99 **For code 730.03:** 015.50-015.56, 015.70-015.76, 015.90-015.96, 017.90-017.96, 730.00, 730.08-730.10, 730.13, 730.18-730.20, 730.23, 730.28-730.30, 730.33, 730.38-730.39, 730.80, 730.83, 730.88-730.90, 730.93, 730.98-730.99: **For code 730.04:** 015.50-015.56, 015.70-015.76, 015.90-015.96, 017.90-017.96, 730.00, 730.08-730.10, 730.14, 730.18-730.20, 730.24, 730.28-730.30, 730.34, 730.38-730.39, 730.80, 730.84, 730.88-730.90, 730.94, 730.98-730.99 **For code 730.05:** 015.10-015.16, 015.50-015.56, 015.70-015.76, 015.90-015.96, 017.90-017.96, 730.00, 730.08-730.10, 730.15, 730.18-730.20, 730.25, 730.28-730.30, 730.35, 730.38-730.39, 730.80, 730.85, 730.88-730.90, 730.95, 730.98-730.99: **For code 730.06:** 015.20-015.56, 015.70-015.76, 015.90-015.96, 017.90-017.96, 730.00, 730.08-730.10, 730.16, 730.18-730.20, 730.26, 730.28-730.30, 730.36, 730.38-730.39, 730.80, 730.86, 730.88-730.90, 730.96, 730.98-730.99 **For code 730.07:** 015.50-015.56, 015.70-015.76, 015.90-015.96, 017.90-017.96, 730.00, 730.08-730.10, 730.17-730.20, 730.27-730.30, 730.37-730.39, 730.80, 730.87-730.90, 730.97-730.99 **For code 730.08:** 015.00-015.06, 015.50-015.56, 015.70-015.76, 015.90-015.96, 017.90-017.96, 730.00-730.39, 730.80-730.99 **For code 730.09:** 015.50-015.56, 015.70-015.76, 015.90-015.96, 017.90-017.96, 730.00-730.39, 730.80-730.99

730.8 CC Excl: **For code 730.80:** see Code
730.09 CC Excl: **For code 730.81:**
015.50-015.56, 015.70-015.76, 015.90-
015.96, 017.90-017.96, 730.00-730.01,
730.08-730.11, 730.18-730.21, 730.28-
730.31, 730.38-730.39, 730.80, 730.88-
730.91, 730.98-730.99 **For code 730.82:**
015.50-015.56, 015.70-015.76, 015.90-
015.96, 017.90-017.96, 730.00, 730.02,
730.08-730.10, 730.12, 730.18-730.20,
730.22, 730.28-730.30, 730.32, 730.38-
730.39, 730.80, 730.88-730.90, 730.92,
730.98-730.99l: **For code 730.83:**
015.50-015.56, 015.70-015.76, 015.90-
015.96, 017.90-017.96, 730.00, 730.03,
730.08-730.10, 730.13, 730.18-730.20,
730.23, 730.28-730.30, 730.33, 730.38-
730.39, 730.80, 730.88-730.90, 730.93,
730.98-730.99: **For code 730.84:**
015.50-015.56, 015.70-015.76, 015.90-
015.96, 017.90-017.96, 730.00, 730.04,
730.08-730.10, 730.14, 730.18-730.20,
730.24, 730.28-730.30, 730.34, 730.38-
730.39, 730.80, 730.88-730.90, 730.94,
730.98-730.99 **For code 730.85:** 015.10-
015.16, 015.50-015.56, 015.70-015.76,
015.90-015.96, 017.90-017.96, 730.00,
730.05, 730.08-730.10, 730.15, 730.18-
730.20, 730.25, 730.28-730.30, 730.35,
730.38-730.39, 730.80, 730.88-730.90,
730.95, 730.98-730.99 **For code
730.86:** 015.20-015.26, 015.50-015.56,
015.70-015.76, 015.90-015.96, 017.90-
017.96, 730.00, 730.06, 730.08-730.10,
730.16, 730.18-730.20, 730.26, 730.28-
730.30, 730.36, 730.38-730.39, 730.80,
730.88-730.90, 730.96, 730.98-730.99
For code 730.87: 015.50-015.56,
015.70-015.76, 015.90-015.96, 017.90-
017.96, 730.00, 730.07-730.10, 730.17-
730.20, 730.27-730.30, 730.37-730.39,
730.80, 730.88-730.90, 730.97-730.99
For code 730.88: 015.00-015.06,
015.50-015.56, 015.70-015.76, 015.90-
015.96, 017.90-017.96, 730.00-730.39,
730.80-730.99: **For code 730.89:**
015.50-015.56, 015.70-015.76, 015.90-
015.96, 017.90-017.96, 730.00-730.39,
730.80-730.99

730.9 CC Excl: **For code 730.90:** see Code
730.89 **For code 730.91:** 015.50-015.56,
015.70-015.76, 015.90-015.96, 017.90-
017.96, 730.00-730.01, 730.08-730.11,
730.18-730.21, 730.28-730.31, 730.38-
730.39, 730.80-730.81, 730.88-730.90,
730.98-730.99 **For code 730.92:** 015.50-
015.56, 015.70-015.76, 015.90-015.96,
017.90-017.96, 730.00, 730.02, 730.08-
730.10, 730.12, 730.18-730.20, 730.22,
730.28-730.30, 730.32, 730.38-730.39,
730.80, 730.82, 730.88-730.90, 730.98-
730.99: **For code 730.93:** 015.50-
015.56, 015.70-015.76, 015.90-015.96,
017.90-017.96, 730.00, 730.03, 730.08-
730.10, 730.13, 730.18-730.20, 730.23,
730.28-730.30, 730.33, 730.38-730.39,
730.80, 730.83, 730.88-730.90, 730.98-
730.99 **For code 730.94:** 015.50-015.56,
015.70-015.76, 015.90-015.96, 017.90-
017.96, 730.00, 730.04, 730.08-730.10,
730.14, 730.18-730.20, 730.24, 730.28-
730.30, 730.34, 730.38-730.39, 730.80,
730.84, 730.88-730.90, 730.98-730.99:
For code 730.95: 015.10-015.16,
015.50-015.56, 015.70-015.76, 015.90-
015.96, 017.90-017.96, 730.00, 730.05,
730.08-730.10, 730.15, 730.18-730.20,
730.25, 730.28-730.30, 730.35, 730.38-
730.39, 730.80, 730.85, 730.88-730.90,
730.98-730.99 **For code 730.96:** 015.20-
015.26, 015.50-015.56, 015.70-015.76,
015.90-015.96, 017.90-017.96, 730.00,
730.06, 730.08-730.10, 730.16, 730.18-
730.20, 730.26, 730.28-730.30, 730.36,
730.38-730.39, 730.80, 730.86, 730.88-
730.90, 730.98-730.99: **For code
730.97:** 015.50-015.56, 015.70-015.76,
015.90-015.96, 017.90-017.96, 730.00,
730.07-730.10, 730.17-730.20, 730.27-
730.30, 730.37-730.39, 730.80, 730.87-
730.90, 730.98-730.99: **For code
730.98:** 015.00-015.06, 015.50-015.56,
015.70-015.76, 015.90-015.96, 017.90-
017.96, 730.00-730.39, 730.80-730.99
For code 730.99: 015.50-015.56,
015.70-015.76, 015.90-015.96, 017.90-
017.96, 730.00-730.39, 730.80-730.99

733.10 CC Excl: 733.10-733.19, 733.93-733.95
733.11 CC Excl: see Code 733.10
733.12 CC Excl: see Code 733.10
733.13 CC Excl: see Code 733.10
733.14 CC Excl: see Code 733.10
733.15 CC Excl: see Code 733.10
733.16 CC Excl: see Code 733.10
733.19 CC Excl: see Code 733.10

733.81   CC Excl: 733.81-733.82
733.82   CC Excl: see Code 733.81
733.93   CC Excl: 733.10-733.19, 733.93-733.95
733.94   CC Excl: see Code 733.93
733.95   CC Excl: see Code 733.93
741.0   CC Excl: 741.00-741.93, 742.59, 742.8-742.9, 759.7-759.89
741.9   CC Excl: see Code 741.0
745.0   CC Excl: 429.71, 429.79, 745.0-745.9, 746.89, 746.9, 747.83, 747.89, 747.9, 759.7-759.89
745.10   CC Excl: see Code 745.0
745.11   CC Excl: see Code 745.0
745.12   CC Excl: see Code 745.0
745.19   CC Excl: see Code 745.0
745.2   CC Excl: see Code 745.0
745.3   CC Excl: see Code 745.0
745.4   CC Excl: see Code 745.0
745.60   CC Excl: see Code 745.0
745.69   CC Excl: see Code 745.0
745.7   CC Excl: see Code 745.0
746.01   CC Excl: 746.00-746.09, 746.89, 746.9, 747.83, 747.89, 747.9, 759.7-759.89
746.02   CC Excl: see Code 746.01
746.1   CC Excl: 746.1-746.7, 746.89, 746.9, 747.83, 747.89, 747.9, 759.7-759.89
746.2   CC Excl: see Code 746.1
746.3   CC Excl: see Code 746.1
746.4   CC Excl: see Code 746.1
746.5   CC Excl: see Code 746.1
746.6   CC Excl: see Code 746.1
746.7   CC Excl: see Code 746.1
746.81   CC Excl: 746.81-746.84, 746.89, 746.9, 747.83, 747.89, 747.9, 759.7-759.89
746.82   CC Excl: see Code 746.81
746.83   CC Excl: see Code 746.81
746.84   CC Excl: see Code 746.81
746.86   CC Excl: see Code 746.81
747.11   CC Excl: 747.10-747.22, 747.83, 747.89, 747.9, 759.7-759.89
747.22   CC Excl: see Code 747.11
748.4   CC Excl: 748.4-748.9
748.5   CC Excl: see Code 748.4
748.61   CC Excl: 494.0-494.1, 496, 506.1, 506.4, 506.9, 748.61
765.0x   CC Excl: 764.00-765.29, 767.8-767.9, 779.81-779.89
767.0   CC Excl: 531.31, 767.0, 767.8-767.9, 779.81-779.89
767.11   **CC Excl:** 767.0, 767.11, 767.8-767.9, 779.81-779.89
768.5   CC Excl: 532.61, 768.5-768.9, 769, 770.0-770.9, 779.81-779.89
769   CC Excl: see Code 768.5

770.0   CC Excl: see Code 768.5
770.1   CC Excl: see Code 768.5
770.2   CC Excl: see Code 768.5
770.3   CC Excl: see Code 768.5
770.4   CC Excl: see Code 768.5
770.5   CC Excl: see Code 768.5
770.7   CC Excl: see Code 768.5
770.84   CC Excl: 768.5-768.6, 768.9, 769, 770.0-770.7, 770.81-770.84, 770.89, 770.9, 779.81-779.89
771.0   CC Excl: 771.0-771.2, 779.81-779.89
771.1   CC Excl: see Code 771.0
771.3   CC Excl: 534.10, 771.3, 779.81-779.89
771.81   CC Excl: 534.10, 771.4-771.7, 771.81-771.83, 771.89, 776.0-776.9, 779.81-779.89
771.82   CC Excl: 771.81, 771.83
771.83   CC Excl: 534.10, 771.4-771.7, 771.81-771.83, 771.89, 776.0-776.9, 779.81-779.89
771.89   CC Excl: 771.81, 771.83
772.10   CC Excl: 772.0-772.2, 772.8-772.9, 776.0-776.9, 779.81-779.89
772.11   CC Excl: see Code 772.10
772.12   CC Excl: see Code 772.10
772.13   CC Excl: see Code 772.10
772.14   CC Excl: see Code 772.10
772.2   CC Excl: 772.0-772.2, 772.8-772.9, 776.0-776.9, 779.7, 779.81-779.89
772.4   CC Excl: 772.0, 772.4-772.5, 772.8-772.9, 776.0-776.9, 779.81-779.89
772.5   CC Excl: see Code 772.4
773.0   CC Excl: 773.0-773.5, 779.81-779.89
773.1   CC Excl: see Code 773.0
773.2   CC Excl: see Code 773.0
773.3   CC Excl: see Code 773.0
773.4   CC Excl: see Code 773.0
774.0   CC Excl: 774.0-774.7, 779.81-779.89
774.1   CC Excl: see Code 774.0
774.2   CC Excl: see Code 774.0
774.30   CC Excl: see Code 774.0
774.31   CC Excl: see Code 774.0
774.39   CC Excl: see Code 774.0
774.4   CC Excl: see Code 774.0
774.5   CC Excl: see Code 774.0
774.7   CC Excl: see Code 774.0
775.1   CC Excl: 775.0-775.9, 779.81-779.89
775.2   CC Excl: see Code 775.1
775.3   CC Excl: see Code 775.1
775.4   CC Excl: see Code 775.1
775.5   CC Excl: see Code 775.1
775.6   CC Excl: see Code 775.1
775.7   CC Excl: see Code 775.1

776.0 CC Excl: 771.81, 771.83, 776.0-776.9, 779.81-779.89
776.1 CC Excl: see Code 776.0
776.2 CC Excl: see Code 776.0
776.3 CC Excl: see Code 776.0
777.1 CC Excl: 777.1-777.9, 779.81-779.89
777.2 CC Excl: see Code 777.1
777.5 CC Excl: see Code 777.1
777.6 CC Excl: see Code 777.1
778.0 CC Excl: 778.0, 779.81-779.89
779.0 CC Excl: 779.0-779.1, 779.81-779.89
779.1 CC Excl: see Code 779.0
779.3 CC Excl: 779.3
779.4 CC Excl: 779.4-779.5
779.7 CC Excl: 772.0, 772.10-772.14, 772.2, 772.8, 772.9, 776.0-776.9, 779.7, 779.81-779.89
780.01 CC Excl: 070.0-070.9, 250.00-250.93, 251.0-251.3, 348.8-348.9, 349.89, 349.9, 430-431, 432.0-432.9, 572.2, 780.01-780.09, 780.2, 780.4, 780.91-780.99, 799.81-799.89, 800.00-800.99, 801.00-801.99, 803.00-803.99, 804.00-804.96, 850.0-850.9, 851.00-851.99, 852.00-852.19, 852.21-852.59, 853.00-853.19, 854.00-854.19,
780.03 CC Excl: see Code 780.01
780.1 CC Excl: 780.1, 780.4, 780.91-780.99, 799.8
780.31 CC Excl: 345.00-345.01, 345.10-345.11, 345.2-345.3, 345.40-345.41, 345.50-345.51, 345.60-345.61, 345.70-345.71, 345.80-345.81, 345.90-345.91, 348.8-348.9, 349.89, 349.9, 779.0-779.1, 780.31, 780.39, 780.91-780.99, 799.81-799.89
780.39 CC Excl: see Code 780.31, 537.84
781.7 CC Excl: 037, 332.0-332.1, 333.0-333.99, 334.0-334.4, 342.10-342.12, 771.3, 780.91-780.99, 781.7, 799.81-799.89
785.4 CC Excl: 440.24, 537.84, 780.91-780.99, 785.4, 799.8
785.50 CC Excl: 780.91-780.99, 785.50-785.59, 785.9, 799.8
785.51 CC Excl: see Code 785.50
785.52 CC Excl: see Code 785.50
785.59 CC Excl: see Code 785.50
786.03 CC Excl: 518.81-518.84, 519.8, 519.9, 786.03, 786.04, 799.1
786.04 CC Excl: 518.81-518.84, 519.8, 519.9, 786.03, 786.04, 799.1
786.3 CC Excl: 780.91-780.99, 786.3-786.4, 786.9, 799.81-799.89

788.20 CC Excl: 274.11, 344.61, 593.3-593.5, 596.0, 596.4-596.59, 596.8-596.9, 599.6, 600.1-600.9, 601.0-601.9, 602.0-602.9, 753.0, 753.1, 753.20-753.23, 753.29, 753.3-753.9, 780.91-780.99, 788.20-788.29, 788.61-788.69, 788.9, 799.81-799.89
788.29 CC Excl: see Code 788.20
789.5 CC Excl: 780.91-780.99, 789.30-789.5, 789.9, 799.81-799.89
790.7 CC Excl: 780.91-780.99, 790.7-790.99, 799.81-799.89
791.1 CC Excl: 780.91-780.99, 791.1, 791.9, 799.81-799.89
791.3 CC Excl: 780.91-780.99, 791.2-791.3, 791.9, 799.81-799.89
799.1 CC Excl: 518.81-518.84, 780.91-780.99, 798.0, 799.0-799.1, 799.81-799.89
799.4 CC Excl: 780.91-780.99, 799.3-799.4, 799.81-799.89
800.0x CC Excl: 800.00-801.99, 803.00-804.99, 829.0-829.1, 850.0-852.19, 852.21-854.19, 873.8-873.9, 879.8-879.9, 905.0, 925.1-925.2, 929.0-929.9, 958.8, 959.01, 959.09, 959.8-959.9
800.1x CC Excl: see Code 800.0
800.2x CC Excl: see Code 800.0
800.3x CC Excl: see Code 800.0
800.4x CC Excl: see Code 800.0
800.5x CC Excl: see Code 800.0
800.6x CC Excl: see Code 800.0
800.7x CC Excl: see Code 800.0
800.8x CC Excl: see Code 800.0
800.9x CC Excl: see Code 800.0
801.0x CC Excl: see Code 800.0
801.1x CC Excl: see Code 800.0
801.2x CC Excl: see Code 800.0
801.3x CC Excl: see Code 800.0
801.4x CC Excl: see Code 800.0
801.5x CC Excl: see Code 800.0
801.6x CC Excl: see Code 800.0
801.7x CC Excl: see Code 800.0
801.8x CC Excl: see Code 800.0
801.9x CC Excl: see Code 800.0
802.1 CC Excl: 800.00-800.99, 801.00-801.99, 802.0-802.1, 803.00-803.99, 804.00-804.99, 829.0-829.1, 850.0-850.9, 851.00-851.99, 852.00-852.19, 852.21-852.59, 853.00-853.19, 854.00-854.19, 873.8-873.9, 879.8-879.9, 905.0, 925.1-925.2, 929.0, 929.9, 958.8, 959.01, 959.09, 959.8-959.9

802.20 CC Excl: 800.00-800.99, 801.00-801.99, 802.20-802.5, 803.00-803.99, 804.00-804.99, 829.0-829.1, 830.0-830.1, 850.0-850.9, 851.00-851.99, 852.00-852.19, 852.21-852.59, 853.00-853.19, 854.00-854.19, 873.8-873.9, 879.8-879.9, 905.0, 925.1, 925.2, 929.0, 929.9, 958.8, 959.01, 959.09, 959.8-959.9

802.21 CC Excl: see Code 802.20
802.22 CC Excl: see Code 802.20
802.23 CC Excl: see Code 802.20
802.24 CC Excl: see Code 802.20
802.25 CC Excl: see Code 802.20
802.26 CC Excl: see Code 802.20
802.27 CC Excl: see Code 802.20
802.28 CC Excl: see Code 802.20
802.29 CC Excl: see Code 802.20
802.30 CC Excl: see Code 802.20
802.31 CC Excl: see Code 802.20
802.32 CC Excl: see Code 802.20
802.33 CC Excl: see Code 802.20
802.34 CC Excl: see Code 802.20
802.35 CC Excl: see Code 802.20
802.36 CC Excl: see Code 802.20
802.37 CC Excl: see Code 802.20
802.38 CC Excl: see Code 802.20
802.39 CC Excl: see Code 802.20
802.4   CC Excl: see Code 802.20
802.5   CC Excl: see Code 802.20
802.6   CC Excl: 800.00-800.99, 801.00-801.99, 802.6-802.9, 803.00-803.99, 804.00-804.99, 829.0-829.1, 850.0-850.9, 851.00-851.99, 852.00-852.19, 852.21-852.59, 853.00-853.19, 854.00-854.19, 873.8-873.9, 879.8-879.9, 905.0, 925.1-925.2, 929.0, 929.9, 958.8, 959.01, 959.09, 959.8-959.9

802.7   CC Excl: see Code 802.6
802.8   CC Excl: see Code 802.6
802.9   CC Excl: see Code 802.6
803.0x CC Excl: 800.00-800.99, 801.00-801.99, 803.00-803.99, 804.00-804.99, 829.0-829.1, 850.0-850.9, 851.00-851.99, 852.00-852.19, 852.21-852.59, 853.00-853.19, 854.00-854.19, 873.8-873.9, 879.8-879.9, 905.0, 925.1-925.2, 929.0, 929.9, 958.8, 959.01, 959.09, 959.8-959.9

803.1x CC Excl: see Code 803.0
803.2x CC Excl: see Code 803.0
803.3x CC Excl: see Code 803.0
803.4x CC Excl: see Code 803.0
803.5x CC Excl: see Code 803.0
803.6x CC Excl: see Code 803.0

803.7x CC Excl: see Code 803.0
803.8x CC Excl: see Code 803.0
803.9x CC Excl: see Code 803.0
804.0x CC Excl: see Code 803.0
804.1x CC Excl: see Code 803.0
804.2x CC Excl: see Code 803.0
804.3x CC Excl: see Code 803.0
804.4x CC Excl: see Code 803.0
804.5x CC Excl: see Code 803.0
804.6x CC Excl: see Code 803.0
804.7x CC Excl: see Code 803.0
804.8x CC Excl: see Code 803.0
804.9x CC Excl: see Code 803.0
805.0x CC Excl: 805.00-805.18, 805.8-805.9, 806.00-806.19, 806.8-806.9, 829.0-829.1, 839.00-839.18, 839.40, 839.49-839.50, 839.59, 839.69, 839.79, 839.8-839.9, 847.0, 847.9, 848.8-848.9, 879.8-879.9, 905.1, 926.11, 929.0, 929.9, 952.00-952.09, 952.8-952.9, 958.8, 959.11-959.19, 959.8-959.9

805.1x CC Excl: see Code 805.0
805.2   CC Excl: 805.2-805.3, 805.8-805.9, 806.20-806.39, 806.8-806.9, 829.0-829.1, 839.21, 839.31, 839.40, 839.49-839.50, 839.59, 839.69, 839.79, 839.8-839.9, 847.1, 847.9, 848.8-848.9, 879.8-879.9, 905.1, 926.11, 929.0, 929.9, 952.10-952.19, 952.8-952.9, 958.8, 959.11-959.19, 959.8-959.9

805.3   CC Excl: see Code 805.2
805.4   CC Excl: 805.4-805.5, 805.8-805.9, 806.4-806.5, 806.8-806.9, 829.0-829.1, 839.20, 839.30, 839.40, 839.49-839.50, 839.59, 839.69, 839.79, 839.8-839.9, 847.2, 847.9, 848.8-848.9, 879.8-879.9, 905.1, 926.11, 929.0, 929.9, 952.2, 952.8-952.9, 958.8, 959.11-959.19, 959.8-959.9

805.5   CC Excl: see Code 805.4
805.6   CC Excl: 805.6-805.9, 806.60-806.9, 829.0-829.1, 839.40-839.59, 839.69, 839.79, 839.8-839.9, 846.0-846.9, 847.3-847.9, 848.5-848.9, 879.8-879.9, 905.1, 926.11, 929.0, 929.9, 952.3-952.9, 958.8, 959.11-959.19, 959.8-959.9

805.7   CC Excl: see Code 805.6
805.8   CC Excl: 733.10-733.19, 733.93-733.95, 805.00-805.9, 806.00-806.9, 829.0-829.1, 839.00-839.59, 839.69, 839.79, 839.8-839.9, 846.0-846.9, 847.0-847.9, 848.5-848.9, 879.8-879.9, 905.1, 926.11, 929.0, 929.9, 952.00-952.9, 958.8, 959.11-959.19, 959.8-959.9

805.9   CC Excl: see Code 805.8

806.00 CC Excl: 733.10-733.19, 733.93-733.95,
805.00-805.18, 805.8-805.9, 806.00-
806.19, 806.8-806.9, 829.0-829.1,
839.00-839.18, 839.40, 839.49-839.50,
839.59, 839.69, 839.79, 839.8-839.9,
847.9, 848.8-848.9, 879.8-879.9, 905.1,
926.11, 929.0, 929.9, 952.00-952.09,
952.8-952.9, 958.8, 959.11-959.19,
959.8-959.9
806.01 CC Excl: see Code 806.00
806.02 CC Excl: see Code 806.00
806.03 CC Excl: see Code 806.00
806.04 CC Excl: see Code 806.00
806.05 CC Excl: see Code 806.00
806.06 CC Excl: see Code 806.00
806.07 CC Excl: see Code 806.00
806.08 CC Excl: see Code 806.00
806.09 CC Excl: see Code 806.00
806.10 CC Excl: see Code 806.00
806.11 CC Excl: see Code 806.00
806.12 CC Excl: see Code 806.00
806.13 CC Excl: see Code 806.00
806.14 CC Excl: see Code 806.00
806.15 CC Excl: see Code 806.00
806.16 CC Excl: see Code 806.00
806.17 CC Excl: see Code 806.00
806.18 CC Excl: see Code 806.00
806.19 CC Excl: see Code 806.00
806.20 CC Excl: 733.10-733.19, 733.93-733.95,
805.2-805.3, 805.8-805.9, 806.20-
806.39, 806.8-806.9, 829.0-829.1,
839.21, 839.31, 839.40, 839.49-839.50,
839.59, 839.69, 839.79, 839.8-839.9,
847.1, 847.9, 848.8-848.9, 879.8-879.9,
905.1, 926.11, 929.0, 929.9, 952.10-
952.19, 952.8-952.9, 958.8, 959.11-
959.19, 959.8-959.9
806.21 CC Excl: see Code 806.20
806.22 CC Excl: see Code 806.20
806.23 CC Excl: see Code 806.20
806.24 CC Excl: see Code 806.20
806.25 CC Excl: see Code 806.20
806.26 CC Excl: see Code 806.20
806.27 CC Excl: see Code 806.20
806.28 CC Excl: see Code 806.20
806.29 CC Excl: see Code 806.20
806.30 CC Excl: see Code 806.20
806.31 CC Excl: see Code 806.20
806.32 CC Excl: see Code 806.20
806.33 CC Excl: see Code 806.20
806.34 CC Excl: see Code 806.20
806.35 CC Excl: see Code 806.20
806.36 CC Excl: see Code 806.20
806.37 CC Excl: see Code 806.20
806.38 CC Excl: see Code 806.20

806.39 CC Excl: see Code 806.20
806.4 CC Excl: 733.10-733.19, 733.93-733.95,
805.4-805.5, 805.8-805.9, 806.4-806.5,
806.8-806.9, 829.0-829.1, 839.20,
839.30, 839.40, 839.49-839.50, 839.59,
839.69, 839.79, 839.8-839.9, 847.2,
847.9, 848.8-848.9, 879.8-879.9, 905.1,
926.11, 929.0, 929.9, 952.2, 952.8-
952.9, 958.8, 959.11-959.19, 959.8-
959.9
806.5 CC Excl: see Code 806.4
806.60 CC Excl: 733.10-733.19, 733.93-733.95,
805.6-805.9, 806.60-806.9, 829.0-
829.1, 839.40-839.59, 839.69, 839.79,
839.8-839.9, 846.0-846.9, 847.0, 847.3-
847.9, 848.5-848.9, 879.8-879.9, 905.1,
926.11, 929.0, 929.9, 952.3-952.9,
958.8, 959.11-959.19, 959.8-959.9
806.61 CC Excl: see Code 806.60
806.62 CC Excl: see Code 806.60
806.69 CC Excl: see Code 806.60
806.70 CC Excl: see Code 806.60
806.71 CC Excl: see Code 806.60
806.72 CC Excl: see Code 806.60
806.79 CC Excl: see Code 806.60
806.8 CC Excl: 733.10-733.19, 733.93-733.95,
805.00-805.09, 806.00-806.9, 829.0-
829.1, 839.00-839.59, 839.69, 839.79,
839.8-839.9, 846.0-846.9, 847.0-847.9,
848.5-848.9, 879.8-879.9, 905.1,
926.11, 929.0, 929.9, 952.00-952.9,
958.8, 959.11-959.19, 959.8-959.9
806.9 CC Excl: see Code 806.8
807.0 CC Excl: **For codes 807.04-807.09:**
807.00-807.19, 807.4, 819.0-819.1,
828.0-828.1, 829.0-829.1, 848.8-848.9,
879.8-879.9, 929.0, 929.9, 958.8,
959.8-959.9
807.1x CC Excl: see Code 807.0
807.2 CC Excl: 807.2-807.4, 829.0-829.1,
848.8-848.9, 879.8-879.9, 929.0, 929.9,
958.8, 959.8-959.9
807.3 CC Excl: see Code 807.2
807.4 CC Excl: 807.00-807.4, 829.0-829.1,
848.8-848.9, 879.8-879.9, 929.0, 929.9,
958.8, 959.8-959.9
807.5 CC Excl: 807.5-807.6, 829.0-829.1,
848.8-848.9, 879.8-879.9, 929.0, 929.9,
958.8, 959.8-959.9
807.6 CC Excl: see Code 807.5

CC Exclusion List

808.0 CC Excl: 733.10-733.19, 733.93-733.95, 808.0-808.1, 808.43, 808.49, 808.53, 808.59, 808.8-808.9, 809.0-809.1, 829.0-829.1, 835.00-835.13, 843.0-843.9, 846.0-846.9 848.5-848.9, 879.8-879.9, 929.0, 929.9, 958.8, 959.6, 959.8-959.9

808.1 CC Excl: 808.0-808.1, 808.43, 808.49, 808.53, 808.59, 808.8-808.9, 809.0-809.1, 829.0-829.1, 835.00-835.13, 843.0-843.9, 846.0-846.9, 848.5-848.9, 879.8-879.9, 929.0, 929.9, 958.8, 959.6, 959.8-959.9

808.2 CC Excl: 733.10-733.19, 733.93-733.95, 808.2-808.3, 808.43, 808.49, 808.53, 808.59, 808.8-808.9, 809.0-809.1, 829.0-829.1, 835.00-835.13, 843.0-843.9, 846.0-846.9, 848.5-848.9, 879.8-879.9, 929.0, 929.9, 958.8, 959.6, 959.8-959.9

808.3 CC Excl: see Code 808.2

808.43 CC Excl: 733.10-733.19, 733.93-733.95, 808.0-808.9, 809.0-809.1, 829.0-829.1, 835.00-835.13, 843.0-843.9, 846.0-846.9, 848.5-848.9, 879.8-879.9, 929.0, 929.9, 958.8, 959.6, 959.8-959.9

808.49 CC Excl: see Code 808.43

808.51 CC Excl: 733.10-733.19, 733.93-733.95, 808.41, 808.43, 808.49, 808.51, 808.53, 808.59, 808.8-808.9, 809.0-809.1, 829.0-829.1, 835.00-835.13, 843.0-843.9, 846.0-846.9, 848.5-848.9, 879.8-879.9, 929.0, 929.9, 958.8, 959.6, 959.8-959.9

808.52 CC Excl: 733.10-733.19, 733.93-733.95, 808.42-808.49, 808.52-808.59, 808.8-808.9, 809.0-809.1, 829.0-829.1, 835.00-835.13, 843.0-843.9, 846.0-846.9, 848.5-848.9, 879.8-879.9, 929.0, 929.9, 958.8, 959.6, 959.8-959.9 "

808.53 CC Excl: 733.10-733.19, 733.93-733.95, 808.0-808.9 809.0-809.1, 829.0-829.1, 835.00-835.13, 843.0-843.9, 846.0-846.9, 848.5-848.9, 879.8-879.9, 929.0, 929.9, 958.8, 959.6, 959.8-959.9

808.59 CC Excl: see Code 808.53
808.8 CC Excl: see Code 808.53
808.9 CC Excl: see Code 808.53

820.00 CC Excl: 733.10-733.19, 733.93-733.95, 820.00-820.9 821.00-821.39, 827.0-827.1, 828.0-828.1, 829.0-829.1, 843.0-843.9, 848.8-848.9, 879.8-879.9, 929.0, 929.9, 958.8, 959.6, 959.8-959.9

820.01 CC Excl: see Code 820.00
820.02 CC Excl: see Code 820.00
820.03 CC Excl: see Code 820.00

820.09 CC Excl: see Code 820.00
820.10 CC Excl: see Code 820.00
820.11 CC Excl: see Code 820.00
820.12 CC Excl: see Code 820.00
820.13 CC Excl: see Code 820.00
820.19 CC Excl: see Code 820.00
820.20 CC Excl: see Code 820.00
820.21 CC Excl: see Code 820.00
820.22 CC Excl: see Code 820.00
820.30 CC Excl: see Code 820.00
820.31 CC Excl: see Code 820.00
820.32 CC Excl: see Code 820.00
820.8 CC Excl: see Code 820.00
820.9 CC Excl: see Code 820.00
821.00 CC Excl: see Code 820.00
821.01 CC Excl: see Code 820.00
821.10 CC Excl: see Code 820.00
821.11 CC Excl: see Code 820.00

839.00 CC Excl: 805.00-805.18, 806.00-806.19, 806.8-806.9, 839.00-839.18, 847.0, 848.8-848.9, 879.8-879.9, 929.0, 929.9, 952.00-952.09, 958.8, 959.8-959.9

839.01 CC Excl: see Code 839.00
839.02 CC Excl: see Code 839.00
839.03 CC Excl: see Code 839.00
839.04 CC Excl: see Code 839.00
839.05 CC Excl: see Code 839.00
839.06 CC Excl: see Code 839.00
839.07 CC Excl: see Code 839.00
839.08 CC Excl: see Code 839.00
839.10 CC Excl: see Code 839.00
839.11 CC Excl: see Code 839.00
839.12 CC Excl: see Code 839.00
839.13 CC Excl: see Code 839.00
839.14 CC Excl: see Code 839.00
839.15 CC Excl: see Code 839.00
839.16 CC Excl: see Code 839.00
839.17 CC Excl: see Code 839.00
839.18 CC Excl: see Code 839.00

850.0 CC Excl: 800.00-800.99, 801.00-801.99, 803.00-803.99, 804.00-804.99, 850.0-850.9, 851.00-851.99, 852.00-852.19, 852.21-852.59, 853.00-853.19, 854.00-854.19, 873.8-873.9, 879.8-879.9, 905.0, 925.1-925.2, 929.0, 929.9, 958.8, 959.01, 959.09, 959.8-959.9

850.1 CC Excl: see Code 850.0
850.2 CC Excl: see Code 850.0
850.3 CC Excl: see Code 850.0
850.4 CC Excl: see Code 850.0
850.5 CC Excl: see Code 850.0
850.9 CC Excl: see Code 850.0
851.0 CC Excl: see Code 850.0
851.1 CC Excl: see Code 850.0

851.2	CC Excl: see Code 850.0
851.3	CC Excl: see Code 850.0
851.4	CC Excl: see Code 850.0
851.5	CC Excl: see Code 850.0
851.6	CC Excl: see Code 850.0
851.7	CC Excl: see Code 850.0
851.8	CC Excl: see Code 850.0
851.9	CC Excl: see Code 850.0
852.0	CC Excl: see Code 850.0
852.1	CC Excl: see Code 850.0

852.2 CC Excl: **For code 852.20:** 800.00-800.99, 801.00-801.99, 803.00-803.99, 804.00-804.99, 850.0-850.9, 851.00-851.99, 852.00-852.59, 853.00-853.19, 854.00-854.19, 873.8-873.9, 879.8-879.9, 905.0, 925.1-925.2, 929.0, 929.9, 958.8, 959.01, 959.09, 959.8-959.9 **For code 852.21:** 800.00-800.99, 801.00-801.99, 803.00-803.99, 804.00-804.99, 850.0-850.9, 851.00-851.99, 852.00-852.19, 852.21-852.59, 853.00-853.19, 854.00-854.19, 873.8-873.9, 879.8-879.9, 905.0, 925.1-925.2, 929.0, 929.9, 958.8, 959.01, 959.09, 959.8-959.9 For codes 852.22-852.29: see Code 852.21

852.3	CC Excl: see Code 852.21
852.4	CC Excl: see Code 852.21
852.5	CC Excl: see Code 852.21
853.0	CC Excl: see Code 852.21
853.1	CC Excl: see Code 852.21
854.0	CC Excl: see Code 852.21
854.1	CC Excl: see Code 852.21

860.0 CC Excl: 860.0-860.5, 861.20-861.32, 862.29, 862.39, 862.8-862.9, 875.0-875.1, 879.8-879.9, 929.0, 929.9, 958.7-958.8, 959.8-959.9

860.1	CC Excl: see Code 860.0
860.2	CC Excl: see Code 860.0
860.3	CC Excl: see Code 860.0
860.4	CC Excl: see Code 860.0
860.5	CC Excl: see Code 860.0

861.01 CC Excl: 861.00-861.13, 862.29, 862.39, 862.8-862.9, 875.0-875.1, 879.8-879.9, 929.0, 929.9, 958.7-958.8, 959.8-959.9

861.02	CC Excl: see Code 861.01
861.03	CC Excl: see Code 861.01
861.10	CC Excl: see Code 861.01
861.11	CC Excl: see Code 861.01
861.12	CC Excl: see Code 861.01
861.13	CC Excl: see Code 861.01

861.22 CC Excl: 861.20-861.32, 862.29, 862.39, 862.8-862.9, 875.0-875.1, 879.8-879.9, 929.0, 929.9, 958.7-958.8, 959.8-959.9

861.30	CC Excl: see Code 861.22
861.31	CC Excl: see Code 861.22
861.32	CC Excl: see Code 861.22

862.1 CC Excl: 862.0-862.1, 862.29, 862.39, 862.8-862.9, 875.0-875.1, 879.8-879.9, 929.0, 929.9, 958.7-958.8, 959.8-959.9

862.21 CC Excl: 862.21, 862.29, 862.31, 862.39, 862.8-862.9, 875.0-875.1, 879.8-879.9, 929.0, 929.9, 958.7-958.8, 959.8-959.9

862.22 CC Excl: 862.22, 862.29, 862.32, 862.39, 862.8-862.9, 875.0-875.1, 879.8-879.9, 929.0, 929.9, 958.7-958.8, 959.8-959.9

862.29 CC Excl: 862.29, 862.39, 862.8-862.9, 875.0-875.1, 879.8-879.9, 929.0, 929.9, 958.7-958.8, 959.8-959.9 "

862.31 CC Excl: 862.21, 862.29, 862.31, 862.39, 862.8-862.9, 875.0-875.1, 879.8-879.9, 929.0, 929.9, 958.7-958.8, 959.8-959.9

862.32 CC Excl: 862.22, 862.29, 862.32, 862.39, 862.8-862.9, 875.0-875.1, 879.8-879.9, 929.0, 929.9, 958.7-958.8, 959.8-959.9

862.39 CC Excl: 862.29, 862.39, 862.8-862.9, 875.0-875.1, 879.8-879.9, 929.0, 929.9, 958.7-958.8, 959.8-959.9 "

862.9 CC Excl: see Code 862.39

863.1 CC Excl: 863.0-863.1, 863.80, 863.89-863.90, 863.99, 868.00, 868.03-868.10, 868.13-868.19, 869.0-869.1, 879.2-879.9, 929.0, 929.9, 958.8, 959.8-959.9

863.30 CC Excl: 863.20-863.39, 863.80, 863.89-863.90, 863.99, 868.00, 868.03-868.10, 868.13-868.19, 869.0-869.1, 879.2-879.9, 929.0, 929.9, 958.8, 959.8-959.9

863.31 CC Excl: 863.21, 863.31, 863.39, 863.80, 863.89-863.90, 863.99, 868.00, 868.03-868.10, 868.13-868.19, 869.0-869.1, 879.2-879.9, 929.0, 929.9, 958.8, 959.8-959.9

863.39 CC Excl: 863.20-863.39, 863.80, 863.89-863.90, 863.99, 868.00, 868.03-868.10, 868.13-868.19, 869.0-869.1, 879.2-879.9, 929.0, 929.9, 958.8, 959.8-959.9

863.50 CC Excl: 863.40-863.59, 863.80, 863.89-863.90, 863.99, 868.00, 868.03-868.10, 868.13-868.19, 869.0-869.1, 879.2-879.9, 929.0, 929.9, 958.8, 959.8-959.9

863.51	CC Excl: see Code 863.50
863.52	CC Excl: see Code 863.50
863.53	CC Excl: see Code 863.50

863.54 CC Excl: see Code 863.50
863.55 CC Excl: see Code 863.50
863.56 CC Excl: see Code 863.50
863.59 CC Excl: see Code 863.50
863.90 CC Excl: 863.80-863.84, 863.89-863.94,
        863.99, 868.00, 868.03-868.10, 868.13-
        868.19, 869.0-869.1, 879.2-879.9,
        929.0, 929.9, 958.8, 959.8-959.9
863.91 CC Excl: 863.80-863.84, 863.91-863.94,
        863.99, 868.00, 868.03-868.10, 868.13-
        868.19, 869.0-869.1, 879.2-879.9,
        929.01, 929.9, 958.8, 959.8-959.9
863.92 CC Excl: see Code 863.91
863.93 CC Excl: see Code 863.91
863.94 CC Excl: see Code 863.91
863.95 CC Excl: 863.80, 863.85, 863.95,
        863.99, 868.00, 868.03-868.10, 868.13-
        868.19, 869.0-869.1, 879.2-879.9,
        929.0, 929.9, 958.8, 959.8-959.9
863.99 CC Excl: 863.80, 863.99, 868.00,
        868.03-868.10, 868.13-868.19, 869.0-
        869.1, 879.2-879.9, 929.0, 929.9, 958.8,
        959.8-959.9
864.0   CC Excl: 863.80, 863.99, 864.00-
        864.19, 868.00, 868.03-868.10, 868.13-
        868.19, 869.0-869.1, 879.2-879.9,
        929.0, 929.9, 958.8, 959.8-959.9
864.1   CC Excl: see Code 864.0
865.0   CC Excl: 865.00-865.19, 868.00,
        868.03-868.10, 868.13-868.19, 869.0-
        869.1, 879.2-879.9, 929.0, 929.9, 958.8,
        959.8-959.9
865.1   CC Excl: see Code 865.0
866.0   CC Excl: 866.00-866.13, 868.00,
        868.03-868.10, 868.13-868.19, 869.0-
        869.1, 879.2-879.9, 929.0, 929.9, 958.8,
        959.8-959.9
866.1   CC Excl: see Code 866.0
867.0   CC Excl: 867.0-867.1, 867.6-867.9,
        868.00, 868.03-868.10, 868.13-868.19,
        869.0-869.1, 879.2-879.9, 929.0, 929.9,
        958.8, 959.8-959.9
867.1   CC Excl: see Code 867.0
867.2   CC Excl: 867.2-867.3, 867.6-867.9,
        868.00, 868.03-868.10, 868.13-868.19,
        869.0-869.1, 879.2-879.9, 929.0, 929.9,
        958.8, 959.8-959.9
867.3   CC Excl: see Code 867.2
867.4   CC Excl: 867.4-867.9, 868.00, 868.03-
        868.10, 868.13-868.19, 869.0-869.1,
        879.2-879.9, 929.0, 929.9, 958.8,
        959.8-959.9
867.5   CC Excl: see Code 867.4

867.6   CC Excl: 867.6-867.9, 868.00, 868.03-
        868.10, 868.13-868.19, 869.0-869.1,
        879.2-879.9, 929.0, 929.9, 958.8,
        959.8-959.9
867.7   CC Excl: see Code 867.6
867.8   CC Excl: see Code 867.6
867.9   CC Excl: see Code 867.6
868.0   CC Excl: **For code 868.00:** 868.00,
        868.03-868.10, 868.13-868.19, 869.0-
        869.1, 879.2-879.9, 929.0, 929.9, 958.8,
        959.8-959.9 **For code 868.01:** 868.00,
        868.01, 868.03-868.11, 868.13-868.19,
        869.0-869.1, 879.2-879.9, 929.0, 929.9,
        958.8, 959.8-959.9 **For code 868.02:**
        868.00, 868.02-868.10, 868.13-868.19,
        869.0-869.1, 879.2-879.9, 929.0, 929.9,
        958.8, 959.8-959.9 For codes 868.03-
        868.09: 868.00, 868.03-868.10, 868.13-
        868.19, 869.0-869.1, 879.2-879.9,
        929.0, 929.9, 958.8, 959.8-959.9
868.1   CC Excl: **For code 868.10:** see Code
        868.03 **For code 868.11:** 868.00, 868.01,
        868.03-868.11, 868.13-868.19, 869.0-
        869.1, 879.2-879.9, 929.0, 929.9, 958.8,
        959.8-959.9 **For code 868.12:** 868.00,
        868.03-868.10, 868.12-868.19, 869.0-
        869.1, 879.2-879.9, 929.0, 929.9, 958.8,
        959.8-959.9 For codes 868.13-868.19:
        868.00, 868.03-868.10, 868.13-868.19,
        869.0-869.1, 879.2-879.9, 929.0, 929.9,
        958.8, 959.8-959.9
869.0   CC Excl: see Code 868.13
869.1   CC Excl: see Code 868.13
870.3   CC Excl: 870.0-870.9, 871.0-871.9,
        879.8-879.9, 929.0, 929.9, 958.8,
        959.8-959.9
870.4   CC Excl: see Code 870.3
870.8   CC Excl: see Code 870.3
870.9   CC Excl: see Code 870.3
871.0   CC Excl: see Code 870.3
871.1   CC Excl: see Code 870.3
871.2   CC Excl: see Code 870.3
871.3   CC Excl: see Code 870.3
871.4   CC Excl: see Code 870.3
871.9   CC Excl: see Code 870.3
872.72 CC Excl: 872.00-872.9, 879.8-879.9,
        929.0, 929.9, 958.8, 959.8-959.9
872.73 CC Excl: see Code 872.72
872.74 CC Excl: see Code 872.72
873.33 CC Excl: 873.20-873.39, 879.8-879.9,
        929.0, 929.9, 958.8, 959.8-959.9
873.9   CC Excl: 847.0, 873.40-873.79, 873.9,
        874.8-874.9, 879.8-879.9, 929.0, 929.9,
        958.8, 959.8-959.9

874.00   CC Excl: 847.0, 874.00-874.12, 874.8-874.9, 879.8-879.9, 929.0, 929.9, 958.8, 959.8-959.9

874.01   CC Excl: see Code 874.00

874.02   CC Excl: see Code 874.00

874.10   CC Excl: see Code 874.00

874.11   CC Excl: see Code 874.00

874.12   CC Excl: see Code 874.00

874.3   CC Excl: 847.0, 874.2-874.3, 874.8-874.9, 879.8-879.9, 929.0, 929.9, 958.8, 959.8-959.9

874.5   CC Excl: 847.0, 874.4-874.9, 879.8-879.9, 929.0, 929.9, 958.8, 959.8-959.9

875.0   CC Excl: 847.1, 862.29, 862.39, 862.8-862.9, 875.0-875.1, 879.8-879.9, 929.0, 929.9, 958.7-958.8, 959.8-959.9

875.1   CC Excl: see Code 875.0

887.0   CC Excl: 880.00-880.29, 881.00-881.22, 882.0-882.2, 883.0-883.2, 884.0-884.2, 885.0-885.1, 886.0-886.1, 887.0-887.7, 929.0, 929.9, 958.8, 959.8-959.9

887.1   CC Excl: see Code 887.0

887.2   CC Excl: see Code 887.0

887.3   CC Excl: see Code 887.0

887.4   CC Excl: see Code 887.0

887.5   CC Excl: see Code 887.0

887.6   CC Excl: see Code 887.0

887.7   CC Excl: see Code 887.0

896.0   CC Excl: 890.0-890.2, 891.0-891.2, 892.0-892.2, 893.0-893.2, 894.0-894.2, 895.0-895.1, 896.0-896.3, 897.0-897.7, 929.0, 929.9, 958.8, 959.8-959.9

896.1   CC Excl: see Code 896.0

896.2   CC Excl: see Code 896.0

896.3   CC Excl: see Code 896.0

897.0   CC Excl: see Code 896.0

897.1   CC Excl: see Code 896.0

897.2   CC Excl: see Code 896.0

897.3   CC Excl: see Code 896.0

897.4   CC Excl: see Code 896.0

897.5   CC Excl: see Code 896.0

897.6   CC Excl: see Code 896.0

897.7   CC Excl: see Code 896.0

900.00   CC Excl: 900.00, 900.82, 900.89, 900.9, 904.9, 929.0, 929.9, 958.8, 959.8-959.9

900.01   CC Excl: see Code 900.00

900.02   CC Excl: see Code 900.00

900.03   CC Excl: see Code 900.00

900.1   CC Excl: 900.82, 900.89, 900.9, 904.9, 929.0, 929.9, 958.8, 959.8-959.9

900.81   CC Excl: see Code 900.1

900.82   CC Excl: see Code 900.1

900.89   CC Excl: see Code 900.1

900.9   CC Excl: see Code 900.1

901.0   CC Excl: 901.0, 904.9, 929.0, 929.9, 958.8, 959.8-959.9

901.1   CC Excl: 901.1, 904.9, 929.0, 929.9, 958.8, 959.8-959.9

901.2   CC Excl: 901.2, 904.9, 929.0, 929.9, 958.8, 959.8-959.9

901.3   CC Excl: 901.3, 904.9, 929.0, 929.9, 958.8, 959.8-959.9

901.41   CC Excl: 901.40, 901.41, 904.9, 929.0, 929.9, 958.8, 959.8-959.9

901.42   CC Excl: 901.40, 901.42, 904.9, 929.0, 929.9, 958.8, 959.8-959.9

901.83   CC Excl: 904.9, 929.0, 929.9, 958.8, 959.8-959.9

902.0   CC Excl: 902.0, 902.87, 902.89, 902.9, 904.9, 929.0, 929.9, 958.8, 959.8-959.9

902.10   CC Excl: 902.10, 902.87, 902.89, 902.9, 904.9, 929.0, 929.9, 958.8, 959.8-959.9

902.11   CC Excl: 902.11, 902.87, 902.89, 902.9, 904.9, 929.0, 929.9, 958.8, 959.8-959.9

902.19   CC Excl: 902.19, 902.87, 902.89, 902.9, 904.9, 929.0, 929.9, 958.8, 959.8-959.9

902.20   CC Excl: 902.20, 902.87, 902.89, 902.9, 904.9, 929.0, 929.9, 958.8, 959.8-959.9

902.22   CC Excl: 902.22, 902.87, 902.89, 902.9, 904.9, 929.0, 929.9, 958.8, 959.8-959.9

902.23   CC Excl: 902.23, 902.87, 902.89, 902.9, 904.9, 929.0, 929.9, 958.8, 959.8-959.9

902.24   CC Excl: 902.24, 902.87, 902.89, 902.9, 904.9, 929.0, 929.9, 958.8, 959.8-959.9

902.25   CC Excl: 902.25, 902.87, 902.89, 902.9, 904.9, 929.0, 929.9, 958.8, 959.8-959.9

902.26   CC Excl: 902.26, 902.87, 902.89, 902.9, 904.9, 929.0, 929.9, 958.8, 959.8-959.9

902.27   CC Excl: 902.7, 902.87, 902.89, 902.9, 904.9, 929.0, 929.9, 958.8, 959.8-959.9

902.29   CC Excl: 902.29, 902.87, 902.89, 902.9, 904.9, 929.0, 929.9, 958.8, 959.8-959.9

902.31   CC Excl: 902.31, 902.87, 902.89, 902.9, 904.9, 929.0, 929.9, 958.8, 959.8-959.9

902.32   CC Excl: 902.32, 902.87, 902.89, 902.9, 904.9, 929.0, 929.9, 958.8, 959.8-959.9

902.33   CC Excl: 902.33, 902.87, 902.89, 902.9, 904.9, 929.0, 929.9, 958.8, 959.8-959.9

902.34   CC Excl: 902.34, 902.87, 902.89, 902.9, 904.9, 929.0, 929.9, 958.8, 959.8-959.9

902.39   CC Excl: 902.39, 902.87, 902.89, 902.9, 904.9, 929.0, 929.9, 958.8, 959.8-959.9

902.40   CC Excl: 902.40, 902.87, 902.89, 902.9, 904.9, 929.0, 929.9, 958.8, 959.8-959.9

902.41   CC Excl: 902.41, 902.87, 902.89, 902.9, 904.9, 929.0, 929.9, 958.8, 959.8-959.9

902.42   CC Excl: 902.42, 902.87, 902.89, 902.9, 904.9, 929.0, 929.9, 958.8, 959.8-959.9

902.49 CC Excl: 902.49, 902.87, 902.89, 902.9, 904.9, 929.0, 929.9, 958.8, 959.8-959.9

902.50 CC Excl: 902.50, 902.53-902.54, 902.59, 902.87, 902.89, 902.9, 904.9, 929.0, 929.9, 958.8, 959.8-959.9

902.51 CC Excl: 902.51, 902.87, 902.89, 902.9, 904.9, 929.0, 929.9, 958.8, 959.8-959.9

902.52 CC Excl: 902.52, 902.87, 902.89, 902.9, 904.9, 929.0, 929.9, 958.8, 959.8-959.9

902.53 CC Excl: 902.50, 902.53, 902.59, 902.87, 902.89, 902.9, 904.9, 929.0, 929.9, 958.8, 959.8-959.9

902.54 CC Excl: 902.50, 902.54, 902.59, 902.87, 902.89, 902.9, 904.9, 929.0, 929.9, 958.8, 959.8-959.9

902.59 CC Excl: 902.50, 902.53-902.54, 902.59, 902.87, 902.89, 902.9, 904.9, 929.0, 929.9, 958.8, 959.8-959.9

902.87 CC Excl: 902.87, 902.89, 902.9, 904.9, 929.0, 929.9, 958.8, 959.8-959.9

904.0 CC Excl: No exclusions

925.1 CC Excl: 873.8-873.9, 905.0, 925.1-925.2, 929.0, 929.9, 958.8, 959.01, 959.09, 959.8-959.9

925.2 CC Excl: 873.8-873.9, 905.0, 925.1-925.2, 929.0, 929.9, 958.8, 959.01, 959.09, 959.8-959.9

929.0 CC Excl: 929.0, 929.9, 958.8, 959.8-959.9

952.00 CC Excl: 805.00-805.18, 805.8-805.9, 806.00-806.19, 806.8-806.9, 839.00-839.18, 839.40, 839.49-839.50, 839.59, 839.69, 839.79, 839.8-839.9, 847.9, 905.1, 926.11, 952.00-952.09, 952.8-952.9, 958.8, 959.11-959.19, 959.8-959.9

952.01 CC Excl: see Code 952.00

952.02 CC Excl: see Code 952.00

952.03 CC Excl: see Code 952.00

952.04 CC Excl: see Code 952.00

952.05 CC Excl: see Code 952.00

952.06 CC Excl: see Code 952.00

952.07 CC Excl: see Code 952.00

952.08 CC Excl: see Code 952.00

952.09 CC Excl: see Code 952.00

952.10 CC Excl: 805.8-805.9, 806.20-806.39, 839.40, 839.49-839.50, 839.59, 839.69, 839.79, 839.8-839.9, 847.9, 905.1, 926.11, 952.10-952.19, 952.8-952.9, 958.8, 959.11-959.19, 959.8-959.9

952.11 CC Excl: see Code 952.10

952.12 CC Excl: see Code 952.10

952.13 CC Excl: see Code 952.10

952.14 CC Excl: see Code 952.10

952.15 CC Excl: see Code 952.10

952.16 CC Excl: see Code 952.10

952.17 CC Excl: see Code 952.10

952.18 CC Excl: see Code 952.10

952.19 CC Excl: see Code 952.10

952.2 CC Excl: 805.8-805.9, 806.4-806.5, 839.40, 839.49-839.50, 839.59, 839.69, 839.79, 839.8-839.9, 847.9, 905.1, 926.11, 952.2, 952.8-952.9, 958.8, 959.11-959.19, 959.8-959.9

952.3 CC Excl: 805.8-805.9, 806.60-806.79, 839.40, 839.49-839.50, 839.59, 839.69, 839.79, 839.8-839.9, 847.9, 905.1, 926.11, 952.3-952.4, 952.8-952.9, 958.8, 959.11-959.19, 959.8-959.9

952.4 CC Excl: see Code 952.3

952.8 CC Excl: 805.8-805.9, 839.40, 839.49-839.50, 839.59, 839.69, 839.79, 839.8-839.9, 847.9, 905.1, 926.11, 952.8-952.9, 958.8, 959.11-959.19, 959.8-959.9

952.9 CC Excl: 805.8-805.9, 839.40, 839.49-839.50, 839.59, 839.69, 839.79, 839.8-839.9, 847.9, 905.1, 926.11, 952.8-952.9, 958.8, 959.11-959.19, 959.8-959.9

953.0 CC Excl: 953.8-953.9, 958.8, 959.8-959.9

953.1 CC Excl: see Code 953.0

953.2 CC Excl: see Code 953.0

953.3 CC Excl: see Code 953.0

953.4 CC Excl: see Code 953.0

953.5 CC Excl: see Code 953.0

953.8 CC Excl: see Code 953.0

953.9 CC Excl: see Code 953.0

958.0 CC Excl: 958.0, 958.8, 959.8-959.9, 997.91, 997.99, 998.81, 998.83-998.9, 999.1

958.1 CC Excl: 958.1, 958.8, 959.8-959.9, 997.91, 997.99, 998.81, 998.83-998.9

958.2 CC Excl: 958.2, 958.8, 959.8-959.9, 997.91, 997.99, 998.81, 998.83-998.9

958.3 CC Excl: 958.3, 958.8, 959.8-959.9, 997.91, 997.99, 998.81, 998.83-998.9

958.4 CC Excl: 958.4, 958.8, 959.8-959.9, 997.91, 997.99, 998.81, 998.83-998.9

958.5 CC Excl: 958.5, 958.8, 959.8-959.9, 995.4, 997.91, 997.99, 998.0, 998.11-998.13, 998.81, 998.83-998.9

958.7 CC Excl: 860.0-860.5, 861.20-861.32, 862.0-862.1, 862.29, 862.31-862.9, 875.0-875.1, 958.7-958.8, 959.8-959.9, 997.91, 997.99, 998.81, 998.83-998.9

995.4 CC Excl: 958.4, 995.4, 997.91, 997.99, 998.0, 998.11-998.13, 998.81, 998.83-998.9

995.86 CC Excl: 958.4, 995.4, 995.86, 997.91, 997.99, 998.0, 998.11-998.13, 998.81, 998.83-998.9

995.90 CC Excl: 003.1, 020.2, 036.2, 038.0, 038.10-038.11, 038.19, 038.2, 038.3, 038.40-038.44, 038.49, 038.8, 038.9, 040.82, 040.89, 041.00-041.05, 041.09, 041.10-041.11, 041.19, 041.2-041.7, 041.81-041.86, 041.89, 041.9, 054.5, 139.8, 995.90-995.94, V09.0-V09.4, V09.50-V09.51, V09.6, V09.70-V09.71, V09.80-V09.81, V09.90-V09.91

995.91 CC Excl: 003.1, 020.2, 036.2, 038.0, 038.10-038.11, 038.19, 038.2, 038.3, 038.40-038.44, 038.49, 038.8, 038.9, 040.82, 040.89, 041.00-041.05, 041.09, 041.10-041.11, 041.19, 041.2-041.7, 041.81-041.86, 041.89, 041.9, 054.5, 139.8, 995.90-995.94, V09.0-V09.4, V09.50-V09.51, V09.6, V09.70-V09.71, V09.80-V09.81, V09.90-V09.91

995.92 CC Excl: 003.1, 020.2, 036.2, 038.0, 038.10-038.11, 038.19, 038.2, 038.3, 038.40-038.44, 038.49, 038.8, 038.9, 040.82, 040.89, 041.00-041.05, 041.09, 041.10-041.11, 041.19, 041.2-041.7, 041.81-041.86, 041.89, 041.9, 054.5, 139.8, 995.90-995.94, V09.0-V09.4, V09.50-V09.51, V09.6, V09.70-V09.71, V09.80-V09.81, V09.90-V09.91

995.93 CC Excl: 003.1, 020.2, 036.2, 038.0, 038.10-038.11, 038.19, 038.2, 038.3, 038.40-038.44, 038.49, 038.8, 038.9, 040.82, 040.89, 041.00-041.05, 041.09, 041.10-041.11, 041.19, 041.2-041.7, 041.81-041.86, 041.89, 041.9, 054.5, 139.8, 995.90-995.94, V09.0-V09.4, V09.50-V09.51, V09.6, V09.70-V09.71, V09.80-V09.81, V09.90-V09.91

995.94 CC Excl: 003.1, 020.2, 036.2, 038.0, 038.10-038.11, 038.19, 038.2, 038.3, 038.40-038.44, 038.49, 038.8, 038.9, 040.82, 040.89, 041.00-041.05, 041.09, 041.10-041.11, 041.19, 041.2-041.7, 041.81-041.86, 041.89, 041.9, 054.5, 139.8, 995.90-995.94, V09.0-V09.4, V09.50-V09.51, V09.6, V09.70-V09.71, V09.80-V09.81, V09.90-V09.91

996.00 CC Excl: 996.00, 996.04, 996.61-996.62, 996.70-996.74, 997.91, 997.99, 998.81, 998.83-998.9

996.01 CC Excl: 996.01, 997.91, 997.99, 998.81, 998.83-998.9

996.02 CC Excl: 996.02, 997.91, 997.99, 998.81, 998.83-998.9

996.03 CC Excl: 996.03, 997.91, 997.99, 998.81, 998.83-998.9

996.04 CC Excl: 996.04, 997.91, 997.99, 998.81, 998.83-998.9

996.09 CC Excl: 996.09, 997.91, 997.99, 998.81, 998.83-998.9

996.1 CC Excl: 996.1, 997.91, 997.99, 998.81, 998.83-998.9

996.2 CC Excl: 996.2, 996.63, 996.75, 997.91, 997.99, 998.81, 998.83-998.9

996.30 CC Excl: 996.30, 996.64-996.65, 996.76, 997.91, 997.99, 998.81, 998.83-998.9

996.39 CC Excl: 996.39, 996.64-996.65, 996.76, 997.91, 997.99, 998.81, 998.83-998.9

996.4 CC Excl: 996.4, 996.66-996.67, 996.77-996.78, 997.91, 997.99, 998.81, 998.83-998.9

996.51 CC Excl: 996.51, 997.91, 997.99

996.52 CC Excl: 996.52, 996.55, 997.91, 997.99

996.53 CC Excl: 996.53, 997.91, 997.99

996.54 CC Excl: 996.54, 997.91, 997.99

996.55 CC Excl: 996.52, 996.55-996.60, 996.68-996.69, 996.70, 996.79, 997.91, 997.99

996.56 CC Excl: 996.56, 996.59-997.99

996.57 CC Excl: 996.00-996.2, 996.30, 996.39, 996.4, 996.51-996.79, 997.91-997.99, 998.81, 998.83-998.9

996.59 CC Excl: 996.59-997.99

996.60 CC Excl: 996.00-996.30, 996.39-996.79, 997.91, 997.99, 998.81, 998.83-998.9

996.61 CC Excl: 996.00-996.1, 996.52, 996.55-996.62, 996.68-996.74, 996.79, 997.91, 997.99, 998.81, 998.83-998.9

996.62 CC Excl: see Code 996.61

996.63 CC Excl: 996.2, 996.52, 996.55-996.60, 996.63, 996.68-996.70, 996.75, 996.79, 997.91, 997.99, 998.81, 998.83-998.9

996.64 CC Excl: 599.0, 996.30, 996.39, 996.56-996.60, 996.64-996.65, 996.68-996.70, 996.76, 996.79, 997.91, 997.99, 998.81, 998.83-998.9

996.65 CC Excl: 996.30, 996.39, 996.52, 996.55-996.60, 996.64-996.65, 996.68-996.70, 996.76, 996.79, 997.91, 997.99, 998.81, 998.83-998.9

996.66 CC Excl: 996.4, 996.52, 996.55-996.60, 996.66-996.70, 996.77-996.79, 997.91, 997.99, 998.81, 998.83-998.9

996.67 CC Excl: see Code 996.66

996.68 CC Excl: 996.56, 996.59, 996.60, 996.68-996.70, 996.79, 997.91, 997.99

996.69 CC Excl: 996.00-996.30, 996.39-996.79, 997.91, 997.99, 998.81, 998.83-998.9

996.70 CC Excl: see Code 996.69

996.71 CC Excl: 996.00, 996.02, 996.09, 996.1, 996.52, 996.55-996.62, 996.68-996.74, 996.79, 997.91-997.99, 998.81, 998.83-998.9

996.72 CC Excl: 996.00-996.02, 996.04, 996.09, 996.1, 996.52, 996.55-996.62, 996.68-996.74, 996.79, 997.91-997.99, 998.81, 998.83-998.9

996.73 CC Excl: 996.1, 996.52, 996.55-996.60, 996.68-996.70, 996.73, 996.79, 997.91, 997.99, 998.81, 998.83-998.9

996.74 CC Excl: 996.00-996.1, 996.52, 996.55-996.62, 996.68-996.74, 996.79, 997.91, 997.99, 998.81, 998.83-998.9

996.75 CC Excl: 996.2, 996.52, 996.55-996.60, 996.63, 996.68-996.70, 996.75, 996.79, 997.91, 997.99, 998.81, 998.83-998.9

996.76 CC Excl: 996.30, 996.39, 996.52, 996.55-996.60, 996.64-996.65, 996.68-996.70, 996.76, 996.79, 997.91, 997.99, 998.81, 998.83-998.9

996.77 CC Excl: 996.4, 996.52, 996.55-996.60, 996.66-996.67, 996.69-996.70, 996.77-996.79, 997.91, 997.99, 998.81, 998.83-998.9

996.78 CC Excl: see Code 996.77

996.79 CC Excl: 996.00-996.30, 996.39, 996.4-996.79, 997.91, 997.99, 998.81, 998.83-998.9

996.80 CC Excl: 996.80, 996.87, 997.91, 997.99

996.81 CC Excl: 996.81, 997.91, 997.99

996.82 CC Excl: 996.82, 997.91, 997.99

996.83 CC Excl: 996.83, 997.91, 997.99

996.84 CC Excl: 996.84, 997.91, 997.99

996.85 CC Excl: 996.85, 997.91, 997.99

996.86 CC Excl: 996.86, 997.91, 997.99

996.87 CC Excl: 996.80, 996.87, 997.91, 997.99

996.89 CC Excl: 996.89, 997.91, 997.99

996.90 CC Excl: 996.90, 997.91, 997.99, 998.81, 998.83-998.9

996.91 CC Excl: 996.91, 997.91, 997.99, 998.81, 998.83-998.9

996.92 CC Excl: 996.92, 997.91, 997.99, 998.81, 998.83-998.9

996.93 CC Excl: 996.93, 997.91, 997.99, 998.81, 998.83-998.9

996.94 CC Excl: 996.94, 997.91, 997.99, 998.81, 998.83-998.9

996.95 CC Excl: 996.95, 997.91, 997.99, 998.81, 998.83-998.9

996.96 CC Excl: 996.96, 997.91, 997.99, 998.81, 998.83-998.9

996.99 CC Excl: 996.99, 997.91, 997.99, 998.81, 998.83-998.9

997.0 CC Excl: For codes 997.00-997.09: 997.00-997.09, 997.91, 997.99, 998.81, 998.83, 998.89, 998.9

997.1 CC Excl: 997.1, 997.91, 997.99, 998.81, 998.83-998.9

997.2 CC Excl: 997.2, 997.79, 997.91, 997.99, 998.81, 998.83-998.9

997.3 CC Excl: 997.3, 997.91, 997.99, 998.81, 998.83-998.9

997.4 CC Excl: 536.40-536.49, 997.4, 997.71, 997.91, 997.99, 998.81, 998.83-998.9

997.5 CC Excl: 997.5, 997.72, 997.91, 997.99, 998.81, 998.83-998.9

997.62 CC Excl: 997.60, 997.62, 997.69, 997.91, 997.99, 998.81, 998.83-998.9

997.71 CC Excl: 997.2, 997.71-997.79, 997.91, 997.99, 998.81, 998.83-998.9

997.72 CC Excl: see Code 997.71

997.79 CC Excl: see Code 997.71

997.99 CC Excl: 997.91, 997.99, 998.81, 998.83-998.9

998.0 CC Excl: 958.4, 995.4, 997.91, 997.99, 998.0, 998.11-998.13, 998.81, 998.83-998.9

998.11   CC Excl: 456.0, 456.20, 530.81-530.83, 530.89, 531.00-531.01, 531.20-531.21, 531.40-531.41, 531.60-531.61, 532.00-532.01, 532.20-532.21, 532.40-532.41, 532.60-532.61, 533.00-533.01, 533.20-533.21, 533.40-533.41, 533.60-533.61, 534.00-534.01, 534.20-534.21, 534.40-534.41, 534.60-534.61, 535.01, 535.11, 535.21, 535.31, 535.41, 535.51, 535.61, 537.83, 562.02-562.03, 562.12-562.13, 569.3, 569.85, 578.0-578.1, 578.9, 772.4, 997.91, 997.99, 998.0, 998.11-998.13, 998.81, 998.89, 998.9

998.12   CC Excl: see code 998.11

998.13   CC Excl: see Code 998.11

998.2   CC Excl: 997.91, 997.99, 998.2, 998.81, 998.83-998.9

998.31   CC Excl: 997.91, 997.99, 998.31, 998.32, 998.81, 998.83, 998.89, 998.9

998.32   CC Excl: 997.91, 997.99, 998.31, 998.32, 998.81, 998.83, 998.89, 998.9

998.4   CC Excl: 997.91, 997.99, 998.4, 998.81, 998.83-998.9

998.51   CC Excl: 997.91, 997.99, 998.51-998.59, 998.81, 998.83-998.9

998.59   CC Excl: see Code 998.51

998.6   CC Excl: 997.91, 997.99, 998.6, 998.81, 998.83-998.9

998.7   CC Excl: 997.91, 997.99, 998.7-998.81, 998.83-998.9

998.83   CC Excl: 997.91, 997.99, 998.81, 998.83, 998.89, 998.9

998.89   CC Excl: see code 998.83

998.9   CC Excl: see code 998.83

999.1   CC Excl: 958.0, 999.1

999.2   CC Excl: 999.2

999.3   CC Excl: 999.3

999.4   CC Excl: 999.4

999.5   CC Excl: 999.5

999.6   CC Excl: 999.6

999.7   CC Excl: 999.7

999.8   CC Excl: 999.8

V23.7   CC Excl: V22.0- V23.9

V23.81   CC Excl: see Code V23.7

V23.82   CC Excl: see Code V23.7

V23.83   CC Excl: see Code V23.7

V23.84   CC Excl: see Code V23.7

V23.89   CC Excl: see Code V23.7

V23.9   CC Excl: see Code V23.7

V42.0   CC Excl: 996.80-996.81, 996.87, V42.0, V42.89-V42.9

V42.1   CC Excl: 996.80, 996.83, 996.87, V42.1, V42.89-V42.9

V42.2   CC Excl: 996.71, V42.2, V42.89-V42.9

V42.6   CC Excl: 996.80, 996.84, 996.87, V42.6, V42.89-V42.9

V42.7   CC Excl: 996.80, 996.82, 996.87, V42.7, V42.89-V42.9

V42.81   CC Excl: 996.80, 996.85, 996.87, V42.9

V42.82   CC Excl: 996.80, 996.87, V42.9

V42.83   CC Excl: 996.80, 996.86-996.87, V42.83, V42.9

V42.84   CC Excl: 996.80, 996.89, V42.84-V42.9

V42.89   CC Excl: 996.80, 996.87-996.89, V42.89-V42.9

V43.2x   CC Excl: 996.80, 996.83, 996.87, V42.1, V43.22

V45.1   CC Excl: 996.73, V45.1

V46.1   CC Excl: V46.0- V46.9

CC Exclusion List

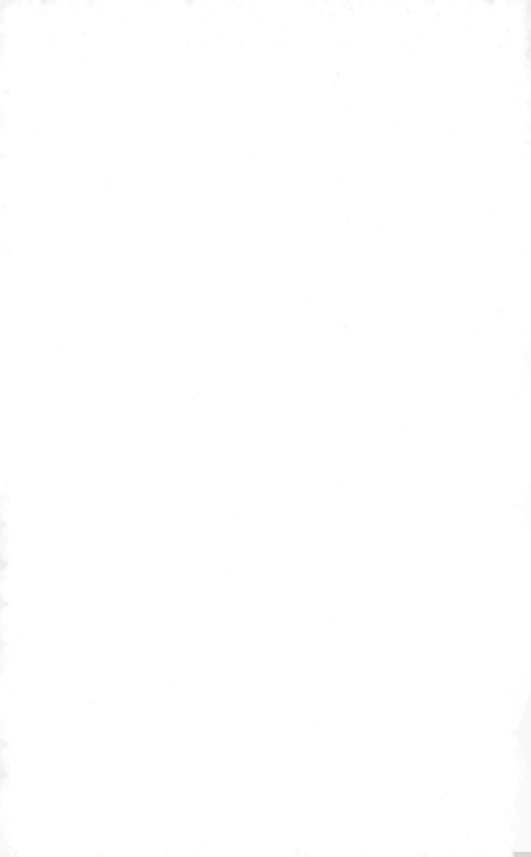

Abnormal EKGs

Abnormal Tracing Documentation

Arrhythmias	**Atrioventricular (AV) block, third-degree** **Definition:** sometimes called complete heart block with (possible) angina pectoris **Signs and Symptoms:** Dizziness, syncope, dyspnea **Drugs:** Treatment is insertion of a pacemaker. However, drugs like atropine, epinephrine and isoproterenol may be used temporarily until a pacemaker is placed. **Trifascicular block** **Signs and Symptoms:** Dizziness, syncope, dyspnea **Drugs:** Treatment is insertion of a pacemaker. However, drugs like atropine, epinephrine and isoproterenol may be used temporarily until a pacemaker is placed.
Arrhythmias, atrial premature ventricular contractions (PVCs), right bundle branch block, cor pulmonale, right axis deviation	**Cor pulmonale** **Definition:** is a term applied to enlargement of the right ventricle resulting from pulmonary hypertension, most often due to chronic obstructive pulmonary disease (COPD). **Signs and Symptoms:** Patients usually exhibit a long course of slowly deteriorating exercise tolerance due to shortness of breath and edema. Sudden decompensation is known as acute cor pulmonale and is most often due to a massive pulmonary embolus. **Drugs:** Bronchodilators, steroids, diuretics, digitalis, antibiotics; occasionally heparin or tissue plasminogen activator (TPA) are given if pulmonary embolus is present
Arrhythmias of all types due to electrolyte imbalance	**Acute renal failure** **Signs and Symptoms:** Lethargy, fatigue, anorexia, nausea, dyspnea, weakness, thirst, oliguria, bradycardia, or tachycardia; can develop as a complication of congestive heart failure, shock, or sepsis **Drugs:** Type of arrhythmia dictates specific drug prescribed
Arrhythmias; ST segment changes, cardiac monitoring usually necessary	**Intermediate coronary syndrome** **Signs and Symptoms:** Anginal pain, history of chronic coronary insufficiency, possible exacerbation of previously stable angina; pending infarction also may be called preinfarction syndrome **Drugs:** Varies per physician discretion
Beats, premature atrial, abnormally shaped P waves, regular rhythm at 150-220 beats per minute	**Paroxysmal supraventricular tachycardia** **Signs and Symptoms:** Abrupt onset and termination of palpitations; often asymptomatic, although patient may be aware of rapid heartbeat; some patients complain of throbbing vessels of the throat, dyspnea, sweating, dizziness, syncope, weakness, polyuria **Drugs:** Digoxin, inderal, metoprolol, esmolol, verapamil, diltiazem, adenocard, quinidine, procainmide, norpace, soltolol, or mexiletine

Abnormal EKGs

Beats, uninterrupted series	Paroxysmal tachycardia **Signs and Symptoms:** Fluttering sensation in chest, weakness, faintness, nausea **Drugs:** May include quinidine, procainamide, tambocor, or disopyramide
Bradycardia (shown in changes prior to arrest), tachycardia or other arrhythmias, fibrillation or asystole	Cardiac arrest **Signs and Symptoms:** Sudden unexpected cessation of cardiac action, absence of heart sounds and/or blood pressure; cardiopulmonary resuscitation (CPR) performed **Drugs:** May include isoproterenol, atropine, sodium bicarbonate, epinephrine, and calcium gluconate
Changes, junction J, ST, T interval, TU segment and U wave	Rupture of papillary muscle **Signs and Symptoms:** Contraction of papillary muscle, possible chest pain, and hemoptysis; deterioration usually sudden and severe; often a manifestation of congestive heart failure with cyanosis and sometimes shock **Drugs:** May include lasix or diuril
Changes, ST segment, inversion or flattening of T waves	Ischemia **Signs and Symptoms:** Arteriosclerotic heart disease, elevated cholesterol disease of aortic valve, thoracic pain, anemia, dizziness, syncope, dyspnea, angina, palpation, neck or jaw pain, or diaphoresis **Drugs:** Nitroglycerin, oxygen, beta-blockers, calcium channel blockers, vasodilators
Complexes, QRS, chaotic and rapid ventricular rhythm	Ventricular fibrillation **Signs and Symptoms:** Absence of effective cardiac action resulting in loss of pulse, respiration and blood pressure; a life-threatening cardiac emergency seizure, death can occur **Drugs:** Lidocaine, procainamide, bretylium tosylate, epinephrine
Complex, QRS, lasting 0–12 seconds or longer, T wave essentially normal in all leads except V1–V3, left anterior fascicular block	Right bundle branch block and left anterior fascicular block **Signs and Symptoms:** Usually asymptomatic **Drugs:** Varies per physician discretion
Complexes, QRS, wide	Paroxysmal ventricular tachycardia **Signs and Symptoms:** Associated with ischemic heart disease, especially myocardial infarction (MI); precordial pain, sudden onset usually preceded by premature ventricular beats, pulse rate of 150–210 beats per minute **Drugs:** May include antiarrhythmic medication (e.g., lidocaine, pronestyl)

Contractions, premature atrial	Functional disturbances following cardiac surgery
	Signs and Symptoms: History of cardiac surgery (may have occurred previously or during the present admission); functional disturbances may be indicated by arrhythmias, level of consciousness, diaphoresis or drop in blood pressure (diastolic pressure less than 60)
	Drugs: May include quinidine, lidocaine, or pronestyl
Deviation, axis features of right or left ventricular failure, hypertrophy	Rupture of chordae tendonae
	Signs and Symptoms: Usually sudden in onset with chest pain, possibly dyspnea and weakness; caused by bacterial endocarditis, trauma, or sudden compression of thorax
	Drugs: May include use of diuretics for congestive heart failure (e.g., lasix)
Deviation, ST segment, bradycardia, tachycardia, fibrillation or asystole	Cardiac arrest
	Signs and Symptoms: Sudden cessation of cardiac action, absence of heart sounds or blood pressure
	Drugs: Isoproterenol, atropine, sodium bicarbonate, epinephrine, lidocaine
Disassociation, AV, sudden onset; block may be 2 to 1, 3 to 1, or 4 to 1	Atrioventricular block, Mobitz type II; also called partial or incomplete heart block
	Signs and Symptoms: Attack of syncope related to sudden cessation of circulation in upright or recumbent position
	Drugs: Atropine for bradycardia; discontinuation of digitalis
Elevation, S-T segment T wave changes, bundle branch abnormality	Aneurysm of heart wall
	Signs and Symptoms: Palpitations, severe dyspnea, generalized edema (may occur after an MI)
	Drugs: Varies per physician discretion
Fibrillation, atrial	Functional disturbances following cardiac surgery
	Signs and Symptoms: History of cardiac surgery (may have occurred previously or during the present admission); functional disturbances may be indicated by arrhythmias, level of consciousness, diaphoresis or drop in blood pressure (diastolic pressure less than 60)
	Drugs: May include the ongoing use of digoxin, diuretics, and quinidine; calan, cardizem, coumadin
	Hypertensive and arteriosclerotic heart disease, MI
	Signs and Symptoms: Palpitations, near-syncope, pallor, nausea, weakness, lightheadedness, and fatigue
	Drugs: Digitalis, quinidine sulfate, procainamide, verapamil

Fibrillation, ventricular	Cardiogenic shock
	Definition: Hypotensive with poor perfusion usually results from massive myocardial infarction leading to severe left ventricular dysfunction, hypotension, pulmonary edema. Prognosis is very poor with mortality rate of 50%.
	Drugs: Lidocaine, procainamide, calan, cardizem, digitalis
	Functional disturbances following cardiac surgery
	Signs and Symptoms: History of cardiac surgery (may have occurred previously or during the present admission); functional disturbances may be indicated by arrhythmias, level of consciousness, diaphoresis or drop in blood pressure (diastolic pressure less than 60)
	Drugs: May include quinidine, lidocaine, or pronestyl
Fibrillation, ventricular and/or conduction defect	Hypovolemic or septic shock
	Definition: Septic shock due to management of underlying disease;
	Signs and Symptoms: Onset of abrupt chills, nausea, vomiting, diarrhea; extreme exhaustion (prostration), hypotension, fever, chills
	Drugs: IV antibiotics
Flutter, atrial	Functional disturbances following cardiac surgery
	Signs and Symptoms: History of cardiac surgery (may have occurred previously or during the present admission); functional disturbances may be indicated by arrhythmias, level of consciousness, diaphoresis, or drop in blood pressure (diastolic pressure less than 60)
	Drugs: May include digoxin, quinidine, propranolol, calan, cardizem, digitalis
	Infarction, rheumatic heart disease
	Signs and Symptoms: Atrial rate between 240 and 400%; palpitations, near-syncope, pallor, nausea, weakness, lightheadedness, and fatigue
	Drugs: Digitalis, quinidine sulfate, procainamide, verapamil
Flutter, ventricular, regular rapid rate over 250 beats per minute	Ventricular flutter
	Signs and Symptoms: Palpitations, dyspnea; possibly a transition between ventricular tachycardia and fibrillation
	Drugs: Lidocaine, procainamide, bretylium
Hypertrophy, left ventricular	Endocardial fibroelastosis
	Signs and Symptoms: Cardiac hypertrophy with documentation of peripheral edema; usually occurs in ages six weeks to six months; in older children, there are usually poor heart sounds and often tachycardia; in patients over 50, history of six to 15 years of heart disease; possible relationship to mumps virus
	Drugs: May include diuretics or digoxin

Infarction, myocardial, acute, PVCs, ventricular tachycardia	Shock **Signs and Symptoms:** Hypotensive with poor perfusion usually results from massive myocardial infarction leading to severe left ventricular dysfunction, hypotension, pulmonary edema. Prognosis is very poor with mortality rate of 50%. **Drugs:** Epinephrine, norepinephrine, dopamine, isoproterenol **Postmyocardial infarction syndrome, called Dressler syndrome** **Signs and Symptoms:** Chest pain usually sharp and stabbing as that caused by infarction; aggravated by change in position and deep inspirations; usually follows an acute infarction by two to 11 weeks (appears to be like pleural effusion, pneumonitis with fever); pericardial friction rub present on auscultation
P waves irregular rhythm (250 to 350 per minute), prolonged PR interval, varying with degree of AV block	Atrial flutter **Signs and Symptoms:** Palpitations, dyspnea, apprehension, dizziness, fainting; result of other conditions, such as acute myocardial infarction, angina, congestive heart failure and sepsis, or after bypass surgery **Drugs:** Digoxin, inderal, metoprolol, esmolol, verapamil, diltiazem, adenocard, quinidine, procainamide, norpace, soltolol, or mexiletine
Patterns producing an irregularly dropped beat that can be determined by cardiac auscultation or palpation of the pulse	Atrioventricular block **Signs and Symptoms:** Dizziness, syncope, dyspnea **Drugs:** Treatment is insertion of a pacemaker; how ever, drugs like atropine, epinephrine, and isoproterenol may be used temporarily until a pacemaker is placed.
QRS 0.14 seconds with R-R1 in the leads V1 + 2 and V5 + 6	Bilateral bundle branch block **Signs and Symptoms:** Usually asymptomatic **Drugs:** No specific therapy
QRS 0.14 seconds with R-R1 morphology in the lateral lead of electrocardiogram (ECG)	Left bundle branch block **Signs and Symptoms:** Usually asymptomatic; can be secondary to coronary artery disease or hypertension; makes the diagnosis of acute myocardial infarction more difficult **Drugs:** No specific therapy
Rate, atrial more than 400 beats per minute with a variable ventricular rate; P waves absent	Atrial fibrillation **Signs and Symptoms:** Palpitations, dyspnea, apprehension, dizziness, fainting; result of other conditions, such as acute myocardial infarction, angina, congestive heart failure and sepsis, or after bypass surgery **Drugs:** Digoxin, inderal, metoprolol, esmolol, verapamil, diltiazem, adenocard, quinidine, procainamide, norpace, soltolol, or mexiletine

Rhythm, ventricular, irregular regular atrial rhythm; often called Wenckebach pause	Atrioventricular block, Mobitz I, second degree; also called partial or incomplete heart block **Signs and Symptoms:** Weakness, faintness, palpitations, dyspnea, transient when in upright position; usually transient in nature and requires no treatment **Drugs:** Atropine for bradycardia
ST, T wave abnormal	Aneurysm of coronary vessels **Signs and Symptoms:** Palpitations, severe dyspnea, heart murmur, generalized edema **Drugs:** Varies per physician discretion
T waves, low to inverted in most leads	Acute pericarditis in diseases classified elsewhere **Signs and Symptoms:** Often a history of recent respiratory infection; precordial pain made worse by change of position, swallowing, coughing, and deep breathing; dyspnea, chills, malaise are usually present; onset is sudden; the underlying condition (e.g., tuberculosis) also must be treated Acute pericarditis **Signs and Symptoms:** Onset is usually abrupt and often preceded by sharp precordial or substernal pain radiating to the neck (precordial pain is distinguished from ischemic coronary pain because it usually is not aggravated by thoracic motion); fever, chills, weakness are common Hemopericardium **Signs and Symptoms:** Results from a perforating trauma or cardiac rupture after myocardial infarction; symptoms include precordial pain, substernal oppression, dyspnea; death can result if emergency measures are not taken immediately **Drugs:** As required to resuscitate patient
Tachycardia, atrial enlargement	Congestive heart failure **Signs and Symptoms:** Dyspnea present with orthopnea and paroxysmal nocturnal dyspnea in more advanced failure; other symptoms include peripheral edema, irritability, weakness, sometimes cyanosis, irregular heart rate, moist rales in base of lungs with productive cough, confusion (usually present) **Drugs:** Digoxin, diuretics, vasodilators Left heart failure **Signs and Symptoms:** Hypertension, fatigue, cough, frothy sputum, pulmonary edema, dyspnea; possible cyanosis **Drugs:** Diuretics, digoxin, vasodilators, dobutamine, amrinone Heart failure **Signs and Symptoms:** Hypertension, fatigue, cough, frothy sputum, pulmonary edema, dyspnea; possible cyanosis **Drugs:** Diuretics, digoxin, vasodilators, dobutamine, amrinone

Tachycardia, bradycardia or PVCs	**Hypertensive heart disease (benign) with congestive heart failure**
	Signs and Symptoms: Hypertension, fatigue, cough, frothy sputum, pulmonary edema, dyspnea; possible cyanosis
	Drugs: Diuretics, digoxin, vasodilators, dobutamine, amrinone
	Hypertensive heart disease (malignant) with congestive heart failure
	Signs and Symptoms: Hypertension, fatigue, cough, frothy sputum, pulmonary edema, dyspnea; confusion is usually present; possible cyanosis
	Drugs: Diuretics, digoxin, vasodilators, dobutamine, amrinone
Tachycardia, intraventricular or bundle branch abnormalities, ST segment changes, ventricular arrhythmias	**Myocarditis, acute in diseases classified elsewhere**
	Signs and Symptoms: Associated with acute pericarditis, influenza, tuberculosis; precordial, substernal discomfort, severe dyspnea, pain in right upper quadrant of abdomen
	Drugs: May include antiarrhythmic drugs to control arrhythmias, antibiotics for underlying infection and anti-inflammatory drugs
	Acute myocarditis
	Signs and Symptoms: Usually persistent fever, fatigue, dyspnea, palpitations, chest discomfort, neck vein distention in the presence of accompanying congestive heart failure; rapidly progressive clinical course can be complicated by congestive heart failure
	Drugs: May include antiarrhythmic drugs to control arrhythmias, antibiotics for underlying infection and anti-inflammatory drugs
	Acute myocarditis; may be termed interstitial
	Signs and Symptoms: Precordial, substernal discomfort, dyspnea, pain, fever; predominant physical findings are friction rub, leukocytosis, rapid sedimentation; there also may be evidence of generalized edema and/or ascites
	Drugs: May include antiarrhythmic drugs to control arrhythmias, antibiotics for underlying infection and anti-inflammatory drugs
	Idiopathic myocarditis
	Signs and Symptoms: MI, acute, possibly viral and parasitic infections, chills, weakness, discomfort in chest (precordial or substernal), onset of persistent fever
	Drugs: May include antiarrhythmic drugs to control arrhythmias, antibiotics for underlying infection and anti-inflammatory drugs
	Septic myocarditis
	Signs and Symptoms: Viral strains, influenza viruses, bacteria
	Drugs: May include antiarrhythmic drugs to control arrhythmias, antibiotics for underlying infection, and anti-inflammatory drugs
	Toxic myocarditis
	Signs and Symptoms: May be caused by chemical poisons such as arsenic, excessive doses of drugs, excessive radiation exposure
	Drugs: May include antiarrhythmic drugs to control arrhythmias, antibiotics for underlying infection, and anti-inflammatory drugs

Tachycardia, PVCs, ventricular hypertrophy	Heart failure, left side **Signs and Symptoms:** Hypertension, fatigue, cough, frothy sputum, pulmonary edema, dyspnea; confusion is usually present; possible cyanosis **Drugs:** Diuretics, digoxin, vasodilators, dobutamine, amrinone
Tachycardia, ST segment elevation, atrial arrhythmias	Idiopathic acute pericarditis **Signs and Symptoms:** Precordial pain intensified by change in position, swallowing, coughing, and deep breathing; dyspnea, chills, malaise, and anorexia; onset is sudden in all ages; physical findings show pericardial friction rub; fever is usually greater than 102 **Drugs:** IV antibiotics corticosteroids, anti-inflammatory drugs such as aspirin
Tachycardia, sinus	Hyperkinetic heart disease **Signs and Symptoms:** Features of congestive heart failure such as cardiac enlargement, gallop rhythm, tachycardia; pulse pressure may be elevated (the difference between diastolic and systolic blood pressure is greater than 100) **Drugs:** All types of antianginal medications and hypertensive drugs are possibilities
Tachycardia, sinus, all forms of heart block (i.e., first, second and third degree), junctional tachycardias	Infectious endocarditis **Definition:** both acute and subacute, is due to infection of the lining of the heart manifested by development of fever, heart murmurs, and persistent bacteremia. Collections of bacteria and inflammatory cells known as vegetations form on the heart lining and heart valves. Pieces of vegetations break loose and embolize to various organs (i.e., kidneys, nailbeds, lungs, etc.) causing damage to these organs and sometimes infection in these organs. Acute endocarditis is a clinical picture as described above accompanied by rapid destruction of heart valves with rapid deterioration of valve function leading to hemodynamic instability and heart failure. It is most often caused by Staphylococcus aureus infection of the heart. Its rapid progression is a result of the virulence of the Staphylococcus aureus organism. Subacute endocarditis represents a partially compensated form of infectious endocarditis, in which hemodynamic deterioration occurs very slowly, often over a period of weeks or months. It is most often due to infection with Streptococcus viridans, which is a much less virulent (or destructive) organism. **Drugs:** IV antibiotics

Tachycardia, sinus, atrial enlargement, PVCs, atrial fibrillation, or ventricular hypertrophy	Primary cardiomyopathy
	Signs and Symptoms: Usually occurs in elderly patients; evidenced by loss of consciousness, palpitations and/or dyspnea (palpitations may be indicated by bounding or rapid pulse, skipped heartbeats); edema and paroxysmal nocturnal dyspnea may be present; may include congestive and restrictive cardiomyopathies
	Drugs: Antianginal medications, antihypertensives, presser agents, digoxin, diuretics
	Secondary cardiomyopathy
	Signs and Symptoms: Dyspnea, paroxysmal nocturnal dyspnea, fatigue, edema, palpitations, hypertrophy of heart; occurs as a complication of cardiovascular disease or other systemic disease
	Drugs: Digoxin, pronestyl, diuretics, and vasodilators
	Alcoholic cardiomyopathy
	Signs and Symptoms: Excessive alcohol intake, exertional dyspnea, cough, fatigue, hemoptysis and edema; frequently found in patients between the ages of 23 and 50
	Nutritional and metabolic cardiomyopathy
	Signs and Symptoms: Dyspnea, paroxysmal nocturnal dyspnea, fatigue, edema, palpitations, high output heart failure; underlying disease is thyrotoxicosis, beriberi, amyloidosis
	Cardiomyopathy in other diseases classified elsewhere
	Signs and Symptoms: Increase in diastolic blood pressure, loss of consciousness, hypertrophy of heart and/or history of heart disease, dyspnea, paroxysmal nocturnal dyspnea, fatigue, edema, palpitations
Tachycardia, strain patterns, LVH	Hypertensive heart and renal disease, malignant
	Signs and Symptoms: History of renal disease, headache, fatigue, irritability, evidence of renal failure, elevated blood pressure (systolic greater than 160 and diastolic greater than 100), confusion may be present
	Drugs: Nipride, vasodilators, nitroglycerin, B-blockers, procardia
Tachycardia, ventricular, atrial flutter, supraventricular tachycardia (SVT)	Functional disturbances following cardiac surgery
	Signs and Symptoms: History of cardiac surgery (may have occurred previously or during the present admission); functional disturbances may be indicated by arrhythmias, level of consciousness, diaphoresis, or drop in blood pressure (diastolic pressure less than 60)
	Drugs: May include quinidine, lidocaine, or Pronestyl

Abnormal Laboratory Values

Acetones or Ketones-Blood-Increased Level

Reference Range: 0.3-2.0 mg/dL Negative (A); 2-4 mg/dL Negative (K)
Hospital Range:_____

Condition	Signs & Symptoms	Treatment
Ketoacidosis **CC**	Excessive thirst, polyuria, irritability, weakness, coma, stupor, dehydration, fruity breath odor	Restricted diet, monitoring of blood sugar levels
Ketosis, alcoholic **CC**	Vomiting and dehydration in association with other symptoms of alcoholism such as delirium tremens and cirrhosis	Intravenous infusion of normal saline and glucose

Acid Phosphatase-Blood-Increased Level

Reference Range: 0-0.8 Units/L
Hospital Range:_____

Condition	Signs & Symptoms	Treatment
Cancer of prostate	Urinary retention, urinary tract infections, palpable lesion of prostate; bone pain is present with metastatic disease	Surgery, hormone therapy, radiation therapy, and chemotherapy may all be employed depending on the stage of the disease
Cirrhosis of liver **CC**	Abdominal pain or distention, fever, ascites, jaundice, anorexia, polyuria	Sodium-restricted diet, intravenous fluids, treatment for relief of symptoms
Failure, renal, chronic **CC**	Bruising, dyspnea, lethargy, weakness, anorexia, polyuria, hematuria	Fluid restrictions, dialysis, transfusion(s) of blood and blood components

Albumin-Blood-Decreased Level

Reference Range: 3.5-5.0 g/dL
Hospital Range:_____

Condition	Signs & Symptoms	Treatment
Burns	Can result from thermal, electrical, or chemical injuries; severity is determined by the size and depth of the burn	Reverse isolation, skin grafts, intravenous fluids, invasive monitoring, high protein/high calorie diet
Cirrhosis of liver **CC**	Abdominal pain or distention, fever, ascites, jaundice, anorexia, polyuria	Sodium-restricted diet, intravenous fluids, treatment for relief of symptoms
Syndrome, nephrotic **CC**	Edema, lethargy, anorexia, orthostatic hypotension	Diuretics, steroid therapy, sodium-restricted high protein diet, frequent urine protein monitoring

---

CC Complication/Comorbidity   **MC** Major Cardiovascular Condition   **CD** Complex Diagnosis

Albumin-Blood-Increased Level

Reference Range: 4.0-6.0 g/dL
Hospital Range:_____

Condition	Signs & Symptoms	Treatment
Dehydration **CC**	Confusion, weakness, poor skin turgor, dry mucous membranes	Monitoring of electrolyte levels, intravenous therapy, force fluids, intake and output monitoring

Aldosterone-Blood-Increased Level

Reference Range: 8.1-15.5 ng/dL
Hospital Range:_____

Condition	Signs & Symptoms	Treatment
Failure, **CC MC CD** heart, congestive, unspecified	Peripheral edema, shortness of breath; cyanosis is present on occasion; heart rate is irregular; moist rales at base of lungs with productive cough; confusion is usually present	Sodium-restricted diet, digitalis regulation, O_2 therapy, diuretics
Hypokalemia	Cardiac arrhythmias, leg cramps, nausea and vomiting, anorexia	Potassium supplement, intravenous fluids

Alkaline Phosphatase-Blood-Increased Level

Reference Range: 30-120 Units/L
Hospital Range:_____

Condition	Signs & Symptoms	Treatment
Calculus of bile **CC** duct	Epigastric pain, nausea and vomiting, jaundice	Intravenous fluids and medications, surgery
Cancer of liver **CC**	Weakness, fever, weight loss, right upper quadrant mass, pain	Chemotherapy, radiation, surgery
Cirrhosis of **CC** liver	Abdominal pain or distention, fever, ascites, jaundice, anorexia, polyuria	Sodium-restricted diet, intravenous fluids, treatment for relief of symptoms
Leukemia **CC**	Weight loss, anorexia, pain in extremities, listlessness	Chemotherapy, intravenous fluids, transfusion(s) of blood and blood components, antibiotic therapy
Pulmonary **CC** embolism **MC CD**	Dyspnea, rales in lungs, sudden onset of substernal pain, dizziness, pallor	Heparin, diuretics

---

Amylase-Blood-Increased Level

Reference Range: 0-130 Units/L
Hospital Range: _____

Condition		Signs & Symptoms	Treatment
Pancreatitis, acute	`CC`	Epigastric pain, nausea, vomiting, fever, sweats, dizziness, confusion	Intravenous fluids, pain medication, replacement of calcium and magnesium, if indicated
Failure, renal, acute	`CC`	Thirst, dyspnea, lethargy, weakness, anorexia, nausea	Management of diet, fluid, and electrolytes; possible dialysis
Failure, renal, chronic	`CC`	Bruising, dyspnea, lethargy, weakness, anorexia, polyuria, hematuria	Fluid restrictions, dialysis, transfusion(s) of blood and blood components
Ketoacidosis	`CC`	Excessive thirst, polyuria, irritability, weakness, coma, stupor, dehydration, fruity breath odor	Restricted diet, monitoring of blood sugar levels

Arterial Blood Gases (ABGs)-Bicarbonate (HCO₃)-Decreased Level

Reference Range: 24-28 mEq/L
Hospital Range: _____

Condition		Signs & Symptoms	Treatment
Acidosis, metabolic	`CC`	Hypotension, weakness, pallor, pulmonary edema	Fluid balance, electrolyte monitoring
Failure, renal, chronic	`CC`	Bruising, dyspnea, lethargy, weakness, anorexia, polyuria, hematuria	Fluid restrictions, dialysis, transfusion(s) of blood and blood components
Infarction, acute myocardial	`CC` `MC` `CD`	Severe chest pain, gallop rhythm and other cardiac arrhythmias, shortness of breath, diaphoresis	Continuous monitoring, O₂ therapy, pain medication, intravenous fluids, intravenous medications, possible resuscitation
Ketoacidosis	`CC`	Excessive thirst, polyuria, irritability, weakness, coma, stupor, dehydration, fruity breath odor	Restricted diet, monitoring of blood sugar levels

ABGs-pCO₂-Decreased Level

Reference Range: 35-45 mm Hg
Hospital Range: _____

Condition		Signs & Symptoms	Treatment
Acidosis, metabolic	`CC`	Hypotension, weakness, pallor, pulmonary edema	Fluid balance, electrolyte monitoring
Alkalosis, respiratory	`CC`	Retention of CO₂ and increasing pCO₂; hypoventilation, dyspnea, drowsiness, weakness, malaise, and nausea due to conditions such as spinal cord injury, pulmonary disease, or drugs such as narcotics	Sedation, prevention of further hyperventilation

`CC` Complication/Comorbidity   `MC` Major Cardiovascular Condition   `CD` Complex Diagnosis

ABGs-pCO$_2$-Increased Level

Reference Range: 35-45 mm Hg
Hospital Range:_____

Condition		Signs & Symptoms	Treatment
Alkalosis, metabolic	CC	Nausea, vomiting, anorexia	Administration of aluminum chloride, respiratory therapy
Alkalosis, respiratory	CC	Retention of CO$_2$ and increasing pCO$_2$; hypoventilation, dyspnea, drowsiness, weakness, malaise, and nausea due to conditions such as spinal cord injury, pulmonary disease, or drugs such as narcotics	Establishment of airway, O$_2$ therapy, artificial ventilation, bicarbonate administration
Disease, chronic obstructive pulmonary	CC	Wheezing, productive cough, shortness of breath	Intermittent positive pressure breathing (IPPB) therapy, intravenous fluids, bronchodilators, antibiotics, physical therapy, artificial ventilation

ABGs-pH-Decreased Level

Reference Range: 7.35-7.45
Hospital Range:_____

Condition		Signs & Symptoms	Treatment
Acidosis, metabolic	CC	Hypotension, weakness, pallor, pulmonary edema	Fluid balance, electrolyte monitoring
Acidosis, respiratory	CC	Retention of CO$_2$ and increasing pCO$_2$; hypoventilation, dyspnea, drowsiness, weakness, malaise, and nausea due to conditions such as spinal cord injury, pulmonary disease, or drugs such as narcotics	Establishment of airway, O$_2$ therapy, artificial ventilation, bicarbonate administration
Ketoacidosis	CC	Excessive thirst, polyuria, irritability, weakness, coma, stupor, dehydration, fruity breath odor	Restricted diet, monitoring of blood sugar levels, fluid replacement, insulin administration

ABGs-pO$_2$-Decreased Level

Reference Range: 75-100 mm Hg
Hospital Range:_____

Condition		Signs & Symptoms	Treatment
Disease, chronic obstructive pulmonary	CC	Wheezing, productive cough, shortness of breath	IPPB therapy, intravenous fluids, bronchodilators, antibiotics, physical therapy, artificial ventilation
Cor pulmonale, acute	CC MC	Wheezing, marked fatigue, persistent cough, dyspnea	IPPB therapy, bronchodilators
Edema, pulmonary	CC	Increased respiration and pulse rate, shortness of breath, cough, anxiety, cyanosis, diaphoresis	Decreased rate of intravenous fluids, diuretics, intake and output monitoring, O$_2$ therapy, mechanical ventilation

---

CC Complication/Comorbidity   MC Major Cardiovascular Condition   CD Complex Diagnosis

Bilirubin-Indirect-Increased Level

Reference Range: 0.1-1.0 mg/dL
Hospital Range:_____

Condition	Signs & Symptoms	Treatment
Anemia, hemolytic **CC**	Vomiting, anorexia, weight loss	Transfusion(s) of blood and blood components, chemotherapy, iron therapy, O$_2$ therapy
Cirrhosis of liver **CC**	Abdominal pain or distention, fever, ascites, jaundice, anorexia, polyuria	Sodium-restricted diet, intravenous fluids, treatment for relief of symptoms
Failure, **CC MC CD** heart, congestive, unspecified	Peripheral edema, shortness of breath; cyanosis is present on occasion; heart rate is irregular; moist rales at base of lungs with productive cough; confusion is usually present	Sodium-restricted diet, digitalis regulation, O$_2$ therapy, diuretics
Hyperbilirubinemia (neonatal jaundice)	Jaundice may be the only symptom as in physiologic jaundice. If caused by pathological jaundice, lack of treatment may result in kernicterus, a condition with severe neurological symptoms.	Phototherapy, exchange transfusion, administration of albumin

Bilirubin-Total/Direct-Increased Level

Reference Range: 0.1-0.5 mg/dL (D); 0.1-1.2 mg/dL (T)
Hospital Range:_____

Condition	Signs & Symptoms	Treatment
Calculus of bile duct **CC**	Epigastric pain, nausea and vomiting, jaundice	Intravenous fluids and medications, surgery
Cancer of liver **CC**	Weakness, fever, weight loss, right upper quadrant mass, pain	Chemotherapy, radiation, surgery
Cirrhosis of liver **CC**	Abdominal pain or distention, fever, ascites, jaundice, anorexia, polyuria	Sodium-restricted diet, intravenous fluids, treatment for relief of symptoms
Hepatitis **CC**	Jaundice, anorexia, dark urine, pruritis, light-colored stools	Rest, force fluids, antiemetics for nausea, isolation precautions for blood and other body fluids

---

CC Complication/Comorbidity   **MC** Major Cardiovascular Condition   **CD** Complex Diagnosis

Bleeding Time-Increased Level
Reference Range: 2-10 minutes
Hospital Range:_____

Condition	Signs & Symptoms	Treatment
Anemia, aplastic **CC**	Weakness, fatigue, shortness of breath, bruising, nosebleeds	Reverse isolation, transfusion(s) of blood and blood components
Coagulation, intravascular disseminated **CC**	Occurs as a complication of other conditions such as infection, neoplastic disease, burns, and obstetric complications. Characterized by abnormal bleeding such as from the gastrointestinal tract and small wounds such as intravenous sites. Bruising is also present.	Transfusion of plasma or platelets; intravenous heparin administration; intake and output monitoring
Disease, Von Willebrand **CC**	Bruising, menorrhagia, epistaxis and possible hemorrhage as a result of surgery	Increased level of factor viii through infusion of cryoprecipitate or fresh frozen plasma prior to surgery or during bleeding episodes

Blood Urea Nitrogen (BUN)-Blood-Increased Level
Reference Range: 9-22 mg/dL
Hospital Range:_____

Condition	Signs & Symptoms	Treatment
Dehydration **CC**	Confusion, weakness, poor skin turgor, dry mucous membranes	Monitoring of electrolyte levels, intravenous therapy, force fluids, intake and output monitoring
Infarction myocardial, acute **CC** **MC**	Severe chest pain, gallop rhythm and other cardiac arrhythmias, shortness of breath, diaphoresis	Continuous monitoring, O_2 therapy, pain medication, intravenous fluids, intravenous medications, possible resuscitation
Failure, renal, acute **CC**	Thirst, dyspnea, lethargy, weakness, anorexia, nausea	Transfusion(s) of blood and blood components, dialysis, fluid restrictions
Shock, cardiogenic **CC** **MC** **CD**	Rapidly developing mental confusion, physical weakness, cold extremities, moist and cool skin, rapid and weak pulse, oliguria, pulmonary edema, hypotension	Fluid balance, O_2 therapy, cardiac monitoring

---

CC Complication/Comorbidity   **MC** Major Cardiovascular Condition   **CD** Complex Diagnosis

Calcium-Blood-Increased Level

Reference Range: 8.5-10.5 mg/dL
Hospital Range:_____

Condition		Signs & Symptoms	Treatment
Cancers that metastasize to bone	CC	Lung and breast cancer	Surgery, chemotherapy, radiation therapy
Failure, renal, acute	CC	Thirst, dyspnea, lethargy, weakness, anorexia, nausea	Transfusion(s) of blood and blood components, dialysis, fluid restriction
Hyperparathyroidism		Muscle weakness, epigastric pain, recurrent renal calculi, hypertension	Hydration with intravenous saline, diuresis with furosemide (lasix), surgery for parathyroid adenoma or hyperplasia

Carbon Dioxide (CO$_2$)-Decreased Level

Reference Range: 22-30 mEq/L
Hospital Range:_____

Condition		Signs & Symptoms	Treatment
Acidosis, metabolic	CC	Hypotension, weakness, pallor, pulmonary edema	Fluid balance, electrolyte monitoring
Dehydration	CC	Confusion, weakness, poor skin turgor, dry mucous membranes	Monitoring of electrolyte levels, intravenous therapy, force fluids, intake and output monitoring
Ketoacidosis	CC	Excessive thirst, polyuria, irritability, weakness, coma, stupor, dehydration, fruity breath odor	Restricted diet, monitoring of blood sugar levels

Complete Blood Count (CBC)- Hematocrit (Hct)-Decreased Level

Reference Range: Male 40-54%; Female 36-46%
Hospital Range:_____

Condition		Signs & Symptoms	Treatment
Anemia, aplastic	CC	Weakness, fatigue, shortness of breath, bruising, nosebleeds	Reverse isolation, transfusion(s) of blood and blood components
Anemia, hypochromic	CC	Tingling of extremities, dyspnea	Iron therapy, transfusion(s) of blood and blood components, O$_2$ therapy
Cirrhosis of liver	CC	Abdominal pain or distention, fever, ascites, jaundice, anorexia, polyuria	Sodium-restricted diet, intravenous fluids, treatment for relief of symptoms
Failure, chronic renal	CC	Bruising, dyspnea, lethargy, weakness, anorexia, polyuria, hematuria	Sodium-restricted diet, digitalis regulation, O$_2$ therapy, diuretics
Hemorrhage, not otherwise specified	CC	Pallor, rapid and shallow respirations, unstable vital signs, melena, hemoptysis, weakness, hematemesis	Intravenous therapy, transfusion(s) of blood and blood components, vitamin K therapy, iron therapy
Leukemia	CC	Weight loss, anorexia, pain in extremities, listlessness	Chemotherapy, intravenous fluids, transfusion(s) of blood and blood components, antibiotic therapy

---

CC Complication/Comorbidity   MC Major Cardiovascular Condition   CD Complex Diagnosis

CBCHematocrit (Hct)Increased Level

Reference Range: Male 40-54%; Female 36-46%
Hospital Range:_____

Condition	Signs & Symptoms	Treatment
Dehydration `CC`	Confusion, weakness, poor skin turgor, dry mucous membranes	Monitoring of electrolyte levels, intravenous therapy, force fluids, intake and output monitoring
Disease, chronic `CC` obstructive pulmonary	Wheezing, productive cough, shortness of breath	IPPB therapy, intravenous fluids, bronchodilators, antibiotics, physical therapy, artificial ventilation
Polycythemia vera	Fatigue, pruritis, vertigo, dizziness, cerebrovascular accident (CVA), transient ischemic attack (TIA)	Phlebotomy
Shock, `CC` hypovolemic	Cold clammy skin, tachycardia, shallow respirations, hypotension, weak thready pulse, confusion	Intravenous therapy, frequent monitoring of vital signs, intake and output monitoring

CBC-Hemoglobin (Hgb)-Decreased Level

Reference Range: Male 13.5-18 g/dL; Female 12-16 g/dL
Hospital Range:_____

Condition	Signs & Symptoms	Treatment
Anemia, aplastic `CC`	Weakness, fatigue, shortness of breath, bruising, nosebleeds	Reverse isolation, transfusion(s) of blood and blood components
Anemia, hypochromic	Tingling of extremities, dyspnea	Iron therapy, transfusion(s) of blood and blood components, O_2 therapy
Cancer: `CC` Large Intestine Liver Rectum Small Intestine	Pain, change in bowel or bladder habit, diarrhea, constipation Melena, weight loss, clay-colored stools, digestive disturbances Pain, incomplete bowel movement, bleeding of rectum Weight loss, vomiting, fever, chills, melena	Chemotherapy, radiation therapy, surgery Chemotherapy, radiation therapy, surgery Chemotherapy, radiation therapy, surgery Chemotherapy, radiation therapy, surgery
Cirrhosis of `CC` liver	Abdominal pain or distention, fever, ascites, jaundice, anorexia, polyuria	Sodium-restricted diet, intravenous fluids, treatment for relief of symptoms
Failure, chronic `CC` renal	Bruising, dyspnea, lethargy, weakness, anorexia, polyuria, hematuria	Fluid restrictions, dialysis, transfusion(s) of blood and blood components
Hemorrhage, `CC` not otherwise specified	Pallor, rapid and shallow respirations, unstable vital signs, melena, hemoptysis, weakness, hematemesis	Intravenous therapy, vitamin K therapy, iron therapy, transfusion(s) of blood and blood components
Kidney disease	Lethargy, weakness, nausea and vomiting, thirst, dyspnea, convulsions	Transfusion(s) of blood and blood components, dialysis, fluid restrictions
Leukemia `CC`	Weight loss, anorexia, pain in extremities, listlessness	Chemotherapy, intravenous fluids, transfusion(s) of blood and blood components, antibiotic therapy

---

`CC` Complication/Comorbidity   `MC` Major Cardiovascular Condition   `CD` Complex Diagnosis

CBC-Hemoglobin (Hgb)-Increased Level
Reference Range: Male 13.5-18 g/dL; Female 12-16 g/dL
Hospital Range:_____

Condition	Signs & Symptoms	Treatment
Dehydration **CC**	Confusion, weakness, poor skin turgor, dry mucous membranes	Monitoring of electrolyte levels, intravenous therapy, force fluids, intake and output monitoring
Disease, chronic **CC** obstructive pulmonary	Wheezing, productive cough, shortness of breath	IPPB therapy, intravenous fluids, bronchodilators, antibiotics, physical therapy, artificial ventilation
Failure, **CC** congestive heart, unspecified	Peripheral edema, shortness of breath; cyanosis is present on occasion; heart rate is irregular; moist rales at base of lungs with productive cough; confusion is usually present; paroxysmal nocturnal dyspnea, wheezing	Sodium-restricted diet, digitalis regulation, O_2 therapy, diuretics

CBC-Mean Corpuscular Hemoglobin (MCH)-Decreased Level
Reference Range: 27-31 pg
Hospital Range:_____

Condition	Signs & Symptoms	Treatment
Anemia, hypochromic	Tingling of extremities, dyspnea	Iron therapy, transfusion(s) of blood and blood components, O_2 therapy
Hemorrhage, **CC** not otherwise specified	Pallor, rapid and shallow respirations, unstable vital signs, melena, hemoptysis, weakness, hematemesis	Intravenous therapy, transfusion(s) of blood and blood components, vitamin K therapy, iron therapy

CBC-Mean Corpuscular Hemoglobin Concentration (MCHC)-Decreased Level
Reference Range: 32-36%
Hospital Range:_____

Condition	Signs & Symptoms	Treatment
Anemia, hypochromic	Tingling of extremities, dyspnea	Iron therapy, transfusion(s) of blood and blood components, O_2 therapy
Thalassemia **CC**	Depending on type, symptoms range from severe anemia, skeletal malformation, hepatomegaly, and bleeding tendencies to mild anemia	Folic acid supplements, transfusion of packed red blood cells

---

CBC-Mean Corpuscular Volume (MCV)-Decreased Level

Reference Range: Male 80-94 μm^3; Female 78-97 μm^3
Hospital Range:_____

Condition	Signs & Symptoms	Treatment
Anemia, hypochromic	Tingling of extremities, dyspnea	Iron therapy, transfusion(s) of blood and blood components, O_2 therapy
Failure, chronic **CC** renal	Bruising, dyspnea, lethargy, weakness, anorexia, polyuria, hematuria	Fluid restrictions, dialysis, transfusion(s) of blood and blood components
Thalassemia **CC**	Depending on type, symptoms range from severe anemia, skeletal malformation, hepatomegaly and bleeding tendencies to mild anemia	Folic acid supplements, transfusion of packed red blood cells

CBC-Red Blood Count (RBC)-Decreased Level

Reference Range: Male 4.4-6.0 $10^6/mm^3$; Female 4.2-5.5 $10^6/mm^3$
Hospital Range:_____

Condition	Signs & Symptoms	Treatment
Aplastic anemia **CC**	Weakness, fatigue, shortness of breath	Reverse isolation, transfusion(s) of blood and blood components
Anemia, **CC** posthemorrhagic	Weight loss, weakness, pain, anorexia	B12, folic acid supplement, iron therapy, transfusion(s) of blood and blood components
Failure, chronic **CC** renal	Bruising, dyspnea, lethargy, weakness, anorexia, polyuria, hematuria	Fluid restrictions, dialysis, transfusion(s) of blood and blood components
Hemorrhage, **CC** not otherwise specified	Pallor, rapid and shallow respirations, unstable vital signs, melena, hemoptysis, weakness, hematemesis	Intravenous therapy, transfusion(s) of blood and blood components, vitamin K therapy, iron therapy
Overhydration **CC**	Irritability, weakness, muscle cramps	Restriction of fluid intake

CBC-RBC-Increased Level

Reference Range: Male 4.4-6.0 $10^6/mm^3$; Female 4.2-5.5 $10^6/mm^3$
Hospital Range:_____

Condition	Signs & Symptoms	Treatment
Cor **CC** **CD** pulmonale, acute	Wheezing, marked fatigue, persistent cough, dyspnea	IPPB therapy, bronchodilators
Dehydration **CC**	Confusion, weakness, poor skin turgor, dry mucous membranes	Monitoring of electrolyte levels, intravenous therapy, force fluids, intake and output monitoring
Polycythemia vera	Fatigue, pruritis, vertigo, dizziness, CVA, TIA	Phlebotomy, radiophosphorus (32P)

CBC-White Blood Count (WBC)-Above 10,000

Reference Range: 5,000-10,000 cells/µL
Hospital Range:_____

Condition	Signs & Symptoms	Treatment
Chronic renal failure **CC**	Bruising, dyspnea, lethargy, weakness, anorexia, polyuria	Fluid restrictions, dialysis, transfusion(s) of blood and blood components
Cirrhosis of liver **CC**	Abdominal pain or distention, fever, ascites, jaundice, anorexia, polyuria	Sodium-restricted diet, intravenous fluids, treatment for relief of symptoms
Embolism, pulmonary **CC MC CD**	Dyspnea, rales in lungs, sudden onset of substernal pain, dizziness, pallor, hemoptysis	Heparin, diuretics
Failure, renal acute **CC MC**	Thirst, dyspnea, lethargy, weakness, anorexia, nausea and vomiting	Management of diet, fluid, electrolytes. Possible dialysis
Infarction, myocardial acute **CC MC**	Severe chest pain, gallop rhythm and other cardiac arrhythmias, shortness of breath, diaphoresis	Continuous monitoring, O_2 therapy, pain medication, intravenous fluids, intravenous medications, possible resuscitation, drug therapy
Infections, acute	Fever, malaise, chills	Intravenous fluids, antibiotic therapy
Leukemia **CC**	Weight loss, anorexia, pain in extremities, listlessness	Chemotherapy, intravenous fluids, transfusion(s) of blood and blood components, antibiotic therapy
Leukocytosis	Increase in the number of leukocytes in the blood; can result from hemorrhage, inflammation, or infection	Diagnostic investigations to determine cause of leukocytosis
Pneumonia **CC**	Dyspnea, chills, chest pain, cough, fever, headache	Intravenous fluids, O_2 therapy, antibiotic therapy
Pneumonia, aspiration **CC**	Cyanosis, cough, dyspnea	Intravenous fluids, O_2 therapy, antibiotic therapy
Pneumonia, pneumococcal **CC**	Cough, severe chest pain, shortness of breath	Intravenous fluids, O_2 therapy, antibiotic therapy
Pneumonia, E. coli/proteus **CC**	Chest pain, shortness of breath, malaise	Intravenous fluids, O_2 therapy, antibiotic therapy
Pneumonia, staphylococcal **CC**	Headache, chest pain, cough	Intravenous fluids, O_2 therapy, antibiotic therapy
Pyelonephritis **CC**	Nausea and vomiting, frequency of urination, dysuria, flank pain, chills	Sulfonamides, intravenous fluids, force fluids, antibiotic therapy
Urinary tract infection **CC**	Fever, dysuria, frequency, burning on urination, hematuria	Urinary antiseptics, antibiotic therapy, intravenous fluids, force fluids

CC Complication/Comorbidity   **MC** Major Cardiovascular Condition   **CD** Complex Diagnosis

CBC-WBC-Below 5,000

Reference Range: 5,000-10,000 cells/μL
Hospital Range:_____

Condition	Signs & Symptoms	Treatment
Anemia, aplastic **CC**	Weakness, fatigue, shortness of breath, bruising, nosebleeds	Reverse isolation, transfusion(s) of blood and blood components
Leukopenia **CC**	Headache, weakness, shortness of breath on exertion	Transfusion(s) of blood and blood components, intravenous fluids

Chloride (Cl)-Blood, Electrolytes-Decreased Level

Reference Range: 95-105 mEq/L
Hospital Range:_____

Condition	Signs & Symptoms	Treatment
Burns	Can result from thermal, electrical, or chemical injuries; severity is determined by the size and depth of the burn	Reverse isolation, skin grafts, intravenous fluids, invasive monitoring, high protein/high calorie diet
Hyponatremia **CC**	Weakness, muscle cramps and spasms, confusion, irritability	Intravenous fluids, sodium concentrate
Ketoacidosis **CC**	Excessive thirst, polyuria, irritability, weakness, coma, stupor, dehydration, fruity breath odor	Restricted diet, monitoring of blood sugar levels

Chloride (Cl)-Blood, Electrolytes-Increased Level

Reference Range: 95-105 mEq/L
Hospital Range:_____

Condition	Signs & Symptoms	Treatment
Acidosis, metabolic **CC**	Hypotension, weakness, pallor, pulmonary edema	Fluid balance, electrolyte monitoring
Dehydration **CC**	Confusion, weakness, poor skin turgor, dry mucous membranes	Monitoring of electrolyte levels, intravenous therapy, force fluids, intake and output monitoring
Failure, renal, acute **CC**	Thirst, dyspnea, lethargy, weakness, anorexia, nausea	Management of diet, fluid and electrolytes; possible dialysis
Hypernatremia **CC**	Poor skin turgor, dry mucous membranes, confusion, stupor, coma	Intravenous fluids, force fluids, administration of H_2O

CC Complication/Comorbidity   **MC** Major Cardiovascular Condition   **CD** Complex Diagnosis

Cholesterol-Increased Level

Reference Range: 150-250 mg/dL
Hospital Range:_____

Condition	Signs & Symptoms	Treatment
Calculus of bile CC duct	Epigastric pain, nausea and vomiting, jaundice	Intravenous fluids and medications, surgery
Cirrhosis of CC liver	Abdominal pain or distention, fever, ascites, jaundice, anorexia, polyuria	Sodium-restricted diet, intravenous fluids, treatment for relief of symptoms
Diabetes CC mellitus, uncontrolled	Excessive thirst, polyuria, irritability, weakness	Restricted diet, monitoring of blood sugar levels, treatment for symptomatology
Failure, renal, CC acute	Thirst, dyspnea, lethargy, weakness, anorexia, nausea	Transfusion(s) of blood and blood components, dialysis, fluid restriction
Infarction, CC myocardial acute	Severe chest pain, gallop rhythm and other cardiac arrhythmias, shortness of breath, diaphoresis	Continuous monitoring, O_2 therapy, pain medication, intravenous fluids, intravenous medications, possible resuscitation

Cold Agglutinins-Increased Level

Reference Range: 1: 15 Titer or less
Hospital Range:_____

Condition	Signs & Symptoms	Treatment
Anemia, CC hemolytic	Vomiting, anorexia, weight loss	Transfusion(s) of blood and blood components, chemotherapy, iron and O_2 therapy
Cirrhosis of CC liver	Abdominal pain or distention, fever, ascites, jaundice, anorexia, polyuria	Sodium-restricted diet, intravenous fluids, treatment for relief of symptoms
Hepatitis CC	Jaundice, anorexia, dark urine, pruritus, light-colored stools	Rest, force fluids, antiemetics for nausea, isolation precautions for blood and other body fluids
Pneumonia CC	Dyspnea, chills, chest pain, cough, fever, headache	Intravenous fluids, O_2 therapy, antibiotic therapy

Creatinine-Blood-Increased Level

Reference Range: 0.6-1.2 mg/dL
Hospital Range:_____

Condition	Signs & Symptoms	Treatment
Failure, renal, `CC` acute	Thirst, dyspnea, lethargy, weakness, anorexia, nausea	Management of diet, fluid and electrolytes; possible dialysis
Glomerulonephriti, chronic	Hypertension, hematuria, azotemia, fatigue	Diuretics, dietary restrictions, antibiotics, dialysis or surgical transplantation
Urinary tract `CC` infection	Fever, dysuria, frequency, burning on urination, hematuria	Urinary antiseptics, antibiotic therapy, intravenous fluids, force fluids

Creatinine Phosphokinase (CPK) (CK)-Blood-Increased Level

Reference Range: 0-150 Units/L
Hospital Range:_____

Condition	Signs & Symptoms	Treatment
Infarction, `CC` `MC` myocardial, acute	Severe chest pain, gallop rhythm and other cardiac arrhythmias, shortness of breath, diaphoresis	Continuous monitoring, O$_2$ therapy, pain medication, intravenous fluids, intravenous medications, possible resuscitation
Muscular `CC` dystrophy	Predominant symptom is weakness; as disease progresses, muscle atrophy, abnormal gait, and cardiac symptoms, such as tachycardia appear	Physical therapy, orthopaedic appliances, surgery to release contractures
Pulmonary `CC` `MC` embolism `CD`	Dyspnea, rales in lungs, sudden onset of substernal pain, dizziness, pallor	Heparin, diuretics

Creatinine Phosphokinase MB-Fraction (CPK-MB) (CK-MB)-Increased Level 1

Reference Range: < 3%
Hospital Range:_____

Condition	Signs & Symptoms	Treatment
Infarction, `CC` myocardial, `MC` acute	Severe chest pain, gallop rhythm and other cardiac arrhythmias, shortness of breath, diaphoresis	Continuous monitoring, O$_2$ therapy, pain medication, intravenous fluids, intravenous medications, possible resuscitation
Muscular `CC` dystrophy	Predominant symptom is weakness; as disease progresses, muscle atrophy, abnormal gait, and cardiac symptoms, such as tachycardia appear	Physical therapy, orthopaedic appliances, surgery to release contractures

---

`CC` Complication/Comorbidity   `MC` Major Cardiovascular Condition   `CD` Complex Diagnosis

White Blood Cell Differential (WBC-DIFF)-Basophils-Increased Level

Reference Range: 0.4-1%
Hospital Range:_____

Condition		Signs & Symptoms	Treatment
Anemia, hemolytic	CC	Vomiting, anorexia, weight loss	Transfusion(s) of blood and blood components, chemotherapy, iron therapy, O_2 therapy
Leukemia	CC	Weight loss, anorexia, pain in extremities, listlessness	Chemotherapy, intravenous fluids, transfusion(s) of blood and blood components, antibiotic therapy
Polycythemia vera		Fatigue, pruritis, vertigo, dizziness, CVA, TIA	Phlebotomy, radiophosphorus (32P)

Differential (WBC-DIFF)-Eosinophils-Increased Level

Reference Range: 1-3%
Hospital Range:_____

Condition		Signs & Symptoms	Treatment
Cancer, lung	CC	Cough, dyspnea, chest and shoulder pain, fever, weight loss, hemoptysis	Surgery, chemotherapy, radiation therapy
Disease, Addison's	CC	Features of crisis include anorexia, headache, weakness, nausea, vomiting, apprehension, diarrhea, abdominal pain, and syncope; chronic Addison's disease may show indications resembling hypoglycemia (i.e., hunger, sweating, irritability, nervousness, depression)	Glucocorticoid and mineralocorticoid replacement
Leukemia	CC	Weight loss, anorexia, pain in extremities, listlessness	Chemotherapy, intravenous fluids, transfusion(s) of blood and blood components, antibiotic therapy
Parasitism, intestinal		Diarrhea, abdominal pain, nausea and vomiting	Fluid replacement (intravenous or by mouth), antibiotics, symptomatic treatment, such as Kaopectate
Reaction, allergic		Can assume a variety of forms from contact dermatitis to anaphylactic shock; most reactions occur on the skin or in the respiratory or gastrointestinal tract	Maintenance of airway, epinephrine, aminophylline

Differential (WBC-DIFF)-Lymphocytes-Decreased Level

Reference Range: 25-35%
Hospital Range:_____

Condition	Signs & Symptoms	Treatment
Anemia, aplastic **CC**	Weakness, fatigue, shortness of breath, bruising, nosebleeds	Reverse isolation, transfusion(s) of blood and blood components
Burns	Can result from thermal, electrical or chemical injuries; severity is determined by depth and size of burn	Reverse isolation, skin grafts, intravenous fluids, invasive monitoring, high protein/high-calorie diet
Disease, **CC** Hodgkin's	Lymphadenopathy, infections, purpura, fatigue	Reverse isolation, radiation therapy, chemotherapy
Lymphocytopenia	Can result from radiation or chemotherapy, renal failure or terminal cancer; symptoms include enlarged lymph nodes and spleen	Treatment of underlying condition; reverse isolation

Differential (WBC-DIFF)-Lymphocytes-Increased Level

Reference Range: 25-35%
Hospital Range:_____

Condition	Signs & Symptoms	Treatment
Leukemia **CC**	Weight loss, anorexia, pain in extremities, listlessness	Chemotherapy, intravenous fluids, transfusion(s) of blood and blood components, antibiotic therapy
Leukemia, **CC** acute lymphoblastic	Lymphadenopathy, infections, purpura, fatigue	Reverse isolation, chemotherapy, bone marrow transplantation
Lymphocytosis	May be relative or absolute; associated with bacterial and viral conditions such as mumps, measles, and tuberculosis. Infectious lymphocytosis is a mild childhood disease	Treatment of underlying condition
Mononucleosis infectious	Fever, lymphadenopathy, fatigue	Bed rest, antibiotics, aspirin or acetaminophen for discomfort
Pneumonia **CC**	Dyspnea, chills, chest pain, cough, fever, headache	Intravenous fluids, O_2 therapy, antibiotic therapy

Differential (WBC-DIFF)-Segmented Neutrophils (Segs)-Decreased Level

Reference Range: 51-67%
Hospital Range:_____

Condition	Signs & Symptoms	Treatment
Anemia, aplastic **CC**	Weakness, fatigue, shortness of breath, bruising, nosebleeds	Reverse isolation, transfusion(s) of blood and blood components
Disease, Addison's **CC**	Features of crisis include anorexia, headache, weakness, nausea, vomiting, apprehension, diarrhea, abdominal pain, and syncope; chronic Addison's disease may show indications resembling hypoglycemia (i.e., hunger, sweating, irritability, nervousness, depression)	Glucocorticoid and mineralocorticoid replacement

Differential (WBC-DIFF)-Segmented Neutrophils (Segs)-Increased Level

Reference Range: 51-67%
Hospital Range:_____

Condition	Signs & Symptoms	Treatment
Infarction, acute myocardial **CC** **MC**	Severe chest pain, gallop rhythm and other cardiac arrhythmias, shortness of breath, diaphoresis	Continuous monitoring, O_2 therapy, pain medication, intravenous fluids, intravenous medications, possible resuscitation
Leukemia **CC**	Weight loss, anorexia, pain in extremities, listlessness	Chemotherapy, intravenous fluids, transfusion(s) of blood and blood components, antibiotic therapy
Pneumonia **CC**	Dyspnea, chills, chest pain, cough, fever, headache	Intravenous fluids, O_2 therapy, antibiotic therapy

Gamma Glutamyl Transferase (GT, GGT)-Increased Level

Reference Range: 0-30 Units/L
Hospital Range:_____

Condition	Signs & Symptoms	Treatment
Alcoholism **CC**	Inability to control alcohol consumption; symptoms can include maladaptive behavior, flushed face, and delirium tremens (DTs)	Antianxiety drugs, B vitamins, psychotherapy
Calculus of bile duct **CC**	Epigastric pain, nausea and vomiting, jaundice	Intravenous fluids and medications, surgery
Cirrhosis of liver **CC**	Abdominal pain or distention, fever, ascites, jaundice, anorexia, polyuria	Sodium-restricted diet, intravenous fluids, treatment for relief of symptoms
Pancreatitis, acute **CC**	Epigastric pain, nausea, vomiting, fever, sweats, dizziness, confusion	Intravenous fluids, pain medication, replacement of calcium and magnesium, if indicated

CC Complication/Comorbidity   **MC** Major Cardiovascular Condition   **CD** Complex Diagnosis

Glucose (Fasting Blood Sugar [FBS])-Blood-Decreased Level

Reference Range: 70-115 mg/dL
Hospital Range:_____

Condition		Signs & Symptoms	Treatment
Cancer of pancreas	CC	Diarrhea, weight loss, abdominal pain, jaundice, nausea, anorexia	Surgery, chemotherapy, radiation therapy
Failure, renal, chronic	CC	Bruising, dyspnea, lethargy, weakness, anorexia, polyuria, hematuria	Fluid restrictions, dialysis, transfusion(s) of blood and blood components
Hepatitis	CC	Jaundice, anorexia, dark urine, pruritus, light-colored stools	Rest, force fluids, antiemetics for nausea, isolation precautions for blood and other body fluids
Reaction, hypoglycemia	CC	Sudden onset of sweating, pale skin, blurred vision, possible loss of consciousness	Withhold insulin, food or juice given with sugar, glucose injection

Glucose (FBS)-Blood-Increased Level

Reference Range: 70-115 mg/dL
Hospital Range:_____

Condition		Signs & Symptoms	Treatment
Diabetes mellitus, uncontrolled	CC	Excessive thirst, polyuria, irritability, weakness	Diet restriction, monitoring of blood sugar, treatment for symptomatology
Failure, heart, congestive, unspecified	CC MC CD	Peripheral edema, shortness of breath; cyanosis is present on occasion; heart rate is irregular, moist rales at base of lungs with productive cough; confusion is usually present	Sodium-restricted diet, digitalis regulation, O_2 therapy, diuretics
Failure, renal, acute	CC	Thirst, dyspnea, lethargy, weakness, anorexia, nausea	Transfusion(s) of blood and blood components, dialysis, fluid restrictions
Infarction, myocardial, acute	CC MC	Severe chest pain, gallop rhythm, and other cardiac arrhythmias, shortness of breath, diaphoresis	Continuous monitoring, O_2 therapy, pain medication, intravenous fluids, intravenous medications, possible resuscitation
Infections (acute)		Fever, malaise, chills	Intravenous fluids, antibiotic therapy
Ketoacidosis	CC	Excessive thirst, polyuria, irritability, weakness, coma, stupor, dehydration, fruity breath odor	Restricted diet, monitoring of blood sugar levels

---

Lactic Dehydrogenase (LDH) (LD)-Increased Level

Reference Range: 50-150 Units/L

Hospital Range:_____

Condition	Signs & Symptoms	Treatment
Cirrhosis of liver **CC**	Abdominal pain or distention, fever, ascites, jaundice, anorexia, polyuria	Sodium-restricted diet, intravenous fluids, treatment for relief of symptoms
Failure, **CC** **MC** **CD** heart, congestive, unspecified	Peripheral edema, shortness of breath; cyanosis is present on occasion; heart rate is irregular; moist rales at base of lungs with productive cough; confusion is usually present	Sodium-restricted diet, digitalis regulation, O_2 therapy, diuretics
Hemolytic anemia **CC**	Vomiting, anorexia, weight loss	Transfusion(s) of blood and blood components, chemotherapy, iron therapy, O_2 therapy
Infarction, **CC** **MC** myocardial, acute	Severe chest pain, gallop rhythm and other cardiac arrhythmias, shortness of breath, diaphoresis	Continuous monitoring, O_2 therapy, pain medication, intravenous fluids, intravenous medications, possible resuscitation
Pernicious anemia	Paresthesia, weakness, nausea, vomiting, ataxia	Parenteral administration of B_{12}
Pulmonary **CC** **MC** embolism **CD**	Dyspnea, rales in lungs, sudden onset of substernal pain, dizziness, pallor	Heparin, diuretics

Lactic Dehydrogenase-1 (LD-1)-Increased Level

Reference Range: 15-40%

Hospital Range:_____

Condition	Signs & Symptoms	Treatment
Anemia, hemolytic **CC**	Vomiting, anorexia, weight loss	Transfusion(s) of blood and blood components, chemotherapy, iron therapy, O_2 therapy
Anemia, megaloblastic	Paresthesia, ataxia, memory loss	Parenteral administration of B_{12}; folic acid supplements
Infarction, **CC** **MC** myocardial, acute	Severe chest pain, gallop rhythm and other cardiac arrhythmias, shortness of breath, diaphoresis	Continuous monitoring, O_2 therapy, pain medication, intravenous fluids, intravenous medications, possible resuscitation

Lipase-Increased Level

Reference Range: 0-1.5 Units/dL
Hospital Range:_____

Condition		Signs & Symptoms	Treatment
Cirrhosis of liver	CC	Abdominal pain or distention, fever, ascites, jaundice, anorexia, polyuria	Sodium-restricted diet, intravenous fluids, treatment for relief of symptoms
Failure, renal, acute	CC	Thirst, dyspnea, lethargy, weakness, anorexia, nausea	Management of diet, fluid and electrolytes; possible dialysis
Pancreatitis, acute	CC	Epigastric pain, nausea, vomiting, fever, sweats, dizziness, confusion	Intravenous fluids, pain medication, replacement of calcium and magnesium, if indicated

Magnesium-Blood-Increased Level

Reference Range: 1.5-2.5 mmole/L
Hospital Range:_____

Condition		Signs & Symptoms	Treatment
Dehydration	CC	Confusion, weakness, poor skin turgor, dry mucous membranes	Monitoring of electrolyte levels, intravenous therapy, force fluids, intake and output monitoring
Failure, renal, chronic	CC	Bruising, dyspnea, lethargy, weakness, anorexia, polyuria, hematuria	Fluid restrictions, dialysis, transfusion(s) of blood and blood components
Leukemia	CC	Weight loss, anorexia, pain in extremities, listlessness	Chemotherapy, intravenous fluids, transfusion(s) of blood and blood components, antibiotic therapy

Osmolality-Blood-Decreased Level

Reference Range: 280-300 mOsm/kg
Hospital Range:_____

Condition		Signs & Symptoms	Treatment
Cancer of bronchus	CC	Productive cough, shortness of breath, dyspnea	Chemotherapy, intravenous fluids
Cancer of lung	CC	Congestion, shortness of breath, productive cough	Chemotherapy, intravenous fluids, surgery, radiation therapy
Deficiency, ADH	CC	Polydipsia, polyuria, headaches, fatigue	Antidiuretic hormone replacement therapy, intake and output monitoring, daily weights
Hyponatremia	CC	Weakness, muscle cramps and spasms, confusion, anorexia, nausea	Intravenous fluids, sodium concentrate

---

Osmolality-Blood-Increased Level

Reference Range: 280-300 mOsm/kg
Hospital Range:_____

Condition		Signs & Symptoms	Treatment
Cirrhosis of liver	CC	Abdominal pain or distention, fever, ascites, jaundice, anorexia, polyuria	Sodium-restricted diet, intravenous fluids, treatment for relief of symptoms
Dehydration	CC	Confusion, weakness, poor skin turgor, dry mucous membranes	Monitoring of electrolyte levels, intravenous therapy, force fluids, intake and output monitoring
Hypernatremia	CC	Irritability, lethargy, weakness, confusion, stupor, coma	Intravenous fluids, force fluids, administration of H_2O

Platelet Count-Decreased Level

Reference Range: 150,000-400,000 cells/µL
Hospital Range:_____

Condition		Signs & Symptoms	Treatment
Anemia, aplastic	CC	Weakness, fatigue, shortness of breath, bruising, nosebleeds	Reverse isolation, transfusion(s) of blood and blood components
Disease, kidney	CC	Lethargy, weakness, nausea and vomiting, thirst, dyspnea, convulsions	Transfusion(s) of blood and blood components, dialysis, fluid restrictions
Leukemia	CC	Weight loss, anorexia, pain in extremities, listlessness	Chemotherapy, intravenous fluids, transfusion(s) of blood and blood components, antibiotic therapy
Reaction, drug, to antineoplastic agents and other medications such as heparin		Spontaneous bleeding such as bruising, epistaxis and gastrointestinal bleeding	Discontinuation of offending drug; platelet transfusion for acute hemorrhage
Thrombocytopenia	CC	Can be due to decreased production of platelets or increased destruction; symptoms include spontaneous bleeding in the skin or any mucous membrane	Treatment of underlying condition; may include corticosteroids and transfusion of blood and blood components, such as platelets

---

CC Complication/Comorbidity   MC Major Cardiovascular Condition   CD Complex Diagnosis

Platelet Count-Increased Level

Reference Range: 150,000-400,000 cells/μL
Hospital Range:_____

Condition		Signs & Symptoms	Treatment
Cirrhosis of liver	CC	Abdominal pain or distention, fever, ascites, jaundice, anorexia, polyuria	Sodium-restricted diet, intravenous fluids, treatment for relief of symptoms
Hemorrhage, not otherwise specified	CC	Pallor, rapid and shallow respirations, unstable vital signs, melena, hemoptysis, weakness, hematemesis	Intravenous therapy, transfusion(s) of blood and blood components, vitamin K therapy, iron therapy
Infections (acute)		Fever, malaise, chills	Intravenous fluids, antibiotic therapy
Thrombocytosis		Can occur as a result of many conditions such as trauma, cancer, anemia, and heart disease	Treatment of underlying condition

Potassium (K)-Blood-Decreased Level

Reference Range: 3.5-5.0 mEq/L
Hospital Range:_____

Condition		Signs & Symptoms	Treatment
Dehydration	CC	Confusion, weakness, poor skin turgor, dry mucous membranes	Monitoring of electrolyte levels, intravenous therapy, force fluids, intake and output monitoring
Failure, renal, acute	CC	Thirst, dyspnea, lethargy, weakness, anorexia, nausea	Management of diet, fluid and electrolytes; possible dialysis
Hypokalemia	CC	Cardiac arrhythmias, leg cramps, nausea and vomiting, anorexia	Administration of potassium chloride orally or intravenously
Ketoacidosis	CC	Excessive thirst, polyuria, irritability, weakness, coma, stupor, dehydration, fruity breath odor	Restricted diet, monitoring of blood sugar levels
Leukemia	CC	Weight loss, anorexia, pain in extremities, listlessness	Chemotherapy, intravenous fluids, transfusion(s) of blood and blood components, antibiotic therapy

Potassium (K)-Blood-Increased Level

Reference Range: 3.5-5.0 mEq/L
Hospital Range:_____

Condition		Signs & Symptoms	Treatment
Anemia, hemolytic	CC	Vomiting, anorexia, weight loss	Transfusion(s) of blood and blood components, chemotherapy, iron therapy, O_2 therapy
Disease, Addison's	CC	Features of crisis include anorexia, headache, weakness, dizziness, nausea, vomiting, apprehension, diarrhea, abdominal pain, and syncope; chronic Addison's disease may show indications resembling hypoglycemia (i.e., hunger, sweating, irritability, nervousness and depression)	Glucocorticoid and mineralocorticoid replacement
Failure, renal, acute	CC	Thirst, dyspnea, lethargy, weakness, anorexia, nausea	Management of diet, fluid and electrolytes; possible dialysis
Hyperkalemia	CC	Weakness and flaccid paralysis may occur; often caused by renal insufficiency	Diagnostic investigations to determine cause of hyperkalemia

Protein-Blood-Decreased Level

Reference Range: 6.0-8.5 g/dL
Hospital Range:_____

Condition		Signs & Symptoms	Treatment
Burns		Can result from thermal, electrical, or chemical injuries; severity is determined by the size and depth of the burn	Reverse isolation, skin grafts, intravenous fluids, invasive monitoring, high protein/high-calorie diet
Cirrhosis of liver	CC	Abdominal pain or distention, fever, ascites, jaundice, anorexia, polyuria	Sodium-restricted diet, intravenous fluids, treatment for relief of symptoms
Hypernatremia	CC	Irritability, lethargy, weakness, confusion, stupor, coma	Intravenous fluids, force fluids, administration of H_2O
Malnutrition	CC	Can be due to a number of diseases and can be a result of socioeconomic factors; symptoms include muscle and fat wasting, edema, and electrolyte imbalances	Nutritional therapy including oral dietary supplements and total parenteral nutrition (TPN)

Prothrombin Time-Increased Level

Reference Range: 11-13 seconds or 70-100%
Hospital Range:_____

Condition	Signs & Symptoms	Treatment
Cirrhosis of liver **CC**	Abdominal pain or distention, fever, ascites, jaundice, anorexia, polyuria	Sodium-restricted diet, intravenous fluids, treatment for relief of symptoms
Disseminated intravascular coagulation (DIC) **CC**	Occurs as a complication of other conditions such as infection, neoplastic disease, burns, and obstetric complications; characterized by abnormal bleeding such as from the gastrointestinal tract and small wounds such as intravenous sites; bruising is also present	Transfusion of plasma or platelets; intravenous heparin administration; intake and output monitoring
Failure, **CC** **MC** **CD** heart, congestive, unspecified	Peripheral edema, shortness of breath; cyanosis is present on occasion; heart rate is irregular; moist rales at base of lungs with productive cough; confusion is usually present	Sodium-restricted diet, digitalis regulation, O_2 therapy, diuretics
Hemophilia **CC**	Symptoms range from asymptomatic to severe bleeding as a result of minor trauma; bleeding into joints and muscles can occur, with resultant swelling and pain	Nonaspirin oral analgesia for pain; deficient factor replacement required prior to even minor surgical procedures

Reticulocyte Count-Decreased Level

Reference Range: 0.5-1.5%
Hospital Range:_____

Condition	Signs & Symptoms	Treatment
Anemia, aplastic **CC**	Weakness, fatigue, shortness of breath, bruising, nosebleeds	Reverse isolation, transfusion(s) of blood and blood components
Anemia, hemolytic **CC**	Vomiting, anorexia, weight loss	Transfusion(s) of blood and blood components, chemotherapy, iron therapy, O_2 therapy
Anemia, hypochromic	Tingling of extremities, dyspnea	Iron therapy, transfusion(s) of blood and blood components, O_2 therapy
Cirrhosis of liver **CC**	Abdominal pain or distention, fever, ascites, jaundice, anorexia, polyuria	Sodium-restricted diet, intravenous fluids, treatment for relief of symptoms

---

CC Complication/Comorbidity   **MC** Major Cardiovascular Condition   **CD** Complex Diagnosis

Reticulocyte Count-Increased Level
Reference Range: 0.5-1.5%
Hospital Range:_____

Condition	Signs & Symptoms	Treatment
Anemia, aplastic `CC`	Weakness, fatigue, shortness of breath, bruising, nosebleeds	Reverse isolation, transfusion(s) of blood and blood components
Anemia, hemolytic `CC`	Vomiting, anorexia, weight loss	Transfusion(s) of blood and blood components, chemotherapy, iron therapy, O_2 therapy
Hemorrhage, not otherwise specified `CC`	Pallor, rapid shallow respirations, unstable vital signs, melena, hemoptysis, weakness, hematemesis	Intravenous therapy, transfusion(s) of blood and blood components, vitamin K therapy, iron therapy

Sedimentation Rate-Increased Level
Reference Range: Male 0-20 mm/hr; Female 0-30 mm/hr
Hospital Range:_____

Condition	Signs & Symptoms	Treatment
Cancer of stomach `CC`	Weakness, constipation, abdominal pain, anorexia, weight loss, hematemesis, melena	Chemotherapy, radiation therapy, surgery, pain medications
Endocarditis, bacterial `CC` `MC`	Skin lesions, weight loss, weakness, sweating, fever, heart murmur	Intravenous fluids, antibiotic therapy
Infarction, acute myocardial `CC` `MC`	Severe chest pain, gallop rhythm and other cardiac arrhythmias, shortness of breath, diaphoresis	Continuous monitoring, O_2 therapy, pain medication, intravenous fluids, intravenous medications, possible resuscitation
Infections (acute)	Fever, malaise, chills	Intravenous fluids, antibiotic therapy

Serum Glutamic-Oxaloacetic Transminase (SGOT)-Increased Level
Reference Range: 0-35 Units/L
Hospital Range:_____

Condition	Signs & Symptoms	Treatment
Cirrhosis of liver `CC`	Abdominal pain or distention, fever, ascites, jaundice, anorexia, polyuria	Sodium-restricted diet, intravenous fluids, treatment for relief of symptoms
Embolism, pulmonary `CC` `MC` `CD`	Dyspnea, rales in lungs, sudden onset of substernal pain, dizziness, pallor	Heparin, diuretics
Failure, heart, congestive, unspecified `CC` `MC` `CD`	Peripheral edema, shortness of breath; cyanosis is present on occasion; heart rate is irregular; moist rales at base of lungs with productive cough; confusion is usually present	Sodium-restricted diet, digitalis regulation, O_2 therapy, diuretics
Infarction, myocardial, acute `CC` `MC`	Severe chest pain, gallop rhythm and other cardiac arrhythmias, shortness of breath, diaphoresis	Continuous monitoring, O_2 therapy, pain medication, intravenous fluids, intravenous medications, possible resuscitation

`CC` Complication/Comorbidity   `MC` Major Cardiovascular Condition   `CD` Complex Diagnosis

Serum Glutamic-Pyruvic Transminase (SGPT) (ALT)-Increased Level

Reference Range: 0-35 Units/L
Hospital Range:_____

Condition		Signs & Symptoms	Treatment
Infarction, myocardial, acute	CC MC	Severe chest pain, gallop rhythm and other cardiac arrhythmias, shortness of breath, diaphoresis	Continuous monitoring, O_2 therapy, pain medication, intravenous medications, possible resuscitation
Cirrhosis of liver	CC	Abdominal pain or distention, fever, ascites, jaundice, anorexia, polyuria	Sodium-restricted diet, intravenous fluids, treatment for relief of symptoms
Failure, heart, congestive, unspecified	CC MC CD	Peripheral edema, shortness of breath; cyanosis is present on occasion; heart rate is irregular; moist rales at base of lungs with productive cough; confusion is usually present	Sodium-restricted diet, digitalis regulation, O_2 therapy, diuretics

Sodium (Na)-Blood, Electrolytes-Decreased Level

Reference Range: 135-145 mEq/L
Hospital Range:_____

Condition		Signs & Symptoms	Treatment
Cirrhosis of liver	CC	Abdominal pain or distention, fever, ascites, jaundice, anorexia, polyuria	Sodium-restricted diet, intravenous fluids, treatment for relief of symptoms
Disease, Addison's	CC	Features of crisis include anorexia, headache, weakness, dizziness, nausea, vomiting, apprehension, diarrhea, abdominal pain, and syncope; chronic Addison's disease may show indications resembling hypoglycemia (i.e., hunger, sweating, irritability, nervousness and depression)	Glucocorticoid and mineralocorticoid replacement
Failure, renal, chronic	CC	Bruising, dyspnea, lethargy, weakness, anorexia, polyuria, hematuria	Fluid restrictions, dialysis, transfusion(s) of blood and blood components
Hyponatremia	CC	Weakness, muscle cramps and spasms, confusion, irritability	Intravenous fluids, sodium concentrate
Ketoacidosis	CC	Excessive thirst, polyuria, irritability, weakness, coma, stupor, dehydration, fruity breath odor	Restricted diet, monitoring of blood sugar levels

Sodium (Na)-Blood, Electrolytes-Increased Level

Reference Range: 135-145 mEq/L
Hospital Range:_____

Condition	Signs & Symptoms	Treatment
Dehydration `CC`	Confusion, weakness, poor skin turgor, dry mucous membranes	Monitoring of electrolyte levels, intravenous therapy, force fluids, intake and output monitoring
Failure, `CC` `MC` `CD` heart, congestive, unspecified	Peripheral edema, shortness of breath; cyanosis is present on occasion; heart rate is irregular; moist rales at base of lungs with productive cough; confusion is usually present	Sodium-restricted diet, digitalis regulation, O_2 therapy, diuretics
Failure, renal, `CC` acute	Thirst, dyspnea, lethargy, weakness, anorexia, nausea	Management of diet, fluid and electrolytes; possible dialysis
Hypernatremia `CC`	Poor skin turgor, dry mucous membranes, confusion, stupor, coma	Intravenous fluids, force fluids, administration of H_2O

Sodium (Na)-Urine-Decreased Level

Reference Range: 40-220 mEq/24 hr
Hospital Range:_____

Condition	Signs & Symptoms	Treatment
Failure, `CC` `MC` `CD` heart, congestive, unspecified	Peripheral edema, shortness of breath; cyanosis is present on occasion; heart rate is irregular; moist rales at base of lungs with productive cough; confusion is usually present	Sodium-restricted diet, digitalis regulation, O_2 therapy, diuretics
Failure, renal, `CC` chronic	Bruising, dyspnea, lethargy, weakness, anorexia, polyuria, hematuria	Fluid restrictions, dialysis, transfusion(s) of blood and blood components

Sodium (Na)-Urine-Increased Level

Reference Range: 40-220 mEq/24 hr
Hospital Range:_____

Condition	Signs & Symptoms	Treatment
Disease, `CC` Addison's	Features of crisis include anorexia, headache, weakness, dizziness, nausea, vomiting, apprehension, diarrhea, abdominal pain, and syncope; chronic Addison's disease may show indications resembling hypoglycemia (i.e., hunger, sweating, irritability, nervousness and depression)	Glucocorticoid and mineralocorticoid replacement
Dehydration `CC`	Confusion, weakness, poor skin turgor, dry mucous membranes	Monitoring of electrolyte levels, intravenous therapy, force fluids, intake and output monitoring

---

`CC` Complication/Comorbidity   `MC` Major Cardiovascular Condition   `CD` Complex Diagnosis

Total Iron Binding Capacity (TIBC)-Decreased Level
Reference Range: 220-370 µg/dL
Hospital Range:_____

Condition	Signs & Symptoms	Treatment
Anemia, aplastic CC	Weakness, fatigue, shortness of breath, bruising, nosebleeds	Reverse isolation, transfusion(s) of blood and blood components
Anemia, sickle cell CC	Enlarged heart, tachycardia, heart murmurs, fatigue, dyspnea, joint and bone pain	Supportive care such as rest, analgesics, warm compresses. Transfusion of packed red blood cells may be necessary
Cirrhosis of liver CC	Abdominal pain or distention, fever, ascites, jaundice, anorexia, polyuria	Sodium-restricted diet, intravenous fluids, treatment for relief of symptoms
Failure, renal, chronic CC	Bruising, dyspnea, lethargy, weakness, anorexia, polyuria, hematuria	Fluid restriction, dialysis, transfusion(s) of blood and blood components
Infections (chronic) CC	Symptoms vary with area of localization of infection; can include fever, nausea, vomiting	Antibiotics, culture, and sensitivity studies including blood cultures

Total Iron Binding Capacity (TIBC)-Increased Level
Reference Range: 220-370 µg/dL
Hospital Range:_____

Condition	Signs & Symptoms	Treatment
Anemia, hypochromic	Tingling of extremities, dyspnea	Iron therapy, transfusion(s) of blood and blood components, O_2 therapy
Anemia, iron deficiency	Exertional dyspnea, fatigue, tachycardia	Iron supplements administered orally or parenterally
Loss, blood acute/chronic CC	Weakness, lethargy, shortness of breath pain	Intravenous fluids, transfusion(s) of blood and blood components, iron therapy
Polycythemia vera	Fatigue, pruritis, vertigo, dizziness, CVA, TIA	Phlebotomy, radiophosphorus (32P)

Uric Acid-Blood-Decreased Level
Reference Range: 3-7 mg/dL
Hospital Range:_____

Condition	Signs & Symptoms	Treatment
Burns	Can result from thermal, electrical, or chemical injuries; severity is determined by the size and depth of the burn	Reverse isolation, skin graphs, intravenous fluids, invasive monitoring, high-protein/high-calorie diet
Cirrhosis of liver CC	Abdominal pain or distention, fever, ascites, jaundice, anorexia, polyuria	Sodium-restricted diet, intravenous fluids, treatment for relief of symptoms

Uric Acid-Blood-Increased Level

Reference Range: 3-7 mg/dL
Hospital Range:_____

Condition		Signs & Symptoms	Treatment
Cirrhosis of liver	CC	Abdominal pain or distention, fever, ascites, jaundice, anorexia, polyuria	Sodium-restricted diet, intravenous fluids, treatment for relief of symptoms
Failure, renal, acute	CC	Thirst, dyspnea, lethargy, fatigue, anorexia, nausea	Management of diet, fluid and electrolytes; possible dialysis
Gout		Severe pain in joints, most usually affecting the metatarsophalangeal (MTP) joint	Colchicine, nonsteroidal anti-inflammatory drugs, sometimes glucocorticoids, low protein diet
Infarction, myocardial, acute	CC MC	Severe chest pain, gallop rhythm and other cardiac arrhythmias, shortness of breath, diaphoresis	Continuous monitoring, O_2 therapy, pain medication, intravenous fluids, intravenous medications, possible resuscitation
Leukemia, myelogenous, chronic	CC	Anorexia, weight loss, weakness, fatigue, bruising, epistaxis, low-grade fever	Chemotherapy is primary treatment; other treatments may include allopurinol to prevent increased uric acid and antibiotics for infections

Urinalysis-Bile-Increased Level

Reference Range: Negative
Hospital Range:_____

Condition		Signs & Symptoms	Treatment
Calculus of bile duct	CC	Epigastric pain, nausea and vomiting, jaundice	Intravenous fluids and medications, surgery
Cirrhosis of liver	CC	Abdominal pain or distention, fever, ascites, jaundice, anorexia, polyuria	Sodium restricted diet, intravenous fluids, treatment for relief of symptoms
Hepatitis	CC	Jaundice, anorexia, dark urine, pruritis, light-colored stools	Rest, force fluids, antiemetics for nausea, isolation precautions for blood and other body fluids

Urinalysis-Ketones or Acetones-Increased Level

Reference Range: Negative
Hospital Range:_____

Condition		Signs & Symptoms	Treatment
Ketoacidosis	CC	Excessive thirst, polyuria, irritability, weakness, coma, stupor, dehydration, fruity breath odor	Restricted diet, monitoring of blood sugar levels
Ketosis, alcoholic	CC	Vomiting and dehydration in association with other symptoms of alcoholism such as delirium tremens and cirrhosis	Intravenous infusion of normal saline and glucose

---

CC Complication/Comorbidity   MC Major Cardiovascular Condition   CD Complex Diagnosis

Urinalysis-pH-Decreased Level

Reference Range: 4.5-8
Hospital Range:_____

Condition		Signs & Symptoms	Treatment
Acidosis, metabolic	CC	Hypotension, weakness, pallor, pulmonary edema	Fluid balance, electrolyte monitoring
Acidosis, respiratory	CC	Retention of CO_2 and increasing pCO_2; hypoventilation, dyspnea, drowsiness, weakness, malaise, nausea	Establishment of airway, O_2 therapy, artificial ventilation
Dehydration	CC	Confusion, weakness, poor skin turgor, dry mucous membranes	Monitoring of electrolyte levels, intravenous therapy, force fluids, intake and output monitoring

Urinalysis-pH-Increased Level

Reference Range: 4.5-8
Hospital Range:_____

Condition		Signs & Symptoms	Treatment
Failure, renal, chronic	CC	Bruising, dyspnea, lethargy, weakness, anorexia, polyuria, hematuria	Fluid restrictions, dialysis, transfusion(s) of blood and blood components
Urinary tract infection	CC	Fever, dysuria, frequency, burning on urination, hematuria	Urinary antiseptics, antibiotic therapy, intravenous fluids, force fluids
Overdose, salicylate	CC	Tinnitus, diaphoresis, nausea, hyperventilation	Gastric lavage, activated charcoal, alkaline diuresis, may require dialysis

Urinalysis-Protein (Albumin)-Increased Level

Reference Range: Negative
Hospital Range:_____

Condition		Signs & Symptoms	Treatment
Disease, renal (glomerular, tubular, interstitial)	CC MC	Fatigue, vomiting, anorexia, polyuria	Fluid restrictions, dialysis
Hematuria	CC	Blood in the urine	Treatment of underlying cause (i.e., infection or trauma)
Urinary tract infection	CC	Fever, dysuria, frequency, burning on urination, hematuria	Urinary antiseptics, antibiotic therapy, intravenous fluids, force fluids
Toxemia of pregnancy	CC	Develops in the late second trimester or third trimester of pregnancy; symptoms include hypertension, edema, and weight gain; in severe eclampsia, seizures and coma can occur	Sedatives, bed rest, frequent monitoring of blood pressure, intake and output, daily weight; cesarean section or induction of labor may be necessary

---

CC Complication/Comorbidity   MC Major Cardiovascular Condition   CD Complex Diagnosis

Urinalysis-Specific Gravity-Decreased Level

Reference Range: 1.005-1.030
Hospital Range:_____

Condition	Signs & Symptoms	Treatment
Disease, **CC** **MC** renal (glomerular, tubular, interstitial)	Fatigue, vomiting, anorexia, polyuria	Fluid restrictions, dialysis
Hypokalemia	Cardiac arrhythmias, leg cramps, nausea and vomiting, anorexia	Potassium supplement, intravenous fluid

Urinalysis-Specific Gravity-Increased Level

Reference Range: 1.005-1.030
Hospital Range:_____

Condition	Signs & Symptoms	Treatment
Dehydration **CC**	Confusion, weakness, poor skin turgor, dry mucous membranes	Monitoring of electrolyte levels, intravenous therapy, force fluids, intake and output monitoring
Failure, **CC** **MC** **CD** heart, congestive, unspecified	Peripheral edema, shortness of breath; cyanosis is present on occasion; heart rate is irregular; moist rales at base of lungs with productive cough; confusion is usually present	Sodium-restricted diet, digitalis regulation, O_2 therapy, diuretics

Urinalysis-Urobilinogen-Increased Level

Reference Range: 0-4.0 mg/24 hr
Hospital Range:_____

Condition	Signs & Symptoms	Treatment
Anemia, **CC** hemolytic	Vomiting, anorexia, weight loss	Transfusion(s) of blood and blood components, chemotherapy, iron therapy, O_2 therapy
Cirrhosis of **CC** liver	Abdominal pain or distention, fever, ascites, jaundice, anorexia, polyuria	Sodium-restricted diet, intravenous fluids, treatment for relief of symptoms

---

CC Complication/Comorbidity   **MC** Major Cardiovascular Condition   **CD** Complex Diagnosis

Urinalysis-Microscopic Exam-Cast Hyaline-Increased Level

Reference Range: 0-4/lp
Hospital Range:_____

Condition	Signs & Symptoms	Treatment
Failure, **CC** **MC** **CD** heart, congestive, unspecified	Peripheral edema, shortness of breath; cyanosis is present on occasion; heart rate is irregular; moist rales at base of lungs with productive cough; confusion is usually present	Sodium-restricted diet, digitalis regulation, O_2 therapy, diuretics
Disease, **CC** **MC** renal (glomerular, tubular, interstitial)	Fatigue, vomiting, anorexia, polyuria	Fluid restrictions, dialysis

Urinalysis-Microscopic Exam-White Blood Cells (WBCs)-Increased Level

Reference Range: 0-4/hpf
Hospital Range:_____

Condition	Signs & Symptoms	Treatment
Pyelonephritis **CC**	Nausea and vomiting, frequency of urination, dysuria, flank pain, chills	Antibiotic therapy, urinary analgesics, surgery if obstruction is present, force fluids
Urinary tract infection **CC**	Fever, dysuria, frequency, burning on urination, hematuria	Urinary antiseptics, antibiotic therapy, intravenous fluids, force fluids

Urine Culture-Presence of Pathogens

Reference Range: Negative
Hospital Range:_____

Condition	Signs & Symptoms	Treatment
Urinary tract infection **CC**	Fever, dysuria, frequency, burning on urination, hematuria	Urinary antiseptics, antibiotic therapy, intravenous fluids, force fluids

---

CC Complication/Comorbidity   **MC** Major Cardiovascular Condition   **CD** Complex Diagnosis

Drug Usage

Drug	Drug Action	Indications
Accupril [quinapril]	ACE inhibitors; antihypertensive	Congestive heart failure; essential hypertension
Acetaminophen/ codeine	Analgesic	Pain, moderate to severe Therapeutic level: 2 mcg/ml. Toxic level: 120 mcg/ml.
Adalat [nifedipine]	Calcium channel blocker	Vasospastic angina; chronic stable angina; essential hypertension
Albuterol Inhalation [butamol, proventil, ventolin]	Antiasthmatics / bronchodilators	Asthma
Aldoril [hydrochlorothiazide and methyldopa]	Antihypertensive, diuretic	Moderate to severe hypertension, particularly in patients with edema and renal dysfunction
Allegra [fexofenadine/ pseudoephedrine]	Antihistamines	Seasonal allergic rhinitis
Allopurinol [zyloprim]	Antigout	Gouty arthritis, renal calculus, hyperuricemia, hyperuricemia secondary to leukemia, hyperuricemia secondary to lymphoma
Alphagan [brimonidine]	Antiglaucoma agent (ophthalmic) antihypertensive, ocular	Glaucoma or another condition in which pressure in the eye is too high (ocular hypertension)
Alprazolam [xanax]	Antianxiety; sedatives/ hypnotics	Anxiety disorders with panic disorder and depression
Altace [ramipril]	Inhibitors; antihypertensives	Congestive heart failure, essential hypertension
Amaryl [glimepiride]	Blood glucose regulators	Diabetes mellitus
Ambien [zolpidem]	Sedatives/hypnotics	Insomnia
Amikin, Amikacin [amikacin sulfate]	Aminoglycoside antibiotic	Active in treatment of gram-negative bacterial infections such as *Pseudomonas, Escherichia coli (E. coli), Proteus, Klebsiella-Enterobacter-Serratia.* Therapeutic level: peak: 1530 mcg/ml; trough: 510 mcg/ml. Toxic level: peak: 35mcg/ml; trough: 10mcg/ml.
Aminophylline [theophylline ethylenediamine]	Bronchodilator, pulmonary vasodilator, smooth muscle relaxant	Relief and/or prevention of symptoms from asthma and reversible bronchospasms in bronchitis and emphysema Therapeutic level: 1020 mcg/ml. Toxic level: 20 mcg/ml.

Drug	Drug Action	Indications
Amoxicillin [trimox/amoxil]	Penicillins	Effective for infections with a broad spectrum of bactericidal activity against many gram-positive and gram-negative micro-organisms; otitis media, gonorrhea, skin, respiratory, gastrointestinal, and genitourinary infections
Ancef	Semisynthetic cephalosporin antibiotic	Respiratory tract infections due to *Streptococcus pneumoniae*, *Klebsiella species*, *Haemophilus infuenzae* (*H. influenzae*), *Staphylococcus aureus*, and group A betahemolytic streptococci; urinary tract infections due to *E. coli*, *Proteus mirabiis*, *Klebsiella* species and some strains of Enterobacter and enterococci; skin and skin structure infections, biliary tract infections, bone and joint infections, genital infections, septicemia, and endocarditis
Antabuse [disulfiram]	Alcohol treatment	Alcoholism
Antivert	Antihistamine	Management of nausea and vomiting, and dizziness associated with motion sickness
Aricept [donepezil hydrochloride]	Dementia symptoms treatment adjunct	Used to treat the symptoms of mild to moderate Alzheimer's disease; it can improve thinking ability in some patients
Arthrotec [diclofenac/ misoprostol]	Analgesic	Used for patients with arthritis who may develop stomach ulcers from taking nonsteroidal anti-inflammatory drugs (NSAIDs) alone; used to help relieve some symptoms of arthritis, such as inflammation, swelling, stiffness, and joint pain
Atenolol [tenormin]	Antianginals; antihypertensives; beta blockers	Chronic stable angina pectoris; essential hypertension; reduces cardiovascular mortality in those with definite or suspected acute myocardial infarction
Atrovent [ipratropium bromide]	Antiasthmatics / bronchodialator	Chronic bronchitis, emphysema; bronchial asthma
Augumentin [amoxicillin/ clavulanate]	Penicillins	Middle ear, lower respiratory, sinus, skin and skin structures, and urinary tract infections
Avapro [irbesartan]	Antihypertensive	Hypertension
Axid [nizatidine]	Acid/peptic disorders	Acid/peptic disorder; gastroesophageal reflux; duodenal, gastric, and peptic ulcers

Drug	Drug Action	Indications
Azmacort [triamcinolone aerosol]	Corticosteroid	Acute and chronic adrenal insufficiency; congenital adrenal hyperplasia; adrenal insufficiency secondary to pituitary insufficiency Nonendocrine disorders: arthritis, rheumatoid carditis, allergic, collagen, intestinal tract, liver, ocular, renal and skin diseases, bronchial asthma, cerebral edema, malignancies
Bactrim [trimethoprim sulfamethoxazole]	Antibacterial	Treatment of urinary tract infections, acute otitis media, acute exacerbation of chronic bronchitis, shigellosis, and pneumocystis carinii
Bactroban [mupirocin]	Dermatologics; topical anti-infectives	Topical treatment of impetigo
Beclovent [beclomethasone dipropionate]	Corticosteroids; antiasthmatics	Bronchial asthma, prevention of nasal polyps, perennial allergic, seasonal allergic and vasomotor rhinitis
Betoptic	Cardioselective beta-adrenergic receptor blocking agent	Lowers intraocular pressure; also used for treatment of ocular hypertension and chronic open-angle glaucoma
Biaxin [clarithromycin]	Macrolides	Acid/peptic disorder or ulcer, acute exacerbation chronic bronchitis, human immunodeficiency virus, lower and upper respiratory tract infection, sinus infection, prophylaxis mycobacterium avium complex, pharyngitis, pneumonia, tonsillitis
BuSpar [buspirone hydrochloride]	Antianxiety	Generalized anxiety disorder
Butazolidin [phenylbutazone]	Nonsteroidal anti-inflamatory	Gout, spondylitis, psoriasis, rheumatoid arthritis, osteoarthritis and postoperative and post-traumatic inflammation
Calan [verapamil hydrochloride]	Antianginals; antiarrhythmics, antiarthritics, antihypertensives, calcium channel blockers	Angina pectoris at rest and chronic stable, arrhythmia, atrial fibrillation, atrial flutter, paroxysmal supraventricular tachycardia, ventricular arrhythmia, essential hypertension
Cardilate [erythrol tetranitrate]	Coronary vasodilator	Long-term management of angina rather than for short-term relief, has slower onset but sustained duration of action similar to nitroglycerin
Cardizem CD/Tiazac [diltiazem hydrochloride]	Antianginals, antiarrhythmics, antihypertensives, channel blockers, coronary vasodilators	Chronic stable angina, atrial fibrillation, atrial flutter, essential hypertension, paroxysmal supraventricular tachycardia

Drug Usage

Drug	Drug Action	Indications
Cardura [doxazosin mesylate]	Antihypertensives	Benign prostatic hyperplasia, essential hypertension
Ceftin [cefuroxime Axetil]	Antibiotic: second generation cephalosporins	Acute exacerbation and chronic bronchitis, middle ear infection, sexually transmitted gonorrhea infection, upper respiratory tract infection, urinary tract infection, pharyngitis, tonsillitis
Cefzil [cefprozil]	Antiobiotic: second generation cephalosporins	Acute exacerbation and chronic bronchitis, lower respiratory tract infection, upper respiratory tract infection, pharyngitis, tonsillitis
Celebrex [celecoxib]	Antirheumatic, nonsteroidal anti-inflammatory	Used to relieve some symptoms caused by arthritis, such as inflammation, swelling, stiffness, and joint pain
Celexa [citalopram]	Antidepressant	Depression
Cipro [ciprofloxacin]	Anti-infective; quinolones	Cystitis, infectious diarrhea, gonorrhea, bone and joint infection, gastrointestinal tract infection, lower and upper respiratory tract infection, sinus infection, urinary tract infection, nosocomial pneumonia, chronic prostatitis
Claritin [loratadine/ pseudoephedrine]	Antihistamines	Seasonal allergic rhinitis, chronic idiopathic urticaria
Clonazepam [klonopin]	Anticonvulsants	Absence, akinetic and myoclonic epilepsy, Lennox-Gastaut syndrome. Therapeutic level: 1050 ng/ml. Toxic level: 100ng/ml.
Clonidine [catapres-TTS]	Antihypertensives	Hypertension
Cogentin [benztropine mesylate]	Antiparkinsonism	Parkinson's disease
Combivent [ipratropium bromide and albuterol sulfate]	Antiasthmatics / bronchodialator	Chronic bronchitis, emphysema; bronchial asthma
Compazine [prochlor-perazine]	Antiemetic, antipsychotic	Nausea, vomiting, and manic phase of bipolar syndrome
Cortisporin [hydrocortisone acetate; neomycin sulfate]	Topical anti-infectives, topical steroids	Dermatosis

Drug	Drug Action	Indications
Coumadin [sodium warfarin]	Thrombolytic agent/ anticoagulant	Used in prophylaxis and treatment of venous thrombosis, treatment of atrial fibrillation with embolization (pulmonary embolism), arrhythmias, myocardial infarction, and stroke prevention
Cozaar [losartan]	Antihypertensives	Essential hypertension
Cytomel	Thyroid hormone	Treatment of hypothyroidism or prevention of euthyroid goiters
Daypro [oxaprozin]	Nonsteroidal anti-inflammatory drug (NSAID)	Osteoarthritis and rheumatoid arthritis
Depakote [divalproex]	Anticonvulsants	Bipolar affective disorder; complex absence, complex partial and mixed pattern epilepsy; migraine headache
Desogen [desogestrel andethinyl estradiol]	Contraceptives; estrogens/ progestins	Contraception
Detrol [tolterodine tartrate]	Muscarinic receptor antagonist	Overactive bladders in patients with urinary frequency, urgency, or urge incontinence
Diflucan [fluconazole]	Antifungal agent	Oropharyngeal and esophageal candidiasis and cryptococcal meningitis in AIDS patients
Digitalis	Cardiotonic glycoside	Heart failure, atrial flutter, atrial fibrillation and supraventricular tachycardia
Dilantin [phenytoin sodium]	Anticonvulsant	Used for control of grand mal and psychomotor seizures Therapeutic level: 1020 mcg/ml. Toxic level: 30 mcg/ml.
Diovan [valsartan]	Ace inhibitors	Essential hypertension
Effexor XR [venlafaxine]	Antidepressants	Depression
Elavil [amitriptyline hydrochloride]	Anorexiants/CNS stimulants; antidepressants	Depression Therapeutic level: 75225 ng/ml. Toxic level: 500 ng/ml.
Entex LA/Contuss-XT [guaifenesin and phenylpropanol-amine]	Antitussives/ expectorants; cold remedies; decongestants, nasal	Nasal congestion
Epinephrine [adrenaline hydrochloride]	Bronchodilator, cardiotonic	Most commonly used to relieve respiratory distress due to bronchospasm and to restore cardiac rhythm in cardiac arrest

Drug	Drug Action	Indications
Erythromycin [erytab]	Acne products; macrolides; ocular anti-infective; topical anti-infectives	Acne vulgaris, intestinal amebiasis, infectious conjunctivitis, diphtheria, endocarditis, prevention, erythrasma treatment of infections: endocervical, gynecologic, lower and upper respiratory tract, ophthalmic, rectal; skin and skin structures, and urethral; Legionnaires' disease, pelvic inflammatory disease, pertussis, pneumonia, rheumatic fever, prophylaxis, syphilis
Estrace [estradiol]	Estrogen therapy	Used to treat menopausal symptoms, functional uterine bleeding, amenorrhea, inoperable prostatic cancer; postpartum breast engorgement, vagina and vulva atrophy, breast cancer, prostate cancer, hypoestrogenism, hypogonadism, female, kraurosis vulvae, menopause, osteoporosis prevention, ovarian failure, atrophic vaginitis
Evista [raloxifene hydrochloride]	Estrogen receptor modulator, selective osteoporosis prophylactic	Used to help prevent thinning of the bones (osteoporosis) only in postmenopausal women
Flexeril [cyclobenzaprine hydrochloride]	Muscle relaxant	Used as adjunct to rest and physical therapy for muscle spasms
Flomax [tamsulosin hydrochloride]	Benign prostatic hypertrophy therapy agent	Used to treat the signs and symptoms of benign enlargement of the prostate (benign prostatic hyperplasia or BPH)
Flonase [fluticasone]	Corticosteroids-inhalation/nasal; topical steroids	Corticosteroid-responsive dermatosis; perennial allergic and seasonal allergic rhinitis
Flovent [fluticasone propionate]	Corticosteroids-inhalation/nasal; topical steroids	Corticosteroid-responsive dermatosis, perennial allergic and seasonal allergic rhinitis
Follutein [chorionic gonadotropin]	Gonadotropic hormone	Prepubital cryptorchidism, hypogonadism, corpus luteum insufficiency and infertility
Fosamax [alendronate]	Calcium metabolism	Osteoporosis; Paget's disease
Furosemide [lasix]	Antihypertensives; diuretics	Used for management of edema associated with congestive heart failure, renal disease, including nephrotic syndrome and hypertension
Glucophage [metformin HCl]	Blood glucose regulators	Diabetes mellitus antihyperglycemic drug used in the management of non-insulin-dependent diabetes mellitus (NIDDM)

Drug	Drug Action	Indications
Glucotrol [glipizide]	Oral blood-glucose-lowering agent	Used as an adjunct to diet for the control of hyperglycemia in patients with noninsulin dependent diabetes mellitus (NIDDM, type II)
Glyburide [micronase]	Blood glucose regulators	Diabetes mellitus
Heparin [heparin sodium]	Anticoagulant	Prophylaxis and treatment of venous thrombosis, pulmonary embolism; prevention of cerebral thrombosis, and treatment of consumptive coagulopathies
Hydrochlorothiazide	Diuretic, antihypertensive	Used in management of hypertension and in adjunctive therapy for edema associated with congestive heart failure, hepatic cirrhosis, corticosteroid, and estrogen therapy
Hydrocodone and acetaminophen	Analgesics, general; analgesics-narcotic; antitussives/expectorants	Pain, moderate to severe
Hytrin [terazosin hydrochloride]	Alphablockers; antihypertensives; diuretics	Benign prostatic hypertrophy; essential hypertension
Hyzaar [losartan/HCTZ]	Antihypertensive	Hypertension
Imdur/ISMO [isosorbide mononitrate]	Antianginals; coronary vasodilators	Angina pectoris
Imitrex [sumatriptan Succinate]	Antimigraine	Migraine headache
Inderal [propranolol hydrochloride]	Beta-adrenergic blocking agent	Management of hypertension, long-term management of angina pectoris due to coronary atherosclerosis, cardiac arrhythmias
Isordil [isosorbide dinitrate]	Smooth muscle relaxant	Acute anginal attacks
Isuprel [isoproterenol sulfate]	Adrenergic agent	Bronchodilator for asthma, chronic pulmonary emphysema, bronchitis, and other conditions accompanied by bronchospasm; can be used in cardiogenic shock cases
K-Dur [potassium chloride]	Repl/regs of electrolytes/ water balance; vitamins/minerals	Hypokalemia
Keflex [cephalexin]	Cephalosporins	Bone, middle ear, skin and skin structures, upper respiratory tract and urinary tract infections; acute prostatitis
Lamisil [terbinafine hydrochloride]	Antifungal	Tinea cruris (jock itch), T. pedis (athlete's foot), T. corporis (ringworm)

Drug	Drug Action	Indications
Lanoxin [digoxin]	Cardiotonic	Used in the treatment of congestive heart failure Therapeutic level: 0.92 ng/ml Toxic level: 2 ng/ml
Lescol [fluvastatin]	Hyperlipidemia	Hypercholesterolemia; hyperlipidemia; hyperlipoproteinemia
Levaquin [levofloxacin]	Quinolones/derivatives	Acute exacerbation chronic bronchitis; cellulitis; furuncle; impetigo; infections of the lower and upper respiratory tract, sinus, skin and skin structures, and urinary tract; pneumonia, community-acquired; pyoderma
Levoxyl [levothyroxine]	Thyroid	Euthyroid goiter; hypothyroidism
Librium [chlordiazepoxide]	Antianxiety agent	Acute withdrawal symptoms, especially from alcohol, or for other anxiety-producing conditions. Therapeutic level: 510 mcg/ml Toxic level: 15 mcg/ml
Lidocaine [lidocaine hydrochloride]	Antiarrhythmic	Management of ventricular arrhythmias or during cardiac manipulation, such as cardiac surgery Therapeutic level: 25 mcg/ml Toxic level: 6 mcg/ml
Lipitor [atorvastatin calcium]	Antilipemic	Hypercholesterolemia, hyperlipidemia, hyperproteinemia
Lithium	Antipsychotic	Used to control manic episodes in bipolar syndrome
Lomotil [diphenoxylate hydrochloride with atropine]	Antidiarrheal	Used to treat symptoms of chronic and functional diarrhea
Lopid [gemfibrozil]	Hyperlipidemia	Hypercholesterolemia, hyperlipidemia, hyperlipoproteinemia, hypertriglyceridemia
Lopressor [metoprolol tartrate]	Antihypertensive, betablocker antianginals; antihypertensives; betablockers	Esstential hypertension therapy, angina pectoris, and myocardial infarction
Lorazepam [ativan]	Antianxiety; sedatives/ hypnotics	Anxiety disorder associated with depressive symptoms; controls tension, aggitation, irritability, and insomnia
Lorfan [levallorphan tartrate]	Narcotic antagonist	Used to overcome respiratory depression induced by drug overdose
Lotensin [benazepril]	ACE inhibitors; antihypertensives	Essential hypertension

Drug	Drug Action	Indications
Lotrel [amlodipine/ benazepril]	Antihypertensive	Hypertension
Lotrisone [clotrimazole/ betamethasone]	Antifungal-corticosteroid, topical	Used to help relieve redness, swelling, itching, and other discomfort of fungus infections
Macrodantin [nitrofurantoin]	Antibacterials, miscellaneous; antiseptics, urinary tract	Urinary tract infection; prophylaxis
Medrol [methylprednisolone]	Corticosteroids; antiarthritics	Acute/chronic adrenal insufficiency, congenital adrenal hyperplasia, adrenal insufficiency secondary to pituitary insufficiency; nonendocrine disorders include: arthritis, rheumatic carditis, bronchial asthma, cerebral edema, and diseases of allergic, collagen, intestinal tract, liver, ocular, renal, and skin
Methergine [methylergonovine maleate]	Oxytocic agent	Used for routine management of postpartum hemorrhage after delivery of placenta
Mevacor [lovastatin]	Hyperlipidemia	Hypercholesterolemia; hyperlipidemia, hyperlipoproteinemia
Miacalcin [calcitonin salmon]	Calcium metabolism	Hypercalcemia, osteoporosis, postmenopausal, Paget's disease
Monopril [fosinopril]	ACE inhibitors; antihypertensives	Essential hypertension
Motrin [ibuprofen]	Analgesics, general; analgesics, non-narcotic; antiarthritics; antigout; antipyretics; NSAID	Osteoarthritis and rheumatoid arthritis, dysmenorrhea, fever; pain, mild to moderate
Naprosyn [naproxen]	Anti-inflammatory analgesics, general; analgesics, non-narcotic; antiarthritics; antigout; NSAID	Used for rheumatoid, gouty arthritis and osteoarthritis; ankylosing spondylitis; bursitis; dysmenorrhea; pain, mild to moderate; tendonitis
Nembutal [pentobarbital sodium]	Sedative, hypnotic	Used as adjunct medication in diagnostic procedures or for emergency use with convulsive disorders
Neurontin [gabapentin]	Anticonvulsants	Epilepsy, partial
Nipride [sodium nitroprusside]	Antihypertensive	Used for potent, rapid action in reducing blood pressure in hypertensive crisis or for controlling bleeding during anesthesia by producing controlled hypotension
Nitrostat [Nitroglycerin] [glyceryltrinitrate]	Muscle relaxant antianginals; antihypertensives; coronary vasodilators; homeopathic products	Used for prophylaxis and treatment of angina pectoris; heart failure associated with myocardial infarction; hypertension, perioperative; surgery, adjunct

Drug	Drug Action	Indications
Nolvadex [tamoxifen citrate]	Antineoplastics; hormonal/ biological response modifiers	Breast cancer
Norflex [orphenadrine citrate]	Muscle relaxant	Used for acute spasms, tension, and post-trauma cases.
Norpace [disopyramide]	Antiarrhythmic	Used for coronary artery disease, for prevention, recurrence and control of unifocal, multifocal, and paired PVCs
Norvasc [amlodipine besylate]	Calcium channel blocker	Used in hypertension, chronic stable angina, and vasospastic angina
Ortho-Novum [norethindrone/ ethinyl estradiol]	Contraceptives; estrogens/ progestins	Contraception
Pavabid [papaverine hydrochloride]	Cerebral, vasodilator	Used for relief of cerebral and peripheral ischemia
Paxil [paroxetine]	Antidepressants	Anxiety with panic disorder and depression; obsessive-compulsive disorder
Pepcid [famotidine]	Acid/peptic disorders	Acid/peptic disorder; adenoma, secretory; gastroesophageal reflux; duodenal and gastric ulcer; Zollinger-Ellison syndrome
Percocet/Roxicet [oxycodone and acetaminophen]	Analgesics, general; analgesics-narcotic	Pain, moderate to severe
Persantine [dipyridamole]	Coronary vasodilator	Therapy for chronic angina pectoris
Phenergan [promethazine hydrochloride]	Anesthesia, adjuncts to; antiemetics; antihistamines; antitussives/expectorants; sedatives/hypnotics; vertigo/ motion sickness/vomiting	Anesthesia; adjunct; angioedema; conjunctivitis; dermographism; hypersensitivity, motion sickness; pain; perennial, seasonal, and allergic rhinitis; sedation, obstetrical; urticaria
Phenobarbital	Sedative, anticonvulsant, antiepileptic	Used for grand mal epilepsy
Pitocin [oxytocin citrate]	Oxytocic agent	Used to induce or stimulate labor at term
Plasmanate [plasma, plasma protein fraction]	Blood volume expander	Used for hypovolemic shock, burn patients and hemorrhages when whole blood is unavailable
Plavix [clopidogrel bisulfate]	Antithrombotic platelet aggregation inhibitor	Used to lessen the chance of heart attack or stroke
Plendil [felodipine]	Antihypertensives; calcium channel blockers	Essential hypertension
Pravachol [pravastatin]	Hyperlipidemia	Hypercholesterolemia, hyperlipidemia, hyperlipoproteinemia

Drug	Drug Action	Indications
Prednisone [prednisolone]	Glucocorticoid corticosteroids; antiarthritics; antineoplastics; ocular anti-inflammatory	Used for its immunosuppressant effects and for relief of inflammations; used in arthritis, polymyositis and other systemic diseases
Premarin [conjugated estrogens]	Antineoplastics; estrogens	Vasomotor symptoms associated with menopause; atrophic vaginitis; raurosis vulvae, female hypogonadism; primary ovarian failure
Prempro [conjugated estrogens/medroxyprogesteron]	Estrogens/progestins	Menopause, osteoporosis, atrophic vaginitis
Prevacid [lansoprazole]	Disorders, acid/peptic	Acid/peptic disorder, erosive esophagitis, duodenal ulcer, Zollinger-Ellison syndrome
Prinivil [lisinopril]	Inhibitors; antihypertensives	Congestive heart failure, essential hypertension
Prilosec [omeprazole]	Gastric acid pump inhibitor	Acid/peptic disorder; endocrine adenoma; erosive esophagitis; systemic mastocytosis; gastroesophageal reflux; duodeanl, peptic and gastric ulcer; Zollinger-Ellison syndrome
Procardia [nifedipine]	Antianginal agent; calcium channel blocker	Used for management of vasospastic angina and chronic stable angina, essential hypertension
Pronestyl [procainamide hydrochloride]	Depresses excitability of cardiac muscle	Used in treatment of PVCs, ventricular tachycardia, atrial fibrillation, and premature atrial tachycardia (PAT)
Propoxyphene hydrochloride	Analgesics, general; analgesics-narcotic	Pain Therapeutic level: 0.20.5 mcg/ml Toxic level: 2 mcg/ml
Prostin [dinoprost tromethamin]	Abortifacient	Used for late second trimester abortion
Provera/Depo-Provera/Cycrin [medroxyproges-terone acetate]	Antineoplastics; contraceptives; progestins	Amenorrhea; carcinoma, endometrium, adjunct; carcinoma, renal; contraception; hemorrhage
Prozac [fluoxetine hydrochloride]	Antidepressants	Bulimia nervosa; depression; obsessive-compulsive disorder
Quinidine, Quinaglute [quinidine gluconate]	Antiarrhythmic	Used for management of cardiac arrhythmias Therapeutic level: 25 mcg/ml Toxic level: 6 mcg/ml
Relafen [nabumetone]	Antiarthritics	Osteoarthritis and rheumatoid arthritis
Restoril [temazepam]	Sedatives/hypnotics	Insomnia

Drug Usage

Drug	Drug Action	Indications
Retrovir (Zidovudine)	Antiretroviral drug	Indicated in symptomatic HIV infection
Risperdal [risperidone]	Antipsychotics / antimanics	Psychosis; schizophrenia
Ritalin [methyl-phenidate hydrochloride]	Central nervous system (CNS) stimulant	Used to overcome depression and hyperkinetic activity in children
Septra [sulfameth-oxazol e-trimethoprim]	Antibacterial	Used for treatment of urinary tract infections, acute otitis media, acute exacerbations of chronic bronchitis, and shigellosis
Serax [oxazepam]	Antianxiety	Used for anxiety, tension, and alcohol withdrawal
Serevent [salmeterol]	Bronchodilators	Asthma
Serzone [nefazodone]	Antidepressants	Depression
Sinemet [carbidopa, levodopa]	Antiparkinsonian	Used to treat Parkinson's disease
Singulair [Montelukast]	Antiasthmatic, leukotriene receptor antagonist	Used in mild to moderate asthma to decrease the symptoms of asthma and the number of acute asthma attacks
Slow-K [potassium chloride]	Repl/regs of electrolytes/water balance; vitamins/minerals	Hypokalemia
Solu-Medrol [methylprednisol one sodium succinate]	Adrenocortico-steroid	Used as anti-inflammatory and antiallergenic for shock and ulcerative colitis
Sparine [promazine hydrochloride]	Antipsychotic	Used for DTs, alcoholic hallucinations and drug withdrawal symptoms
Stadol [butorphanol-tartrate]	Narcotic analgesic	Used for moderate to severe postsurgical pain
Synthroid/Levot hroid [levothyroxine sodium]	Thyroid preparation	Used for treatment of hypothyroidism
Tagamet [cimetidine]	Histamine antagonist	Used for treatment of active duodenal ulcer, short-term treatment of active, benign gastric ulcer and treatment of pathological hypersecretory conditions
Tegretol [carbamazepine]	Anticonvulsant	Used for epilepsy, especially with complex symptomatology Therapeutic level: 210 mcg/ml Toxic level: 12mcg/ml
TheoDur, Theolair [theophylline]	Bronchodilator, pulmonary vasodilator, smooth muscle relaxant	Used for treatment of bronchial obstruction in asthma and chronic obstructive pulmonary disease Therapeutic level: 1020 mcg/ml Toxic level: 20 mcg/ml

Drug	Drug Action	Indications
Tobradex [tobramycin and cexamethasone]	Aminoglycosides; ocular anti-infective/ anti-inflammatory	Infectious conjunctivits; dermatosis, corticosteroid-responsive with secondary infection; foreign body in eye; corneal inflammation; uveitis
Toprol-XL [Metoprolol]	Antianginals; antihypertensives; beta blockers	Angina pectoris, essential hypertension
Trazodone HCl [Desyrel]	Analgesics, general; antianxiety; antiarthritics; antidepressants	Depression Therapeutic level: 5001100mcg/ml Toxic level: 1500 mcg/ml
Triamterene/HC TZ	Antihypertensives, diuretics	Edema; essential hypertension
Trimethoprim/Sulfa [trimeth/sulfam eth]	Sulfonamides antimicrobials	Acute exacerbation chronic bronchitis; travelers' diarrhea; Infections of the middle, lower respiratory tract, and urinary tract; pneumonia, pneumocystis; shigellosis
Trinsicon [ferrous fumarate]	Antianemic preparation	Used for treatment of anemias
Triphasil [L-norgestrel/ethinyl estradiol]	Antineoplastics, contraceptives, estrogens/ progestins	Contraception
Ultram [tramadol]	Analgesics, non-narcotic	Pain, moderate to moderately severe
Urispas (flavoxate HCL)	Urinary tract spasmolytic	Used for relief of dysuria; urgency; nocturia, spurapubic pain, frequency, and incontinence associated with cystitis, prostatitis, urethritis, and urethrocystitis/urethrotrigonitis
Valium [diazepam]	Antianxiety, muscle relaxant, anticonvulsant adjuncts to, antianxiety, anticonvulsant, skeletal muscle hyperactivity	Used for anxiety, tension, withdrawal from alcohol, muscle spasms and anticonvulsant therapy; epilepsy, generalized tonic-clonic; status epilepticus; stiff-man syndrome; tetanus
Vasotec [enalapril]	ACE inhibitors, antihypertensives	Congestive heart failure; essential hypertension
Veetids [penicillin VK]	Penicillins	Chorea, prevention; endocarditis, prevention, secondary to tooth extraction; erysipelas; infections of the skin and skin structures, upper respiratory tract; rheumatic fever, prophylaxis; scarlet fever; Vincent's gingivitis; Vincent's pharyngitis

Drug	Drug Action	Indications
Verapamil [calan]	Antianginals, antiarrhythmics, antiarthritics, antihypertensives, calcium channel blockers	Angina pectoris; chronic stable angina; atrial fibrillation; atrial flutter; paroxysmal supraventricular tachycardia; ventricular arrhythmia; essential hypertension Therapeutic level: 50–200 ng/ml Toxic level: 400 ng/ml
Viagra [sildenafil citrate]	Impotence	Erectile dysfunction
Vistaril [hydroxyzine pamoate]	Antianxiety agent, antiemetic	Used for treating nausea and vomiting, for reducing narcotic requirement in surgery and as tranquilizer for tension, anxiety or agitation states
Vioxx [rofecoxib]	Antirheumatic, nonsteroidal anti-inflammatory analgesic antidysmenorrheal	Used to relieve some symptoms caused by arthritis, such as inflammation, swelling, stiffness, and joint pain
Wellbutrin SR [bupropion HCl]	Antidepressants; CNS	Depression; smoking cessation
Xalatan [latanoprost]	Glaucoma	Glaucoma, open-angle; ocular hypertension
Yutopar [ritodrine hydrochloride]	Inhibition of contractility of uterine smooth muscles	Used in management of labor in preterm patients
Zantac [ranitidine]	Antihistamines; acid/peptic disorders	Acid/peptic disorder; erosive esophagitis; gastrointestinal hypersecretion; mastocytosis; gastroesophageal reflux; peptic ulcer; Zollinger-Ellison syndrome
Zestoreti [lisinopril and hydrochlorothiazide]	ACE inhibitors; antihypertensives	Congestive heart failure; essential hypertension
Zestril [lisinopril]	ACE inhibitors; antihypertensives	Congestive heart failure; essential hypertension
Ziac [bisoprolol/ HCTZ]	Antihypertensives	Essential hypertension
Zithromax [azithromycin]	Macrolides	Infections of the cervix, lower respiratory tract, skin and skin structures, urethra, nongonococcal; mycobacterium avium complex; pharyngitis, streptococcal; pneumonia; tonsillitis
Zocor [simvastatin]	Hyperlipidemia	Hypercholesterolemia, hyperlipidemia, hyperlipoproteinemia, hypertriglyceridemia
Zoloft [sertraline HCl]	Antidepressants	Anxiety with panic disorder and depression; obsessive-compulsive disorder

Drug	Drug Action	Indications
Zoviraz [acyclovir]	Antiviral	Used in treatment of genital herpes and herpes zoster infections.
Zyprexa [olanzapine]	Antipsychotics/antimanics	Psychotic disorders; schizophrenia
Zyrtec [cetirizine]	Antihistamines	Perennial allergic and seasonal allergic rhinitis; chronic urticaria

Organisms

Specimen Site Normal Flora/Possible Pathogens

Bladder	**Normal Condition of Flora:** Specimen is normally sterile and free of organism growth. **Possible Pathogens:** Any organism; common contaminants are *Enterobacter, Escherichia (E. coli), Klebsiella,* and *Staphylococcus epidermidis*
Blood (multiple cultures usually performed)	**Normal Condition of Flora:** Specimen is normally sterile and free of organism growth. **Possible Pathogens:** Any organism; common contaminant is Staphylococcus epidermidis. Most common pathogens are *Bacteroides* species, *Haemophilus influenzae (H. influenzae), Staphylococcus aureus* and *Streptococcus pyogenes, E. coli, Pseudomonas, Streptococcus pneumoniae.* Opportunistic fungi include *Candida, Nocardia, Blastomyces dermatitidis, Histoplasma capsulatum.*
Cerebrospinal fluid	**Normal Condition of Flora:** Specimen is normally sterile and free of organism growth. **Possible Pathogens:** Any organism; common contaminant is Staphylococcus epidermidis. Pathogens include *Haemophilus influenzae, E. coli, Neisseria meningitidis* and *Streptococci agalactiae.* Viruses include coxsackie A and B, echovirus, HSV, mumps, HIV, adenovirus. Fungi include *Histoplasma capsulatum, Cryptococcus neoformans, Coccidioides immitis.*
Cervix	**Normal Condition of Flora:** Diphtheroids, *E. coli,* lactobacilli, nonhemolytic *Streptococcus,* and *Staphylococcus epidermidis* **Possible Pathogens:** *Candida albicans* (in large numbers), *Gardnerella vaginalis, Neisseria gonorrhoeae,* and *Trichomonas*
External ear	**Normal Condition of Flora:** Bacillus species, diphtheroids, *Saprophytic fungi,* alphahemolytic streptococci, and *Staphylococcus epidermis* **Possible Pathogens:** *Streptococcus pneumoniae* is the most significant. *Candida albicans, Haemophilus influenzae, Proteus* species, *Pseudomonas* species, *Staphylococcus aureus,* and *Papovavirus*
Middle ear	**Normal Condition of Flora:** Specimen is normally sterile and free of organism growth. **Possible Pathogens:** Acute otitis media common contaminants include *H. influenzae, Streptococcus pneumoniae,* beta-hemolytic streptococci. Chronic otitis media common contaminants include *Staphylococcus aureus, Pseudomonas, Proteus,* and influenza virus.

Organisms

Specimen Site Normal Flora/Possible Pathogens (continued)

Eye	**Normal Condition of Flora:** Diptheroids, *Moraxella* species, *Neisseria* species, and *Staphylococcus epidermis* **Possible Pathogens:** Any organisms; common pathogens include *H. influenzae, Staphylococcus aureus,* and *Streptococcus viridans*
Joints	**Normal Condition of Flora:** Specimen is normally sterileand free of organism growth. **Possible Pathogens:** Common contaminants include *Staphylococcus aureus, Staphylococcus epidermidis, Streptococcus pneumoniae, H. influenzae,* group B, *Klebsiella pneumoniae.* Viruses include mumps, rubella, parvovirus. Fungi include *Candida, Blastomyces dermatitidis, Coccidioides immitis.*
Kidney	**Normal Condition of Flora:** Specimen is normally sterile and free of organism growth. **Possible Pathogens:** Any organism; most common are *Staphylococcus* and streptococci
Large intestine, colon and rectum	**Normal Condition of Flora:** *Aspergillus, Bacillus subtilis, Bacteroides, Candida, Clostridium species,* diphtheroids, *Enterobacter,* enterococci, *E. coli, Fusobacterium, Klebsiella,* lactobacilli, *Peptococcus, Peptostreptococcus, Proteus* species, *Pseudomonas* species, staphylococci, and yeasts **Possible Pathogens:** *Campylobacter species, Chlamydia, Neisseria gonorrhoeae, Candida albicans* in large numbers, *Salmonella* species, *Shigella* species, *Vibrio cholera,* and *Yersinia* species. Viruses include rotavirus, CMV.
Lower ileum	**Normal Condition of Flora:** *Clostridium perfringens, Enterococcus,* occasionally *E. coli,* lactobacilli, staphylococci, *Streptococcus* of viridans group **Possible Pathogens:** *Salmonella* species and *Shigella* species
Mouth	**Normal Condition of Flora:** (After newborn period) bacteroids, *Branhamella catarrhalis, Candida albicans,* diphtheroids, *E. coli, Haemophilus* species, *Neisseria murosa, Peptostreptococcus lactobacillus, Staphylococcus epidermidis* and *Streptococcus* of viridans group **Possible Pathogens**: *Candida albicans* in large numbers, *Haemophilus influenzae* and *Haemophilus parainfluenzae, Staphylococcus aureus* (in large numbers), *Streptococcus* group A

Specimen Site Normal Flora/Possible Pathogens (continued)

Nasal passages	**Normal Condition of Flora:** Diphtheroids, *Enterobacter* species, gram-positive bacilli, *Klebsiella* species, *Staphylococcus* species and *Streptococcus* species **Possible Pathogens:** *H. influenzae*; acute sinusitiscommon contaminants include *Staphylococcus aureus, Streptococcus pneumoniae, Klebsiella enterobacter*, alphahemolytic streptococci, *Moraxella catarrhalis*; chronic sinusitis common contaminants include *Staphylococcus aureus, Streptococcus pneumoniae*, alphahemolytic streptococci, *Mucor, Aspergillus*
Nasopharynx	**Normal Condition of Flora:** (Sterile at birth) Bacteroids, diphtheroids, *E. coli*, gram-positive bacilli, *H. influenzae, Neisseria* species, staphylococci, streptococci, *Streptococcus pneumoniae* and *Proteus* species. Marked predominance of any of these organisms may be clinically significant even if it is a normal inhabitant. **Possible Pathogens:** *Bordetella pertussis, Corynebacterium diptheriae*; in large numbers: *E. coli*, gram-negative bacilli, *Haemophilus* species, *Proteus* species, *Pseudomonas* species, *Staphylococcus aureus*, and *Streptococcus pneumoniae*
Pericardium	**Normal Condition of Flora:** Specimen is usually sterile and free of organism growth. **Possible Pathogens:** Any organism; common contaminants are *Staphylococcus aureus, Streptococcus pneumoniae, Enterobacteriaceae, Pseudomonas, H. influenzae, Candida, Actinomyces.*
Peritoneal fluid	**Normal Condition of Flora:** Specimen is usually sterile and free of organism growth. **Possible Pathogens:** Any organism; common contaminants are *E. coli*, enterococci, *Streptococcus pneumoniae, Clostridium, Staphylcoccus aureus*, alphahemolytic streptococci.
Pleural fluid	**Normal Condition of Flora:** Specimen is usually sterile and free of organism growth. **Possible Pathogens:** Any organism; common contaminants are *Staphylococcus aureus, Staphylococcus epidermidis, Streptococcus pneumoniae, H. influenzae, E. coli, Klebsiella pneumoniae.*
Skin	**Normal Condition of Flora:** *Acinetobacter*, alphahemolytic streptococci, *Candida albicans*, diphtheroids, enterococci, enterococci propioni-bacterium, *Proteus, Staphylococcus epidermidis*, and *Staphylococcus* species **Possible Pathogens:** *Clostridium* species, *Corynebacterium diphtheriae, E. coli, Klebsiella, Neisseria, Staphylococcus aureus, Staphylococcus pyogenes*. Viruses include papillomavirus, varicella-simplex. Fungi include: *Trichophyton, Actinomyces, Norcardia, Microsporum*

Specimen Site Normal Flora/Possible Pathogens (continued)

Sputum	**Normal Condition of Flora:** Specimen is normally free of organism growth **Possible Pathogens:** Any organism; common contaminants are oral bacteria. The greater the number of squamous epithelial cells,the greater the contamination by oral-pharynx materials. Most common pathogens include gram negative bacilli or *Staphylococcus aureus*. Others are *H. influenzae* and *Streptococcus pneumoniae*.
Stomach, small Intestine	**Normal Condition of Flora:** Specimen is normally free of organism growth. Scant bacteria in two-thirds to include *E. coli*, *Klebsiella enterobacter*, enterococci, alphahemolytic streptococci, *Staphylococcus epidermidis*, diphtheroids. **Possible Pathogens:** *Helicobacter pylori*, *Campylobacter jejuni*
Stool, feces	**Normal Condition of Flora:** Bacteroids, *Clostridium albicans* (in large numbers), diphtheroids, *Enterobacter* species, *E. coli*, *Fusobacterium*, *Klebsiella* species, *Lactobacillus* species, *Peptococcus* species, *Peptostreptococcus* species, *Proteus* species, *Pseudomonas* species, *Staphylococcus* species, *Streptococcus* species, and yeast **Possible Pathogens:** *Campylobacter* species, *Candida albicans* (in large numbers), *Salmonella* species, *Shigella* species, *Vibrio cholera*, and *Yersenia* species. *Candida albicans* can be pathogenic when preceded by antibiotic therapy.
Throat	**Normal Condition of Flora:** Diphtheroids, *E. coli*, *Haemophilus* species, *Staphylococcus* species, *Streptococcus* species **Possible Pathogens:** *Bordetella pertussis*, *Corynebacterium* diphtheria, *Haemophilus* species; in large numbers: *E. coli*, *Proteus* species, *Pseudomonas* species, *Staphylococcus aureus*, *Streptococcus pneumoniae*, *Streptococcus pyogenes* group A
Trachea, bronchi, lungs, sinus cavities	**Normal Condition of Flora:** Specimen is normally sterile and free of organism growth. **Possible Pathogens:** *Candida albicans*, *Coccidioides*, *E. coli* or *Proteus mirabilis*, *H. influenzae*, *Klebsiella*, *Mycoplasma pneumoniae*, parainfluenza virus, Pneumocystis, Pseudomonas, *Salmonella*, staphylococci, *Streptococcus pneumoniae*; viruses include influenza, rhinovirus, coronavirus, adenovirus
Ureter	**Normal Condition of Flora:** Specimen is normally sterile and free of organism growth. **Possible Pathogens:** Any organism; most common pathogen is *E. coli.*, *Proteus*, *Pseudomonas*, and *Staphylococcus aureus* are others.

Specimen Site Normal Flora/Possible Pathogens (continued)

Urethra	**Normal Condition of Flora:** Diphtheroids, *Enterococcus*, *Mycoplasma*, *Staphylococcus epidermidis*
	Possible Pathogens: Common contaminants for males are *Neisseria gonorrhoeae*, *Chlamydia*, *Gardnerella vaginalis*, *E. coli*, and *Klebsiella enterobacter*. Common contaminants for females include *Candida albicans*, *Neisseria gonorrhoeae*, *Trichomonas*, *Clostridiumperfringens*, *Gardnerella vaginalis*, *Chlamydia*, and yeasts.
Urine, clean catch	**Normal Condition of Flora:** Specimen is normally sterile and free of organism growth.
	Possible Pathogens: Any organism count greater than 100,000 organisms per milliliter. Chronic infection may have repeatedly lower colony counts. Common contaminant is *Staphylococcus epidermidis*. Most common pathogen is *E. coli*. Others include *Proteus*, *Pseudomonas*, *Staphylococcus aureus*, *Klebsiella enterobacter*, *Candida albicans*, beta-hemolytic streptococci.
Vagina	**Normal Condition of Flora:** (Adult) *Candida albicans*, *Clostridium sporogenes*, diphtheroids, *E. coli*, lactobacilli, nonhemolytic and alphahemolytic *Streptococcus* species, *Staphylococcus epidermidis*, and yeasts
	Possible Pathogens: *Candida albicans* (in large numbers), *Gardnerella vaginalis*, *Neisseria gonorrhoeae*, and *Trichomonas*
Wound or abscess	**Normal Condition of Flora:** Specimen is normally sterile and free of organism growth.
	Possible Pathogens: *Clostridium* species, *E. coli*, *Pseudomonas* species, *Proteus* species, *Staphylococcus aureus*, *Streptococcus pyogenes* group A; a common contaminant is *Staphylococcus epidermidis*

Organisms

Major Cardiovascular Complications & Complex Diagnosis List

The following is a list of conditions considered to be major complications and complex diagnoses that when present as a secondary diagnosis may affect DRG assignment for DRG 121 Circulatory Disorders with Acute Myocardial Infarction and Major Complications, Discharged Alive and DRG 124 Circulatory Disorders Except Acute Myocardial Infarction with Cardiac Catheterization and Complex Diagnosis. An asterisk (*) indicates a code range is represented.

Code	Title		
398.91	Failure, heart, congestive, rheumatic	CD	MC
402.01	Hypertensive heart disease, malignant, with heart failure	CD	MC
402.11	Hypertensive heart disease, benign, with heart failure	CD	MC
402.91	Hypertensive heart disease, unspecified, with heart failure	CD	MC
404.01	Hypertensive heart and renal disease, malignant with failure, heart	CD	MC
404.03	Hypertensive heart and renal disease, malignant, with failure, heart and renal	CD	MC
404.11	Hypertensive heart and renal disease, benign, with failure, heart	CD	MC
404.13	Hypertensive heart and renal disease, benign, with failure, heart and renal	CD	MC
404.91	Hypertensive heart and renal disease, unspecified with failure, heart	CD	MC
404.93	Hypertensive heart and renal disease, unspecified, with failure, heart and renal	CD	MC
411.0	Syndrome, postmyocardial infarction	CD	MC
411.1	Syndrome, intermediate coronary	CD	
*411.8	Disease, heart, ischemic, acute and subacute forms, other	CD	
*414.1	Aneurysm, heart		MC
415.0	Cor pulmonale, acute	CD	
*415.1	Embolism and infarction, pulmonary	CD	MC
416.0	Hypertension, pulmonary, primary		MC
420.0	Pericarditis, acute, in diseases classified elsewhere	CD	
*420.9	Pericarditis, acute, unspecified	CD	
*421	Endocarditis, acute, subacute	CD	
422.0	Myocarditis, acute, in diseases classified elsewhere	CD	
*422.9	Myocarditis, acute, unspecified	CD	
423.0	Hemopericardium	CD	
424.90	Endocarditis, valve unspecified, unspecified cause	CD	
424.91	Endocarditis, in diseases classified elsewhere	CD	

MC Major Cardiovascular Condition   CD Complex Diagnosis

425.2	Cardiomyopathy, obscure, of Africa	CD
425.3	Fibroelastosis, endocardial	CD
425.4	Cardiomyopathy, other, primary	CD
425.5	Cardiomyopathy, alcoholic	CD
425.7	Cardiomyopathy, nutritional and metabolic, classified elsewhere	CD
425.8	Cardiomyopathy, other diseases classified elsewhere	CD
425.9	Cardiomyopathy, secondary, unspecified	CD
426.0	Block, complete, atrioventricular	MC
426.10	Block, unspecified, atrioventricular	MC
426.12	Block, Mobitz, type II, atrioventricular	MC
426.13	Block, other second-degree, atrioventricular	MC
426.3	Block, other, bundle branch, left	MC
426.51	Block, bundle branch, right, and left fascicular block, posterior	MC
426.52	Block, bundle branch, right, and left fascicular block, anterior	MC
426.53	Block, other, bundle branch, bilateral	MC
426.54	Block, trifascicular	MC
427.0	Tachycardia, paroxysmal, supraventricular	MC
427.1	Tachycardia, paroxysmal, ventricular	CD MC
427.2	Tachycardia, paroxysmal, unspecified	MC
*427.3	Fibrillation and flutter, atrial	MC
*427.4	Fibrillation and flutter, ventricular	MC
427.5	Arrest, cardiac	CD MC
*428	Failure, heart	CD MC
429.4	Disturbance, heart, functional, following cardiac surgery	CD
429.5	Rupture, chordae tendinae	CD MC
429.6	Rupture, papillary muscle	CD MC
*429.7	Sequelae, of myocardial infarction, not elsewhere classified	CD
429.81	Disorders, other, papillary muscle	CD MC
429.82	Disease, hyperkinetic, heart	CD
430	Hemorrhage, subarachnoid	MC
431	Hemorrhage, intracerebral	MC
*432	Hemorrhage, intracranial, other and unspecified	MC
433.01	Occlusion, stenosis, with cerebral infarction, artery, basilar	MC
433.11	Occlusion, stenosis, with cerebral infarction, artery, carotid	MC
433.21	Occlusion, stenosis, with cerebral infarction, artery, vertebral	MC
433.31	Occlusion, stenosis, with cerebral infarction, arteries, multiple and bilateral, precerebral	MC
433.81	Occlusion, stenosis, with cerebral infarction, arteries, other specified, precerebral	MC

MC Major Cardiovascular Condition   CD Complex Diagnosis

©2003 Ingenix, Inc.

433.91	Occlusion, stenosis, with cerebral infarction, arteries, unspecified, precerebral	MC
*434	Thrombosis, arteries, cerebral	MC
436	Disease, acute, but ill-defined, cerebrovascular	MC
*441.0	Aneurysm, dissecting, aorta, unspecified site	MC
458.8	Hypotension, other specified	MC
458.9	Hypotension, unspecified	MC
481	Pneumonia, pneumococcal	MC
482.0	Pneumonia, bacterial, due to *Klebsiella pneumoniae*	MC
482.1	Pneumonia, bacterial, due to *Pseudomonas*	MC
482.2	Pneumonia, bacterial, due to *Hemophilus influenzae*	MC
*482.3	Pneumonia, bacterial, due to *Streptococcus*	MC
*482.4	Pneumonia, bacterial, *Staphylococcus*	MC
482.81	Pneumonia, bacterial, due to anaerobes	MC
482.82	Pneumonia, bacterial, due to *Escherichia coli* (E. coli)	MC
482.83	Pneumonia, bacterial, due to gram-negative bacteria, other	MC
482.89	Pneumonia, bacterial, other specified	MC
482.9	Pneumonia, bacterial, unspecified	MC
*483	Pneumonia due to *Mycoplasma pneumoniae*	MC
*484	Pneumonia, in infectious diseases classified elsewhere	MC
485	Bronchopneumonia, organism unspecified	MC
486	Pneumonia, organism unspecified	MC
487.0	Influenza, with pneumonia	MC
*507	Pneumonitis, due to inhalation, solids, liquids	MC
518.0	Collapse, pulmonary	MC
518.5	Insufficiency, pulmonary, following trauma and surgery	MC
518.81	Failure, respiratory, acute	MC
518.83	Failure, respiratory, chronic	MC
518.84	Failure, respiratory, acute and chronic	MC
*584	Failure, renal, acute	MC
707.0	Ulcer, decubitus	MC
785.50	Shock, unspecified, without mention of trauma	CD MC
785.51	Shock, cardiogenic	CD MC
996.62	Complication, infection, inflammatory reaction, vascular device, implant and graft, other	MC
996.72	Complication, other, cardiac device, implant and graft, other	MC

MC Major Cardiovascular Condition   CD Complex Diagnosis

Implications of Complex Cardiovascular Diagnoses

Aneurysm of aorta, dissecting, any part 441.00 441.01 441.02 441.03	**Signs and Symptoms:** Severe pain in anterior part of chest, possibly back, lumbar area and abdomen; nausea, weakness of legs, unconsciousness and intermittent claudication; condition is an extreme emergency necessitating emergency surgery and invasive monitoring and intensive stabilizing measures **History and Physical Exam:** Pulsation of lower extremities **Nurse's Notes:** Documentation of increased blood pressure; oxygen therapy blood transfusion and invasive monitoring **Procedures:** Pulmonary capillary wedge pressure and central venous pressure **Radiology:** CAT scan to confirm size and location, aortography, MRI; widening of aortic shadow; arteriography-calcification
Aneurysm of coronary vessels 414.11	**Signs and Symptoms:** Distressing cardiac palpitation; severe dyspnea; generalized edema **Radiology:** Chest x-ray-cardiac enlargement; arteriography-calcifications
Aneurysm of heart 414.10 414.19	**Signs and Symptoms:** Distressing cardiac palpitation; severe dyspnea; generalized edema; shock can occur after myocardial infarction **Drug Therapy:** May include antiarrhythmics such as procainamide, quinidine or calan, cardizem **EKG:** Bundle branch abnormality, possible T wave changes; S-T segment elevated **Nurse's Notes:** Frequent monitoring of vital signs and intake and output, and cardiopulmonary resuscitation **Procedures:** Cardioversion **Radiology:** Chest x-ray-enlarged heart with dilation, possibly localized calcification Ventriculography reduced cardiac output and hypertrophy of left ventricle

Arrest, cardiac 427.5	**Signs and Symptoms:** Sudden unexpected cessation of cardiac action, absence of heart sounds and/or blood pressure; loss of consciousness, rapid, shallow breathing; cardiopulmonary resuscitation performed **Drug Therapy:** May include isoproterenol, atropine, sodium bicarbonate, epinephrine, and calcium gluconate **EKG:** Changes prior to arrest may show bradycardia, tachycardia or other arrhythmias, fibrillation, such as ventricular fibrillation, or asystole **Nurse's Notes:** Resuscitative efforts recorded in notes or "code sheet" **Procedures:** May include intubation and artificial ventilation; may also include defibrillation
Atelectasis 518.0	**Signs and Symptoms:** Known as lung collapse; symptomatologies vary with amount of parenchyma involved; dyspnea, cough, and possibly orthopnea **Nurse's Notes:** Deep breathing and coughing; postural drainage (often done by physical therapist) **Procedures:** Bronchoscopy, spirometry, and nebulizer treatments **Radiology:** Chest x-ray-clinically diagnostic; CT scan of thorax
Block, atrioventricular 426.10	**Signs and Symptoms:** Dyspnea, faintness, and weakness **Drug Therapy:** Atropine may be given; in addition, antiarrhythmics such as calan, cardizem, or lidocaine **EKG:** Various patterns producing an irregularly dropped beat can be determined by cardiac auscultation or palpation of the pulse
Block, atrioventricular, complete (third-degree block) 426.0	**Signs and Symptoms:** Also called "complete" heart block; atrioventricular disassociation, complete; possible angina pectoris; exertional dyspnea, dizziness, palpitation and possible syncope **Drug Therapy:** Antiarrhythmics such as calan, cardizem, or lidocaine **EKG:** Focus below bifurcation; premature ventricular beats **Procedures:** Insertion of temporary pacemaker followed by a permanent pacemaker
Block, atrioventricular, Mobitz type I, second degree 426.13	**Signs and Symptoms:** Also called "partial" or "incomplete" heart block; weakness, faintness, palpitation, and dyspnea transient when in upright position; usually transient in nature and requires no treatment **Drug Therapy:** Atropine for bradycardia; in addition, antiarrhythmics such as calan, cardizem, or lidocaine **EKG:** Often documented as "Wenckebach" pause; irregular ventricular rhythm, regular atrial rhythm **Procedures:** Temporary pacemaker

Block, atrioventricular, Mobitz type II 426.12	**Signs and Symptoms:** Also called "partial" or "incomplete" heart block; attack of syncope related to sudden cessation of circulation in upright or recumbent position **Drug Therapy:** Atropine for bradycardia; discontinue digitalis; antiarrhythmics such as calan, cardizem, or lidocaine **EKG:** Block may be documented as 2:1, 3:1, or 4:1; sudden onset of AV disassociation **Procedures:** Temporary pacemaker and permanent pacemaker, if necessary
Block, bilateral bundle branch 426.53	**Signs and Symptoms:** Symptoms are usually absent **EKG:** QRS duration of 0.12 seconds or more; diastolic gallop rhythm
Block, left bundle branch 426.3	**Signs and Symptoms:** Symptoms are usually absent; usually secondary to coronary artery disease or hypertension; makes the diagnosis of acute myocardial infarction more difficult **EKG:** QRS duration of 0.12 seconds or more and contour of complex is distorted; diastolic gallop rhythm
Block, right bundle branch and left anterior fascicular block 426.52	**Signs and Symptoms:** Symptoms are usually absent **EKG:** Left anterior fascicular block; QRS complex lasting 0.12 seconds or longer; T-wave essentially normal in all leads except V1-V3
Block, right bundle branch and left posterior fascicular block 426.51	**Signs and Symptoms:** Symptoms are usually absent; occurs less frequently than left anterior fascicular block **EKG:** Left posterior fascicular block; QRS complex lasting 0.12 seconds or longer; T-wave essentially normal in all leads except V1-V3
Block, trifascicular 426.54	**Signs and Symptoms:** Dizziness, syncope, dyspnea, and weakness **EKG:** Combined arrhythmias
Cardiomyopathy in other diseases classified elsewhere 425.8	**Signs and Symptoms:** Increase in diastolic blood pressure; loss of consciousness, hypertrophy of heart and/or history of heart disease; symptoms include dyspnea, paroxysmal nocturnal dyspnea, fatigue, edema, and palpitations; can occur with sarcoidosis, hypertension, or muscular dystrophy **Drug Therapy:** May include digoxin, pronestyl, diuretics, vasodilators, calan, or nitrostat **EKG:** May show atrial enlargement, sinus tachycardia, premature ventricular contractions, atrial fibrillation, or ventricular hypertrophy **Nurse's Notes:** Intake and output, daily weights, frequent vital signs, and documentation of complete bed rest; oxygen therapy **Procedures:** Cardiac catheterization, echocardiogram, and possible heart transplant **Radiology:** Chest x-ray may show cardiac hypertrophy or pleural effusion

Cardiomyopathy of Africa, obscure 425.2	**Signs and Symptoms:** Viral in etiology; destroys heart muscle and tissue; probable heart failure **Drug Therapy:** May include digoxin, pronestyl, diuretics, vasodilators, calan, or nitrostat **EKG:** May show atrial enlargement, sinus tachycardia, premature ventricular contractions, atrial fibrillation, or ventricular hypertrophy **Nurse's Notes:** Intake and output, daily weights,frequent vital signs, and documentation of complete bed rest; oxygen therapy **Procedures:** Cardiac catheterization, echocardiogram, and possible heart transplant **Radiology:** Chest x-ray may show cardiac hypertrophy or pleural effusion
Cardiomyopathy, alcoholic 425.5	**Signs and Symptoms:** Documentation of excessive alcohol intake, exertional dyspnea, cough, fatigue, hemoptysis, and edema This condition is frequently found in patients between 23 and 50 years of age. **Drug Therapy:** May include digoxin, pronestyl, diuretics, vasodilators, calan, or nitrostat **EKG:** May show atrial enlargement, sinus tachycardia, premature ventricular contractions, atrial fibrillation, or ventricular hypertrophy **Nurse's Notes:** Intake and output, daily weights, frequent vital signs, and documentation of complete bed rest; oxygen therapy **Procedures:** Cardiac catheterization, echocardiogram, and possible heart transplant **Radiology:** Chest x-ray may show cardiac hypertrophy or pleural effusion
Cardiomyopathy, nutritional and metabolic 425.7	**Signs and Symptoms:** Underlying disease: thyrotoxicosis, beriberi, amyloidosis; symptoms include dyspnea, paroxysmal nocturnal dyspnea, fatigue, edema, and palpitations **Drug Therapy:** May include digoxin, pronestyl, diuretics, vasodilators, calan, or nitrostat **EKG:** May show atrial enlargement, sinus tachycardia, premature ventricular contractions, atrial fibrillation, or ventricular hypertrophy **Nurse's Notes:** Intake and output, daily weights, frequent vital signs, and documentation of complete bed rest; oxygen therapy **Procedures:** Cardiac catheterization, echocardiogram, and possible heart transplant **Radiology:** Chest x-ray may show cardiac hypertrophy or pleural effusion

Cardiomyopathy, primary 425.4	**Signs and Symptoms:** Usually demonstrated in elderly patients with loss of consciousness, palpitations, and/or dyspnea; palpitations may be evident by bounding or rapid pulse and skipped heartbeats; edema and paroxysmal nocturnal dyspnea also may be present; may include congestive and restrictive cardiomyopathies
	Drug Therapy: May include digoxin, pronestyl, diuretics, vasodilators, calan, or nitrostat
	EKG: May show atrial enlargement, sinus tachycardia, premature ventricular contractions, atrial fibrillation, or ventricular hypertrophy
	Nurse's Notes: Intake and output, daily weights, frequent vital signs, and documentation of complete bed rest; oxygen therapy
	Procedures: Cardiac catheterization, echocardiogram, and possible heart transplant
	Radiology: Chest x-ray may show cardiac hypertrophy or pleural effusion
Cardiomyopathy, secondary 425.9	**Signs and Symptoms:** Hypertrophy of heart; occurs as a complication of cardiovascular disease or other systemic disease; symptoms include dyspnea, paroxysmal nocturnal dyspnea, fatigue, edema, and palpitations
	Drug Therapy: May include digoxin, pronestyl, diuretics, vasodilators, calan, or nitrostat
	EKG: May show atrial enlargement, sinus tachycardia, premature ventricular contractions, atrial fibrillation, or ventricular hypertrophy
	Nurse's Notes: Intake and output, daily weights, frequent vital signs, and documentation of complete bed rest; oxygen therapy
	Procedures: Cardiac catheterization, echocardiogram, and possible heart transplant
	Radiology: Chest x-ray may show cardiac hypertrophy or pleural effusion
Cerebrovascular disease, acute, ill-defined 436	**Signs and Symptoms:** Hemiplagia, hemiparesis, vertigo, numbness, aphasia, dysarthria. CVA lacks specificity and is dependent upon ischemic or hemorrhagic lesions. The effects reflect the damaged area of the brain and the specific artery affected.
	Drug therapy: May include thrombolytic agents for treatment; anticoagulants and antiplatelet agents for prevention
	Procedures: Vascular surgery such as thromboendarterectomy
	Radiology: CT scan and MRI may help to determine ischemic versus hemorrhagic. Angiography can identify site. Arteriography may be indicated for suspected diagnosis.

Implications of Complex
Cardiovascular Diagnoses

Congestive heart failure (CHF), unspecified 428.0	**Signs and Symptoms:** Dyspnea is present with orthopnea and paroxysmal nocturnal dyspnea present in more advanced failure; other symptoms include peripheral edema, irritability weakness and neck (jugular) vein distention; cyanosis is present on occasion; heart rate is irregular; moist rales are present in bases of lungs with productive cough; confusion is usually present
	Drug Therapy: May include digoxin, diuretics and vasodilators (e.g., altrace, aldoril, vasotec, zestril)
	EKG: Tachycardia and atrial enlargement Laboratory: Possible increase in plasma volume above 5% of body weight
	Nurse's Notes: Frequent monitoring of vital signs, intake and output, antiembolism hose, low-sodium diet, oxygen therapy, daily weights, fluid restriction, and rotating tourniquets
	Procedures: Echocardiography, cardiac blood pool imaging, pulmonary artery monitoring and cardiac catheterization
	Radiology: Chest x-ray-may show cardiac hypertrophy, pleural effusion or pulmonary venous congestion; S3 chest sound and pulmonary edema or pulmonary vascular congestion on chest x-ray
Cor pulmonale, acute 415.0	**Signs and Symptoms:** Progressive dyspnea, substernal discomfort or pain, persistent cough, wheezing, fatigue, and edema; documentation of infection; most commonly results from chronic obstructive pulmonary disease (COPD); pulmonary hypertension results within hours of onset
	Drug Therapy: May include bronchodilators (e.g., alupent, brethine, aminophylline, bronkosol, epinephrine or theophylline and diuretics, vasodilators, digoxin, antibiotics)
	EKG: Cardiac arrhythmias such as premature atrial and ventricular contractions
	Laboratory: Arterial blood gas: may show poor air exchange (pO_2 75100); hypoxemia indicated by low O_2 saturation (O_2 less than 80); hematocrit often more than 50%; spirometry
	Nurse's Notes: Intake and output, daily weights, fluid restriction, and low-salt diet
	Procedures: Echocardiography or cardiac angiography demonstrating right ventricular hypertrophy
	Respiratory Therapy: May include IPPB treatment, use of O_2 (in low concentrations for patients with COPD) and/or use of bronchodilators; pulmonary function studies

Coronary occlusion, acute, without myocardial infarction 411.81	**Signs and Symptoms:** Arteriosclerotic heart disease, elevated cholesterol, disease of aortic valve, thoracic pain, chest pain with or without exertion, anemia, dizziness, syncope, and dyspnea **Drug Therapy:** May include nitroglycerin, lidocaine, pronestyl, digoxin, quinidine, and potassium supplement administered intravenously **EKG:** Documentation may indicate subacute ischemia **Laboratory:** Potassium level may be decreased, indicating cardiac damage. enzymes may be slightly elevated; cholesterol level may be greater than 250; anemia (hemoglobin less than 8 and hematocrit less than 28) may be present **Nurse's Notes:** May document cardiac monitoring or coronary care unit services **Procedures:** Cardiac catheterization, PTCA **Radiology:** Echocardiogram, myocardial perfusion studies, =gated blood pool imaging; chest x-ray may show cardiac enlargement =and increased hilar markings
Defect, cardiac, septal, acquired and other 429.71 429.79	**Signs and Symptoms:** S2 sounds normally split in small ventricular defect; soft, early systolic ejection murmur **EKG:** P waves normal or peaked; P3 may be inverted in sinus venosus defect **Radiology:** Chest x-ray normal or light LVE; little or no increase in pulmonary vasculature in ventricular defects
Disturbances, heart, functional, following cardiac surgery 429.4	**Signs and Symptoms:** History of cardiac surgery (may have occurred previously or during the present admission); functional disturbances may be indicated by arrhythmias, level of consciousness, diaphoresis, or a drop in blood pressure (diastolic pressure less than 60) **Drug Therapy:** May include quinidine, lidocaine, or pronestyl **EKG:** Ventricular tachycardia or fibrillation and premature atrial contractions (PACs) **Nurse's Notes:** Monitoring of vital signs and dietary restrictions
Endocardial fibroelastosis 425.3	**Signs and Symptoms:** Cardiac hypertrophy with documentation of peripheral edema; usually occurs in ages six weeks to six months; in older children, there is usually documentation of poor heart sounds and often tachycardia; in patients over 50, documentation of six to 15 years of heart disease; possible relationship to mumps virus **EKG:** Left ventricular hypertrophy **Procedures:** Angiocardiography; fluoroscopy: may be clinically diagnostic **Radiology:** Chest x-ray may show extreme left ventricle enlargement

Endocarditis in diseases classified elsewhere 424.91	**Signs and Symptoms:** Underlying cause may be documented as blastomycosis (116.0), Q fever (083.0), or typhoid fever (002.0); excludes bacterial endocarditis; patient may have arthralgia and possibly purpura; may show elevated temperature (greater than 102-) **Drug Therapy:** Antibiotic therapy in large doses intravenously **EKG:** Atrial arrhythmias **Laboratory:** Positive blood cultures for 85–95% of patients; most common pathogens include Streptococcus viridans with subgroups; enterococcus or Streptococcus faecalis; coagulase negative Staphylococci; white blood cell count may be increased or decreased; ESR rate is elevated; urinalysis may show hematuria **Nurse's Notes:** Monitoring of intake and output and documentation of bed rest **Procedures:** Echocardiogram; surgery may be performed for infection of a cardiac prosthesis or for severe damage to the heart valves **Radiology:** Abdominal x-ray: possible spleen enlargement
Endocarditis, acute 421.0	**Signs and Symptoms:** Onset of abrupt chills, sweats, weakness, anorexia, malaise, arthralgia, and hematuria; chest pain and possible fever; painless red-blue lesions on palms or soles and splinter hemorrhages of nail beds; heart murmur may be present **Drug Therapy:** Antibiotic therapy in large doses administered intravenously **EKG:** Atrial arrhythmias **Laboratory:** Positive blood cultures for 85–95% of patients. Most common pathogens include Streptococcus viridans with subgroups; enterococcus or Streptococcus faecalis; coagulase negative staphylococci; white blood cell count may be increased or decreased; erythrocyte sedimentation rate (ESR) is elevated; urinalysis may show hematuria **Nurse's Notes:** Monitoring of intake and output and documentation of bed rest **Procedures:** Echocardiogram; surgery may be performed for infection of a cardiac prosthesis or for severe damage to the heart valves **Radiology:** Abdominal x-ray: possible spleen enlargemen

Endocarditis, bacterial 421.9	**Signs and Symptoms:** Onset is insidious depending upon pre-existing damage to the cardiovascular system; documentation may show malaise; cough; sweating; weakness; history of weight loss; and pain in chest, abdomen, and extremities; fever (over 102°); other indications are skin lesions, increased paresthesia, and hematuria; bacterial endocarditis usually follows rheumatic fever; heart murmur usually present in subacute endocarditis, but may not be evident in acute endocarditis **Drug Therapy:** Antibiotic therapy in large doses intravenously **EKG:** Atrial arrhythmias **Laboratory:** Positive blood cultures for 85–95% of patients; most common pathogens include Streptococcus viridans with subgroups; enterococcus or Streptococcus faecalis; coagulase negative staphylococci; white blood cell count may be increased or decreased; ESR is elevated; urinalysis may show hematuria **Nurse's Notes:** Monitoring of intake and output and documentation of bed rest **Procedures:** Echocardiogram; surgery may be performed for infection of a cardiac prosthesis or for severe damage to the heart valves **Radiology:** Abdominal x-ray: possible spleen enlargement
Endocarditis, infective, acute and subacute, in diseases classified elsewhere 421.1	**Signs and Symptoms:** Underlying cause may be documented as blastomycosis, Q fever, or typhoid fever; excludes bacterial endocarditis; patient may have arthralgia and possibly purpura; may show elevated temperature (greater than 102°) **Drug Therapy:** Antibiotic therapy in large doses administrated intravenously **EKG:** Atrial arrhythmias **Laboratory:** Positive blood cultures for 85–95% of patients; most common pathogens include Streptococcus viridans with subgroups; enterococcus or Streptococcus faecalis; coagulas negative staphylococci; white blood cell count may be increased or decreased; ESR is elevated; urinalysis may show hematuria **Nurse's Notes:** Monitoring of intake and output and documentation of bed rest **Procedures:** Echocardiogram; surgery may be performed for infection of a cardiac prosthesis or for severe damage to the heart valves **Radiology:** Abdominal x-ray: possible spleen enlargement

Endocarditis, valve unspecified, unspecified cause 424.90	**Signs and Symptoms:** incompetence and insufficiency of heart valve; valvulitis; nonbacterial thrombotic stenosis of valve; regurgitation of mitral valve; inflammatory conditions of heart valve; symptoms include heart murmur, weakness, intermittent fever, petechiae, arthralgia, and confusion
	Drug Therapy: IV antibiotics
	EKG: May reveal tachycardia
	Laboratory: Blood: anemia (hemoglobin less than 8 and hematocrit less than 28); urinalysis may show red blood cells; blood cultures: positive in 85–95% of patients
	Nurse's Notes: Monitoring of intake and output
	Procedures: Echocardiogram may be diagnostic; blood transfusion, surgery for infection of cardiac prosthesis or severe damage to the heart valves
	Radiology: Chest x-ray may show cardiac enlargement
Failure, heart 428.9	**Signs and Symptoms:** Documentation of cardiac insufficiency, fatigue, or dyspnea
	Radiology: Chest x-ray-cardiac enlargement
Fibrillation, atrial 427.31	**Signs and Symptoms:** Occurs as a result of other conditions, such as congestive heart failure and sepsis, or after bypass or valve replacement surgery; symptoms include palpitations, dyspnea, dizziness, fainting and apprehension
	Drug Therapy: May include the ongoing use of digoxin, diuretics, and quinidine, calan, cardizem, and coumadin
	EKG: Atrial rate over 400/minute with a variable ventricular rate; absence of P waves
	Procedures: Cardioversion and echocardiography
Fibrillation, ventricular 427.41	**Signs and Symptoms:** A life-threatening cardiac emergency; absence of effective cardiac action resulting in loss of pulse, respirations, and blood pressure; seizures and death can occur
	Drug Therapy: Lidocaine, procainamide, calan, cardizem, and digitalis
	EKG: Bizarre (QRS) complexes; ventricular rhythm chaotic and rapid
	Nurse's Notes: CPR and oxygen therapy
	Procedures: Cardiopulmonary resuscitation and defibrillation; withdrawal and documentation of withdrawal symptomatology
	Procedures: Detoxification and group and/or individual therapy
	Radiology: Liver scan and abdominal series

Flutter, atrial 427.32	**Signs and Symptoms:** Palpitation, weakness, dizziness, syncope, anxiety and feeling of impending death **Drug Therapy:** May include digoxin, quinidine, propranolol, calan, cardizem, digitalis **EKG:** P waves in regular rhythm (250–350 per minute) and PR interval prolonged, varying with degree of AV block **Nurse's Notes:** Documentation of rapid, regular atrial rate between 220 and 360 per minute **Procedures:** Cardioversion, atrial pacemaker, and vagal stimulation
Flutter, ventricular 427.42	**Signs and Symptoms:** Palpitations and dyspnea; possible transition between ventricular tachycardia and fibrillation **EKG:** Evidence of ventricular flutter, regular rapid rate over 250/ minute
Heart failure, unspecified 428.9	**Signs and Symptoms:** Documentation of cardiac insufficiency, fatigue, or dyspnea **Radiology:** Chest x-ray-cardiac enlargement
Hemopericardium 423.0	**Signs and Symptoms:** Results from a perforating trauma or cardiac rupture after myocardial infarction; symptoms include precordial pain, substernal oppression, and dyspnea; death can result if emergency measures are not taken immediately **EKG:** May show low to inverted T waves in most leads **Nurse's Notes:** Monitoring of vital signs, intake and output and chest tube care (for patient on whom a thoracotomy was performed) **Procedures:** Pulmonary artery catheterization; aspiration of pericardium; echocardiography **Radiology:** Chest x-ray may indicate increase in acuity of cardiophrenic angle; shape of heart more globular in recumbent position; widening of the base
Hyperkinetic heart 429.82	**Signs and Symptoms:** Features of congestive heart failure such as cardiac enlargement, gallop rhythm, and tachycardia; pulse pressure may be elevated (the difference between diastolic and systolic blood pressure is greater than 100) **Drug Therapy:** May include lasix **EKG:** Sinus tachycardia **Radiology:** Chest x-ray: cardiac enlargement and increased hilar marking

Hypertensive heart and renal disease 404.01 404.03 404.11 404.13 404.91 404.93	**Signs and Symptoms:** History of renal disease, headache, fatigue and irritability; evidence of renal failure; elevated blood pressure (systolic greater than 160 and diastolic greater than 100); malignant hypertension diastolic pressure above 140 mm hg, or lower diastolic pressure described as rising and irregular, or accompanied by focal neurological deficits **Drug Therapy:** Parenteral antihypertensive therapy, with a rapid acting agent such as the vasodilator Nitrostat **EKG:** Possible tachycardia **Laboratory:** BUN level greater than 20 and creatinine above 2.5 **Nurse's Notes:** Frequent monitoring of vital signs, intake and output, and low-sodium diet **Procedures:** Possible kidney transplant and dialysis; arteriogram, bicycle stress testing, echocardiography **Radiology:** Renal scan, and urography
Hypertensive heart disease, benign, with heart failure 402.11	**Signs and Symptoms:** Elevated blood pressure (systolic greater than 160 and diastolic greater than 100); symptoms may include headache, fatigue, irritability, dyspnea and cardiac arrhythmia **Drug Therapy:** May include hydrochlorothiazide, aldoril, altrace, lopressor, or lasix **EKG:** Tachycardia, bradycardia, or PVCs **Nurse's Notes:** Frequent monitoring of vital signs, intake and output, and oxygen therapy **Procedures:** Ophthalmoscopy: retinopathy; spirometry; arteriogram, bicycle stress testing, echocardiography, swan-ganz catheterization **Radiology:** Chest x-ray-may indicate cardiac enlargement
Hypertensive heart disease, malignant, with heart failure 402.01	**Signs and Symptoms:** Atherosclerosis, history of uncontrolled blood pressure and history of oliguria with varying degrees of renal insufficiency; onset of elevated blood pressure is usually sudden in nature; malignant hypertension diastolic pressure above 140 mm hg, or lower diastolic pressure described as rising and irregular, or accompanied by focal neurological deficits **Drug Therapy:** Parenteral antihypertensive therapy, with a rapid acting agent such as the vasodilator nitrostat; may include hydrochlorothiazide, aldoril, altrace, lopressor, or lasix **Laboratory:** BUN greater than 20 and creatinine greater than 2.5 **Nurse's Notes:** Frequent monitoring of vital signs with evidence of rapidly accelerated high blood pressure (diastolic greater than 100, systolic greater than 140) and sodium-restricted diet **Procedures:** Ophthalmoscopyretinopathy; arteriogram, bicycle stress testing, echocardiography, swan-ganz catheterization **Radiology:** Chest x-ray heart failure

Hypertensive heart disease, unspecified, with heart failure 402.91	**Signs and Symptoms:** Atherosclerosis, obesity, ischemic heart disease, headaches, features of myocardial infarction and paroxysmal nocturnal dyspnea **Drug Therapy:** May include hydrochlorothiazide, aldoril, altrace, lopressor, or lasix **Nurse's Notes:** Frequent monitoring of vital signs with evidence of high blood pressure (diastolic greater than 100, systolic greater than 140) **Procedures:** Ophthalmoscopy-retinopathy and papilledema; arteriogram, bicycle stress testing, echocardiography, swan-ganz catheterization **Radiology:** Chest x-ray heart failure and cardiac enlargement
Hypotension 458.8 458.9	**Signs and Symptoms:** Weakness, fatigue, dizziness, impairment and blurred vision, and syncope; can be caused by a vasovagal response or by drugs that cause orthostatic hypotension such as antihypertensive drugs and antidepressants **Drug Therapy:** Fluid challenge **Nurse's Notes:** Blood pressures taken while patient is lying, sitting, and standing; support hose
Infection and inflammatory reaction due to other vascular device, implant and graft 996.62	**Signs and Symptoms:** At the site of entry, skin erythema or tenderness. Skin is red, hot, and edematous. Borders may reveal cellulitis or petechiae. Systemic manifestations such as sepsis may result. Leukocytosis is common **Drug Therapy:** May include antibiotic therapy dependent upon culture results **Laboratory:** Wound culture by aspiration or skin biopsy; blood culture for systemic involvement **Nurse's Notes:** Frequent monitoring of vital signs and dressing changes
Influenza with pneumonia 487.0	**Signs and Symptoms:** Cough, fever, chills, muscle aches, malaise **Drug Therapy:** Appropriate antibiotic therapy is usually given **Laboratory:** Blood: elevated WBCs; culture (sputum) is positive for influenza virus **Nurse's Notes:** Oxygen therapy and analgesics **Procedures:** May include bronchoscopy **Radiology:** Chest x-ray-may show infiltrates

Intermediate coronary syndrome 411.1	**Signs and Symptoms:** Patients present with anginal pain; history of chronic coronary insufficiency and possible exacerbation of previous stable angina; "pending infarction" ; also may be called "preinfarction syndrome"
	EKG: Cardiac monitoring: usually necessary; S-T segment changes and arrhythmias may be present
	Laboratory: Enzyme studies: normal or not diagnostic
	Nurse's Notes: Usually anginal pain is unrelieved by nitrates and onset of pain is nonexertional
	Procedures: Holter monitor, stress test, percutaneous transluminal angioplasty, and bypass surgery
	Radiology: Angiography may show coronary artery disease
Intracerebral hemorrhage 431	**Signs and Symptoms:** Abrupt headache, followed by steadily increasing neurologic deficits, hemiparesis, cerebellar or brain stem dysfunction (conjugate eye deviation or ophthalmoplegia, stertorous breathing, pinpoint pupils), nausea, vomiting, delirium, seizures and coma.
	Drug therapy: Narcotics may be needed to relieve headache, severe nausea or vomiting may require IV fluid administration
	Procedures: Trephination to evacuate blood and relieve pressure
	Radiology: CAT scan, MRI also helps distinguish hemorrhagic from ischemic strokes
Intracranial hemorrhage, other and unspecified 432.0 432.1 432.9	**Signs and Symptoms:** Recent history of head trauma, daily headache, fluctuating drowsiness or changes in consciousness, intracranial swelling and pressure, motor dysfunction, and papillary changes
	Drug therapy: May include thrombolytic agents for treatment. Anticoagulants and antiplatelet agents for prevention.
	Procedures: Drill burr holes for evacuation of clot. Continuous intracranial pressure measurements. CSF for presence of blood.
	Radiology: CT scan, MRI to detect surgically treatable lesions. Cerebral angiography may be indicated after CT, MRI

Ischemia, coronary, acute and subacute, other 411.89	**Signs and Symptoms:** Arteriosclerotic heart disease, elevated cholesterol, disease of aortic valve, thoracic pain, chest pain with or without exertion, anemia, dizziness, syncope, and dyspnea
	Drug Therapy: May include nitroglycerin, lidocaine, pronestyl, digoxin, quinidine, and potassium supplement administered intravenously
	EKG: Documentation may indicate subacute ischemia
	Laboratory: Potassium level may be decreased, indicating cardiac damage. enzymes may be slightly elevated; cholesterol level may be greater than 250; anemia (hemoglobin less than 8 and hematocrit less than 28) may be present
	Nurse's Notes: May document cardiac monitoring or coronary care unit services
	Procedures: Stress EKG and cardiac catheterization
	Radiology: Echocardiogram, myocardial perfusion studies, gated blood pool imaging; chest x-ray may show cardiac enlargement and increased hilar markings
Left heart failure 428.1	**Signs and Symptoms:** Hypertension, fatigue, cough, frothy sputum, pulmonary edema and dyspnea; confusion is usually present; documentation may state that the patient is cyanotic
	Drug Therapy: May include digoxin, diuretics and vasodilators; (e.g., altrace, aldoril, vasotec, zestril)
	Laboratory: Blood gases: oxygen saturation reduced; CO_2 tension: less than normal
	Nurse's Notes: Rotation of tourniquets, daily weights, intake and output, and frequent vital signs
	Procedures: Pulmonary artery monitoring, pulmonary capillary wedge pressure and echocardiography
	Radiology: Chest x-ray-pulmonary congestion and pleural effusion
Myocarditis, acute, in diseases classified elsewhere 422.0	**Signs and Symptoms:** Associated with acute pericarditis, influenza and tuberculosis; precordial and substernal discomfort; severe dyspnea and pain in the right upper quadrant of abdomen
	Drug Therapy: May include antiarrhythmic drugs to control arrhythmias, antibiotics for underlying infection and anti-inflammatory drugs
	EKG: Tachycardia, intraventricular or bundle branchabnormalities
	Laboratory: CPK, SGOT, and LDH may be elevated; viral antibody titers, WBC, and ESR are also elevated
	Nurse's Notes: Oxygen therapy, frequent vital signs, and documentation of bed rest
	Procedures: Endomyocardial biopsy and echocardiogram
	Radiology: Chest x-ray: cardiac enlargement

Myocarditis, acute, other, unspecified and idiopathic 422.90 422.91 422.99	**Signs and Symptoms:** May be termed "interstitial"; acute form presents with precordial and substernal discomfort, dyspnea, pain, and fever; the predominant physical findings are a friction rub, leukocytosis and rapid sedimentation rate; there may also be evidence of generalized edema and/or ascites; may be complicated by congestive heart failure **Drug Therapy:** May include antiarrhythmic drugs to control arrhythmias, antibiotics for underlying infection and anti-inflammatory drugs **EKG:** Tachycardia, intraventricular, or bundle branch abnormalities **Laboratory:** CPK, SGOT, and LDH may be elevated; viral antibody titers, WBCs, and ESR are also elevated **Nurse's Notes:** Oxygen therapy, frequent vital signs, and documentation of bed rest **Procedures:** Endomyocardial biopsy and echocardiogram **Radiology:** Chest x-ray: cardiac enlargement
Myocarditis, septic 422.92	**Signs and Symptoms:** Viral strains; influenza viruses; bacteria **Drug Therapy:** May include antiarrhythmic drugs to control arrhythmias, antibiotics for underlying infection and anti-inflammatory drugs **EKG:** Tachycardia, intraventricular, or bundle branch abnormalities **Laboratory:** CPK, SGOT, and LDH may be elevated; viral antibody titers, WBCs, and ESR are also elevated; blood culture: positive **Nurse's Notes:** Oxygen therapy, frequent vital signs, and documentation of bed rest **Procedures:** Endomyocardial biopsy and echocardiogram **Radiology:** Chest x-ray: cardiac enlargement
Myocarditis, toxic 422.93	**Signs and Symptoms:** May be caused by one of the following: chemical poisons such as arsenic, excessive doses of drugs, or excessive radiation exposure **Drug Therapy:** May include antiarrhythmic drugs to control arrhythmias, antibiotics for underlying infection, and anti-inflammatory drugs **EKG:** Tachycardia, intraventricular, or bundle branch abnormalities **Laboratory:** CPK, SGOT, and LDH may be elevated; viral antibody titers, WBC, and ESR are also elevated **Nurse's Notes:** Oxygen therapy, frequent vital signs and documentation of bed rest **Procedures:** Endomyocardial biopsy and echocardiogram **Radiology:** Chest x-ray: cardiac enlargement

Occlusion and stenosis of precerebral arteries, with cerebral infarction 433.01 433.11 433.21 433.31 433.81 433.91	**Signs and Symptoms:** Aphasia, hemiplegia, motor or sensory impairment, changes in consciousness. Neurological symptoms vary by site of the occlusion. Symptoms can be transient dependent upon blood supply, infarction results in permanent neurological damage. **Drug therapy:** May include heparin may stabilize symptoms. Anticoagulants for prevention **Procedures:** Thromboendarterectomy, rehabilitation therapy for long-term effects. **Radiology:** CT scan and MRI may help to determine ischemic versus hemorrhagic. Angiography can identify site. Arteriography may be indicated for suspected diagnosis.
Occlusion of cerebral arteries 434.00 434.01 434.10 434.11 434.90 434.91	**Signs and Symptoms:** Aphasia, hemiplegia, motor or sensory impairment, changes in consciousness. Neurological symptoms vary by site of the occlusion. Symptoms can be transient dependent upon blood supply, infarction results in permanent neurological damage. **Drug therapy:** Heparin may stabilize symptoms; anticoagulants for prevention **Procedures:** Thromboendarterectomy, rehabilitation therapy for long-term effects **Radiology:** CT scan and MRI may help to determine ischemic versus hemorrhagic. Angiography can identify site. Arteriography may be indicated for suspected diagnosis
Other complication due to other cardiac device, implant and graft 996.72	**Signs and Symptoms:** Presence of device may cause vascular embolism, fibrosis, hemorrhage, pain, stenosis, thrombosis **Drug Therapy:** May include analgesics, antibiotics, antithrombotic therapy, thrombolytics, and IV therapy **Procedures:** Angioplasty, bypass grafting **Radiology:** Arteriography, angiography, venography, Doppler ultrasonography
Papillary muscle disorders 429.81	**Signs and Symptoms:** Sudden development of pulmonary edema; shortness of breath, edema and severe chest pain; normally occurs within 10 days of an acute myocardial infarction; patient usually dies within 24 hours, and 90% die within two weeks **Nurse's Notes:** Frequent monitoring of vital signs and intake and output **Procedures:** Emergency mitral valve or cardiac catheterization using intra-aortic balloon pump; aortocoronary saphenous vein bypass is usually performed; mitral valve replacement may be performed Radiology: Ultrasound of heart or angiography may confirm clinical diagnosis

Pericarditis, acute, in diseases classified elsewhere 420.0	**Signs and Symptoms:** Often a history of recent respiratory infection; precordial pain made worse by change of position, swallowing, coughing, and deep breathing; dyspnea, chills and malaise are usually present; onset is sudden; the underlying condition (e.g., tuberculosis) must also be treated **Drug Therapy:** Intravenous antibiotics, corticosteroids, and anti-inflammatory drugs such as aspirin **EKG:** Tachycardia, S-T segment elevation, and atrial arrhythmias **Laboratory:** WBCs 15,000–20,000, SGOT increased (above40 units) and PPD skin test is positive if caused by tuberculosis; positive gram stain and positive culture **Nurse's Notes:** Documentation of complete bed rest, frequent monitoring of vital signs, and oxygen therapy **Procedures:** Pericardiocentesis: fluid may be hemorrhagic or straw-colored; echocardiogram if pericardial effusion is present **Radiology:** Chest x-ray: usually serial for the purpose of ruling out cause of pleuritic chest pain; may show slight cardiac hypertrophy
Pericarditis, acute, other, unspecified and idiopathic 420.90 420.91 420.99	**Signs and Symptoms:** Sudden onset of sharp precordial pain, not aggravated by thoracic motion; chills, fever, weakness, and dyspnea **Drug Therapy:** Intravenous antibiotics, corticosteroids, and anti-inflammatory drugs such as aspirin **EKG:** Tachycardia, S-T segment elevation, and atrial arrhythmias **Laboratory:** WBCs 15,000–20,000, SGOT increased (above 40 units) and PPD skin test is positive if caused by tuberculosis; positive gram stain and positive culture **Nurse's Notes:** Documentation of complete bed rest, frequent monitoring of vital signs, and oxygen therapy **Procedures:** Pericardiocentesis: fluid may be hemorrhagic or straw-colored; echocardiogram if pericardial effusion is present **Radiology:** Chest x-ray: usually serial for the purpose of ruling out cause of pleuritic chest pain; may show slight cardiac hypertrophy
Pneumonia 481 482.0 482.1 482.2 482.30 482.31 482.32 482.39 482.40 482.41 482.49 482.81 482.82 482.83 482.89 482.9 483.0 483.1 483.8 484.1 484.3 484.5 484.6 484.7 484.8 485 486	**Signs and Symptoms:** Lung infection may be due to a number of organisms that may cause the infection; symptoms include cough, fever, chills, and sometimes general aching **Drug Therapy:** Appropriate antibiotic therapy is usually given according to organism **Laboratory:** Blood: elevated WBCs; culture (sputum) is positive for *Haemophilus influenzae, Klebsiella, Pseudomonas, Staphylococcus, Streptococcus*, or other specified bacteria **Nurse's Notes:** Oxygen therapy and analgesics for chest pain **Procedures:** May include bronchoscopy **Radiology:** Chest x-ray-may show infiltrates

Pneumonitis due to solids and liquids 507.0 507.1 507.8	**Signs and Symptoms:** Rales, dyspnea, cyanosis, hypotension, may have history of feeding disorder
	Drug Therapy: Appropriate antibiotic therapy is usually given
	Laboratory: ABGs suggest hypoxia, sputum gross exam may show blood, culture (sputum) may be positive if infective nasopharyngeal organisms were aspirated
	Procedures: Suction, oxygen therapy, chest physiotherapy
	Radiology: Chest x-ray-may show infiltrates
Postmyocardial infarction syndrome 411.0	**Signs and Symptoms:** Called "Dressler syndrome"; chest pain is usually sharp and stabbing in nature and often as severe as that caused by infarction; aggravated by change in position and deep inspirations; usually follows an acute infarction of two to 11 weeks; (symptoms similar to pleural effusion, pneumonitis with fever) pericardial friction rub present on auscultation
	Drug Therapy: May include a short intensive course of corticosteroids. Intensive anti-inflammatory therapy may be documented
	Laboratory: May show increased WBC of 10,000 to 20,000
	Procedures: Echocardiography to determine extent of pericardial effusion; pericardiocentesis may be necessary
	Radiology: Chest x-ray-may reveal pericardial and pleural effusion; may show enlargement of silhouette with later reduction or evidence of pulmonary infiltrates
Pulmonary embolism and infarction 415.11 415.19	**Signs and Symptoms:** Manifestations of embolism with infarction include cough, hemoptysis, pleuritic chest pain, fever and signs of pulmonary consolidation of pleural fluid; indications of an embolism develop abruptly over a period of minutes; those of an infarction over a period of hours; may follow a major surgical procedure after which the patient may have been confined to bed rest
	Drug Therapy: Includes low doses of heparin, analgesics, thrombolytic drugs, and dextran administered intravenously
	Laboratory: Arterial blood gas may show poor air exchange; sputum may show red blood cells; LDH may be elevated
	Nurse's Notes: Checking of pedal pulses, range of motion exercises, encouragement of ambulation and oxygen therapy
	Procedures: Pulmonary arteriography may confirm diagnosis
	Radiology: Chest x-ray-may show pleural effusion or infiltrates; radioisotope perfusion lung scanning often accompanies ventilation scanning

Pulmonary hypertension, primary 416.0	**Signs and Symptoms:** Diffuse narrowing of the pulmonary arterioles, formation of pulmonary thrombi and emboli, raised pulmonary vascular resistance, cough, hemoptysis, pleuritic chest pain, progressive exertional dyspnea **Drug Therapy:** Includes low doses of heparin, analgesics, thrombolytic drugs, vasodilators (e.g., prostacyclin, nifedipine) **Laboratory:** Arterial blood gas may show poor air exchange; LDH may be elevated, prothrombin time **Procedures:** Ventilation/perfusion scanning, pulmonary function testing, unilateral or bilateral lung transplantation **Radiology:** Chest x-ray-may show pleural effusion or infiltrates; radioisotope perfusion lung scanning. Pulmonary angioscopy may reveal chronic mural thrombi
Pulmonary insufficiency following trauma and surgery 518.5	**Signs and Symptoms:** Dyspnea, intercostal and suprasternal retraction on inspiration. Skin may appear cyanotic. May develop within 24 to 48 hours following trauma to the thoracic cavity. Hypoxemia and cardiac arrest may result. **Drug Therapy:** May include IV fluids **Laboratory:** Arterial blood gases for acute respiratory alkalosis **Procedures:** Swan-Ganz catheter to monitor pulmonary pressure; oxygen therapy, endotracheal intubation, mechanical ventilation **Radiology:** Chest x-ray
Renal failure, acute 584.9	**Signs and Symptoms:** Lethargy, fatigue, anorexia, nausea, dyspnea, weakness, thirst, oliguria, bradycardia or tachycardia, and hematuria **EKG:** Arrhythmias of all types due to electrolyte imbalance **Laboratory:** Urinalysis: low specific gravity, high specific gravity if due to prerenal or postrenal factors, RBC, protein; traces of glucose, casts, epithelial cells; Blood: increase in WBCs during infection; increase of BUN and creatinine **Nurse's Notes:** Daily weights and intake and output; Often with acute failure urine output is less than 500 ml per day **Procedures:** Dialysis; renal scan, ultrasound of kidney, kidney biopsy
Renal failure, acute, with lesion of renal cortical necrosis 584.6	**Signs and Symptoms:** Lethargy, fatigue, anorexia, nausea, dyspnea, weakness, thirst, oliguria, bradycardia, or tachycardia **EKG:** Evidence of arrhythmias (e.g., bradycardia or tachycardia) **Laboratory:** Urinalysis: low specific gravity; high specific gravity if due to prerenal or postrenal factors; RBC; protein; traces of glucose; casts; epithelial cells; Blood: increased BUN and creatinine **Nurse's Notes:** Intake and output, daily weights **Radiology:** Kidney x-ray-evidence of cortical necrosis; IVP-clinically diagnostic

Renal failure, acute, with lesion of renal medullary (papillary) necrosis 584.7	**Signs and Symptoms:** Lethargy, fatigue, anorexia, dyspnea, weakness, nausea, thirst, oliguria, bradycardia or tachycardia; seen most commonly in association with conditions such as liver disease and diabetes **EKG:** Evidence of arrhythmias (e.g., bradycardia or tachycardia) **Laboratory:** Urinalysis; low specific gravity; high specific gravity if due to prerenal or postrenal factors; Blood: increased RBC, protein, BUN, and creatinine **Nurse's Notes:** Intake and output, daily weights **Radiology:** X-ray-may show renal medullary (papillary) lesion; IVP-clinically diagnostic
Renal failure, acute, with lesion of tubular necrosis 584.5	**Signs and Symptoms:** Lethargy, fatigue, anorexia, nausea, dyspnea, weakness, thirst, bradycardia or tachycardia; can be associated with other conditions such as shock, sepsis, renal artery surgery, and heavy metal poisoning **EKG:** Evidence of arrhythmias (e.g., bradycardia or tachycardia) **Laboratory:** Urinalysis: low specific gravity; high specific gravity if due to prerenal or postrenal factors; Blood: increased BUN and creatinine **Nurse's Notes:** Intake and output, daily weights **Radiology:** X-ray-evidence of lesion of tubular necrosis; IVP-clinically diagnostic
Renal failure, acute, with specified pathological lesion in kidney 584.8	**Signs and Symptoms:** Lethargy, fatigue, anorexia, nausea, dyspnea, weakness, thirst, bradycardia, or tachycardia **EKG:** Evidence of arrhythmias (e.g., bradycardia or tachycardia) **Laboratory:** Urinalysis: low specific gravity; high specific gravity if due to prerenal or postrenal factors; Blood: increased BUN, and creatinine **Nurse's Notes:** Intake and output, daily weights **Radiology:** X-ray-evidence of pathologic lesion in kidney; IVP-clinically diagnostic
Respiratory failure 518.81 518.83 518.84	**Signs and Symptoms:** Inability of the pulmonary and cardiac systems to maintain an adequate exchange of carbon dioxide and oxygen in the lungs; acute respiratory failure is a life-threatening emergency; symptoms include increase in sputum production, cough and shortness of breath **Laboratory:** Arterial blood gases: increased pCO_2 (greater than 50) and decreased pO_2 (less than 50), pH less than 7.35 could be an indication **Procedures:** O_2 therapy and artificial ventilation **Radiology:** Chest x-ray-may show congestion caused by an infectious process or an obstructive process such as emphysema or chronic obstructive pulmonary disease

Rheumatic heart failure 398.91	**Signs and Symptoms:** Decreased cardiac output, edema, hypertension, valvular stenosis and/or insufficiency, myocardial damage, heart murmur, cardiomegaly
	Drug Therapy: Corticosteroids, methylprednisolone succinate, NSAIDs, cardiotonic drugs such as digoxin
	Procedures: Echocardiography, cardiac blood pool imaging, pulmonary artery monitoring and cardiac catheterization, PR prolongation on EKG
	Radiology: Chest x-ray-may show cardiac hypertrophy, pleural effusion or pulmonary venous congestion
Rupture of chordae tendinae 429.5	**Signs and Symptoms:** Caused by bacterial endocarditis, trauma or sudden compression of thorax; usually sudden in onset, with pain in the chest; patient may have dyspnea and weakness
	Drug Therapy: May include use of diuretics for congestive heart failure (e.g., lasix)
	EKG: Features of right or left ventricular failure, hypertrophy and axis deviation Physician
	Nurse's Notes: Documentation of congestive heart failure
	Radiology: Chest x-ray-cardiac enlargement
Rupture of papillary muscle 429.6	**Signs and Symptoms:** Contraction of papillary muscle, also ischemia of papillary muscle; possible chest pain; there is usually sudden and severe deterioration; possible hemoptysis; often manifestation of congestive heart failure with cyanosis and sometimes shock; occurs in 35% of all myocardial infarction patients
	Drug Therapy: May include lasix or diuril
	EKG: Changes in junction J, S-T, T interval, TU segment and U wave
	Procedures: Mitral valve replacement is often performed
	Radiology: Chest x-ray-cardiac enlargement and pulmonary congestion
Shock 785.50	**Signs and Symptoms:** Noted to be failure of peripheral circulation; this category of shock would include shock caused by anaphalaxis, third-degree burns, extensive tissue trauma or general trauma; may be indicated by documentation of respiratory distress, hypotension, tachycardia, cool moist skin, and reduced urinary output
	EKG: Tachycardia
	Laboratory: Serum potassium lactate, BUN, and specific gravity are increased
	Nurse's Notes: Intravenous blood and fluid replacement, oxygen therapy, frequent monitoring of vital signs, Foley catheter, monitoring of intake and output, and cardiopulmonary resuscitation

Shock, cardiogenic 785.51	**Signs and Symptoms:** A life-threatening emergency requiring intensive stabilizing measures; most often occurs as the result of a myocardial infarction, end-stage cardiomyopathy or possibly a malfunction of the mitral valve; rapidly developing mental confusion with weakness, cyanosis, oliguria, tachycardia and gallop rhythm, systolic pressure drops to 50; skin is cool and moist **Drug Therapy:** May include morphine to control chest pain, dopamine, norepinephrine, and nitroprusside **EKG:** Ventricular fibrillation may be present **Laboratory:** May show serum acidosis; BUN and creatinine are elevated, as are CPK, LDH, SGOT, and SGPT; arterial blood gases demonstrate acidosis, and hypoxia **Nurse's Notes:** May indicate a weak, rapid pulse, cardiac monitoring, and intake and output **Procedures:** Pulmonary artery pressure monitoring and pulmonary capillary wedge pressure; may also include intra-aortic balloon pump **Radiology:** Chest x-ray-may show pulmonary edema
Subarachnoid hemorrhage 430	**Signs and Symptoms:** Sudden, acute headache, nausea and vomiting, loss or impairment of consciousness **Procedures:** Spinal puncture, resection of AV malformations, trephination to evacuate blood and relieve pressure **Radiology:** CT of head, cerebral arteriography, bilateral carotid and vertebral arteriography, MRI
Tachycardia, paroxysmal, supraventricular 427.0	**Signs and Symptoms:** Abrupt onset and termination of palpitations; often asymptomatic although patient may be aware of a rapid heartbeat; some patients complain of throbbing vessels of the throat, dyspnea, sweating, dizziness, syncope, weakness, and polyuria **Drug Therapy:** May include propranolol, quinidine, or calan **EKG:** Premature atrial beats, abnormally shaped P waves; regular rhythm at 150–220 beats per minute **Procedures:** May include intracardiac electrophysiologic studies and vagal stimulation; may also see reduced vital capacity and increased cardiac output and circulation time
Tachycardia, paroxysmal, unspecified 427.2	**Signs and Symptoms:** Fluttering sensation in the chest, weakness, faintness, and nausea **Drug Therapy:** May include quinidine, procainamide, and calan **EKG:** Uninterrupted series of beats

Tachycardia, paroxysmal, ventricular 427.1	**Signs and Symptoms:** Associated with ischemic heart disease, especially myocardial infarction; precordial pain; sudden onset usually preceded by premature ventricular beats; pulse rate of 150–210 per minute **Drug Therapy:** May include quinidine, procainamide, calan **EKG:** Wide QRS complexes **Nurse's Notes:** Cardiopulmonary resuscitation **Procedures:** Cardioversion
Ulcer, decubitus 707.0	**Signs and Symptoms:** Also known as a bedsore or pressure sore; occurs most frequently in debilitated patients who are bed- or wheelchair-confined; is a result of loss of circulation to a susceptible body area, such as a bony prominence **Drug Therapy:** May include topical antibiotic ointments **Nurse's Notes:** May show special mattresses used for treatment and prevention of spread of ulcer, dressing changes, and treatment of decubitus **Procedures:** Fourth stage ulcers may be debrided; whirlpool debridements in physical therapy may be required

Noninvasive Diagnostic Test Outcomes

Cardiology Procedures

Myocardial perfusion imaging (pharmacologic stress testing)	**Signs and Symptoms:** Chest pain suspected to be of cardiac origin (to include tightness, pressure and discomfort), evaluation of the results of coronary bypass or balloon angioplasty, syncope, abnormal exercise EKG, abnormal cardiovascular function study, dyspnea, shortness of breath **Diagnostic Outcomes:** Acute myocardial infarction, ischemic heart disease, ventricular arrhythmia, cardiomyopathy, cardioembolic strokes, postmyocardial infarction, cardiomegaly, angina pectoris, coronary atherosclerosis, congestive heart failure, aortic aneurysm, peripheral angiography, status post heart transplant evaluation, coronary artery bypass or balloon angioplasty
Transesophageal echocardiography (TEE)	**Signs and Symptoms:** Syncope and collapse, fever, shock, persistent febrile state, pre-existent valvular pathology, inadequate defined volume status for ventilator patients, heart mass **Diagnostic Outcomes:** Mitral, tricuspid, and aortic valve disorders; endocarditis; aneurysm of heart; myocarditis; cardiomyopathy; acquired cardiac septal defect; cerebral embolism; cerebrovascular disease; coarctation of aorta; volume depletion; fluid overload; mechanical complication cardiac device; implant or graft (including cardiac pacemaker or heart valve prosthesis); status post heart transplant or valve replacement; malignant or secondary neoplasm of heart; thoracic aorta disruption after blunt trauma; monitor heart function during cardiac surgery; evaluation of left atrial thrombosis and masses; in the evaluation of bacterial endocarditis and its complications; and in the evaluation of intracardiac shunts
Transthoracic echocardiography (TTE)	**Signs and Symptoms:** Syncope and collapse, chest pain, heart murmur, abnormal heart sounds, bacteremia, fever, shock, dyspnea, and shortness of breath **Diagnostic Outcomes:** Hypertensive heart disease, pulmonary hypertension, endocarditis, acute cor pulmonale, atrial fibrillation, pulmonary embolism and infarction, myocarditis, cardiomyopathy, heart failure, systemic lupus erythematosus, acute myocardial infarction, acquired septal defect, angina pectoris, cerebral embolism, poisoning by chemotherapy and immunosuppressive drugs, mechanical complication of cardiac device, implant or graft (including cardiac pacemaker or heart valve prosthesis), malignant or secondary neoplasm of heart

Neurology Procedures

Electromyography (EMG)	**Signs and Symptoms:** Muscle spasms, pain in limb, abnormal involuntary movements, abnormality in gait, lack of coordination, changes in skin sensation (tingling, numbness, burning, or prickling sensation), voice disturbances
	Diagnostic Outcomes: Intervertebral disc disorders, muscular dystrophy, neuropathy, systemic lupus, sarcoidosis, myalgia, neuralgia, neuritis, radiculitis, acquired spondylolisthesis, cervical spinal cord injury, botulism, diabetes with neurogenic manifestations, peripheral nervous system disorders, chronic renal failure, injury to peripheral nerves, malignant neoplasm of spinal cord and meninges, anesthesia and paresthesia, especially of the extremities
Nerve conduction testing (amplitude, latency/velocity, F-wave study)	**Signs and Symptoms:** Muscle spasms, pain in limb, abnormal involuntary movements, abnormality in gait, lack of coordination, changes in skin sensation (tingling, numbness, burning, or prickling sensation), voice disturbances
	Diagnostic Outcomes: Myopathy, radiculopathy, intervertebral disc disorders, myalgia, neuralgia, neuritis, neuropathy, radiculitis, acquired spondylolisthesis, spinal cord injuries, diabetes with neurological manifestations, chronic renal failure, malignant neoplasms of spinal cord and meninges

Pulmonary Function Tests

Spirometry, bronchospasm evaluation, vital capacity, flow volume loop, thoracic gas volume	**Signs and Symptoms:** Sleep disturbances, dyspnea, shortness of breath, cough, hemoptysis, abnormal chest sounds, asphyxia, abnormal findings on x-ray, wheezing
	Diagnostic Outcomes: Sarcoidosis, myasthenia gravis, acute cor pulmonale, pulmonary hypertension, congestive heart failure, cystic fibrosis, asthma, acute bronchitis, stenosis of larynx, pneumonia, chronic obstructive pulmonary disease, emphysema, bronchiectasis, malignant neoplasm of trachea, bronchus or lung, status post lung transplant or surgery

Radiology Procedures

Barium swallow studies	**Signs and Symptoms:** Feeding difficulties and mismanagement, heartburn, dysphasia
	Diagnostic Outcomes: Aspiration pneumonia, esophageal reflux, achalasia and cardiospasm, diverticulum of esophagus, stricture and stenosis of esophagus, malignant neoplasm of oropharynx, hypopharynx, or esophagus

Radiology Procedures (continued)

Bone density measurements	**Signs and Symptoms:** Estrogen deficiency (postmenopausal), low-body weight (25th percentile), smoker, vitamin D deficiency, long-term use of corticosteroids or glucocorticoid therapy, history of anorexia
	Diagnostic Outcomes: Osteoporosis, pathological fractures, hyperthyroidism, hyperparathyroidism, osteomalacia, endometriosis, multiple myeloma, Cushing's disease, osteopenia, postablative ovarian failure, ectopic hormone secretion, vertebral fracture
Cerebrovascular arterial studies (duplex scans, transcranial Doppler, periorbital Doppler)	**Signs and Symptoms:** Syncope and collapse, abnormality in gait, lack of coordination, transient paralysis of limb, changes in skin sensation (numbness, tingling, paresthesia), aphasia, slurred speech, cervical bruits
	Diagnostic Outcomes: Transient ischemic attacks, vasculitis, hemiplegia and hemiparesis, paraplegia, quadriplegia and quadriparesis, transient visual loss, occlusion and stenosis or precerebral and cerebral arteries, cerebral atherosclerosis, cerebrovascular accident, cerebral aneurysm
Chest x-ray	**Signs and Symptoms:** Cough, hemoptysis, dyspnea, fever of unknown origin, alterations of consciousness, syncope and collapse, convulsions, dizziness and giddiness, abnormality of gait, cachexia, edema, bacteremia
	Diagnostic Outcomes: Atelectasis, bronchiectasis, pneumonia, cardiomyopathy, pneumothorax, chronic obstructive bronchitis, pleural effusion, congestive heart failure, emphysema, respiratory failure, fracture of rib(s), sternum, larynx, trachea, foreign body in bronchus or lung, mechanical complication of cardiac device, heart transplant complications, lung abscess, malignant neoplasms, other infections, such as tuberculosis, status post lung surgery or transplant
Computerized axial tomography (CAT) abdomen	**Signs and Symptoms:** Fever, abnormal weight loss, enlargement of lymph nodes, abdominal pain, localized abdominal tenderness, hepatomegaly, splenomegaly, abdominal or pelvic swelling, mass or lump, bacteremia, abnormal results of liver function study, abnormal findings on x-ray
	Diagnostic Outcomes: Gastric; duodenal or peptic ulcers; lymphoma; appendicitis; hernias; ulcerative colitis; abscess of intestines; chronic liver disease and cirrhosis; cholelithiasis; gastrointestinal hemorrhage; hydronephrosis; cystic kidney disease; persistent postoperative fistula; fracture of pelvis; open wound of abdominal organ; injury to spleen, kidney, liver; foreign body of digestive system; complication of kidney, liver, or pancreatic transplant; malignant neoplasms

Radiology Procedures (continued)

Computerized axial tomography (CAT) cranial	**Signs and Symptoms:** Alteration of consciousness, hallucinations, syncope and collapse, dizziness and giddiness, lack of coordination, transient paralysis of limb, headache, speech disturbances
	Diagnostic Outcomes: Senile and presenile dementia, arteriosclerotic dementia, trigeminal nerve disorders, Alzheimer's disease, bipolar disorder, cerebral palsy, subarachnoid and intracerebral hemorrhage, subdural, epidural, or hematoma, brain abscess occlusion and stenosis of cerebral arteries, transient cerebral ischemia, nodular lymphoma, fracture of skull, intracranial injury, injury to face and neck, congenital anomalies of skull and face bones; malignant neoplasms of brain, cranial nerves, cerebral meninges, pituitary gland and pineal gland
Computerized axial tomography (CAT) pelvis	**Signs and Symptoms:** Fever, abdominal pain, localized abdominal tenderness, hepatomegaly, splenomegaly, abdominal or pelvic swelling, mass or lump, bacteremia, abnormal findings on x-ray or abnormal function studies
	Diagnostic Outcomes: Septicemia, sarcoidosis, uterine leiomyoma, abdominal aneurysm, renal failure, appendicitis, hernias, ulcerative colitis, blood in stool, gastrointestinal hemorrhage, hematuria, endometriosis, lipoma of intra-abdominal organs, disseminated candidiasis, open wound of abdominal organ, foreign body in intestinal tract, mechanical complication of genitourinary device, graft, implant, nonhealing surgical wound, malignant and benign neoplasms, ovarian cysts, and ectopic pregnancy
Hemodialysis access examination (duplex scan)	**Signs and Symptoms:** Chronic abnormal functioning of dialysis access site including difficult cannulation, thrombus aspiration, elevated venous pressure greater than 200 mmHg on a 300 cc/min pump, elevated recirculation time of 15% or greater, low urea reduction rate of less than 60% or shunt collapse
	Diagnostic Outcomes: Complication due to renal access device, implant or graft to include occlusion, embolism, hemorrhage, pain, stenosis, thrombosis
Magnetic resonance imaging (MRI) of the brain	**Signs and Symptoms:** Coma, syncope and collapse, convulsions, changes in skin sensation (tingling, numbness, burning, or prickling sensation), headache, aphasia
	Diagnostic Outcomes: Meningitis, encephalitis, Alzheimer's disease, Parkinson's disease, bipolar disorder, cerebral degenerations, hemiplegia and hemiparesis, epilepsy, diplopia, optic neuritis, subarachnoid and intracerebral hemorrhage, occlusion of cerebral arteries, transient cerebral ischemia, multiple sclerosis, malignant primary and secondary neoplasms

Radiology Procedures (continued)

Magnetic resonance angiography (MRA)	**Signs and Symptoms:** Syncope and collapse, dizziness and giddiness, pain in limb, edema, gangrene, dyspnea, shortness of breath, hemoptysis, chest pain, surgery status **Diagnostic Outcomes:** Pulmonary embolism and infarction; thoracic aortic dissection and aneurysm; subarachnoid and intracerebral hemorrhage; occlusion and stenosis of cerebral arteries; arteriovenous malformation; atherosclerosis; phlebitis and thrombophlebitis; mechanical complication of vascular device, graft, or implant
Peripheral arterial studies (Doppler wave-form analysis, volume plethysmography, transcutaneous oxygen tension measurement, duplex scan of extremity arteries or arterial bypass grafts)	**Signs and Symptoms:** Claudication, rest pain, absent pulses in extremities, gangrene, nonhealing or difficult wounds **Diagnostic Outcomes:** Peripheral vascular disease, atherosclerosis of extremities and bypass grafts, arterial embolism and thrombosis, arterial occlusive disease, rupture of artery, injury to blood vessel, ulcer of lower extremity, surgery status
Peripheral venous studies (Doppler wave-form analysis, phleborheography, impedance plethysmography, duplex scan of extremity veins)	**Signs and Symptoms:** Pain in limb, swelling of limb, localized edema, gangrene, hemoptysis, painful respiration, chest pain, abnormal lung scan, apnea, hypoxia **Diagnostic Outcomes:** Deep vein thrombosis; chronic venous insufficiency; pulmonary embolism and infarction; phlebitis and thrombophlebitis; varicose veins; ulcer of lower extremity; injury to blood vessel; mechanical complication of vascular device, implant, or graft
Ultrasound, abdominal	**Signs and Symptoms:** Abdominal pain; localized abdominal tenderness; hepatomegaly; splenomegaly; abdominal or pelvic swelling, mass, or lump; ascites; abnormal serum enzyme levels; nonvisualization of gallbladder; abnormal liver studies **Diagnostic Outcomes:** Abdominal aneurysm; acute appendicitis; Crohn's disease; chronic liver disease and cirrhosis; liver abscess; abdominal abscess; peritonitis; cholelithiasis; kidney infection; injury to spleen; splenic artery or vein; malignant neoplasms of the liver, pancreas, uterus, abdomen, gallbladder; or secondary neoplasms of the intra-abdominal lymph nodes, liver, or digestive system

Radiology Procedures (continued)

Ultrasound, retroperitoneal	**Signs and Symptoms:** Hematuria; oliguria and anuria; renal colic; abdominal pain, swelling, mass, or lump; abnormal function studies of the kidney
	Diagnostic Outcomes: Hodgkin's disease, acute and chronic renal failure, hypertensive renal disease, kidney infections, abdominal aneurysm, aneurysm of renal artery, lymphosarcoma, acute glomerulonephritis, nephritis and nephropathy, hydronephrosis, cyst of kidney, urinary tract infection, complications of transplanted kidney, malignant neoplasm of urinary organs

Durable Medical Equipment (DME) and Supplies

Durable Medical Equipment (DME)

Bandage, elastic	Compression , Ace™, Kendall™, Curity	**Purpose:** To compress, support, or hold/immobilize a dressing, other bandages, or an extremity in place **Indications:** Fracture, dislocation, sprain, wound due to trauma; suture site, lymphedema **Procedures:** Open/closed reduction of a fracture or fracture/dislocation with or without internal fixation; support a sprain or strain, or suture site; to compress an extremity after lymphedema therapy
Bed, hospital	Oscillating, circulating, Stryker™, burn	**Purpose:** To alternate the pressure on a body site and to improve circulation to body sites for patients unable to change position or for patients who are immobile **Indications:** Decubitus ulcer (pressure sore), paralysis, coma, unconsciousness, neuromuscular disorders, burns, cellulitis, abscess, infection, trauma (e.g., fractures and multiple trauma) **Procedures:** Debridement, excision of a decubitus ulcer or wound; dressing change under anesthesia; reduction of fractures; decubitus ulcer, cellulitis, and abscess are frequently missed CCs
Blood pressure monitor		See "monitor, blood pressure"
Brace, neck		**Purpose:** To support and/or immobilize the neck **Indications:** Fractures, fracture/dislocations, neck strain, whiplash injury, multiple trauma **Procedures:** A rigid neck brace sized to the patient is applied to the neck.
Cast material		**Purpose:** To immobilize a bone, muscle, and/or tendons **Indications:** Fractures and fracture/dislocations, multiple trauma **Procedures:** Casting material is wrapped around stocking material or is wrapped in combination with splinting material to immobilize the affected area.

Catheter, intra-aortic balloon and pump	IABC, IABP, intra-aortic balloon counter-pulsation	**Purpose:** To assist circulation, increase stroke volume and decrease preload, cardiac work, or myocardial oxygen demand, and to improve coronary blood flow and perfusion **Indications:** Acute or old myocardial infarction; coronary atherosclerosis; mitral and aortic heart valve disorders; primary cardiomyopathies; complete or secondary degree atrioventricular (AV) block; cardiac arrest; sinoatrial node dysfunction; other cardiac dysrhythmia; congestive and left heart failure; myocardial degeneration; functional disturbances following cardiac surgery; acquired cardiac septal defect; cardiogenic shock; mechanical complication of heart valve prosthesis, device, implant, or graft; complications of cardiac pacemaker; status arotocoronary bypass; or transluminal coronary angioplasty **Procedures:** A balloon catheter is inserted into the ascending aorta through an open or percutaneous route. The balloon is connected to an external pump that inflates and deflates the balloon in rhythm with the diastole and systole. Congestive heart failure, major heart blocks, paroxysmal supraventricular, ventricular ad unspecified tachycardia are frequently missed CCs
Catheter, urinary	Foley, indwelling	**Purpose:** To empty the bladder, prevent urinary incontinence, obtain specimen **Indications:** urinary retention, urinary tract infection (UTI), urosepsis, coma, intraoperativ, postoperative, unconsciousness, spinal cord injuries, and paralysis **Procedures:** Examination of urine; microscopic examination of the urine, culture, and sensitivities; measure urine output Urinary retention and urinary tract infections are frequently missed CCs
Catheter, urinary	French, intermittent	**Purpose:** To empty the bladder, prevent urinary incontinence, obtain specimen **Indications:** Urinary retention, urinary tract infection, spinal cord injuries and paralysis **Procedures:** Examination of urine; microscopic examination of the urine, culture, and sensitivities Urinary retention and urinary tract infections are frequently missed CCs
Continuous positive airway pressure system	CPAP	**Purpose:** To keep the airway patent and/or deliver medication **Indications:** Obstructive sleep apnea (OSA), congestive heart failure (CHF), asthma, chronic obstructive pulmonary disease (COPD), cystic fibrosis, chronic bronchitis, atelectasis, apnea or respiratory distress syndrome of preterm infants, hyponea **Procedures:** As the patient inhales using an oral or nasal mask, the negative inspiratory force signals the machine to deliver a positive-pressure breath of air/oxygen alone or in combination with medication. CHF and COPD are frequently missed CCs

Device, intermittent positive pressure	IPPB	**Purpose:** To inflate the lungs by means of positive pressure to deliver medication **Indications:** Conditions that result in ineffective deep breathing and coughing (e.g., chronic obstructive pulmonary disease (COPD), lung congestion, neuromuscular diseases, pneumonia, and other respiratory infections or chronic respiratory diseases), postsurgical conditions that make it difficult to raise respiratory secretions **Procedures:** As the patient inhales using a breathing tube, the negative inspiratory force signals the machine to deliver a positive-pressure breath of air/ oxygen alone or in combination with medication. COPD is a frequently missed CC.
Device, pneumatic compression (intermittent)	IPC	**Purpose:** To prevention of deep vein thrombosis and pulmonary embolism **Indications:** Leg trauma, surgery (postoperative), venous stasis, venous insufficiency, spinal cord injury **Procedures:** Used with elastic (surgical) stockings, a compartmentalized sleeve placed over a lower extremity sequentially applies pressure by use of a controller and air hoses hooked to the sleeve See also "Stockings, surgical."
Device, traction		See "equipment traction."
Dialysis, equipment and supplies		See "equipment, dialysis."
Dressings, surgical		**Purpose:** To cover a wound or injury **Indications:** Open or surgical wounds, abrasions, abscess, cellulitis, open fractures or fracture dislocations, postoperative, multiple trauma **Procedures:** Dry, wet, or wet-to-dry sterile dressings are applied to the affected area. Abscess and cellulitis are frequently missed CCs
Equipment, traction		**Purpose:** To place a fracture site in traction **Indications:** Open or closed fractures or fracture/ dislocations, muscle, and bone trauma and wounds, multiple trauma **Procedures:** Traction is placed on the affected bone to immobilize, reduce a fracture or fracture dislocation, or to keep a fracture "reduced" and in alignment.
Intra-aortic balloon catheter	IABC	See "Catheter, intra-aortic balloon and pump."
Infusion pump, parenteral and enteral		See "pump, parenteral or enteral."
Intravenous pump		See "pump, intravenous."

Durable Medical
Equipment and Supplies

Mattress	Air, alternating pressure, flotation	**Purpose:** To alternate the pressure on a body site and to improve circulation to body sites for patients unable to change position **Indications:** Decubitus ulcer (pressure sore), paralysis and spinal cord injuries, coma, unconsciousness, neuromuscular disorders, amyotrophic lateral sclerosis (ALS), burns, cellulitis, abscess, infection, trauma, and multiple trauma **Procedures:** Debridement or excision of a decubitus ulcer or wound, dressing change under anesthesia, drainage of an abscess or infection, reduction of fractures, treatment of wounds and other forms of trauma; decubitus ulcer, cellulitis, and abscess are frequently missed CCs
Machine, dialysis	Hemodialysis, peritoneal dialysis	**Purpose:** To partially or completely replace the function of the kidneys; to filter the blood **Indications:** Acute or chronic renal disease, end-stage renal disease, removal of toxic substances from the blood **Procedures:** A dialysis catheter is inserted into the peritoneal space or into a vein or previously placed arteriovenous fistula, cannula, or graft. Renal dialysis status is a frequently missed CC.
Machine, suction		**Purpose:** To remove secretions from upper airway (e.g., nose, and/or trachea); tracheal suctioning is performed when the patient has a tracheostomy or endotracheal tube present because the cough reflex is decreased **Indications:** Malignant neoplasms of the upper gastrointestinal tract; anoxic brain damage; stenosis of larynx; acute respiratory failure; newborn respiratory distress syndrome; chronic respiratory distress; dyspnea; respiratory abnormalities; pulmonary insufficiency following trauma; fractures of the cervical vertebrae; fracture of the larynx; open wound or crush injury of the larynx, trachea, or neck; foreign body in larynx or trachea; burn of the larynx or trachea; respiratory complication of a surgery or procedure; paralysis or unconsciousness due to injury or trauma **Procedures:** A sterile catheter with a specially designed tip is inserted through the nares, mouth, or tracheostomy tube. The opposite end of the catheter is connected to a suction machine, the machine is turned on and secretions are removed.
Monitor, blood glucose	Glucometer	**Purpose:** To monitor blood glucose levels to determine insulin requirements **Indications:** Diabetes mellitus, gestational diabetes **Procedures:** The patient's finger is pierced with a small lancet; a drop of blood is placed on a chemically prepared strip and inserted into the monitor; the monitor reads and displays the blood glucose level

Monitor, blood pressure		**Purpose:** To monitor changes in blood pressure **Indications:** Hypertension, malignant hypertension (arteriolar hypertension), hypertensive crisis, hypotension, shock, toxemia of pregnancy, diabetes with renal manifestations, renal hypertension, acute renal failure **Procedures:** At predetermined intervals the machine inflates a blood pressure cuff. As the cuff deflates the systolic and diastolic blood pressure measurements are taken. Malignant hypertension is a frequently missed CCs
Monitor, cardiac		**Purpose:** To monitor cardiac function (e.g., heart rate, rhythm, conduction, and output) **Indications:** Angina; myocardial infarction; atrial fibrillation; flutter; paroxysmal supraventricular, ventricular, or atrial tachycardia; heart block; CHF; other cardiac arrhythmia's; pericarditis; carditis; myocarditis; Wolfe-Parkinson White syndrome and other aberrant heart conduction abnormalities; heart valve disorders; congenital heart anomalies (e.g., ventricular septal defect, cardiomyopathy) **Procedures:** Percutaneous transluminal coronary angioplasty (PTCA), coronary artery bypass, ablation of aberrant conduction pathways, lidocaine drip, insertion of temporary or permanent pacemaker, pericardiocentesis, myocardial revascularization, heart valve repair or replacement, repair of ventricular septal defect, heart transplant Angina, atrial fibrillation or flutter, major heart blocks, paroxysmal supraventricular, ventricular, or unspecified tachycardia, and CHF are frequently missed CCs
Monitor, central venous pressure	CVP monitor	**Purpose:** Record the pressure within the right atrium of the heart and the great vessels **Indications:** Hypovolemia, shock, ventricular heart failure **Procedures:** Continuous measurement of the central venous pressure by use of a catheter centrally placed into a pulmonary vein
Oxygen and oxygen supplies	O2, portable, stationary, mask, nasal cannula, tubing	**Purpose:** To increase the amount of oxygen available to the patient to a level beyond that ordinarily found in room air **Indications:** Any condition that requires a higher concentration of oxygen than the patient is able to generate on their own with room air, such as shock, cardiac arrest, anemia, lung malignancy, respiratory arrest, respiratory distress syndrome (adult or newborn, COPD, and fetal distress (oxygen delivered to fetus via mother) **Procedures:** Oxygen is delivered in a concentrated form from a stationary or portable oxygen source via tubing, and mask or cannula to the patient. Anemia due to acute and chronic blood loss and COPD are frequently missed CCs

Durable Medical Equipment and Supplies

Pump, enteral nutrition		**Purpose:** To supply nutrients to the body, such as vitamins, minerals, amino acids, fat, and dextrose **Indications:** Cachexia, malnutrition, due to cancer or other wasting diseases **Procedures:** Placement of a feeding gastrostomy, or jejunostomy tube; cachexia and malnutrition are frequently missed CCs
Pump, intra-aortic balloon counter pulsation	IABP, IAB	See "catheter, intra-aortic balloon and pump."
Pump, total parenteral nutrition	TPN, TNA, intravenous hyperalimentation	**Purpose:** To supply nutrients to the body, such as vitamins, minerals, electrolytes, amino acids, fat, and dextrose **Indications:** Burns, malnutrition, cachexia, AIDS, sepsis, cancer, malabsorption disorders, bowel diseases (e.g., Crohn's disease), anorexia nervosa, status post intestinal surgery **Procedures:** Placement of a peripheral, central, or atrial intravenous lines; cachexia and malnutrition are frequently missed CCs
Pump, suction		See "machine, suction."
Sling		**Purpose:** To immobilize a sprain, strain, fracture, wound, or other postoperative site **Indications:** Sprains, strains, fractures, fracture/dislocations, open or postoperative wounds, and trauma **Procedures:** A commercial sling is placed around the affected area.
Splint		**Purpose:** To immobilize a sprain, strain, fracture, wound or other postoperative site **Indications:** Sprains, strains, fractures, fracture/dislocations, open or postoperative wounds, and trauma **Procedures:** A commercial sling is placed around the affected area.
Suction machine		See "machine suction."
Ventilator	Vent, mechanical, volume, negative pressure, positive pressure, stationary, portable	**Purpose:** To maintain ventilation of the lungs and oxygen requirements of the body **Indications:** COPD; shock; multisystem failure; coma; neuromuscular diseases; paralysis; fracture or crush injury to cervical vertebrae or neck; post-thoracic or other surgery; burns of the face, mouth, esophagus, trachea, larynx, or neck; acute respiratory failure; cardiopulmonary arrest; open wounds; and multiple trauma **Procedures:** Tracheostomy, treatment of wounds, burns, or fractures COPD and respiratory ventilator dependence are frequently missed CCs

Supplies

Catheter, central venous	**Purpose:** To maintain continuous venous access for antibiotics, IV fluids, obtain blood specimens, infuse peripheral nutrition, or control pain **Indications:** Cellulitis, abscess, pneumonia, infections, malnutrition, cachexia, dehydration, postoperative or chronic pain **Procedures:** A catheter is inserted into a central vein between anticubital area and the head of the clavicle. Cellulitis, abscess, malnutrition, cachexia, and dehydration are frequently missed CCs.
Garment, pressure	**Purpose:** To prevent scar formation **Indications:** Burns **Procedures:** Excision burn eschar, scar, or contracture
Implant, carpal	**Purpose:** To replace a carpal bone **Indications:** Fracture, fracture/dislocation, nonunion, malunion, arthritis, trauma-crush injuries **Procedures:** Arthroplasty
Implant, hip	**Purpose:** To partially or totally replace the hip joint **Indications:** Fracture, fracture/dislocation, nonunion, malunion, arthritis, trauma-crush injuries **Procedures:** Arthroplasty
Implant, knee	**Purpose:** To partially or totally replace the knee joint **Indications:** Fracture, fracture/dislocation, nonunion, malunion, arthritis, trauma-crush injuries **Procedures:** Arthroplasty
Implant, metacarpal	**Purpose:** To replace a metacarpal bone **Indications:** Fracture, fracture/dislocation, nonunion, malunion, arthritis, trauma-crush injuries **Procedures:** Arthroplasty
Meter, peak expiratory flow rate	**Purpose:** To measure the expiratory flow **Indications:** Asthma, bronchitis, COPD **Procedures:** The patient takes a deep breath and exhales rapidly through a mouthpiece that is attached to the meter.

Durable Medical Equipment and Supplies

Pacemaker, temporary	Transvenous, single chamber, dual chamber	**Purpose:** To restore the normal heart conduction system function **Indications:** Acute myocardial infarction, heart blocks, anomalous artioventricular excitation, atrial fibrillation and flutter, proxysmal supraventricular tachycardia, cardiac arrest, cardiogenic shock, sinoatrial node dysfunction, mechanical complication due to pacemaker, heart valve prosthesis, coronary artery bypass graft, automatic implantable cardiac defibrillator **Procedures:** Pacemaker electrodes are placed transvenously to temporarily restore the heart's conduction system. Atrial fibrillation and flutter, major heart blocks, and paroxysmal supraventricular tachycardia are frequently missed CCs.
Pacemaker, permanent	Atrial, ventricular, atrial and ventricular, epicardial, transvenous, single chamber, dual chamber	**Purpose:** To restore the normal heart conduction system function **Indications:** Heart blocks; anomalous artioventricular excitation; atrial fibrillation; proxysmal supraventricular tachycardia; sinoatrial node dysfunction; mechanical complication due to pacemaker; complications due to other cardiac device, implant, and graft; cardiac pacemaker in situ **Procedures:** Transvenous or thoracotomy insertion of permanent pacemaker electrodes and pulse generator Atrial fibrillation, major heart blocks, and paroxysmal supraventricular tachycardia are frequently missed CCs.
Stent, ureteral		**Purpose:** To keep a ureter patent **Indications:** Ureteral obstruction or anomaly, kidney infection, renal disorders **Procedures:** A stent is placed into a ureter to keep it patent.
Stocking, surgical		**Purpose:** Prevention of deep vein thrombosis and pulmonary embolism **Indications:** Leg trauma, surgery (postoperative), venous stasis, varacosities, venous insufficiency, spinal cord injury **Procedures:** Vein ligation or stripping, graft or bypass of extremity arteries or veins See also. "Device, pneumatic compression (intermittent)."

Supply radioelement	Technitium (Tc 99m tetrofosmin, medronate), thallous chloride (TL-201), indium (IN 111 capromab-pendetide), strontium-89 chloride, samarium (sm 153 lexidronamm)	**Purpose:** To eradicate a malignancy **Indications:** Malignant neoplasms **Procedures:** A solution of radiation seeds are placed intravenously, into a body cavity, or on the surface of a malignant tumor.
Tracheostomy, tube, mask and cuff, collar, cannula, suction catheter		**Purpose:** To bypass upper airway obstruction, which allows removal of secretions, prevents aspiration of secretions from the gastrointestinal tract, and is often used to allow mechanical ventilation. **Indications:** Malignant neoplasm's of the upper gastrointestinal tract; anoxic brain damage; stenosis of larynx; acute respiratory failure; newborn respiratory distress syndrome; chronic respiratory distress; dyspnea; respiratory abnormalities; pulmonary insufficiency following trauma; fractures of the cervical vertebrae; fracture of the larynx; open wound or crush injury of the larynx, trachea, or neck; foreign body in larynx or trachea; burn of the larynx or trachea; respiratory complication of a surgery or procedure **Procedures:** An incision is made through the second or third tracheal cartilage and dissection is taken down to the level of the trachea. A cuffed tracheostomy tube is inserted into the opening. The tracheostomy cuff is inflated to occlude the area between the tracheal wall and the tube.

Developing an Effective DRG Audit Process

Introduction

With increased government scrutiny in detecting aberrant patterns of upcoding, hospitals need to perform regular audits and/or other evaluation techniques to monitor coding, claim development and submission, as suggested in the Officer of Inspector General's (OIG) "Compliance Program Guidance for Hospitals." Every hospital compliance program should include components related to diagnosis-related group (DRG) coding accuracy to ensure minimal variation in coding practices and to improve the billing and accuracy, integrity, and quality of inpatient claims submission and payment.

Internal Corporate Coding Compliance Program

The OIG encourages facilities to establish internal corporate compliance/fraud and abuse programs. One main goal is to establish a culture in the hospital that promotes prevention, detection, and resolution. A compliance program should reflect the facility's commitment to ethical practices. It should be able to identify practices that do not comply with federal and state law, and federal and state private payer health care program requirements. The OIG guidance was initiated to promote voluntary interest from hospitals in establishing good business sense and commitment to accurate coding thus accurate reimbursement by the Medicare program.

In developing your internal coding compliance program, keep in mind the following risk areas:

- upcoding/DRG creep
- unbundling
- billing for items or services not actually rendered
- providing medically unnecessary services
- duplicate billing
- outpatient services rendered in connection with inpatient stays
- billing for discharge in lieu of transfer
- patient dumping
- physician query form review

Additionally, include areas of concern related to internal practice issues that present the greatest potential for abuse or inconsistency as related to coder error or physician documentation. Obtain feedback from the coding staff, physicians or utilization review staff as they frequently encounter problems that exist on a daily basis and may represent gray areas needing clarification or review.

What should coding departments do to ensure compliance?

Use the following up-to-date coding resources for inpatient coding:

- *ICD-9-CM Expert for Hospitals,* volumes 1, 2, and 3, updated every October
- *Coding Clinic for ICD-9-CM*, a quarterly publication from the American Hospital Association
- *DRG Expert*
- *Physician's Desk Reference*

- anatomy illustrations
- medical dictionary
- up-to-date internal coding policies and guidelines

Maintaining an Ongoing Education Program

Ongoing education for coders is vital to the success of any corporate compliance program. Education is required to keep coders up to date on the ever-changing field of coding. This will help to ensure an accurate database for your facility. Maintain a record of attendance to the in-services, and follow-up with staff who may not have participated consistently.

Ongoing education can be achieved in various forms such as

- ongoing educational program with specified time frames, such as bimonthly, with the requirement that all coders attend the educational sessions
- seminar training material
- workshops
- teleconferences
- group study sessions regarding difficult coding topics
- interaction with the local, state, or national health information management association
- annual external coding audits on a noncontingency fee basis in which the consultant will offer feedback and education while at the facility site
- regular internal monitoring of coding with documentation and feedback

Education should include

- official coding guidelines found in the AHA's *Coding Clinic for ICD-9-CM*
- anatomy and physiology
- disease processes commonly coded
- Medicare reimbursement principles
- internal coding policies
- corporate ethics
- coders code of ethics
- fraud and abuse laws
- billing processes

Official Sources for Coding Guidelines

It should be the policy of every health information management (HIM) coding department to adhere to official coding guidelines; however, every coding scenario is not represented. Therefore, other sources of coding guidelines can be acceptable. Coding staff should be accountable in seeking out correct coding guidelines when necessary for determining appropriate code assignment. In the absence of clear coding guidelines, coding staff should seek management approval and support to determine internal policy.

In addition to the AHA's *Coding Clinic for ICD-9-CM*, the following sources are secondary resources for coding staff:

- federal notices such as the *Federal Register*, Medicare program memorandums, Medicare fiscal intermediary (FI) provider bulletins
- quality improvement organizations (QIOs, formerly known as PROs)
- internal hospital policy and procedure manual
- ICD-9-CM coding book instructional notes
- third-party payer guidelines when published and provided by the insurance carrier (may include managed care contracts and may vary from AHA *Coding Clinic* guidelines, depending on the payer)

When billing issues, questions, or discrepancies arise, work closely with your QIO and FI. When the QIO or FI responds verbally to your question, ask for a specific resource you can reference. If the QIO or FI cannot refer you to an existing resource, request that the response be put in writing. Be sure to document and file all interactions with your QIO and FI and their resulting direction.

Impacts of "Undercoding"–Lost Revenue

The risk of upcoding and undercoding are both of equal importance. Due to new scrutiny the coding process is placed under, some hospitals are assigning lower weighted DRGs when under review by the OIG. Facilities overcompensate due to the risk of upcoding and end up undercoding. This, of course, results in under payment for the facility. The goal is to code accurately based on detailed, accurate, and complete documentation by the physician.

An ineffective DRG program results in inaccurate payment to the hospital, either lower or higher reimbursement, and skewed data. The exhibit below represents a DRG report showing potential lost revenues to a hospital.

Exhibit 1: Sample DRG Coding Assessment

There were 65 charts reviewed, 12 of which had DRG changes. This represented $20,130.16 in revenue that the hospital did not receive.

Current DRG Assignment	Revised DRG Assignment	Current Payment	Revised Payment	Increase/ Decrease	Payment Difference
165	164	$3,737.05	$6,720.49	+	$2,983.44
158	157	1,581.00	3,114.88	+	1,533.88
077	076	3,237.33	7,678.70	+	4,441.37
175	174	1,659.74	2,993.67	+	1,333.93
131	130	1,807.61	2,803.02	+	995.41
089	079	3,548.57	5,372.92	+	2,824.35
133	138	1,629.67	2,491.78	+	862.11
311	310	1,613.86	2,791.86	+	1,178.00
122	121	3,510.75	4,965.27	+	1,454.52
183	182	1,640.21	2,361.27	+	721.06
125	124	2,467.60	3,815.17	+	1,347.57
122	121	3,510.75	4,965.27	+	1,454.52

Total Payment Variation	$20,130.16

Frequent Causes of Lost Revenues

The most frequent causes of lost revenue include the following:

- omission of CC conditions that were detectable through evidence of diagnostic and treatment modalities, or physician documentation
- difficulty in selecting principal diagnosis when coexisting reasons for admission and treatment are documented
- inappropriate sequencing of principal/secondary diagnoses
- incomplete documentation, such as a failure to identify organism growth on culture reports
- unidentified major complications associated with myocardial infarctions

- lack of diagnostic conclusions (discharge diagnoses) documented by physician in chart at the time of coding
- medical record department operational issues, such as dictation turnaround time or a high medical record incomplete/delinquency rate for the completion of records

How Omitted CCs Impact Payment

Exhibits 1 and 2 illustrate how lack of accurate DRG coding results in lost payment. Exhibit 3 shows that this revenue is often lost due to unidentified complication/comorbid conditions (CCs).

Exhibit 3: Projected Payment Losses From Missed CCs

Medicare discharges per month	300
Medicare discharges per year	3,600
One sixth of those discharges are DRGs that lack a CC	600
Assumption is that one-half of the CCs are being missed	300
Average of each missed CC (based upon the 12 changed DRGs in exhibit1)	$1,457.62
Anticipated lost revenue per year attributable to missed CCs	$437,286.00

The Basics of Coding Reviews

Establishing an Audit Plan

Before performing an audit, it is important to establish a specific plan for carrying it out. The components of the audit plan should be spelled out clearly. The first step is to determine the frequency with which the audits will be performed and the results to be reported. Many facilities find that reviewing a smaller number of medical records on a more frequent basis enables them to review the specific number of records designated in their sample size. Therefore, a plan might state that retrospective audits would occur weekly with cumulative results compiled monthly and the results reported quarterly to the medical staff.

The plan should also define the audits purpose. For example, the purpose may be to ensure data integrity with emphasis on complete and accurate documentation, appropriate reporting of the principal diagnosis, other (additional) diagnoses and procedures, and accurate ICD-9-CM code and DRG assignment. The sample size should also be defined. Since consideration of data integrity should not be limited to specific payers or initiatives, your plan should address all payers. The sample size should include at least 3 percent of all discharges per month. You may, however, choose to review a larger sample size that is more representative of your patient population. The plan should specify the exact number of Medicare and non-Medicare records to be reviewed per week or month.

External Versus Internal Coding Reviews

As a part of an internal corporate compliance program, the OIG suggests an annual external coding audit. In choosing a company to perform your coding review, first review the company and select on an unbiased basis. Ensure the consultants that will be performing your internal coding review have the expertise required. Ask for a bio of the consultant that details his or her years of coding experience and the credentials he or she holds. Ensure the consultant will offer education to the coding staff while on site. The consultant should allow time to discuss each recommendation while on site. Review the contract for the length of time you can follow up with the company with future coding questions. Test different consulting companies over time to find the company with which you are most comfortable.

When you are prepared to have an external company perform a DRG and coding review, work through your facility's compliance officer and/or hospital attorney. Also, inform the billing department that a coding review will be taking place. DRG bill adjustments are required when a change in the DRG is realized. The facility will have 60 days from the date of the intermediary payment notice to resubmit a claim.

Benefits of an external review are an unbiased third party with outside experiences. Additionally, most outside consulting firms offer education and training programs, which focus on physician documentation improvement and formal coding education tracks.

Internal Data Quality
Consider developing an internal coding validation review program assigned to a data quality coordinator position.

Start by creating the following review criteria:

- what elements will be validated: the DRG, all secondary codes, missed codes, documentation issues, accuracy of all abstracted data, capture of appropriate discharge status, medical necessity issues
- how will you create your sample size or what percentage of records will be reviewed
- what DRGs will you choose for review (see below)
- how often will the review take place: weekly, monthly, quarterly
- will the review include all payers
- how will the results be tracked and documented
- who will be included in the distribution list for your documented findings
- designate a time to offer education to the coding staff based on the findings
- monitor, track, and document the improvement

Selecting an Audit Approach
There are many models used by consultants and hospitals designed for assessing coding quality. The selection of the audit approach is facility dependent based on operational decisions such as available resources, staffing, budget constraints, exposure to outside payer audits, and the severity of the historical trending results of overall and coder specific quality rates. The decision on which approach to select typically revolves around whether a random sample of cases (for example, top 10 DRGs) are needed or whether a problem oriented review for an isolated or widespread, ongoing issue is warranted. For example, if upon review of the case mix a trend analysis identifies a specific shift related to a certain coding practice, a problem-focused review of the DRGs involved may be selected.

Retrospective
The retrospective or rebill process is the most common audit approach, which provides the ability to review the entire revenue process from claim submission to payment. This type of review takes place on the back end after claims submission and payment. In the case of reviewing Medicare DRGs, the reviewer would take the Medicare remittance advice, select the services based on target areas, and verify the DRG assignment matches the coding abstract assignment. The next step is to review the medical documentation and verify coding/DRG accuracy.

Billing errors are typically identified through the retrospective review and may warrant a review of the UB-92 to reconcile whether the codes submitted through the HIM abstract matches the codes submitted for payment. Typically, the retrospective review is most advantageous when the coding error rates are low and require few resubmits. A high rebill or resubmit percentage could trigger concern from the Medicare FI who may initiate further investigation.

Prospective

The prospective or prebill process is the most resource-intensive audit approach; however, the benefits outweigh the disadvantages. The prospective approach involves the review of cases prior to claims submission, the correction of areas identified is immediate. This approach provides the coder with immediate feedback and keeps the case in question fresh on his or her mind. Additionally, if performed on the unit or immediately following discharge of the patient, physician documentation issues can be addressed while the case is still current in the physician's mind.

The disadvantages to prospective review relate to the hold up of account receivables in that accounts are not released for billing until coding or documentation issues are resolved. Most hospitals have a billing requirement that falls within the first four days following discharge; therefore, the prospective review would need to resolve issues quickly. For these reasons, the prospective review is usually reserved for situations where there is a higher error rate that needs correction prior to claims submission to limit exposure of overbilling.

Sample Selection and Using Comparative Data

The review methodology should be clearly documented. Facilities have been known to target DRGs and review methodology may be twofold, with both a targeted and a random review of cases. The Medicare review would be a targeted review based on the DRG assigned. The DRGs targeted should be defined in the compliance plan.

Some hospitals find that comparing their coding and DRG levels with those of other hospitals alerts them to potential areas of miscoding. Comparative norms for coding practices are made on a national, state, or regional basis. For example, data used to target hospitals for national investigations of upcoding can be performed by examining the Centers for Medicare and Medicaid Services (CMS) Medicare Provider Analysis and Review (MedPAR) files. The MedPAR file contains information for 100 percent of Medicare beneficiaries using hospital inpatient services. Data are provided by state and then by DRG for all short stay and inpatient hospitals. The following fields are furnished: total charges, covered charges, Medicare reimbursement, total days, number of discharges, and average total days.

As investigators explain, if your hospital codes more strokes and fewer transient ischemic attacks than most hospitals, there may be a good reason for that. Some coding variances are acceptable but if peer data show outliers, it could be indicative of miscoding. It clearly behooves facilities to look at comparative data and know it's an outlier before the government finds the trend. One standard comparative sample used is the complication and comorbidity (CC) capture rate. This is an area of focus because 40 percent of all Medicare patients fall into a DRG pair where one DRG is weighted higher due to the presence of a CC. A high CC rate could be indicative of aggressive coding and should be validated by an audit.

More hospitals are using both in-house computer programs and the services of consultants to examine their numbers. There are numerous organizations that offer reports to facilities based on their billing data. An example of one product that reports these numbers for hospitals is available from the Center for Healthcare Industry Performance Studies (CHIPS). The report, tailored to an individual hospital, gives a rundown of dozens of DRG pairs, tells the hospital what percentage it coded to the higher-paying DRG, and how this compares to competing hospitals and the national average.

The report also shows the dollar amount each variance from the national average represents. That information helps the facility in deciding which DRG is worth investigating further, either for upcoding or downcoding. This comparison can make your code auditing efforts more effective. It can point you to DRGs you need to examine, whereas a random sample of all your charts may not find those trouble spots.

In addition, the report displays an analysis for each DRG that shows the trends for the hospital's coding over four years, as well as the comparable trends for three other hospitals and the national averages. This kind of look at the numbers can not only reveal conditions for which you're receiving too much reimbursement from Medicare but also highlight cases for which you are receiving too little. If your hospital chooses codes that fall into a higher-paying DRG significantly less frequently than other hospitals, you may want to investigate whether you are losing revenue by not coding to the highest appropriate level.

Audit Criteria

The plan should also address components of review. There should be a written policy and procedure for how the audits will be conducted. For instance, it might state the review will consist of the following components:

- validation of ICD-9-CM codes against the AHA's *Coding Clinic for ICD-9-CM*
- validation of DRG assignments against uniform hospital discharge data set (UHDDS) definitions for principal diagnosis and *Diagnosis Related Groups Definition Manual*
- reconciliation of the coding summary with the physician documentation such as the discharge summary
- ensure the correct codes are on the UB-92 prior to billing
- selection of discharge status
- accuracy of key abstracting fields such as age and admission/discharge dates

It should be noted that reconciliation of the coding summary with the physician documentation, such as, the discharge summary is important for those facilities practicing prospective or retrospective coding methodology. It is necessary to identify discrepancies between the coding summary, which is generated concurrently, and the discharge summary, which in many cases is generated, retrospectively. This is done to identify opportunities for improvement in communication or clarification of clinical conditions on the nursing unit, documentation, and education for both medical and coding staff.

Documentation Review

Strong documentation practices can help to ensure accurate and complete code assignment. This will result in the assignment of the appropriate DRG for reimbursement under the Medicare prospective payment system (PPS) program. The goal of the DRG system is for facilities to assign the appropriate DRG based on severity of patient condition, resource utilization, and length of stay. Incomplete documentation can lead to incomplete or inaccurate coding that may result in an inappropriate DRG assignment, and in turn, inappropriate reimbursement.

Documentation in the medical record by the health care practitioner is required to document pertinent facts, findings, and observations about the patient's medical history including past and present illnesses, examinations, tests, treatments, and outcomes.

The medical record documentation is important in contributing to

- the ability of the health care professional to evaluate and plan the patient's immediate treatment, and to monitor the patient's health care over time
- communication and continuity of care among all health care professionals involved in the patient's care
- accurate and timely claims review and payment
- appropriate utilization review and quality of care evaluations
- collection of data used for research and education
- acting as a legal document to support services and care rendered

The principals of documentation are as follows:

- All efforts should be made by a facility to ensure that documentation is legible. Illegible documentation is of no value.
- Documentation should support severity of illness, length of stay, and choice of setting.
- The documentation should support the intensity of the patient evaluation and/or the treatment, including complexity of medical decision making.
- Each record should include documentation of the date of service, reason for visit, history and physical exam, review of ancillary test data, assessment and plan of care, treatment plan, and discharge plan.
- Past and present diagnoses should be clearly documented for attending and consulting physicians.
- All services, tests, and procedures performed should be supported by documentation reflecting the need for the services, and address any abnormal results.
- Health risk factors should be identified.
- There should be detailed documentation concerning the patient's progress, including response to treatment, change in treatment, or change in diagnosis.
- All entries should be dated and authenticated.

Every facility should have a means by which to educate the medical staff on documentation issues, Medicare rules and regulations, billing issues, coding, and fraud and abuse issues. Better success may be achieved if the medical staff education program includes information on documentation related to their office visits. Also, there should be a means of educating ancillary departments in their documentation, such as respiratory therapy, diabetic educators, medical nutritionists, pharmacy, etc.

Compiling the Results

Individual results should be compiled to identify undesirable coding patterns and trends. A cumulative report of each review should be kept to monitor improvement or worsening of a specific issue identified. A consistent method should be used to determine error rates. Some consultants use two categories of errors, one related to coding accuracy and the other related to documentation. The documentation issues would need further discussion and clarification with the attending physician, which would normally constitute the initiation of the physician query process.

The coding error rate threshold varies amongst facilities and consulting companies. An average of 95 percent accuracy is a standard used. The variances in error rates depend upon if the reviewed classifies errors affecting reimbursement different from those not affecting reimbursement.

Ideally, an expectation of 100 percent would be met; however, a zero percent error rate is not realistic. Most importantly, when problems or opportunities for improvement are identified, corrective action plans should be implemented and monitored to prevent recurrence of future error. Follow-up reviews are indicated to show progress.

Reporting

Reports should be designed for tracking and analyzing coding audit results. These results should present overall accuracy rates as well as individual coder results. A breakdown by DRG and MDC could help focus on areas problematic within a certain clinical specialty or body area. In addition to being shared with the coding manager and staff, the results should be summarized and submitted to the appropriate compliance professional for review and feedback.

DRGs to Review

A DRG target list should be developed based upon each facility's patient population, for example, encompassing high volume, high error, or high revenue producing services. The target list should be reviewed at least annually to re-evaluate process and review methodology. An essential part of developing an internal coding quality program is to determine the DRGs for review. Work closely with your QIOs. Each QIO can determine what DRGs it will review. Include the QIO's focused DRGs in your list of focus DRGs. In addition to the QIO's DRGs, include the DRGs that have been designated by CMS as target DRGs.

Target pairs of DRGs are sets of two DRGs for which some hospitals are coding cases to one when they should go to the other. An example of the distinction between DRG groups is described in the target DRG listing chapter on page 523.

Target DRG listings help administrators pinpoint on areas where problems can occur. Ensuring that the errors do not occur or continue to recur requires reviews of records and the analysis of a facility's benchmark statistics, as well as training of coding staff, and providing standard sources for good coding practices.

Sources: Documents used for the hints on coding include *ICD-9-CM Coding Handbook with Answers*, AHA Publishing; *Coding Clinic for ICD-9-CM*, AHA.

Additional Information TARGET DRGs

The OIG uses computer analysis of Medicare files to flag hospitals for possible upcoding of certain DRGs.

Septicemia

The OIG staff used the MedPAR file to determine that DRG 416, Septicemia, discharges increased from 1.51 percent of all discharges in 1993 to 1.88 percent in 1996. The OIG then identified those hospitals which had two characteristics: in each facility, more than 3 percent of discharges were for DRG 416, and the proportion of DRG 416 discharges had more than doubled in three years.

Of the 120 facilities falling into that category, the percentage of DRG 416 discharges had actually increased from 1.57 percent to 4.33 percent, an almost threefold jump.

A previous record validation study had estimated that, nationally, 13 percent of all DRG 416 discharges were upcoded. Of the sample used by the OIG, 20 percent were labeled as miscoded.

Previous DRG reviews have found that DRG 320, Kidney and Urinary Track Infections, Age > 17 with CC, seems to be the category most vulnerable to being upcoded to DRG 416. Such a miscode can cause an overpayment of about $2,000. OIG analysis shows that for these 120 hospitals, the percentage of discharges coded to DRG 320 fell from 2.17 percent to 1.54 percent during the three years in question.

Reviewers also found that there is upcoding to DRG 416 from about 20 other DRGs, including: 089, Simple Pneumonia and Pleurisy, Age > 17 with CC; 296, Nutritional and Miscellaneous Disorders, Age > 17 with CC; and 144, Other Circulatory System Diagnoses with CC.

Nutritional and Miscellaneous Metabolic Disorders

Additionally, reviewers found that 10 percent of the cases reported as DRG 296, Nutritional and Miscellaneous Metabolic Disorders, Age > 17 with CC, were improperly coded. Of the 43 improperly coded cases, 31 caused overpayments to the hospitals, for a total estimated overpayment by Medicare of $6.7 million.

The OIG actually pinpointed 60 hospitals for which total DRG 296 discharges had more than doubled in recent years. These facilities had average increases of 32 percent annually at a time when the national average remained almost unchanged.

This group of hospitals was also targeted because the proportion of DRG 296 discharges to total discharges nearly doubled, from 2.58 percent in 1993 and 5.08 percent in 1996. The national average decreased.

The diagnoses that the survey found that were most often improperly upcoded to DRG 296 were:

- DRG 182, Esophagitis, Gastroenteritis and Miscellaneous Digestive Disorders, Age > 17 with CC
- DRG 449, Poisoning and Toxic Effects of Drugs, Age > 17 with CC
- DRG 294, Diabetes, Age > 35
- DRG 463, Signs and Symptoms with CC

DRG 475–Respiratory System Diagnosis with Ventilator Support

DRG 475 is now a target DRG, based on the reviews under the OIG. For hospitals that had reported DRG 475, reviewers determined the number of DRG 475 discharges and the total overall number of discharges for each year. They then calculated the proportion of DRG 475 discharges to the total discharges for each hospital in 1996. They then did the same for the year 1993. Between 1993 and 1996, the proportion of DRG 475 to all discharges had increased by more than 100 percent in 14 percent of the hospitals.

For 46 hospitals, the total DRG 475 assignments increased per year by 38 percent. For all other hospitals, the total increased by 7 percent per year. The estimated overpayment could be as high as $11.5 million for 1996. These hospitals have been referred to the OIG.

Coding of Pathologic Fractures

DRG 239, Pathological Fractures and Musculoskeletal and Connective Tissue Malignancy, is the focus of government investigations. The OIG identified that this DRG is one of the 10 DRGs with the highest rates of upcoding.

Pathological Versus Traumatic Fractures

Not all fractures are alike. True, a fracture is a break, rupture, or crack in a bone or cartilage, but there are many etiologies of a fracture other than those frequently encountered with injury or trauma. Determining the etiology of the fracture is an important step for coding professionals when determining the correct ICD-9-CM code assignment for the case. As in all coding scenarios, the medical record documentation must establish and support the appropriate diagnosis code assignment.

Occasionally, fractures are not caused by injury or trauma, but instead occur when the bone has been weakened in one or more areas by a disease process, such as metastatic carcinoma or progressed osteoporosis. These types of fractures are called pathological fractures (i.e., fractures of diseased or weakened bones produced by forces that would not have fractured a healthy bone). Some clinicians broaden this definition to include any fracture through weakened or diseased bone. Certain disease conditions and processes during which gradual demineralization and/or lysis of the osseous tissues takes place over a period of time can be the cause of pathological fractures. Such conditions include osteomalacia, osteomyelitis, tuberculosis, bone cysts, disseminated bone disorders, inflammatory bone disease, Paget's disease, and lytic lesions secondary to neoplasms.

These types of fractures usually occur without an apparent cause, that is, no trauma is associated with the fracture. Often, these fractures occur during normal physical activity such as rolling over in bed, walking up or down stairs, or when there is a sudden but not unusual twisting or turning of a limb at a site within the bone which is weakened by the underlying disease. These fractures also sometimes occur in connection with minimal trauma that, under ordinary circumstances, would not produce a break in a healthy bone. Many pathological fractures occur spontaneously, especially in superattenuated areas of severely diseased bone.

To classify a fracture as pathological, the medical record should document a cause-and-effect relationship between the fracture and the underlying pathology. Fractures not specified as pathological or due to an underlying disease are classified to the category range 800–829 indicating a traumatic injury. A code for a traumatic fracture is never assigned in conjunction with a code for a pathological fracture of the same bone.

In the situation where there is evidence that the fracture was associated with an injury, such as a fall, and the attending physician also has documented the fracture as being pathological, the physician should be contacted for clarification before the case is coded. If the physician confirms that the fracture is pathological, the correct code assignments would be for the underlying disease (e.g., bone cancer) and the site of the pathological fracture. On the other hand, if the physician documents that the patient's fracture was caused by the fall, the correct diagnosis code assignment is for the anatomical site of the fracture.

Targeted DRG Listing

DRG 014 Intracranial Hemorrhage and Stroke with Infarction

DRG 015   Nonspecific Cerebrovascular and Precerebral Occlusion without Infarction

DRG 524   Transient Ischemia

Issue

The issue of coding cerebrovascular disease (430–438) is problematic because of the lack of physician documentation on the known or suspected presence of cerebral infarction and the complexity of ICD-9-CM diagnosis codes and coding guidelines for cerebrovascular disorders. The following represent the major issues affecting the DRG pairs 014 and 015:

- distinguishing between whether the patient has experienced a cerebrovascular accident, or a transient ischemic attack (both produce similar symptoms)
- physician documentation in establishing a relationship between the stroke or cerebrovascular accident and the site of a neurological brain impairment such as a cerebral infarction or cerebral hemorrhage for the current episode of care
- determination of the underlying cause such as hemorrhagic or ischemic, ischemic strokes account for 80 percent of all strokes
- documentation of onset of current acute condition versus residual neurological deficits from previous stroke

Most Common Diagnosis Codes

DRG 014

- 431, Intracranial hemorrhage
- 434.11, Cerebral embolism with cerebral infarction
- 434.91, Cerebral artery occlusion with cerebral infarction
-

DRG 015

- 433.10, Occlusion and stenosis of carotid artery without mention of cerebral infarction
- 436, Cerebrovascular accident **

DRG 524

- 435.9 Transient ischemic attacks**

Note: Effective October 1, 2002, changes to the fiscal year 2003 hospital inpatient prospective payment system produced new titles and movement of codes between DRG 014 (Intracranial Hemorrhage and Stroke with Infarction) and DRG 015 (Nonspecific Cerebrovascular and Precerebral Occlusion without Infarction) as well as the creation of a new DRG 524 (Transient Ischemia).

** Denotes codes that have been reassigned for FY 2003

Coding and Documentation Guidelines

431   Intracerebral hemorrhage   DRG 014

CG: *Do not* classify cerebrovascular accident (CVA) to category 431 without obtaining physician verification and supporting documentation in the medical record

AHA CC: Use code 431 if the physician documents 'new CVA,' indicating a repeat hemorrhage of a new or same site. [*Coding Clinic,* 2Q, '89, 8, effective with discharges July 31, 1989]

AHA CC: Use code 434.11 when the physician documents a diagnosis of right embolic hemorrhagic infarct of the temporal lobe. Do not assign code 431, intracranial hemorrhage, as the hemorrhage is a component of the occlusion. [*Coding Clinic,* 3Q, '97, 11, effective with discharges August 1, 1997]

AHA CC: If the physician documents a diagnosis of RIND, the code assignment depends on the context in which the "reversible ischemic neurologic deficit" is used. Neurologic deficits (e.g., weakness, paralysis of facial muscles, clumsiness, paresthesia or paralysis in one or both limbs on the same side, numbness, loss of sensation, inability to eat or talk, loss of vision or partial vision in one eye, double vision, memory loss and vertigo) are commonly associated with cerebral vascular disease (430–435). The physician may further describe the deficits as either fixed (ongoing) or reversible (of brief duration or recovery occurring within six months or more). Use a code from category 434, occlusion of cerebral arteries, if RIND is used in association with a physician's diagnosis of cerebral artery occlusion. A microthrombosis or microembolism may result in a reversible neurologic deficit if the blood supply to the ischemic region is restored promptly. [*Coding Clinic,* M-A, '85, 7]

DOC: Use code 431 if the physician documents basilar, bulbar, cerebellar, cerebral, cerebramemingeal, cortical, internal capsule, intrapontine, pontine, subcortical, or ventricular hemorrhage.

DOC: Use code 431 if the physician documents a rupture of a blood vessel in the brain.

DOC: Use code 431 if the physician documents "new CVA," indicating a repeat hemorrhage of a new or same site. [*Coding Clinic,* 2Q, '89, 8, effective with discharges July 31, 1989]

434.11   Cerebral embolism with cerebral infarction   DRG 014

CG: Use code 434.11 if the physician documents the obstruction or occlusion of a cerebral artery due to the migration of a blood clot, which can cause the death of brain tissue (cerebral infarction). The cerebral artery is one that supplies the main portion of the brain (right and left cerebral hemispheres), which occupies the upper cranial cavity. The majority of cerebral emboli originate from the carotid bifurcation. Rarely, the embolism may consist of fat, vegetations, air, a mass of bacteria or other foreign material.

CG: *Do not* classify CVA to category 434 without obtaining physician verification and supporting documentation in the medical record.

AHA CC: Use code 431 if the physician documents 'new CVA,' indicating a repeat hemorrhage of a new or same site. [*Coding Clinic,* 2Q, '89, 8, effective with discharges July 31, 1989]

AHA CC: Never assume that an infarction has occurred without this being clearly documented in the medical record. Use the fifth digit '0' to indicate the absence of an infarct during the current episode of care. The fifth digit '0' identifies 'without mention of cerebral infarction.' The 5th digit of "1" for infarction is only applicable to the current episode of care, not previous episodes and only to the infarction of the artery documented by the physician, not any other artery. A direct cause-and-effect relationship between the occlusion and infarction can be made. However it is not correct to identify occlusion in a cerebral artery that resulted in infarction as a precerebral (carotid) artery occlusion with infarction. The coding should be assigned as 434.91, cerebral artery occlusion with cerebral infarction and 433.10 precerebral occlusion without infarction. *Do not* use the fifth digit '1' to identify an 'old' or 'history of' infarct. [*Coding Clinic,* 2Q, '95, 14, effective with discharges April 15, 1995]

434.11   Cerebral embolism with cerebral infarction (continued)   **DRG 014**

AHA CC: Use code 434.11 when the physician documents a diagnosis of right embolic hemorrhagic infarct of the temporal lobe. *Do not* assign code 431, intracranial hemorrhage, as the hemorrhage is a component of the occlusion. [*Coding Clinic,* 3Q, '97, 11, effective with discharges August 1, 1997]

AHA CC: Use code 434.11 if the physician documents an initial onset of CVA with neurologic deficits (hemiplegia, dysphagia, dysphasia, aphasia, and/or other paralysis, such as of eye muscles) if the type of CVA is stated as cerebral artery embolism with cerebral infarction. Code also any neurologic deficit still present at the time of discharge. [*Coding Clinic,* 2Q, '89, 8, effective with discharges July 1, 1989]

AHA CC: Use code 434.11 if the physician documents 'new CVA,' indicating a repeat embolism of a new or same site. [*Coding Clinic,* 2Q, '89, 8, effective with discharges July 1, 1989]

AHA CC: Use Code 433.1 with the fifth digit '0' to indicate a patient who is status post carotid artery occlusion with cerebral infarction six weeks ago and is admitted to have an endarterectomy. [*Coding Clinic,* 2Q, '95, 14, effective with discharges April 15, 1995]

AHA CC: If the physician documents a diagnosis of RIND, the code assignment depends on the context in which the 'reversible ischemic neurologic deficit' is used. Neurologic deficits, e.g., weakness, paralysis of facial muscles, clumsiness, paresthesia or paralysis in one or both limbs on the same side, numbness, loss of sensation, inability to eat or talk, loss of vision or partial vision in one eye, double vision, memory loss and vertigo, are commonly associated with cerebral vascular disease (430-435). The physician may further describe the deficits as either fixed (ongoing) or reversible (of brief duration or recovery occurring within six months or more). Use a code from category 434, occlusion of cerebral arteries, if RIND is used in association with a physician's diagnosis of cerebral artery occlusion. A microthrombosis or microembolism may result in a reversible neurologic deficit if the blood supply to the ischemic region is restored promptly. [*Coding Clinic,* M-A, '85, 7]

434.91   Cerebral artery occlusion, unspecified, with cerebral   **DRG 014**
infarction

CG: Do not classify CVA to category 434 without obtaining physician verification and supporting documentation in the medical record.

AHA CC: Never assume that an infarction has occurred without this being clearly documented in the medical record. Use the fifth digit '0' to indicate the absence of an infarct during the current episode of care. The fifth digit '0' identifies 'without mention of cerebral infarction.' The 5th digit of "1" for infarction is only applicable to the current episode of care, not previous episodes and only to the infarction of the artery documented by the physician, not any other artery. A direct cause-and-effect relationship between the occlusion and infarction can be made. However it is not correct to identify occlusion in a cerebral artery that resulted in infarction as a precerebral (carotid) artery occlusion with infarction. Rather the coding should be assigned as 434.91, cerebral artery occlusion with cerebral infarction and 433.10, precerebral occlusion without infarction. *Do not* use the fifth digit '1' to identify an 'old' or 'history of' infarct. [*Coding Clinic,* 2Q, '95, 14, effective with discharges April 15, 1995]

AHA CC: Use code 434.91 if the physician documents cerebral artery occlusion with cerebral infarction but does not specify the occlusion as either thrombosis (434.01) or embolism (434.11).

AHA CC: Use the fifth digit '0' to indicate a patient who is status post carotid artery occlusion with cerebral infarction six weeks ago and is admitted to have an endarterectomy. [*Coding Clinic,* 2Q, '95, 14, effective with discharges April 15, 1995]

AHA CC: Use code 434.91 if the physician documents a CVA (stroke) due to a cerebral infarction but the site of the infarction is uncertain. Use of this code is permissible when the type of infarct is not specified and the site is not known. [*Coding Clinic,* 2Q, '95, 14, effective with discharges April 15, 1995]

434.91   Cerebral artery occlusion, unspecified, with cerebral   DRG 014
infarction (continued)

AHA CC: Use code 434.91 if the physician documents an initial onset of CVA with neurologic deficits (hemiplegia, dysphagia, dysphasia, aphasia, and/or other paralysis, such as of eye muscles) if the type of CVA is stated as cerebral artery occlusion with cerebral infarction. Code also any neurologic deficit still present at the time of discharge. [*Coding Clinic,* 2Q, '89, 8, effective with discharges July 1, 1989]

AHA CC: Use code 434.91 if the physician documents 'new CVA,' indicating a repeat cerebral occlusion of a new or same site. [*Coding Clinic,* 2Q, '89, 8, effective with discharges July 1, 1989]

AHA CC: If the physician documents a diagnosis of RIND, the code assignment depends on the context in which the 'reversible ischemic neurologic deficit' is used. Neurologic deficits, e.g., weakness, paralysis of facial muscles, clumsiness, paresthesia or paralysis in one or both limbs on the same side, numbness, loss of sensation, inability to eat or talk, loss of vision or partial vision in one eye, double vision, memory loss and vertigo, are commonly associated with cerebral vascular disease (430-435). The physician may further describe the deficits as either fixed (ongoing) or reversible (of brief duration or recovery occurring within six months or more). Use a code from category 434, occlusion of cerebral arteries, if RIND is used in association with a physician's diagnosis of cerebral artery occlusion. A microthrombosis or microembolism may result in a reversible neurologic deficit if the blood supply to the ischemic region is restored promptly. [*Coding Clinic,* M-A, '85, 7]

433.10   Occlusion and stenosis of carotid artery without mention of   DRG 015
cerebral infarction

CG: *Do not* use code 433.10 to describe insufficiency not otherwise specified of the carotid artery (435.8).

CG: *Do not* classify CVA to category 433 without obtaining physician verification and supporting documentation in the medical record.

CG: The usual etiology of the transient ischemic attack (TIA) is embolization from precerebral artery plaque or due to cardiac causes. If a patient has the signs and symptoms of a TIA due to conditions classifiable to category 433, only a code from category 433 should be used.

CG: Use code 433.10 if the physician documents an initial onset of CVA with neurologic deficits (hemiplegia, dysphagia, dysphasia, aphasia, and/or other paralysis, such as of eye muscles) if the type of CVA is stated as carotid artery occlusion without cerebral infarction. Code also any neurologic deficit still present at the time of discharge. [*Coding Clinic,* 2Q, '89, 8, effective with discharges July 31, 1989]

AHA CC: The physician documents that the patient was admitted for a stroke. During the hospitalization the x-ray revealed a 60 percent occlusion of the carotid artery. However, the physician's diagnostic statement is CVA. Before using 433.10, question the physician on the significance of the finding in the x-ray report and the relationship to the stroke. Indication on x-ray of carotid occlusion does not necessarily mean that it was the cause of the stroke. If the physician documents that the stroke occurred as a result of the carotid artery occlusion, assign code 433.11. [*Coding Clinic,* 2Q, '95, 14, effective with discharges April 15, 1995]

AHA CC: Never assume that an infarction has occurred without this being clearly documented in the medical record. Use the fifth digit '0' to indicate the absence of an infarct during the current episode of care. The fifth digit '0' identifies 'without mention of cerebral infarction.' The 5th digit of "1" for infarction is only applicable to the current episode of care, not previous episodes and only to the infarction of the artery documented by the physician, not any other artery. A direct cause-and-effect relationship between the occlusion and infarction can be made. However it is not correct to identify occlusion in a cerebral artery that resulted in infarction as a precerebral (carotid) artery occlusion with infarction. Rather the coding should be assigned as 434.91, cerebral artery occlusion with cerebral infarction and 433.10, precerebral occlusion without infarction. *Do not* use the fifth digit '1' to identify an 'old' or 'history of' infarct. [*Coding Clinic,* 2Q, Õ95, 14, effective with discharges April 15, 1995]

433.10 Occlusion and stenosis of carotid artery without mention of   **DRG 015** cerebral infarction (continued)

AHA CC: ICD-9-CM groups occlusion and stenosis of precerebral arteries together in category 433. Category 433 also includes embolism, narrowing, obstruction, and thrombosis of the precerebral arteries. These are all similar conditions, i.e., they all cause diminished flow of blood through the precerebral arteries. [*Coding Clinic,* 3Q, Ō90, 16, effective with discharges July 15,1990]

AHA CC: Use the fifth digit '0' to indicate a patient who is status post carotid artery occlusion with cerebral infarction six weeks ago and is admitted to have an endarterectomy. [*Coding Clinic,* 2Q, '95, 14, effective with discharges April 15, 1995]

AHA CC: Use code 433.10, occlusion and stenosis of precerebral arteries, carotid artery, without mention of cerebral infarction, as principal diagnosis when occlusion and stenosis of the carotid artery is diagnosed as causing amaurosis fugax. Use code 362.34, transient arterial occlusion, to describe Amaurosis fugax. [*Coding Clinic,* 1Q, '00, 16, effective with discharges January 1, 2000]

AHA CC: If the physician documents a diagnosis of RIND, the code assignment depends on the context in which the 'reversible ischemic neurologic deficit' is used. Neurologic deficits, e.g., weakness, paralysis of facial muscles, clumsiness, paresthesia or paralysis in one or both limbs on the same side, numbness, loss of sensation, inability to eat or talk, loss of vision or partial vision in one eye, double vision, memory loss and vertigo, are commonly associated with cerebral vascular disease (430-435). The physician may further describe the deficits as either fixed (ongoing) or reversible (of brief duration or recovery occurring within six months or more). Use a code from category 434, occlusion of cerebral arteries, if RIND is used in association with a physician's diagnosis of cerebral artery occlusion. A microthrombosis or microembolism may result in a reversible neurologic deficit if the blood supply to the ischemic region is restored promptly. [*Coding Clinic,* M-A, '85, 7]

DOC: Use code 433.10 if the physician documents embolism, narrowing, obstruction or thrombosis of the carotid artery. Occlusion is usually due to atherosclerosis. The internal carotid arteries are paired right and left and are both intra- and extracranial.

436   Acute, but ill-defined, cerebrovascular disease   **DRG 015**

CG: The term 'stroke' is an imprecise descriptor of acute cerebrovascular disease. It is most frequently associated with cerebral thrombosis, embolism or hypotension that results in an infarction of the brain. Code stroke not otherwise specified to category 436.

CG: Do not use code 436 with any condition classifiable to categories 430-435.

AHA CC: *Do not* use code 436 if the physician documents a CVA (stroke) due to a cerebral infarction but the site of the infarction is uncertain. Instead, use code 434.91 when the type of infarct is not specified and the site is not known. [*Coding Clinic,* 2Q, '95, 14, effective with discharges April 15, 1995]

AHA CC: Use code 436 if the physician documents 'new CVA,' indicating a stroke of a new or same site. [*Coding Clinic,* 2Q, '89, 8, effective with discharges July 31, 1989]

AHA CC: Use code 436 if the physician documents an initial onset of CVA with neurologic deficits (hemiplegia, dysphagia, dysphasia, aphasia, and/or other paralysis, such as of eye muscles). Code also the neurologic deficit. [*Coding Clinic,* 2Q, '89, 8, effective with discharges July 31, 1989]

DOC: Use code 436 if the physician documents apoplectic attack, cerebral apoplexy, apoplectic seizure, cerebral seizure, cerebrovascular accident (CVA) or stroke.

Targeted DRG Listing

435.9   Unspecified transient cerebral ischemia   DRG 524

CG: Use code 435.9 if the physician documents impending cerebrovascular accident (CVA), intermittent cerebral ischemia, or transient ischemic attack (TIA). Neurologic symptoms that last less than 24 hours indicate a TIA. A stroke followed by neurologic symptoms that resolve within 24 hours is also considered a TIA. For example, a patient who has had a stroke (436) and cannot move the left arm (344.4x) is readmitted at a later date with slurred speech (784.5) that lasts only three hours. If it was determined that the stroke was the cause of the slurred speech, the admission would be coded as a TIA (435.9) because the slurred speech resolved within 24 hours.

AHA CC: Use code 435.9 if the physician documents drop attack associated with a transient cerebral ischemia. [*Coding Clinic*, N-D, '85, 12]

AHA CC: If the physician documents a diagnosis of RIND, the code assignment depends on the context in which the 'reversible ischemic neurologic deficit' is used. Neurologic deficits (e.g., weakness, paralysis of facial muscles, clumsiness, paresthesia or paralysis in one or both limbs on the same side, numbness, loss of sensation, inability to eat or talk, loss of vision or partial vision in one eye, double vision, memory loss and vertigo) are commonly associated with cerebral vascular disease (430-435). The physician may further describe the deficits as either fixed (ongoing) or reversible (of brief duration or recovery occurring within six months or more). Use code 435.9, unspecified transient cerebral ischemia, if the RIND is associated with a transient ischemic attack. Included in category 435 are neurologic deficits of sudden onset and brief duration due to insufficiency of cerebral circulation. The duration of the neurologic deficit varies and may last from 5 minutes to 24 hours and is designated as reversible. With the possible exception of some 'weakness,' the neurologic deficits will have diminished upon discharge. [*Coding Clinic*, M-A, '85, 7]

DOC: Use code 435.9 if the physician documents cerebrovascular insufficiency with transient focal neurological signs and symptoms.

DRG 079 Respiratory Infections and Inflammations, Age Greater than 17 with CC

DRG 089 Simple Pneumonia and Pleurisy, Age Greater than 17 with CC

Issue

The coding of pneumonia is one of the most frequent problems encountered by hospital inpatient coders today. It is problematic because of the lack of physician documentation on the organism causing the pneumonia when the causative organism is known or suspected and the complexity of the ICD-9-CM diagnosis codes and coding guidelines for pneumonia. The following represent the major issues affecting the DRG pairs 079 and 089:

- failure of the physician documentation in clearly confirming the type (bacterial versus viral) and organism causing pneumonia (gram-negative versus gram-positive) after study
- presence of coexisting conditions such as septicemia on admission, and lack of support of physician documentation to determine sequencing of principal versus secondary diagnoses, which may or may not be equally treated
- symptoms of pneumonia overlap with other chronic forms of respiratory disease such as acute bronchitis and chronic obstructive pulmonary disease

Most Common Diagnosis Codes

DRG 079

- 482.1, Pneumonia due to pseudomonas
- 482.41, Pneumonia due to *Staphylococcus aureus*
- 482.83, Pneumonia due to gram-negative organisms
- 507.0, Pneumonia due to aspiration of food or vomitus

DRG 089

- 486, Pneumonias, organism unspecified

Coding and Documentation Guidelines

482.1 **Pneumonia due to *Pseudomonas*** **DRG 079**

AHA CC: An abnormal finding on a sputum gram stain is not necessarily indicative of a bacterial pathogen and, therefore, should not be coded as a specified cause of bacterial pneumonia without definitive sputum cultures and further chart documentation. Use code 482.9, bacterial pneumonia unspecified, if the physician documents that the patient had a bacterial pneumonia without further specification. Code 486, pneumonia, organism unspecified, is used if the physician does not specify an etiology. [*Coding Clinic*, 1Q, '94, 17, effective with discharges January 1, 1994, and *Coding Clinic*, 2Q, '98, 3,4, effective with discharges July 1, 1998]

AHA CC: *Do not* arbitrarily report a diagnosis code on the basis of an abnormal laboratory finding alone. *Do not* list a diagnosis code on the basis of a single lab value or abnormal diagnostic finding. Many factors influence the value of a lab sample. These include the method used to obtain the sample, the collection device, the method used to transport the sample to the lab, the calibration of the machine that reads the values, and the condition of the patient. Check with the physician and have him or her document the responsible pathogen in the medical record. [*Coding Clinic*, 2Q, '90, 3, effective with discharges April 1, 1990, and *Coding Clinic*, 4Q, '93, 39, effective with discharges August 18, 1993]

482.1   Pneumonia due to *Pseudomonas* (continued)   DRG 079

AHA CC: *Do not* assign a code indicating bacterial pneumonia unless the medical record documentation supports the presence of a bacterial organism. *Do not* assume that pneumonia not specified as viral or bacterial is bacterial. [*Coding Clinic*, 3Q, '94, 10, effective with discharges July 1, 1994]

AHA CC: Use multiple codes when the physician documents that the pneumonia is due to more than one organism or both aspiration and bacterial pneumonia. If sputum culture indicates multiple organisms, verify with the physician the responsible organism(s). *Do not* assign a code(s) based on lab results alone. [*Coding Clinic*, 3Q, '91, 16, effective for discharges July 1, 1991, and *Coding Clinic*, 4Q, '93, 39, effective for discharges August 18, 1993]

DOC: Use code 482.1 when the physician documents a diagnosis of pneumonia due to pseudomonas.

482.41   Pneumonia due to *Staphylococcus aureus*   DRG 079

CG: Effective for discharges on or after October 1, 1998, new codes were created that separately classify pneumonia due to *Staphylococcus*, unspecified (482.40), pneumonia due to *Staphylococcus aureus* (482.41), and other *Staphylococcus* pneumonia (482.49).

AHA CC: An abnormal finding on a sputum gram stain is not necessarily indicative of a *Do not* arbitrarily report a diagnosis code on the basis of an abnormal laboratory finding alone. *Do not* list a diagnosis code on the basis of a single lab value or abnormal diagnostic finding. Many factors influence the value of a lab sample. These include the method used to obtain the sample, the collection device, the method used to transport the sample to the lab, the calibration of the machine that reads the values, and the condition of the patient. Check with the physician and have him or her document the responsible pathogen in the medical record. [*Coding Clinic*, 2Q, '90, 3, effective with discharges April 1, 1990, and *Coding Clinic*, 4Q, '93, 39, effective with discharges August 18, 1993]

AHA CC: *Do not* arbitrarily report a diagnosis code on the basis of an abnormal laboratory finding alone. *Do not* list a diagnosis code on the basis of a single lab value or abnormal diagnostic finding. Many factors influence the value of a lab sample. These include the method used to obtain the sample, the collection device, the method used to transport the sample to the lab, the calibration of the machine that reads the values, and the condition of the patient. Check with the physician and have him or her document the responsible pathogen in the medical record. [*Coding Clinic*, 2Q, '90, 3, effective with discharges April 1, 1990, and *Coding Clinic*, 4Q, '93, 39, effective with discharges August 18, 1993]

AHA CC: Use codes 507.x (with the fourth digit indicating the nature of the substance aspirated) and 482.41 when the physician documents a diagnosis of aspiration pneumonia with a growth of *Staphylococcus aureus*. This situation describes a patient who presented with aspiration pneumonia with superimposed staphylococcal pneumonia. Code 507.0 does not include pneumonia due to aspiration of microorganisms. When both aspiration pneumonia and bacterial pneumonia are documented in the medical record by the physician, assign codes for each. [*Coding Clinic*, 3Q, '91, 16, effective for discharges July 1, 1991, and *Coding Clinic*, 4Q, '98, 40, effective for discharges July 1, 1998]

AHA CC: *Do not* assign a code indicating bacterial pneumonia unless the medical record documentation supports the presence of a bacterial organism. *Do not* assume that pneunonia not specified as viral or bacterial is bacterial. [*Coding Clinic*, 3Q, '94, 10, effective with discharges July 1, 1994]

AHA CC: Use multiple codes when the physician documents that the pneumonia is due to more than one organism. If sputum culture indicates multiple organisms, verify with the physician the responsible organism(s). *Do not* assign a code(s) based on lab results alone. [*Coding Clinic*, 4Q, '93, 39, effective for discharges August 18, 1993]

482.83 Pneumonia due to Gram-negative organisms   DRG 079

AHA CC: A culture of expectorated sputum may be of limited value in the diagnosis of the agent causing acute pneumonia, especially when antibiotics have previously been administered. In the absence of confirmatory cultures (e.g., the culture and smear reveal several organisms, none of which can be identified as the causative agent, the sputum was not obtainable or sputum reveals no growth or normal flora) review the medical record documentation for the following factors:

- a debilitated, chronically ill, or aged patient
- worsening of cough, dyspnea, reduction of oxygen level
- fever
- purulent sputum
- patchy infiltration on chest x-ray (in addition to those previously noted densities caused by a primary underlying disease)
- elevated leukocyte count or a normal count in aged and debilitated patients

If these conditions exist in the patient and the physician documents a diagnosis of gram-negative pneumonia, probable gram-negative pneumonia or mixed bacterial pneumonia, assign code 482.8, pneumonia due to other specified bacteria, with the additional code of 041.8. [*Coding Clinic,* 3Q, '88, 11]

AHA CC: If the results of the sputum culture with gram-stain show the presence of gram-negative bacteria, but the physician documents only pneumonia in the final diagnosis statement, do not assign code 482.83. A gram-stain does not constitute conclusive evidence of gram-negative pneumonia. The physician must document in the medical record a final diagnosis of gram-negative pneumonia before code 482.83 is assigned. [*Coding Clinic,* 2Q, '98, 5, effective with discharges July 1, 1998]

AHA CC: An abnormal finding on a sputum gram stain is not necessarily indicative of a bacterial pathogen and, therefore, should not be coded as a specified cause of bacterial pneumonia without definitive sputum cultures and further chart documentation. Use code 482.9, bacterial pneumonia unspecified, if the physician documents that the patient had a bacterial pneumonia without further specification. Code 486, pneumonia, organism unspecified, is used if the physician does not specify an etiology. [*Coding Clinic,* 1Q, '94, 17, effective with discharges January 1, 1994, and *Coding Clinic,* 2Q, '98, 3,4, effective with discharges July 1, 1998]

AHA CC: *Do not* arbitrarily report a diagnosis code on the basis of an abnormal laboratory finding alone. *Do not* list a diagnosis code on the basis of a single lab value or abnormal diagnostic finding. Many factors influence the value of a lab sample. These include the method used to obtain the sample, the collection device, the method used to transport the sample to the lab, the calibration of the machine that reads the values, and the condition of the patient. Check with the physician and have him or her document the responsible pathogen in the medical record. [*Coding Clinic,* 2Q, '90, 3, effective with discharges April 1, 1990, and *Coding Clinic,* 4Q, '93, 39, effective with discharges August 18, 1993]

AHA CC: If the results of the sputum culture laboratory report provide evidence of a gram-negative type of bacteria but no specific organism is stated and the physician documents in the medical record that the cause or probable cause of the pneumonia is this organism, code 482.83 may be assigned. [*Coding Clinic,* M-A, '85, 3]

AHA CC: Use this code when the physician documents a diagnosis of *Hemophilus parainfluenza* pneumonia. [*Coding Clinic,* 3Q, '94, 9, effective with discharges July 1, 1994]

AHA CC: Use this code when the physician documents a diagnosis of pneumonia due to *Enterobacter cloacae.* [*Coding Clinic,* 4Q, '93, 39, effective with discharges August 18, 1993]

AHA CC: *Do not* assign a code indicating bacterial pneumonia unless the medical record documentation supports the presence of a bacterial organism. *Do not* assume that pneumonia not specified as viral or bacterial is bacterial. [*Coding Clinic,* 3Q, '94, 10, effective with discharges July 1, 1994]

DOC: Use this code when the physician documents a diagnosis of pneumonia due to *Proteus,* pneumonia due to *Serratia marcascens,* pneumonia due to *Bacterium anitratum,* or pneumonia due to *Herellea.*

482.83   Pneumonia due to Gram-negative organisms (continued)   DRG 079

DOC: Use this code when the physician documents a diagnosis of pneumonia due to gram-negative bacteria except gram-negative anerobes, *Bacteroides*, *E. coli*, or Legionnaires' disease.

DOC: *Do not* use this code when the physician documents a diagnosis of pneumonia due to gram-negative anerobes. The correct code to use is 482.81

DOC: *Do not* use this code when the physician documents a diagnosis of pneumonia due to Legionnaires' disease. The correct code to use is 482.84

507.0   Pneumonitis due to inhalation of food or vomitus   DRG 079

AHA CC: If a patient has a documented diagnosis of both aspiration pneumonia and bacterial pneumonia, a code for each should be assigned. Use code 507.x (with the fourth digit indicating the nature of the substance aspirated) and the code for the bacterial pneumonia. Code 507.0 does not include pneumonia due to aspiration of micro-organisms. When both aspiration pneumonia and bacterial pneumonia are documented in the medical record by the physician, assign a code for each. [*Coding Clinic*, 3Q, '91, 16, effective for discharges July 1, 1991]

AHA CC: Assign code 997.3 for postoperative pneumonia if the lung donor aspirates prior to death and the lung transplant recipient subsequently develops 'aspiration pneumonia' Since the aspiration pneumonia resulted following the lung transplant procedure, this should be coded as a postoperative complication. ICD-9-CM does not include a code to identify that the donor had aspirated prior to the lung being removed for transplantation. [*Coding Clinic*, 1Q, '89, 9, effective with discharges July 15, 1989]

DOC: Use code 507.0 when the physician documents pneumonia due to inhalation of food or vomitus. This includes aspiration pneumonia due to food, gastric secretions, milk, saliva, vomitus, or the physician does not specify the inhalant

486   Pneumonia, organism unspecified   DRG 089

CG: Use code 486 when the specific bacteria is not stated.

CG: A culture of expectorated sputum may be of limited value in the diagnosis of the agent causing acute pneumonia, especially when antibiotics have previously been administered. In the absence of confirmatory cultures (e.g., the culture and smear reveal several organisms, none of which can be identified as the causative agent) the sputum was not obtainable or sputum reveals no growth or normal flora, review the medical record documentation for the following factors:

- a debilitated, chronically ill, or aged patient
- worsening of cough, dyspnea, reduction of oxygen level
- fever
- purulent sputum
- patchy infiltration on chest x-ray (in addition to those previously noted densities caused by a primary underlying disease)
- elevated leukocyte count or a normal count in aged and debilitated patients

If these conditions exist in the patient and the physician documents a diagnosis of gram-negative pneumonia, probable gram-negative pneumonia or mixed bacterial pneumonia, assign code 482.8, pneumonia due to other specified bacteria, with the additional code of 041.8. [*Coding Clinic*, 3Q, '88, 11]

AHA CC: An abnormal finding on a sputum gram stain is not necessarily indicative of a bacterial pathogen and, therefore, should not be coded as a specified cause of bacterial pneumonia without definitive sputum cultures and further chart documentation. Use code 482.9, bacterial pneumonia unspecified, if the physician documents that the patient had a bacterial pneumonia without further specification. Code 486, pneumonia, organism unspecified, is used if the physician does not specify an etiology. [*Coding Clinic*, 1Q, '94, 17, effective with discharges January 1, 1994, and *Coding Clinic*, 2Q, '98, 3,4, effective with discharges July 1, 1998]

486   Pneumonia, organism unspecified (continued)   **DRG 089**

AHA CC: *Do not* arbitrarily report a diagnosis code on the basis of an abnormal laboratory finding alone. *Do not* list a diagnosis code on the basis of a single lab value or abnormal diagnostic finding. Many factors influence the value of a lab sample. These include the method used to obtain the sample, the collection device, the method used to transport the sample to the lab, the calibration of the machine that reads the values, and the condition of the patient. Check with the physician and have him or her document the responsible pathogen in the medical record. [*Coding Clinic,* 2Q, '90, 3, effective with discharges April 1, 1990, and *Coding Clinic,* 4Q, '93, 39, effective with discharges August 18, 1993]

AHA CC: Use code 486 when postobstructive pneumonia is documented and the infective organism is not known or is not specified. The presence of a postobstructive process (e.g., tumor, foreign body, etc.) causing the (obstructive) pneumonia has no bearing on the code for the pneumonia. Specificity depends on the causative organism. If the physician documents the obstructive process, assign a code for the condition in addition to the code for the pneumonia. If there is no documentation of the postobstructive process, then assign only the code for the pneumonia. The selection of the principal diagnosis depends upon the particulars of the admission. [*Coding Clinic,* 1Q, '98, 8, effective with discharges January 15, 1998]

AHA CC: Use codes 486 and 491.20 when the patient with chronic obstructive bronchitis is admitted with pneumonia. *Do not* assign code 491.21, obstructive bronchitis with acute exacerbation, as the pneumonia is not an acute exacerbation of COPD. Always code these two conditions separately when they occur together. [*Coding Clinic,* 3Q, 97, 9, effective with discharges August 1, 1997]

AHA CC: *Do not* assign code 482.89 when a patient with pneumonia and a gram stain identifying gram-positive cocci. An abnormal finding on a sputum gram stain is not necessarily indicative of a bacterial pathogen and, therefore, should not be coded as a specified cause of bacterial pneumonia without definitive sputum cultures and further chart documentation. Use code 482.9, bacterial pneumonia unspecified, if the physician documents that the patient had a bacterial pneumonia without further specification. Code 486, pneumonia, organism unspecified, is used if the physician does not specify an etiology. [*Coding Clinic,* 1Q, '94, 17, effective with discharges January 1, 1994]

AHA CC: *Do not* assign code 482.9 as a "default code" when the physician documentation does not specify the organism or type of pneumonia. Code 486 should be assigned in this case. [*Coding Clinic,* 2Q, '98, 4, effective with discharges July 1, 1998]

AHA CC: *Do not* assign code 482.89 when the physician documents mixed bacteria pneumonia and the medical record does not indicate the specific organisms other than mixed. The correct code to use is 482.9. This advice replaces advice published in *Coding Clinic,* third quarter 1988, page 11 (see above). [*Coding Clinic,* 2Q, '97, 6, effective with discharges May 1, 1997]

AHA CC: *Do not* assign a code indicating bacterial pneumonia unless the medical record documentation supports the presence of a bacterial organism. *Do not* assume that pneumonia not specified as viral or bacterial is bacterial. [*Coding Clinic,* 3Q, '94, 10, effective with discharges July 1, 1994]

DOC: *Do not* use this code when the physician documents a diagnosis of influenza with pneumonia. The correct code to use is 487.0

DOC: *Do not* use this code when the physician documents a diagnosis of inhalation or aspiration pneumonia due to foreign materials. The correct code to use is 507.0-507.8.

DOC: *Do not* use this code when the physician documents a diagnosis of pneumonia due to fumes and vapors. The correct code to use is 506.0.

DOC: *Do not* use this code when the physician documents a diagnosis of hypostatic or passive pneumonia. The correct code to use is 514

DRG 087 Pulmonary Edema and Respiratory Failure

DRG 088   Chronic Obstructive Pulmonary Disease

Issue

The coding of respiratory failure and pulmonary edema is problematic because documentation of clinical findings in patients with respiratory disease varies markedly depending upon the stage of the disease. Coders must review the record to determine whether the patient is experiencing an acute episode or has a chronic form of pulmonary disease. Depending on the physician documentation, the complexity of the ICD-9-CM diagnosis code and coding guidelines could have a major impact on hospital reimbursement under the Medicare DRG prospective payment system (PPS).

Most Common Diagnosis Codes

DRG 087

- 518.4, Acute lung edema, unspecified
- 518.81, Acute respiratory failure
- 518.84, Acute and chronic respiratory failure

DRG 088

- 491.21, Chronic obstructive bronchitis with acute exacerbation
- 493.20, Chronic obstructive asthma without mention of status asthmaticus
- 496, Chronic obstructive pulmonary disease (COPD)

Coding and Documentation Guidelines

518.4   Acute edema of lung, unspecified   **DRG 087**

CG: *Do not* assign code 518.4 if the pulmonary edema is due to external agents. The correct code is chosen from the 506.0-506.9 series.

AHA CC: Other forms of acute pulmonary edema include those that are noncardiogenic in origin and those classified to disease of the lung or to trauma. Assign codes as follows for the given situation:

- Assign code 518.4 when the physician documents postoperative pulmonary edema NOS (without adult respiratory distress syndrome) unless the pulmonary edema is stated to be due to left ventricular failure (428.1) or congestive heart failure (428.0).
- Assign code 518.4 and 276.6 when the physician documents postoperative pulmonary edema due to fluid overload.
- *Do not* assign code 518.4 when the physician documents postoperative pulmonary edema with adult respiratory distress syndrome. The correct code is 518.5. Pulmonary edema is included in conditions classified to code 518.5.
- Assign codes 518.4 and 518.82 when the physician documents acute pulmonary edema due to adult respiratory distress syndrome associated with conditions not classifiable to code 518.5.
- Assign code 518.4 when the physician documents acute pulmonary edema due to bacterial pneumonia, 482.0-482.9, or viral pneumonia, 480.0-480.9, except when the physician states that the acute pulmonary edema is due to left ventricular failure (428.1) or congestive heart failure (428.0).

518.4   Acute edema of lung, unspecified (continued)   DRG 087

- *Do not* assign code 518.4 when the physician documents radiation pneumonitis with acute pulmonary edema. Only use code 508.0.
- Use 518.4 when the physician documents endotoxic shock, 785.59, uremia, 586, or septicemia, 038.9, with acute pulmonary edema.
- *Do not* use 518.4 when the physician documents acute pulmonary edema resulting from smoke inhalation. The correct code assignment is 506.1. An E-code should also be assigned to describe the external cause.
- Use code 518.4 when the physician documents that the acute pulmonary edema is noncardiogenic and is caused by venous congestive overloads, such as pulmonary venous fibrosis, 459.89, congenital stenosis of pulmonary veins, 747.49, or pulmonary venous occlusions, 415.1x.
- *Do not* use code 518.4 when the physician documents acute pulmonary edema due to aspiration when water is introduced into the respiratory tract (along with solutes and solids it contains) in cases of near-drowning. The correct code is 994.1, and 518.5 (optional).
- *Do not* use code 518.4 when the physician documents acute pulmonary edema due to high altitude (decreased atmospheric pressure). The correct code is 993.2.
- Use code 518.4 when the physician documents acute pulmonary edema described as neurogenic (neurogenic pulmonary edema) in patients with central nervous system disorders unless there is mention of left ventricular failure. Then assign code 428.1. [*Coding Clinic*, 3Q, '88, 3]

AHA CC: Acute pulmonary edema with congestive heart failure due to or associated with nonrheumatic and nonhypertensive heart disease is assigned to 428.0 (left heart failure followed by right heart failure). For a diagnosis of acute pulmonary edema of cardiogenic origin, the physician would usually reference cardiac enlargement, presence of S-3 gallop, elevated pulmonary artery.

AHA CC: Use code 428.0 when the physician documents acute pulmonary edema with congestive heart failure due to or associated with nonrheumatic and nonhypertensive heart disease. [*Coding Clinic*, 3Q, '88, 3]

AHA CC: Use code 428.1 for acute myocardial infarction, acute or subacute ischemic heart disease, or coronary atherosclerosis (414.0x and 414.8), with mention of acute pulmonary edema, except when pulmonary edema is mentioned with congestive heart failure or decompensated left ventricular failure. In that case, use code 428.0. [*Coding Clinic*, 3Q, '88, 3]

AHA CC: Pulmonary edema, a pathologic state in which there is excessive, diffuse accumulation of fluid in the tissues and alveolar spaces of the lung, can be of cardiac or noncardiac origin. When of cardiac origin, it is a manifestation of heart failure, and, as such, is not coded separately. For example, acute pulmonary edema is included in the following:

- left ventricular failure, 428.1
- congestive heart failure, 428.0
- right heart failure secondary to left heart failure, 428.0
- hypertensive heart disease (see 402.0, 402.1, and 402.9 with fifth digit of "1")
- rheumatic heart disease, acute, 391.8
- rheumatic active chorea, 392.0
- rheumatic heart disease or chorea, inactive, chronic or quiescent, 398.91
- rheumatic disease of heart valve (394-396), code also 398.91 [*Coding Clinic*, 3Q, '88, 3]

DOC: *Do not* assign code 518.4 when the physician documents the diagnosis of acute pulmonary edema and also mentions heart disease or failure. The correct code is 428.1.

DOC: Do not assign code 518.4 if the pulmonary edema is described as chronic or unspecified. The correct code is 514.

DOC: Use code 518.4 when the physician documents the diagnosis of acute pulmonary edema, acute edema of lung or postoperative pulmonary edema wedge pressure, or associated cardiac diseases in the medical record of a patient with acute pulmonary edema of cardiac origin. Pleural effusions and the presence of Kerly B lines would frequently be seen on x-rays. The patient frequently is treated with diuretics and other cardiac medications. [*Coding Clinic*, 3Q, '88, 3]

Targeted DRG Listing

518.81   Acute respiratory failure   DRG 087

AHA CC: Not all cases of respiratory failure require mechanical ventilatory support. Look for documentation in the medical record of mechanical ventilation in a patient with Pa O_2 below 50 mm Hg and/or Pa CO_2 above 50 mm Hg (or in a COPD case with deterioration in the usual state of blood gases) for evidence of the diagnosis of respiratory failure. However, the patient does not need to be managed with mechanical ventilation for the physician to document a diagnosis of respiratory failure. [*Coding Clinic*, 3Q, '88, 7]

AHA CC: Assign code 518.81 as the principal diagnosis when it meets the definition. Management may or may not include intubation and mechanical ventilation and the use of 518.81 as the principal diagnosis is not dependent on this. If acute respiratory failure is supported by the documentation in the medical record, assign acute respiratory failure as the principal diagnosis. [*Coding Clinic*, 3Q, '88, 7]

AHA CC: When the acute exacerbation of COPD is clearly documented by the physician and the medical record indicates that the COPD patient was admitted with acute respiratory failure, assign codes 518.81 and 496. [*Coding Clinic*, 3Q, '88, 5]

AHA CC: Review the following guidelines to determine the principal diagnosis in instances where a patient is admitted in respiratory failure with as associated or an underlying nonrespiratory condition:

- Assign the respiratory failure as the principal diagnosis when the physician documents that a patient is admitted in respiratory failure due to/associated with a chronic nonrespiratory condition.
  Example: A patient with progressive myasthenia gravis leading to acute respiratory failure was admitted. Both the respiratory failure and the myasthenia gravis were treated.
  Principal diagnosis: 518.81 Acute respiratory failure
  Additional diagnosis: 358.0 Myasthenia gravis

- *Do not* assign respiratory failure as the principal diagnosis when a patient is admitted in respiratory failure due to/associated with an acute exacerbation of a chronic nonrespiratory condition.
  Example: Following dietary indiscretion, a patient with compensated congestive heart failure developed paroxysmal nocturnal dyspnea, orthopnea, and pedal edema leading to increased respiratory distress. He was seen in the emergency room. Upon examination, the patient was determined to have cardiogenic pulmonary edema and acute respiratory failure. Treatment involved intubation in the emergency room. Admission followed with treatment for congestive heart failure. During the hospitalization no myocardial infarction was found.
  Principal diagnosis: 428.0 Congestive heart failure
  Additional diagnosis: 518.81 Acute respiratory failure

  For this case, the congestive heart failure was acute and required immediate hospital care. The associated development of acute respiratory failure is coded as an additional complicating factor, but should not be assigned as the principal diagnosis. Assign the acute condition as the principal diagnosis when a patient is admitted with respiratory failure due to/associated with an acute nonrespiratory condition.

  Example A: A patient who was seen in the emergency room with chest pain and shortness of breath was intubated. After admission, the patient was diagnosed as having an acute subendocardial myocardial infarction complicated by acute respiratory failure. Sequence the acute myocardial infarction (AMI) requiring admission as the principal diagnosis, even though the acute respiratory failure developed prior to the admission and required immediate attention.
  Principal diagnosis: 410.71 Acute subendocardial infarction, initial episode
  Additional diagnosis: 518.81 Acute respiratory failure

518.81 Acute respiratory failure (continued)   **DRG 087**

Example B: A patient experienced a cerebrovascular thrombosis. Upon arrival at the hospital the patient was in acute respiratory failure. Once the patient was placed on mechanical ventilation, admission followed to the intensive care unit for further care for management of the respiratory failure and cerebrovascular thrombosis. The reason for admission to the hospital was cerebrovascular thrombosis. The respiratory failure, while requiring additional intensive treatment and present on admission, was a complication of the cerebrovascular thrombosis.
Principal diagnosis: 434.0 Cerebral thrombosis
Additional diagnosis: 518.81 Acute respiratory failure

Example C. A hospitalized patient with a one-week history of progressive muscle weakness and respiratory difficulties was diagnosed as having acute respiratory failure and acute idiopathic polyneuritis (Guillain-Barre syndrome). This condition may begin with some viral illness or immunization and is followed by rapidly spreading weakness, usually beginning in the legs and spreading to involve the muscles of the arms and trunk. Respiratory failure may result and require assisted ventilation. Sequence the acute polyneuritis (Guillain-Barr syndrome) as the principal diagnosis as this was the condition that caused admission.
Principal diagnosis: 357.0 Acute infective polyneuritis
Additional diagnosis: 518.81 Acute respiratory failure
[*Coding Clinic*, 2Q, '91, 3, effective with discharges April 1, 1991]

AHA CC: Respiratory failure, a condition characterized by inadequate exchange of oxygen and carbon dioxide by the lungs, is generally diagnosed when the patient's arterial Pa O2 falls below 60 mm Hg and/or the arterial Pa CO_2 rises above 50 mm Hg. Thus, the physician bases his or her diagnosis on measurements of blood gases. However, for certain types of patients, particularly those with COPD, blood gas determinations are reviewed in light of the patient's usual status before making a diagnosis of respiratory failure. Those patients with COPD have chronically lowered Pa O_2 and increased Pa CO_2. The physician will look at the degree of change from the usual state of the individual and not simply at the levels of Pa O2 and/or Pa CO_2 described above when making a diagnosis of respiratory failure. For example, a physician would not document a diagnosis of respiratory failure in a patient with COPD and Pa CO_2 levels in the range of 50 mm Hg and near normal arterial pH due to renal compensation for chronic hypercapnia. The diagnosis of respiratory failure in such a patient would not be justified solely on a Pa CO_2 blood gas value of 50 mm Hg. However, medical record documentation of an acute decrease in Pa O_2 from a usual mid-70 mm Hg range to the low 60s may be indicative of acute respiratory failure as an acute drop from a chronic mid-50 mm Hg range to the mid-40s would. Also, a drop in Pa O_2 equal to or greater than 10 to 15 mm Hg generally is an indication of an acute respiratory failure. [*Coding Clinic*, 3Q, '88, 7]

AHA CC: Use code 518.81 when the condition that occasions admission to the hospital is respiratory failure due to an underlying respiratory condition. The respiratory failure is assigned as the principal diagnosis, with an additional code for the underlying respiratory disease. [*Coding Clinic*, 2Q, '00, 21]

AHA CC: Effective for discharges on or after October 1, 1998, new codes for respiratory failure were created that separately classify acute respiratory failure (518.81), chronic respiratory failure (518.83), and acute and chronic respiratory failure (518.84). Assign code 518.81 when the respiratory failure is described as respiratory failure, NOS. [*Coding Clinic*, 4Q, '98, 41]

AHA CC: For discharges on or after October 1, 1997, assign code 518.81 for acute or not otherwise specified respiratory failure. Assign respiratory failure when the documentation supports it. There are a number of underlying pulmonary conditions that may lead to respiratory failure. These include

* COPD
* obstructive chronic bronchitis
* emphysema
* asthma
* interstitial pulmonary fibrosis

518.81 Acute respiratory failure (continued)   DRG 087

In addition, severe pneumonitis may culminate in respiratory failure. Nonpulmonary conditions, such as multiple sclerosis, infarction of cerebral arteries, Guillain-Barr syndrome, or congenital kyphoscoliosis may lead to respiratory failure. [*Coding Clinic,* Special Edition, 1987]

AHA CC: *Do not assign* code 518.81 as the principal diagnosis when the physician documents the patient was admitted in repiratory failure due to *Pneumocystis carinii,* which is due to AIDS. The correct principal diagnosis is Human Immunodeficiency Virus [HIV]. Assign 518.81, Acute respiratory failure as an additional diagnosis. [*Coding Clinic,* 1Q, '03, 15]

AHA CC: *Do not* assign code 518.81 as the principal diagnosis when the physician documents that that the patient was admitted in acute respiratory failure and placed on mechanical ventilation after taking an unknown quantity of alcohol along with Elavil and Xanax. The correct principal diagnosis is any one of the three poisoning codes. [*Coding Clinic,* 3Q, '91, 14, effective with discharges July 1, 1991]

AHA CC: *Do not* assign code 518.81 on the basis of arterial blood gases alone. Arterial blood gas determinations are only one of the supportive clinical findings of respiratory failure. The physician will look at other factors before the diagnosis of respiratory failure is determined. Physicians may consider blood gas determinations in light of the patient's usual status (such as with COPD) before a diagnosis of respiratory failure is made. Presenting aspects to acute respiratory failure include increased work of breathing as typified by rapid respiratory rate, use of accessory muscles of respiration (such as intercostal muscle retraction), and possibly paradoxical breathing and/or cyanosis. The physician will closely monitor patients with respiratory failure, a life-threatening disorder. Management of the respiratory failure patient usually includes placement of the patient in a monitored bed, aggressive respiratory therapy, and/or mechanical ventilation. However, the patient does not need to be placed on mechanical ventilation for the physician to make a diagnosis of respiratory failure. If a patient has an arterial blood gas pH of less than 7.35, this is often associated with acute respiratory failure in a patient with known chronic lung disease and this determination will be a factor in the physician diagnosing the patient with acute respiratory failure. [*Coding Clinic,* 2Q, '90, 20, effective with discharges April 1, 1990]

AHA CC: Code 518.81 can be assigned as the principal diagnosis when the acute respiratory failure is due to an underlying disease if it led to hospital admission, or it may be listed as an associated condition if it occurs after admission. Assign code 518.5 when respiratory failure occurs following surgery or trauma. Respiratory failure, a life-threatening condition, is usually regarded as being acute in nature and may occur in the presence of either chronic lung disease or in previously normal lungs. Causes of respiratory failure include

- alveolar hypoventilation in normal lungs related to trauma, drug overdose, neurologic diseases (such as multiple sclerosis or nontraumatic intracranial hemorrhage or infarction), neuromuscular diseases, or respiratory muscle diseases (such as congenital chest abnormalities or muscular dystrophy), and direct chest trauma or other injuries indirectly affecting the lungs
- injury to small capillary and alveolar walls resulting in adult respiratory distress syndrome (ARDS), and due to smoke inhalation, near-drowning, some pesticides, and previous infections
- chronic obstructive lung disease, which is most often seen with chronic emphysema and bronchitis
- chronic intrinsic restrictive lung disease (CIRLD), characterized by stiffness of the lung tissue resulting from changes in the lung's intrinsic elastic properties, which encompasses more than 100 different diseases that share the characteristics of stiffness and chronicity, such as hypersensitivity pneumonitis and pneumoconiosis; and acute major loss of pulmonary vascular bed associated with massive pulmonary embolism [*Coding Clinic* S-O, '87, 1]

DOC: Use code 518.81 when the physician documents the diagnosis of acute respiratory failure or respiratory failure NOS.

DOC: *Do not* use code 518.81 if the physician documents the diagnosis of acute respiratory distress, acute respiratory insufficiency, or adult respiratory distress syndrome (ARDS) NEC. The correct code is 518.82.

518.81   Acute respiratory failure (continued)   DRG 087

DOC: *Do not* use code 518.81 if the physician documents the diagnosis of respiratory arrest or cardiorespiratory failure. The correct code is 799.1.

DOC: *Do not* use code 518.81 if the physician documents the diagnosis of chronic respiratory failure. The correct code is 518.83 (effective October 1, 1998).

DOC: *Do not* use code 518.81 if the physician documents the diagnosis of acute and chronic respiratory failure. The correct code is 518.84 (effective October 1, 1998).

518.84   Acute and chronic respiratory failure   DRG 087

AHA CC: Use code 518.81 when the condition that occasions admission to the hospital is respiratory failure due to an underlying respiratory condition. The respiratory failure is assigned as the principal diagnosis, with an additional code for the underlying respiratory disease. [*Coding Clinic,* 2Q, '00, 21]

AHA CC: Effective for discharges on or after October 1, 1998, new codes for respiratory failure were created that separately classify acute respiratory failure (518.81), chronic respiratory failure (518.83), and acute and chronic respiratory failure (518.84). [*Coding Clinic,* 4Q, '98, 4]

AHA CC: Assign code 581.84 as the principal diagnosis when the condition that occasions admission to the hospital is respiratory failure due to an underlying respiratory condition. [*Coding Clinic,* 2Q, '00, 21]

DOC: Use code 518.84 if the physician documents the diagnosis of acute and chronic respiratory failure.

491.21   Obstructive chronic bronchitis with acute   DRG 088
exacerbation

AHA CC: Use code 491.21 when the physician documents COPD in exacerbation, severe COPD in exacerbation, end-stage COPD in exacerbation, and exacerbation of COPD. [*Coding Clinic,* 3Q, '02, 18]

AHA CC: When the physician documents the acute exacerbations of COPD, the usual and appropriate treatment for acute exacerbations is the same as for COPD, namely antibiotics, intensification of bronchodilator therapy, liquification, evacuation of secretions, and controlled oxygen supplementation. Intravenous, short-term corticosteroids may be used in reducing respiratory symptomatology, and diuretic therapy in the management of associated cor pulmonale. Once clinically symptomatic, the progression of COPD may be relentless, ranging from (a) patients with evidence of decompensation and increased sputum production only, (b) patients with severe dyspnea or purulent bronchitis, or (c) patients whose efforts to expectorate their tenacious sputum is complicated by bronchospasm. [*Coding Clinic,* 3Q, '88, 5]

AHA CC: Use codes 486 and 491.20 when the patient with chronic obstructive bronchitis is admitted with pneumonia. *Do not* assign code 491.21, obstructive bronchitis with acute exacerbation, as the pneumonia is not an acute exacerbation of COPD. Always code these two conditions separately when they occur together. [*Coding Clinic,* 3Q, '97, 9, effective with discharges August 1, 1997]

AHA CC: Use code 491.21 when the physician documents a diagnosis of acute exacerbation of chronic obstructive pulmonary disease with bronchitis secondary to the patient's exposure to tobacco smoke (patient has smoked for the past 25 years). Code 305.1 is assigned as a secondary diagnosis. [*Coding Clinic,* 2Q, '96, 10, effective with discharges May 1, 1996]

AHA CC: Use code 491.21 when the physician documents a diagnosis of acute exacerbation of chronic asthmatic/obstructive bronchitis. *Do not* use code 466.0. To provide for the coding of an acute exacerbation of chronic asthmatic/obstructive bronchitis, ICD-9-CM was revised. This advice replaces advice published in *Coding Clinic,* November-December 1984, page 17 (see above). [*Coding Clinic,* 4Q, '91, 24, effective with discharges October 1, 1991]

Targeted DRG Listing

491.21 Obstructive chronic bronchitis with acute exacerbation (continued)

DRG 088

AHA CC: Assign only code 491.2x when the physician documents COPD further described as chronic obstructive bronchitis with acute respiratory insufficiency. *Do not* assign code 518.82 as an additional code as respiratory insufficiency is an integral part of COPD and is included in any COPD code. [*Coding Clinic*, 2Q, '91, 21, effective with discharges April 1, 1991]

AHA CC: *Do not* use code 496 when the COPD is specified as obstructive chronic bronchitis (491.2), chronic asthmatic bronchitis (491.2), asthma with chronic obstruction (493.0-493.9), or emphysema (492.0-492.8). [*Coding Clinic*, 3Q, '88, 5]

AHA CC: If the physician documents acute exacerbation of chronic asthmatic bronchitis, further specificity by the physician is necessary to identify the acute attack, such as a superimposed infection (purulent) of the bronchial tree, marked or severe respiratory distress, or respiratory failure. [*Coding Clinic*, N-D, '84, 17]

DOC: Use code 491.21 when the physician documents a diagnosis of obstructive chronic bronchitis with acute exacerbation, chronic asthmatic bronchitis with acute exacerbation, obstructive bronchitis with acute exacerbation, bronchitis with chronic airway obstruction with acute exacerbation, bronchitis with emphysema with acute exacerbation, acute bronchitis with COPD, acute and chronic obstructive bronchitis, chronic asthmatic bronchitis with acute exacerbation, or emphysema with both acute and chronic bronchitis.

493.20 Chronic obstructive asthma without mention of status asthmaticus

DRG 088

CG: Effective with discharges beginning October 1, 2000, the ICD-9-CM classification system has been expanded to include a new fifth digit subclassification for use with category 493. Acute exacerbation of chronic obstructive asthma will be indicated with the addition of a fifth digit 2 to subcategory codes under 493. Additionally in October 1, 2001, the fifth digit of 0 was revised to include terms acute exacerbation or unspecified.

493 Asthma

The following fifth-digit subclassification is for use with category 493:

- 0 without mention of status asthmaticus or acute exacerbation or unspecified
- 1 with status asthmaticus
- 2 with acute exacerbation

CG: Status asthmaticus has a variety of definitions, including the following:

- an asthmatic patient with continuous wheezing despite therapy, including (a) stabilized asthmatic patient who wheezes chronically, as well as (b) a patient with severe bronchial asthma who fails to respond to the usual therapy
- an acute asthmatic attack in which the degree of bronchial obstruction is not relieved by the usual treatment, such as by epinephrine or aminophylline, which is the American Thoracic Society's definition of status asthmaticus
- acute pulmonary insufficiency caused by bronchial obstruction sustained for 24 hours or longer that is unresponsive to usual therapy and totally disables the patient.

A case may fall into two groups of status asthmaticus patients where, in either one, the fifth digit '1' would be assigned:

- early stage asthmaticus, representing patients who have refractoriness or failure to respond to the usual therapy
- advanced status asthmaticus, representing patients who show full development of an asthmatic attack that could culminate in respiratory failure with signs and symptoms of hypercapnia (excess carbon dioxide in the blood) [*Coding Clinic*, 3Q, '88, 9]

CG: These definitions cover a range of situations, extending from those chronic asthmatic patients who may present to the physician's office with an acute attack unresponsive to the usual outpatient medications, such as theophyllines (aminophylline) and beta-adrenergic drugs (epinephrine), to those patients requiring intensive care and possibly intubation and controlled ventilation

493.20 Chronic obstructive asthma without mention of status asthmaticus (continued)

AHA CC: If the physician documents acute exacerbation of chronic asthmatic bronchitis, further specificity by the physician is necessary to identify the acute attack, such as a superimposed infection (purulent) of the bronchial tree, marked or severe respiratory distress, or respiratory failure. [*Coding Clinic,* N-D, '84, 17]

AHA CC: Assign only code 493.2x when the physician documents COPD further described as chronic obstructive asthma with acute respiratory insufficiency. *Do not* assign code 518.82 as an additional code as respiratory insufficiency is an integral part of COPD and is included in any COPD code. [*Coding Clinic,* 2Q, '91, 21, effective with discharges April 1, 1991]

AHA CC: *Do not* assume that a patient admitted to the hospital because of asthma must be in status asthmaticus. *Do not* assign the fifth digit "1" unless the physician states "status asthmaticus," indicating a patient's failure to respond to therapy administered during an asthmatic episode. [*Coding Clinic,* 1Q, '91, 13, effective with discharges January 1, 1991]

AHA CC: Use code 493.2x when the physician documents the diagnosis of asthma with COPD. Use this code whether or not the physician states "chronic obstructive" asthma. Code 493.2x was added to distinguish between nonobstructive and obstructive asthma (that in chronic obstructive lung disease). In patients with a diagnosis of COPD with asthma there is continuous obstruction to airflow on expiration, unlike a patient with nonobstructive asthma where the patient wheezes during an asthma attack, but returns to normal breathing once the attack subsides. Use codes 493.0x, 493.1x and 493.9x when the physician documents asthma in patients without chronic obstructive lung disease. [*Coding Clinic,* 2Q, '90, 20, effective with discharges April 1, 1990]

AHA CC: Status asthmaticus constitutes a medical emergency for treatment of acute severe asthma. Other terms the physician may document to describe status asthmaticus include the following:

* intractable asthmatic attack
* refractory asthma
* severe, prolonged asthmatic attack
* airway obstruction (mucous plug) not relieved by bronchodilators
* severe, intractable wheezing [*Coding Clinic,* 3Q, '88, 9]

AHA CC: *Do not* assign a code for bronchospasm as it is a component of an acute asthmatic attack and, as such, is included in the code assignment under category 493, asthma. [*Coding Clinic,* 3Q, '88, 5]

AHA CC: When the acute exacerbation of COPD is clearly documented by the physician and the medical record indicates that the COPD patient was admitted for treatment of asthma or asthma attack, assign a code from the 493.0x-493.9x series. Assign only one code in accordance with the instructions in the alphabetic index and tabular list. [*Coding Clinic,* 3Q, '88, 5]

AHA CC: Documentation of a prolonged, severe asthmatic attack is an indication of "status asthmaticus." The physician may describe the following symptoms in the medical record:

* prolonged, severe intractable wheezing
* prolonged, severe respiratory distress
* asthma with respiratory failure
* asthma attack with absence of breath sounds
* patient in a lethargic or confused state due to prolonged asthmatic attack

Unless the physician documents the presence of any "status asthmaticus," the fifth digit "1" should not be assigned. [*Coding Clinic,* M-A, '85, 7]

AHA CC: Use a code from category 493 when the physician documents steroid-dependent asthma with no mention of side effects due to steroid therapy. There is no ICD-9-CM code for dependency on steroid therapy. If the physician documents side effects, code both the asthma and the side effect of the steroid. [*Coding Clinic,* J-A, '85, 8]

AHA CC: If the physician documents respiratory failure, code also respiratory failure. If respiratory failure is present on admission, assign code 518.81 as the principal diagnosis followed by the code assignment for asthma with status asthmaticus, 493.91. [*Coding Clinic,* 3Q, '88, 9]

493.20   Chronic obstructive asthma without mention of status   **DRG 088**
            asthmaticus (continued)

AHA CC: *Do not* use code 496 when the COPD is specified as obstructive chronic bronchitis (491.2x), chronic asthmatic bronchitis (491.2x), asthma with chronic obstruction (493.0x-493.9x), or emphysema (492.0x-492.8). [*Coding Clinic,* 3Q, '88, 5]

DOC: Use code 493.20 when the physician documents chronic obstructive asthma without status asthmaticus or asthma with chronic obstructive pulmonary disease (COPD) without status asthmaticus

DOC: *Do not* use code 493.20 when the physician documents chronic asthmatic bronchitis. The correct code is 491.2x

DOC: *Do not* use code 493.20 when the physician documents chronic obstructive bronchitis. The correct code is 491.2x.

496   Chronic airway obstruction, not elsewhere classified   **DRG 088**

CG: Use code 496 when the chronic obstructive lung (pulmonary) disease (COPD) is not specified as or with allergic alveolitis, asthma, bronchietasis, bronchitis, or emphysema.

CG: *Do not* use category 496 for chronic obstructive lung disease [COPD] specified (as) (with) bronchiectasis. Use codes 494.0-494.1

CG: *Do not* use code 496 with any other code from categories 491-493.

AHA CC: Assign only code 496 when the physician documents "with acute respiratory insufficiency." *Do not* assign code 518.82 as an additional code as respiratory insufficiency is an integral part of COPD and is included in any COPD code. [*Coding Clinic,* 2Q, '91, 21, effective with discharges April 1, 1991]

AHA CC: *Do not* assign a code for bronchospasm if the physician mentions bronchospasm in conjunction with acute exacerbation of COPD. Assign only code 496. [*Coding Clinic,* 3Q, '88, 5]

AHA CC: Use code 496 where acute exacerbation is not further described, for example:

- the physician mentions the exacerbation as progressive worsening or deterioration with increased shortness of breath, weakness, wheezing, and activity intolerance
- the physician states the exacerbation of COPD relates to periods of heavy air pollution, increases in humidity, or barometric changes that prompt increased stress in breathing and cause bronchospasm
- the physician documents retained airway secretions due to mild dehydration, or ineffective cough exacerbating COPD
- the physician states that the exacerbation of COPD is due to depressed ventilation caused by sedatives or uncontrolled oxygen therapy or failure to continue maintenance bronchodilator medications
- the physician describes the exacerbation of COPD as due to continued employment in occupation that exposes the patient to either organic or inorganic dust, prompting accelerated decline in lung function with increased dyspnea and fatigue [*Coding Clinic,* 3Q, '88, 5]

AHA CC: Use code 496 when the cause of acute exacerbation of COPD is not clearly identified. When the physician does not document the exact nature of the exacerbation a more specific identification of "acute exacerbation" should not be undertaken. [*Coding Clinic,* 3Q, '88, 5]

AHA CC: *Do not* use code 496 when the COPD is specified as obstructive chronic bronchitis (491.2x), chronic asthmatic bronchitis (491.2x), asthma with chronic obstruction (493.0-493.9), or emphysema (492.0-492.8). [*Coding Clinic,* 3Q, '88, 5]

AHA CC: Use code 496 when the physician documents a diagnosis of chronic obstructive lung (or pulmonary) disease (COPD). COPD is a condition in which there is chronic obstruction to airflow due to chronic bronchitis and/or emphysema. Patients may be treated on an outpatient basis for exacerbations of COPD, such as episodes of increased shortness of breath and cough, or they may require hospital admission during more severe exacerbations of their illness, such as that with bronchitis, pneumonia, or other infection. [*Coding Clinic,* 3Q, '88, 5]

496   Chronic airway obstruction, not elsewhere classified (continued)   DRG 088

AHA CC: When the acute exacerbation of COPD is clearly documented by the physician and the medical record indicates that the COPD patient was admitted with respiratory failure, assign codes 518.81 and 496. [*Coding Clinic,* 3Q, '88, 5]

AHA CC: When the acute exacerbation of COPD is clearly documented by the physician and the medical record indicates that the COPD patient was admitted for treatment of asthma or asthma attack, assign a code from the 493.0x-493.9x series. Assign only one code in accordance with the instructions in the alphabetic index and tabular list. [*Coding Clinic,* 3Q, '88, 5]

AHA CC: The physician's use of the term "acute exacerbation of COPD" may refer to respiratory failure (799.1), respiratory distress (alveolar hypoventilation) (786.09), which may lead into respiratory failure (799.1) or refer to cor pulmonale (415.0) in advanced COPD. Acute upper or lower respiratory infections could also be present. Verify with the physician and have him or her document the meaning of this term in the medical record before assigning the code. [*Coding Clinic,* J-A, '84, 17]

AHA CC: Clarify with the physician the meaning behind COPD when used in conjunction with asthma. COPD not further specified as to type of dysfunction with asthma is coded to the 493.0x-493.9x series. [*Coding Clinic,* J-A, '84, 17]

AHA CC: When both asthma (reversible airway obstruction) and COPD (irreversible airway obstruction) appear together in the diagnostic statement, verify with the physician which type of pulmonary dysfunction was involved. Options include the following:

- either asthma or chronic obstructive bronchitis as comorbidity, such as chronic obstructive bronchitis (491.2x) superimposed on intrinsic asthma (493.10)
- chronic pneumothorax (518.8) with extrinsic (493.00) or intrinsic (493.10) asthma
- mediastinal or subcutaneous nontraumatic emphysema (518.1) with asthma (493.00 or 493.10)
- atelectasis (518.0) associated with asthma (493.0-493.9)
- bronchiectasis (494) associated with asthma (493.0-493.9)
- chronic obstructive emphysema (492.8) associated with asthma (493.0- 493.9), such as in a patient who is a tobacco smoker
- wheezing (786.09), which is a symptom common to COPD and asthma [*Coding Clinic,* J-A, '84, 17]

AHA CC: If the diagnosis is COPD and chronic bronchitis, check with the physician before classifying this to obstructive chronic bronchitis or chronic obstructive emphysematous bronchitis, 491.2. [*Coding Clinic,* J-A, '84, 17]

AHA CC: Query the physician if the diagnostic statement is COPD with asthmatic bronchitis to determine whether chronic obstructive pulmonary emphysema (492.8) with chronic pulmonary heart disease (416.8) is the correct classification assignment. [*Coding Clinic,* J-A, '84, 17]

AHA CC: Coding the diagnosis of COPD is not easy, as the physician's use of this term is not compatible in all instances with textbook descriptions of COPD or ICD-9-CM classification of COPD. The physician may use COPD to describe chronic airway obstruction caused by

- chronic bronchitis with or without mention of centrilobular emphysema (code 491.2) (blue bloater)
- predominant emphysema (panacinar) (492.8) (pink puffer)
- coexistence of the two above-mentioned clinical entities (code 496)

Check with the physician and have him or her document which of the above interpretations is correct before assigning a code. [*Coding Clinic,* J-A, '84, 17]

DOC: Use code 496 when the physician documents chronic nonspecific lung disease or chronic obstructive lung disease.

DRG 088 Chronic Obstructive Pulmonary Disease
DRG 096 Bronchitis and Asthma, Age Greater than 17 with CC

Issue

The coding of chronic obstructive pulmonary disease is problematic because documentation of clinical findings in patients with respiratory disease varies markedly depending upon the stage of the disease. Respiratory patients are assigned to the DRG because the principal diagnosis documented describes an 'acute' reversible process as opposed to the 'acute exacerbations' that occur from underlying, irreversible disease processes. Coders must review the record to determine whether the patient is experiencing an acute episode or has a chronic form of pulmonary disease. Depending on the physician documentation, the complexity of the ICD-9-CM diagnosis code and coding guidelines could have a major impact on hospital reimbursement under the Medicare DRG PPS.

Most Common Diagnosis Codes:

DRG 088
- 491.21, Chronic obstructive bronchitis with acute exacerbation
- 493.20, Chronic obstructive asthma without mention of status asthmaticus
- 496, Chronic obstructive pulmonary disease

DRG 096
- 466.0, Acute bronchitis
- 490, Bronchitis, not specified as acute or chronic
- 493.90, Asthma without mention of status asthmaticus
- 493.91, Asthma with status asthmaticus

Coding and Documentation Guidelines

491.21 Obstructive chronic bronchitis with acute exacerbation	DRG 088

See standards on page 562.

493.20 Chronic obstructive asthma, without mention of status asthmaticus	DRG 088

See standards on page 562.

496 Chronic airway obstruction, not elsewhere classified	DRG 088

See standards on page 564.

466.0 Acute bronchitis	DRG 096

CG: *Do not* use code 466.0 for acute bronchitis with: asthmatic bronchitis (493.9x), bronchiectasis (494.1), or chronic obstructive pulmonary disease (491.21).

AHA CC: Assign codes 466.0 and 079.6 when the physician documents acute tracheobronchitis due to RSV. [*Coding Clinic*, 4Q, '96, 28, effective with discharges October 1, 1996]

466.0 Acute bronchitis (continued) DRG 096

AHA CC: Use code 491.21 when the physician documents a diagnosis of acute exacerbation of chronic asthmatic/obstructive bronchitis. *Do not* use code 466.0. To provide for the coding of an acute exacerbation of chronic asthmatic/obstructive bronchitis, ICD-9-CM was revised. This advice replaces advice published in *Coding Clinic,* November-December 1984, page 17 (see above). [*Coding Clinic,* 4Q, '91, 24, effective with discharges October 1, 1991]

AHA CC: When a condition is documented as both acute and chronic and the Alphabetic Index provides separate codes at either the third-digit, fourth-digit, or fifth-digit level for acute and for chronic, code both and sequence the acute condition first. [*Coding Clinic,* M-A, '85, 3].

DOC: Use code 466.0 when the physician documents a diagnosis of acute or subacute bronchitis with or without bronchospasm or obstruction.

DOC: Use code 466.0 when the physician documents a diagnosis of acute or subacute bronchitis further described as fibrinous, membranous, pneumococcal, purulent, septic, or viral.

DOC: Use code 466.0 when the physician documents a diagnosis of acute tracheobronchitis

DOC: Use code 466.0 when the physician documents a diagnosis of croupous bronchitis.

490 Bronchitis, not specified as acute or chronic DRG 096

AHA CC: Use an unspecified code only when neither the diagnostic statement nor a thorough review of the medical record provides adequate information to permit assignment of a more specific code. Assign an unspecified code only when the information at hand does not permit either a more specific or 'other' code assignment. [*Coding Clinic,* J-F, '86, 6]

DOC: Use code 490 when the physician documents a diagnosis of bronchitis not specified as acute or chronic, catarrhal bronchitis, tracheobronchitis, or bronchitis with tracheitis.

DOC: *Do not* use code 490 when the physician documents a diagnosis of allergic bronchitis. The correct code to use is 493.9x

DOC: *Do not* use code 490 when the physician documents a diagnosis of asthmatic bronchitis. The correct code to use is 493.9x.

DOC: *Do not* use code 490 when the physician documents a diagnosis of bronchitis due to fumes and vapors. The correct code is 506.0

DOC: *Do not* use code 490 when the physician documents a diagnosis of obstructive bronchitis. The correct code is 491.2x.

493.90 Asthma, unspecified, without status asthmaticus DRG 096

CG: Effective with discharges beginning October 1, 2000, the ICD-9-CM classification system has been expanded to include a new fifth digit subclassification for use with category 493. Acute exacerbation of chronic obstructive asthma will be indicated with the addition of a fifth digit 2 to subcategory codes under 493. Additionally in October 1, 2001, the fifth digit of 0 was revised to include terms acute exacerbation or unspecified

The following fifth-digit subclassification is for use with category 493:

- 0 without mention of status asthmaticus or acute exacerbation or unspecified
- 1 with status asthmaticus
- 2 with acute exacerbation

AHA CC: If the physician documents acute exacerbation of chronic asthmatic bronchitis, further specificity by the physician is necessary to identify the acute attack, such as a superimposed infection (purulent) of the bronchial tree, marked or severe respiratory distress, or respiratory failure. [*Coding Clinic,* N-D, '84, 17]

493.90   Asthma, unspecified, without status asthmaticus (continued)   DRG 096

AHA CC: If the physician documents acute exacerbation of chronic asthmatic bronchitis, further specificity by the physician is necessary to identify the acute attack, such as a superimposed infection (purulent) of the bronchial tree, marked or severe respiratory distress, or respiratory failure. [*Coding Clinic*, N-D, '84, 17]

AHA CC: *Do not* use code 496 when the COPD is specified as obstructive chronic bronchitis (491.2), chronic asthmatic bronchitis (491.2), asthma with chronic obstruction (493.0-493.9), or emphysema (492.0-492.8). [*Coding Clinic*, 3Q, '88, 5]

AHA CC: Use code 493.90 when the physician documents the diagnosis of acute recurrent asthmatic bronchitis, which may designate a recurrent acute attack of asthmatic bronchitis. When the acute attack is documented in the medical record as severe (stage III or IV) or there is mention of marked or severe respiratory distress, respiratory failure, absence of breath sounds or the presence of lethargy or confusion, assign code 493.91. [*Coding Clinic*, N-D, '84, 17]

AHA CC: *Do not* assume that a patient admitted to the hospital because of asthma must be in status asthmaticus. *Do not* assign the fifth digit '1' unless the physician states 'status asthmaticus,' indicating a patient's failure to respond to therapy administered during an asthmatic episode. [*Coding Clinic*, 1Q, '91, 13, effective with discharges January 1, 1991]

AHA CC: Use code 493.2x when the physician documents the diagnosis of asthma with COPD. Use this code whether or not the physician states 'chronic obstructive' asthma. Code 493.2x was added to distinguish between nonobstructive and obstructive asthma (that in chronic obstructive lung disease). In patients with a diagnosis of COPD with asthma there is continuous obstruction to airflow on expiration, unlike a patient with nonobstructive asthma where the patient wheezes during an asthma attack, but returns to normal breathing once the attack subsides. Use codes 493.0x, 493.1x and 493.9x when the physician documents asthma in patients without chronic obstructive lung disease. [*Coding Clinic*, 2Q, '90, 20, effective with discharges April 1, 1990]

AHA CC: Status asthmaticus constitutes a medical emergency for treatment of acute severe asthma. Other terms the physician may document to describe status asthmaticus include the following:

- intractable asthmatic attack
- refractory asthma
- severe, prolonged asthmatic attack
- airway obstruction (mucous plug) not relieved by bronchodilators
- severe, intractable wheezing [*Coding Clinic*, 3Q, '88, 9]

AHA CC: Status asthmaticus has a variety of definitions, including the following:

- an asthmatic patient with continuous wheezing despite therapy, including (a) a stabilized asthmatic patient who wheezes chronically, as well as (b) a patient with severe bronchial asthma who fails to respond to the usual therapy
- an acute asthmatic attack in which the degree of bronchial obstruction is not relieved by the usual treatment, such as by epinephrine or aminophylline, which is the American Thoracic Society's definition of status asthmaticus
- an acute pulmonary insufficiency caused by bronchial obstruction that is sustained for 24 hours or longer, is unresponsive to usual therapy and totally disables the patient

These definitions cover a range of situations, extending from those chronic asthmatic patients who may present to the physician's office with an acute attack unresponsive to the usual outpatient medications, such as theophyllines (aminophylline) and beta-adrenergic drugs (epinephrine), to those patients requiring intensive care and possibly intubation and controlled ventilation. A case may fall into two groups of status asthmaticus patients where, in either one, the fifth digit '1' would be assigned:

- early stage asthmaticus, representing patients who have refractoriness or failure to respond to the usual therapy
- advanced status asthmaticus, representing patients who show full development of an asthmatic attack that could culminate in respiratory failure with signs and symptoms of hypercapnia (excess carbon dioxide in the blood)

493.90   Asthma, unspecified, without status asthmaticus (continued)   DRG 096

AHA CC: If the physician documents respiratory failure, code also respiratory failure. If respiratory failure is present on admission, assign code 518.81 as the principal diagnosis followed by the code assignment for asthma with status asthmaticus, 493.91. [*Coding Clinic,* 3Q, '88, 9]

AHA CC: *Do not* assign a code for bronchospasm as it is a component of an acute asthmatic attack and, as such, is included in the code assignment under category 493, asthma. [*Coding Clinic,* 3Q, '88, 5]

AHA CC: When a diagnosis documented at the time of discharge is qualified as 'probable,' 'suspected,' 'likely,' '?,' 'possible' or 'still to be ruled out,' code it as if it existed or was established. Medical record documentation would show a diagnostic workup, arrangements for further workup or observation, and an initial therapeutic approach that conform most closely to the established diagnosis. [*Coding Clinic,* M-A, '85, 3]

AHA CC: Use a code from category 493 when the physician documents steroid-dependent asthma with no mention of side effects due to steroid therapy. There is no ICD-9-CM code for dependency on steroid therapy. If the physician documents side effects, code both the asthma and the side effect of the steroid. [*Coding Clinic,* J-A, '85, 8]

AHA CC: Documentation of a prolonged, severe asthmatic attack is an indication of 'status asthmaticus.' The physician may describe the following symptoms in the medical record:

- prolonged, severe intractable wheezing
- prolonged, severe respiratory distress
- asthma with respiratory failure
- asthma attack with absence of breath sounds
- patient in a lethargic or confused state due to prolonged asthmatic attack
- Unless the physician documents the presence of any 'status asthmaticus,' the fifth digit '1' should not be assigned. [*Coding Clinic,* M-A, '85, 7]

DOC: Use code 493.90 when the physician documents (bronchial) (allergic NOS) asthma without status asthmaticus, allergic bronchitis without status asthmaticus, or (acute) asthmatic bronchitis without status asthmaticus.

DOC: *Do not* use code 493.90 when the physician documents chronic asthmatic bronchitis without status asthmaticus. The correct code is 491.2x

493.91   Asthma, unspecified, with status asthmaticus   DRG 096

CG: Effective with discharges beginning October 1, 2000, the ICD-9-CM classification system has been expanded to include a new fifth digit subclassification for use with category 493. Acute exacerbation of chronic obstructive asthma will be indicated with the addition of a fifth digit 2 to subcategory codes under 493. Additionally in October 1, 2001, the fifth digit of 0 was revised to include terms acute exacerbation or unspecified.

493 Asthma

The following fifth-digit subclassification is for use with category 493:

- 0 without mention of status asthmaticus or acute exacerbation or unspecified
- 1 with status asthmaticus
- 2 with acute exacerbation

Status asthmaticus has a variety of definitions including the following:

- an asthmatic patient with continuous wheezing despite therapy, including (a) a stabilized asthmatic patient who wheezes chronically, as well as (b) a patient with severe bronchial asthma who fails to respond to the usual therapy
- an acute asthmatic attack in which the degree of bronchial obstruction is not relieved by the usual treatment, such as by epinephrine or aminophylline, which is the American Thoracic Society's definition of status asthmaticus

493.91   Asthma, unspecified, with status asthmaticus (continued)   DRG 096

- an acute pulmonary insufficiency caused by bronchial obstruction that is sustained for 24 hours or longer, is unresponsive to usual therapy and totally disables the patient

These definitions cover a range of situations extending from those chronic asthmatic patients who may present to the physician's office with an acute attack unresponsive to the usual outpatient medications, such as theophyllines (aminophylline) and beta-adrenergic drugs (epinephrine), to those patients requiring intensive care and possibly intubation and controlled ventilation. A case may fall into two groups of status asthmaticus patients where, in either one, the fifth digit "1" would be assigned:

- early stage asthmaticus, representing patients who have refractoriness or failure to respond to the usual therapy
- advanced status asthmaticus, representing patients who show full development of an asthmatic attack that could culminate in respiratory failure with signs and symptoms of hypercapnia (excess carbon dioxide in the blood)

AHA CC: If the physician documents respiratory failure, code also respiratory failure. If respiratory failure is present on admission, assign code 518.81 as the principal diagnosis followed by the code assignment for asthma with status asthmaticus, 493.91. [*Coding Clinic,* 3Q, '88, 9]

AHA CC: Use code 493.90 when the physician documents the diagnosis of acute recurrent asthmatic bronchitis, which may designate a recurrent acute attack of asthmatic bronchitis. When the acute attack is documented in the medical record as severe (stage III or IV) or there is mention of marked or severe respiratory distress, respiratory failure, absence of breath sounds or the presence of lethargy or confusion, assign code 493.91. [*Coding Clinic,* N-D, '84, 17]

AHA CC: *Do not* assume that a patient admitted to the hospital because of asthma must be in status asthmaticus. *Do not* assign the fifth digit '1' unless the physician states 'status asthmaticus,' indicating a patient's failure to respond to therapy administered during an asthmatic episode. [*Coding Clinic,* 1Q, '91, 13, effective with discharges January 1, 1991]

AHA CC: Use code 493.2x when the physician documents the diagnosis of asthma with COPD. Use this code whether or not the physician states 'chronic obstructive' asthma. Code 493.2x was added to distinguish between nonobstructive and obstructive asthma (that in chronic obstructive lung disease). In patients with a diagnosis of COPD with asthma there is continuous obstruction to airflow on expiration, unlike a patient with nonobstructive asthma where the patient wheezes during an asthma attack, but returns to normal breathing once the attack subsides. Use codes 493.0x, 493.1x, and 493.9x when the physician documents asthma in patients without chronic obstructive lung disease. [*Coding Clinic,* 2Q, '90, 20, effective with discharges April 1, 1990]

AHA CC: Status asthmaticus constitutes a medical emergency for treatment of acute severe asthma. Other terms the physician may document to describe status asthmaticus include the following:

- intractable asthmatic attack
- refractory asthma
- severe, prolonged asthmatic attack
- airway obstruction (mucous plug) not relieved by bronchodilators
- severe, intractable wheezing [*Coding Clinic,* 3Q, '88, 9]

AHA CC: *Do not* assign a code for bronchospasm as it is a component of an acute asthmatic attack and, as such, is included in the code assignment under category 493, asthma. [*Coding Clinic,* 3Q, '88, 5]

AHA CC: *Do not* use code 496 when the COPD is specified as obstructive chronic bronchitis (491.2), chronic asthmatic bronchitis (491.2), asthma with chronic obstruction (493.0-493.9), or emphysema (492.0-492.8). [*Coding Clinic,* 3Q, '88, 5]

AHA CC: When the acute exacerbation of COPD is clearly documented by the physician and the medical record indicates that the COPD patient was admitted for treatment of asthma or asthma attack, assign a code from the 493.0x-493.9x series. Assign only one code in accordance with the instructions in the Alphabetic Index and Tabular List. [*Coding Clinic,* 3Q, '88, 5]

493.91   Asthma, unspecified, with status asthmaticus (continued)   DRG 096

AHA CC: Use a code from category 493 when the physician documents steroid-dependent asthma with no mention of side effects due to steroid therapy. There is no ICD-9-CM code for dependency on steroid therapy. If the physician documents side effects, code both the asthma and the side effect of the steroid. [*Coding Clinic,* J-A, '85, 8]

AHA CC: Documentation of a prolonged, severe asthmatic attack is an indication of 'status asthmaticus.' The physician may describe the following symptoms in the medical record:

- prolonged, severe intractable wheezing
- prolonged, severe respiratory distress
- asthma with respiratory failure
- asthma attack with absence of breath sounds
- patient in a lethargic or confused state due to prolonged asthmatic attack

AHA CC: Unless the physician documents the presence of any 'status asthmaticus,' the fifth digit '1' should not be assigned. [*Coding Clinic,* M-A, '85, 7]

DOC: If the physician documents acute exacerbation of chronic asthmatic bronchitis, further specificity by the physician is necessary to identify the acute attack, such as a superimposed infection (purulent) of the bronchial tree, marked or severe respiratory distress, or respiratory failure. [*Coding Clinic,* N-D, '84, 17]

DOC: Use code 493.91 when the physician documents (bronchial) (allergic NOS) asthma with status asthmaticus, allergic bronchitis with status asthmaticus, or (acute) asthmatic bronchitis with status asthmaticus.

DOC: *Do not* use code 493.91 when the physician documents chronic asthmatic bronchitis. The correct code is 491.2x with status asthmaticus.

DRG 089 Simple Pneumonia and Pleurisy, Age Greater than 17 with CC

DRG 096 Bronchitis and Asthma, Age Greater than 17 with CC

Issue

The coding of pneumonia, bronchitis and asthma is problematic because documentation of clinical findings in patients with respiratory disease varies markedly depending upon the stage of the disease. Coders must review the record to distinguish the difference between those respiratory processes that require fewer resources to manage and those that require costly resources. Such documentation signals can be found in symptomatologies and the physician's choice of clinical treatment. Depending on the physician documentation, the complexity of the ICD-9-CM diagnosis code and coding guidelines have a major an impact on hospital reimbursement under the Medicare DRG PPS.

Most Common Diagnosis Codes

DRG 089

- 486, Pneumonia, organism unspecified

DRG 096

- 466.0, Acute bronchitis
- 490, Bronchitis, not specified as acute or chronic
- 493.90, Asthma without mention of status asthmaticus
- 493.91, Asthma with status asthmaticus

Coding and Documentation Guidelines

486	Pneumonia, organism unspecified	DRG 089
(See standards on page 554.)		

466.0	Acute bronchitis	DRG 096
(See standards on page 566.)		

490	Bronchitis, not specified as acute or chronic	DRG 096
(See standards on page 567.)		

493.90	Asthma, unspecified, without status asthmaticus	DRG 096
(See standards on page 567.)		

493.91	Asthma, unspecified, with status asthmaticus	DRG 096
(See standards on page 569.)		

DRG 121 Circulatory Disorders with Acute Myocardial Infarction and Major Complications, Discharged Alive

DRG 124 Circulatory Disorders Except Acute Myocardial Infarction with Cardiac Catheterization and Complex Diagnosis

Issue

The coding of ischemic heart disease and congestive heart failure is problematic because of the lack of physician documentation and complexity of ICD-9-CM diagnosis codes and coding guidelines. The following represent the major issues affecting the DRG pairs 121 and 124:

- the known or suspected presence of acute myocardial infarction
- determination of the initial or subsequent episode of care for myocardial infarctions, particularly in transfer cases
- the significant impact the presence of a principal and/or secondary complex diagnosis or major complications ICD-9-CM diagnosis code(s) has on targeted DRGs
- whether the patient is experiencing an acute versus chronic form of ischemic heart disease
- final discharge disposition of the patient
- presence of cardiac catherization during episode of care.

Most Common Diagnosis Codes

DRG 121
- 410.11, Acute myocardial infarction of anterolateral wall, initial episode of care
- 410.41, Acute myocardial infarction of other inferior wall, initial episode of care
- 410.71, Acute myocardial infarction of other inferior wall
- 410.91, Acute myocardial infarction of unspecified site
- 428.0, Congestive heart failure, unspecified

DRG 124
- 414.01, Coronary atherosclerosis of native coronary artery disease
- 428.0, Congestive heart failure, unspecified

Coding and Documentation Guidelines

410.11	Acute myocardial infarction of other anterior wall, initial episode of care	**DRG 121**

DOC: Use code 410.11 when the physician documents an initial episode of acute myocardial infarction of the anterior wall, acute anteroapical myocardial infarction, acute anteroseptal myocardial infarction, or coronary (artery) embolism, occlusion, rupture or thrombosis of the anterior wall.

410.41	Acute myocardial infarction of other inferior wall, initial episode of care	**DRG 121**

DOC: Use code 410.41 when the physician documents acute myocardial infarction of the diaphragmatic wall or inferior wall with contiguous portion of intraventricular septum, initial episode of care.

410.71	Acute myocardial infarction, subendocardial infarction, initial episode of care	DRG 121

DOC: Use code 410.71 when the physician documents subendocardial or nontransmural infarction, initial episode of care.

410.91	Acute myocardial infarction, unspecified site, initial episode of care	DRG 121

DOC: Use code 410.91 when the physician documents acute myocardial infarction, NOS, initial episode of care.

DOC: Use code 410.91 when the physician documents coronary (artery) embolism, occlusion, rupture or thrombosis, unspecified site, initial episode of care.

DOC: *Do not* assign code 410.9x when the physician documents the diagnosis as acute myocardial injury and there is no evidence of myocardial infarction, based on cardiac enzymes, and no electrocardiogram changes are noted other than acute myocardial injury. The correct code assignment is 411.89. *Do not* interpret 'acute myocardial injury' to mean infarction. The more synonymous term for acute myocardial injury is acute myocardial ischemia. A review of the index provides codes for acute myocardial ischemia with and without infarction. [*Coding Clinic*, 1Q, '92, 9, effective with discharges January 1, 1992]

410.XX	Acute myocardial infarction category	DRG 121

AHA CC: Assign the appropriate code from category 410 to identify the acute and code 458.8, Other specified hypotension, for the post M.I. hypotension.

[*Coding Clinic*, 4Q, '97, 10, effective with discharges October 1, 1997]

AHA CC: Assign the appropriate code from category 411, Other acute and subacute forms of ischemic heart disease, to identify postmyocardial infarction angina. Do not use the codes from categories 410, Acute myocardial infarction unless the angina leads to a myocardial infarction.

[*Coding Clinic*, 4Q, '94, 55, effective with discharges October 1, 1994]

AHA CC: Use the fifth digit '1' for the episode of care that covers all care provided to a newly diagnosed myocardial infarction patient until the patient is discharged from medical care. Transfers to and from other facilities prior to the patient's discharge and occurring within the eight-week time frame are included. Use the fifth digit '2' for the episode of care involving further observation, evaluation or treatment rendered after the initial treatment (discharge) and occurring within the eight-week time frame. [*Coding Clinic*, 4Q, '92, 24, effective with discharges October 1, 1992]

AHA CC: Assign a code from the 410 series when the physician documents a diagnosis of acute myocardial ischemia and a myocardial infarction has occurred, and code 411.8x if no infarction is documented. Code 411.81 is used if there is evidence of occlusion or thrombosis; otherwise, assign code 411.89. [*Coding Clinic*, 3Q, '91, 18, effective with discharges July 1, 1991]

AHA CC: Fifth-digit subclassifications were added to category 410 effective October 1, 1989. Their definitions are as follows:

- 0 episode of care unspecified
  Use when the source document does not contain sufficient information for the assignment of fifth digit '1' or '2.'
- 1 initial episode of care
  Use to designate the acute phase of care regardless of the location of treatment. Includes cases that are transferred for care and treatment within the acute phase of care. Any subsequent episode of care for another (repeat) myocardial infarction is also assigned the fifth digit of '1.'
- subsequent episode of care
  Use to designate observation, treatment or evaluation of myocardial infarction within eight weeks of onset, but following the acute phase, or in the healing state where the episode of care may be for related or unrelated condition(s).

410.XX   Acute myocardial infarction category (continued)   DRG 121

- Examples illustrating how to use these new fifth digits follow:
- Both hospital A and hospital B would assign code 410.11 in the case where a patient was admitted to hospital A with a diagnosis of acute anteroseptal myocardial infarction and transferred to hospital B two days later for continued care and further diagnostic workup. Hospital B provided diagnostic cardiac catheterization and discharged the patient home following further treatment of the myocardial infarction.
- Use code 410.92 when the medical record documents a patient with an acute myocardial infarction four weeks ago who is now being admitted for diagnostic workup. This included cardiac catheterization followed by a percutaneous transluminal coronary angioplasty (attempted and failed) and a coronary bypass. [*Coding Clinic,* 3Q, '89, 3, effective with discharges October 15, 1989]

AHA CC: If the physician records the diagnosis as 'complete atrioventricular (heart) block in acute myocardial infarction, anterior site,' assign code 410.11 as the principal diagnosis and 426.0 as a secondary condition. [*Coding Clinic,* J-A, '84, 5]

AHA CC: If the physician documents any mitral insufficiency resulting from papillary muscle infarction, assign codes 410.8x and 424.0. [*Coding Clinic,* J-A, '84, 5]

AHA CC: The physician may document the diagnosis of congestive heart failure or shock. These conditions may be present at onset of myocardial infarction or may develop later. Assign a code from the 410 series as the principal diagnosis, with any mention of congestive heart failure, cardiogenic shock, ventricular arrhythmia, or fibrillation being sequenced secondarily. [*Coding Clinic,* J-A, '84, 5]

AHA CC: Pay careful attention to the reason for hospitalization for those patients who are admitted with angina and undergo tissue plasminogen activator (TPA) administration, when despite TPA administration the angina evolves into an acute myocardial infarction. The acute myocardial infarction would be assigned as a principal diagnosis and no additional code for th angina, as it is an inherent part of the condition. [*Coding Clinic,* 2Q, '01, 8]

AHA CC: When documenting the diagnosis at the time of the patient's discharge, the medical staff should be encouraged to include the site of the myocardial infarction. A 'transmural' myocardial infarction involves full thickness of myocardium from endocardium to epicardium. A 'minor' myocardial infarction is not a full-thickness infarction. [*Coding Clinic,* J-A, '84, 5]

AHA CC: Pay careful attention to the reason for hospitalization for those patients who are post-myocardial with a stated duration of 'eight weeks or less.' Admissions or readmissions eight weeks or less from the date of a myocardial infarction do not necessarily constitute a reclassification as acute myocardial infarction. Examples of which code to select for those patients admitted or readmitted eight weeks or less from the time of acute myocardial infarction follow:

- Use the appropriate code from the 410.0-410.8 series if the episode of care is stated to be an extension of the myocardial infarction site, a repeat myocardial infarction, or an infarction of another myocardial site. Code 410.9 should be avoided if possible.
- Use the appropriate code from the 410.0-410.9 series if the diagnosis is stated as an acute ischemia or ischemic attack, post-myocardial infarction.
- In those situations where the patient is admitted six to eight weeks from the time of a myocardial infarction for purposes of diagnostic studies to determine the extent of coronary atherosclerosis or the presence of any sequelae following the myocardial infarction, code the diagnosis as stated by the physician. A physician may admit a patient for diagnostic studies when there are mild or no symptoms of angina, and this may be at six weeks rather than the arbitrary 'eight weeks' stated in the inclusion note under category 410. For example, a patient admitted for purposes of cardiac catheterization, coronary angiogram, and/or ventriculography may result in a diagnosis of coronary atherosclerosis or arteriosclerosis, vessel disease described as 1, 2 or 3, chronic coronary insufficiency, mitral valve insufficiency with coronary atherosclerosis, ventricular aneurysm, or rupture of papillary muscle. Diagnostic studies after a myocardial infarction are usually carried out to determine how extensive

410.XX   Acute myocardial infarction category (continued)   DRG 121

the atherosclerosis is and the need for any operative intervention, such as a coronary bypass. Assign a code from the 410.0-410.9 series if a myocardial infarction occurs during the course of the diagnostic study.

- Use code 411.0 if the post-myocardial diagnosis is pericarditis with friction rub, pericardial effusion, pleurisy, or pleural effusion, and joint pains. [*Coding Clinic,* J-A, '84, 5]

AHA CC: ICD-9-CM directs the coder to use category 410 when the patient's diagnosis is acute ischemia of the coronary artery(ies), heart or myocardium. However, because acute ischemia may not result in a myocardial infarction, the final code assignment depends on the medical record documentation. For example, choose a code from category 411 or 413 when the diagnosis on the medical record is 'acute ischemic (coronary) heart disease' or 'acute myocardial ischemia,' the diagnostic studies show no evidence of a myocardial infarct and the attending physician states or replies that there is no evidence of a myocardial infarction occurring. Ask the physician to clarify the terminology, i.e., which code best represents the patient's condition, 411.1 or 411.8x, or whether the reference is to ischemic angina pain classified to category 413. One form of acute myocardial ischemia is unstable angina. Look in the medical record for documentation that the patient received an antithrombolytic agent (streptokinase) during an angiogram or a transluminal (balloon) coronary angioplasty. These procedures may have prevented an infarction. [*Coding Clinic,* J-A, '84, 5]

AHA CC: Assign code 428.0 as the principal diagnosis when a patient is readmitted four days after being discharged following inferior wall myocardial infarction with substernal chest pressure associated with severe dyspnea. The physician documents the patient's refusal of a coronary artery bypass graft (CABG) during the previous admission and that the patient is now being admitted with congestive heart failure. Assign code 410.42 as a secondary diagnosis and not the principal because the reason for admission was the congestive heart failure. [*Coding Clinic,* 3Q, '97, 10, effective with discharges August 1, 1997]

AHA CC: Use code 411.81 when the physician's documentation in the medical record indicates clinical evidence of coronary occlusion or thrombosis, or the attending physician includes mention of either of these conditions in the diagnostic statement and the patient does not advance to acute myocardial infarction. Today, treatment with thrombolytic agents may dissolve a developing clot so the infarction does not occur although the patient may sustain occlusion or thrombosis. [*Coding Clinic,* 1Q, '91, 14, effective with discharges January 1, 1991, and *Coding Clinic,* 3Q, '91, 24]

AHA CC: *Do not* assign code 411.1 with code 411.8x. In addition, do not use a code from category 411, except code 411.0, when infarction has occurred. This is different than the example given in the third quarter 1989 issue of *Coding Clinic,* page 5. [*Coding Clinic,* 1Q, '91, 14, effective with discharges January 1, 1991, and *Coding Clinic,* 3Q, '91, 24]

AHA CC: Use code 411.1 when the physician documents the patient's diagnosis as unstable angina, crescendo angina, preinfarction angina, or impending myocardial infarction. The patient's admission and treatment is for unstable angina without documentation of infarction, occlusion, or thrombosis. If the patient's angina leads to myocardial infarction, do not assign a code for the angina. Use the appropriate code from category 410. [*Coding Clinic,* 1Q, '91, 14, effective with discharges January 1, 1991, and *Coding Clinic,* 3Q, '91, 24]

DOC: *Do not* use category 410 when the physician documents a diagnosis of mural thrombus when no infarction has occurred. Use code 429.89 for the mural thrombus whether or not a cardiac condition or coronary artery disease is associated with the thrombus. Assign an additional code for the underlying cardiac condition if one exists and is documented. If the physician documents the associated condition as chronic ischemic heart disease, use code 414.8. Assign code 429.79 if the mural thrombus occurs following an earlier myocardial infarction, with an additional code to identify the infarction. [*Coding Clinic,* 1Q, '92, 10, effective with discharges January 1, 1992]

428.0   Congestive heart failure, unspecified   **DRG 121**

CG: Assign code 428.0 as the principal diagnosis in instances where pleural effusion is associated with congestive heart failure. It is common for patients with congestive heart failure with or without pulmonary edema to have pleural effusion. Since the pleural effusion is usually minimal and not specifically addressed other than by more aggressive treatment of the underlying congestive heart failure, it should not be reported as an additional diagnosis. The exception would be if the physician has specifically indicated it should be reported. [*Coding Clinic*, 3Q, '91, 19, effective with discharges July 1, 1991]

AHA CC: Assign code 428.0 in addition to the code for hypertensive heart disease, unspecified with heart failure and the code for diastolic heart failure, unspecified when the physician documentation states congestive heart failure due to diastolic dysfunction due to hypertension. [*Coding Clinic*, 4Q, '02, 52]

AHA CC: Use code 428.0 as a secondary diagnosis in addition to the principal diagnosis code for combined systolic and diastolic heart failure, acute on chronic when the physician documents the patient has a known history of congestive heart failure and is admitted to the hospital for an acute episode of a chronic condition. [*Coding Clinic*, 4Q, '02, 52]

AHA CC: Assign code 428.0 as principal diagnosis when a patient is admitted in congestive heart failure resulting from fluid overload secondary to noncompliance with dialysis treatment. [*Coding Clinic*, 2Q, '01, 13]

AHA CC: Assign code 428.0 in addition to the code for the congenital heart disease when the physician documentation states congestive heart failure secondary to congenital heart disease. [*Coding Clinic*, 1Q, '99, 11, effective with discharges February 15, 1999]

AHA CC: Assign code 996.83 as principal diagnosis and 428.0 as secondary diagnosis when the admission is for congestive heart failure affecting a transplanted heart regardless of whether or not the patient had CHF prior to the transplant. CHF is a complication affecting a transplanted organ. [*Coding Clinic*, 3Q, '98, 5, effective with discharges September 1, 1998]

AHA CC: Assign code 428.0 as the principal diagnosis when a patient is readmitted four days after being discharged following inferior wall myocardial infarction with substernal chest pressure associated with severe dyspnea. The physician documents the patient's refusal of a CABG during the previous admission and that the patient is now being admitted with congestive heart failure. Assign code 410.42 as a secondary diagnosis and not the principal because the reason for admission was the congestive heart failure. [*Coding Clinic*, 3Q, '97, 10, effective with discharges August 1, 1997]

AHA CC: Assign code 428.0 as the principal diagnosis and codes 584.9, 585, and V15.81 as additional diagnoses for the following scenario: A patient with chronic renal failure is noncompliant with dialysis and diet and goes into volume overload due to salt and fluid levels. As a result, the patient develops congestive heart failure and acute renal failure. Physician documentation indicates that the congestive heart failure is due to poor compliance with salt and water restrictions rather than from a primary cardiac dysfunction. [*Coding Clinic* 3Q, '96, 9, effective with discharges August 15, 1996]

AHA CC: When both congestive cardiomyopathy and congestive heart failure are documented by the physician and the patient's treatment is directed at the congestive heart failure (salt restriction, diuretics, and other drugs), assign either code 428.0 or 428.1 as the principal diagnosis. Assign code 425.4 as an additional diagnosis. Congestive cardiomyopathy or 'dilated' cardiomyopathy is a myocardial disease characterized by ventricular dilation, contractile dysfunction, and symptoms of congestive heart failure. [*Coding Clinic*, 2Q, '90, 19, effective with discharges April 1, 1990]

AHA CC: Assign codes 428.0 and 401.9 if the physician states that the patient has congestive heart failure and hypertension but does not indicate that the congestive heart failure is due to hypertension. Before assigning these codes it is best to check with the physician to verify that the patient does not have hypertensive heart disease with congestive heart failure, 401.91, a determination that can be made only by the physician. [*Coding Clinic*, 2Q, '89, 12, effective with discharges July 31, 1989]

AHA CC: Use code 428.0 when the physician documents acute pulmonary edema with congestive heart failure due to or associated with nonrheumatic and nonhypertensive heart disease. [*Coding Clinic*, 3Q, '88, 3]

DRG Desk Reference

DRGs 121, 124

428.0   Congestive heart failure, unspecified (continued)   DRG 121

AHA CC: Use code 428.1 for acute myocardial infarction, acute or subacute ischemic heart disease, or coronary atherosclerosis (414.0x and 414.8) with mention of acute pulmonary edema, except when pulmonary edema is mentioned with congestive heart failure or decompensated left ventricular failure. In that case, use code 428.0. [*Coding Clinic*, 3Q, '88, 3]

AHA CC: Pulmonary edema, a pathologic state in which there is excessive, diffuse accumulation of fluid in the tissues and alveolar spaces of the lung, can be of cardiac and noncardiac origin. When of cardiac origin, it is a manifestation of heart failure and, as such, is not coded separately. For example, acute pulmonary edema is included in the following:

- left ventricular failure, 428.1
- congestive heart failure, 428.0
- right heart failure secondary to left heart failure, 428.0
- hypertensive heart disease (see 402.0, 402.1, and 402.9 with fifth digit of '1')
- rheumatic heart disease, acute, 391.8
- rheumatic active chorea, 392.0
- rheumatic heart disease or chorea, inactive, chronic, or quiescent, 398.91
- rheumatic disease of heart valve (394-396), code also 398.91 [*Coding Clinic*, 3Q, '88, 3]

AHA CC: Heart failure patients may experience symptoms of dyspnea, orthopnea, paroxysmal nocturnal dyspnea, fatigue, weakness and decreased cerebral function. Signs documented by the physician may include pulmonary rales, pedal edema, congestive hepatomegaly and pleural effusions. Evaluation of patients with heart failure include not only the underlying cause of heart disease, but also the precipitating causes of heart failure such as cardiac arrhythmias, hypertension, myocardial infarction, and physical, dietary, environmental, and emotional excesses, including noncompliance with cardiac medications. When an underlying heart disease is not present, these precipitating causes usually do not, by themselves, lead to heart failure. The physician will direct the treatment at removal of the precipitating cause, correction of the underlying heart disease (i.e., surgical treatment of valvular disease or correction of septal defects), and control of the congestive heart failure. There are a variety of forms of heart failure, including:

- *High output versus low output heart failure.* The physician may describe the low cardiac output syndrome with either left-sided or right-sided congestive heart failure. This type of heart failure may be secondary to ischemic heart disease, hypertension, cardiomyopathy, or valvular or pericardial disease. Hyperthyroidism, anemia, arteriovenous fistulas, beri-beri, and Paget's disease may exist with high output heart failure. Left-sided congestive heart failure is manifested by dyspnea, orthopnea, paroxysmal nocturnal dyspnea, cardiac asthma (bronchospasm) and/or acute pulmonary edema due to accumulation of excess fluid behind the left ventricle.
- *Right-sided versus left-sided heart failure.* Manifestations of left-sided congestive heart failure are dyspnea, orthopnea, paroxysmal
- nocturnal dyspnea, cardiac asthma (bronchospasm), and/or acute pulmonary edema due to accumulation of excess fluid behind the left ventricle. Manifestations of right-sided congestive heart failure are systemic venous congestion (distended neck veins), enlarged tender liver, pitting edema of the lower extremities or other dependent portions of the body, and/or ascites due to congestion of fluid behind the right ventricle.
- *Compensated versus decompensated heart failure.* The physician may describe the heart failure in these ways to further indicate the ability or inability of the heart to handle the increased work load.

Follow the alphabetic index when assigning codes to the terms described above. Selection will be from the 428.0-428.9 series, except compensated heart failure, which is currently coded to 429.9. [*Coding Clinic*, 2Q, '90, 16, effective with discharges April 1, 1990]

AHA CC: Acute pulmonary edema with congestive heart failure due to or associated with nonrheumatic and nonhypertensive heart disease is assigned to 428.0 (left heart failure followed by right heart failure). For a diagnosis of acute pulmonary edema of cardiogenic origin, the physician would usually reference cardiac enlargement, presence of S-3 gallop, elevated pulmonary artery wedge pressure, or associated cardiac diseases in the medical record of a patient with acute pulmonary edema of cardiac origin. Pleural effusions and the presence of Kerly B lines would frequently be seen on x-rays. The patient frequently is treated with diuretics and other cardiac medications. [*Coding Clinic*, 3Q, '88, 3]

578

©2003 Ingenix, Inc.

428.0   Congestive heart failure, unspecified (continued)   DRG 121

DOC: Use code 428.0 when the physician documents congestive heart failure or right heart failure secondary to left heart failure.

DOC: Use code 428.0 when the physician documents congestive heart failure resulting from fluid overload. Fluid overload is a component of congestive heart failure and should not be coded separately.

DOC: Do not use 428.0 when the physician documents hypertensive heart disease with congestive heart failure. The correct code is 402.91.

DOC: Do not use 428.0 when the physician documents rheumatic heart failure. The correct code is 398.91.

414.01   Coronary atherosclerosis of native coronary artery   DRG 124

CG: Assign code 414.01 as the principal diagnosis when a patient with an established diagnosis of coronary atherosclerosis, of native artery with a known history of coronary artery disease, status post myocardial infarction, is admitted for treatment of impending myocardial infarction and the acute MI is aborted. The patient was treated with intravenous nitroglycerin and placed on calcium blockers.

CG: As described in *Coding Clinic*, angina pectoris is a condition characterized by chest pain or discomfort, generally exacerbated by exertion, and relieved by medications (nitroglycerin), rest, and/or treatment of the heart disease. Use code 411.1 when the physician documents preinfarction, unstable, initial onset or crescendo angina. For this type of angina, the patient's pain is of longer duration and/or happens more often than stable angina. It is difficult to control unstable angina with medication and the angina can develop into an acute myocardial infarction (AMI). An underlying cardiac condition such as coronary arteriosclerosis or aortic stenosis causes the patient to have angina. The physician also may document ischemic heart disease or CAD that can occur because of an insufficient blood flow caused by the narrowing of the coronary arteries due to the formation of atherosclerotic plaque. The patient may undergo additional diagnostic studies, such as cardiac catheterization, or treatment to arrest the disease process, such as percutaneous transluminal coronary angioplasty of CABG. Use the following information to assist with coding:

- Assign code 413.9 for stable forms of angina or angina of effort. This type of angina occurs in patients at certain levels of exertion or stress and is relieved in an expected way with rest or nitroglycerin. Hospitalization is usually not required.
- When the diagnosis documented is 'angina' without further qualification, the physician should be contacted so that he or she may specify the type of angina. If a patient is hospitalized, it would usually be for preinfarctional or unstable angina. However, without further qualification by the physician, code 'angina' to 413.9.
- Code the underlying cause of the angina as the principal diagnosis when a patient is admitted with angina and diagnostic procedure(s) are carried out, showing that the angina was caused by coronary atherosclerosis, aortic stenosis or some other heart disease.

CG: Code an AMI as the principal diagnosis when a patient is admitted with symptomatic angina that develops into an AMI. Do not assign an additional code for the angina.

AHA CC: Use code 411.1 for the aborted MI as a secondary diagnosis. In the absence of an established diagnosis of coronary atherosclerosis, code assignments for aborted or impending myocardial infarctions should always be based on physician documentation for whether an infarction has occurred. [*Coding Clinic*, 2Q, '01, 9]

AHA CC: Assign code 414.01 for the patient with coronary artery disease and no mention of a past history of CABG. Check with the physician if the documentation is unclear regarding the patient's past history of bypass surgery. [*Coding Clinic*, 3Q, '97, 15, effective with discharges August 1, 1997]

AHA CC: *Do not* assign a code from subcategory 414.0 when a patient has a history of CABG and the physician makes no mention of coronary atherosclerosis during this admission. [*Coding Clinic*, 3Q, '97, 15, effective with discharges August 1, 1997]

Targeted DRG Listing

414.01   Coronary atherosclerosis of native coronary artery (continued)   DRG 124

AHA CC: Assign code 414.00 for the patient with coronary artery disease who had a CABG done years earlier and whose medical record does not specify which vessel is affected by the coronary artery disease (CAD). *Do not* assign code 414.01 to show the native artery bypassed earlier unless the record supports the current existence of CAD in a native coronary vessel. Use code 414.05 if the physician confirmed that CAD had developed over the previous bypass graft. Also, do not assign CAD of bypass graft based solely on the fact that the patient has atherosclerosis and has a history of bypass surgery. [*Coding Clinic,* 3Q, '97, 15, effective with discharges August 1, 1997]

AHA CC: Effective October 1, 1994, fifth digits were added for subcategory code 414.0 to allow for a distinction between a disease process that occurs to a native coronary artery and one affecting a bypass graft. Assign code 414.00 if the physician documents in the medical record coronary atherosclerosis but does not indicate whether this is a native vessel or a graft. Assign code 414.05 if the physician documents in the medical record the diagnosis of coronary atherosclerosis of bypass graft with a patient history of CABG and no further documentation on the bypass graft is available. [*Coding Clinic,* 4Q, '96, 31, effective with discharges October 1, 1996]

AHA CC: A patient is admitted with angina and known CAD. Previously, the patient had a PTCA. Cardiac catheterization performed during this admission identifies that the vessels have reoccluded. Assign code 414.01 as the principal diagnosis and codes 413.9 and V45.82 as additional diagnoses. [*Coding Clinic,* 2Q, '95, 17, effective with discharges April 15, 1995]

AHA CC: Assign code 414.8 for a diagnosis of ischemic cardiomyopathy. However, it is best to check with the physician for clarification on how he or she is using this term. The physician sometimes may utilize this diagnostic term to designate a condition in which ischemic heart disease causes diffuse fibrosis or multiple infarctions and leads to heart failure with left ventricular dilation. There may or may not be an associated angina pectoris. The code series 410-414 classifies all ischemic heart diseases. [*Coding Clinic,* 2Q, '90, 19, effective with discharges April 1, 1990]

AHA CC: Assign code 414.02 when the physician has indicated a redo of a CABG performed 15 years ago where the arteries have occluded due to atherosclerosis. Use code 414.01 as an additional code if the physician has also documented the presence of atherosclerosis in any remaining native vessels. [*Coding Clinic,* 2Q, '95, 17, effective with discharges April 15, 1995]

AHA CC: Assign code 414.02 for atherosclerosis of the graft vessel and code 414.01 for atherosclerosis of the native vessels when a patient with CAD is admitted with unstable angina. History indicates past CABG. Cardiac catheterization was performed on the current admission, showing occlusion in both the graft vessels and a native vessel. Assign code 411.1 as an associated diagnosis. [*Coding Clinic,* 2Q, '95, 17, effective with discharges April 15, 1995]

AHA CC: New codes implemented on October 1, 1994, for subcategory 414.0 have changed previous advice published in *Coding Clinic* November-December 1986 and first quarter 1994 *Coding Clinic* regarding the use of code 996.03. The October 1, 1994 sequencing advice published in Volume 10, Number 5, 1993, and *Coding Clinic* second quarter 1994, page 15, remains unchanged (see above). Assign code 996.03 for conditions such as acute (abrupt) closures and leakage at the anastomosis site. As of October 1, 1994, do not assign code 996.03 when the physician has documented that atherosclerosis has occurred in the bypass graft vessel. Rather, assign a code from subcategory 414.0x since the presence of atherosclerosis in a bypass graft is considered a progression of the disease rather than a mechanical complication. [*Coding Clinic,* 2Q, '95, 17, effective with discharges April 15, 1995]

AHA CC: When a patient is admitted with angina, has known CAD and no previous history of any procedures being done, assign code 414.01. Assign code 413.9 as an additional diagnosis. [*Coding Clinic,* 2Q, '95, 17, effective with discharges April 15, 1995]

AHA CC: Assign code 414.01 when the medical record documentation shows no history of prior coronary artery bypass. When the documentation is unclear concerning prior bypass surgery, verify with the physician and have him or her document in the medical record whether previous surgery has occurred. [*Coding Clinic,* 2Q, '95, 17, effective with discharges April 15, 1995]

414.01 Coronary atherosclerosis of native coronary artery (continued)   DRG 124

AHA CC: Assign code 414.0x as the principal diagnosis for a patient who is status post heart transplant four years ago and suffers from progressive CAD of the transplanted heart. Code V42.1 may be assigned as an additional diagnosis. [*Coding Clinic,* 2Q, '94, 13, effective with discharges April 1, 1994]

AHA CC: Assign code 414.0x for a postpercutaneous transluminal coronary angioplasty (PTCA) reocclusion of the coronary artery. In a PTCA, the coronary artery is left intact, that is, no 'artificial' grafts are involved and treatment is considered complete. When a PTCA is performed, a balloon is used to apply pressure inside the vessel at the location of the arteriosclerotic plaque. The arteriosclerosis is not removed and remains after PTCA. Therefore, reocclusion of an angioplastied vessel may occur either because of the progression of the arteriosclerotic plaque or the re-expansion of the arteriosclerotic plaque within the vessel. When this happens it is considered to be progression of the atherosclerosis unless the physician specifies this as a complication of the procedure. This situation is different than when a coronary artery bypass graft reoccludes. In this case, the graft itself has the problem and is considered to be a complication. Reasons for the reocclusion include thrombus formation, fibrointimal proliferation or atherosclerotic spread. [*Coding Clinic,* 1Q, '94, 6, effective with discharges January 1, 1994

AHA CC: If a patient is admitted with unstable angina and a heart catheterization is done, assign code 414.0x as the principal diagnosis. Angina is a symptom and should not be coded when a related definitive diagnosis has been established. The known diagnosis rather than a symptom should be coded. However, the physician must state the cause and effect relationship between the angina and underlying coronary atherosclerosis or CAD. Sequence the angina as the principal diagnosis when the cause of the angina is not established or documented. When the physician documents the cause of the angina, list that cause (e.g., CAD) as principal. Since the CAD caused the symptom, angina, the definition of principal diagnosis is met. [*Coding Clinic,* 4Q, '93, 44, effective with discharges September 3, 1993]

AHA CC: The physician may use diagnostic study findings such as exercise stress tests and electrocardiographs to determine a diagnosis of asymptomatic or pre-symptomatic atherosclerotic coronary artery disease. Use code 414.0x for symptomatic or presymptomatic coronary heart or artery disease. If the medical record supports the presence of an old 'silent' myocardial infarct in the findings of asymptomatic coronary heart disease, assign codes 414.0x and 412. [*Coding Clinic,* J-A, '84, 5]

AHA CC: Code 414.0x includes arteriosclerotic coronary artery disease and atherosclerosis of the coronary artery. Arteriosclerosis, a generic term, may be further delineated as to type. For example, atherosclerosis or atheroma is arteriosclerosis of the muscular arteries, including the aortic, coronary, femoral, iliac, internal carotid, and cerebral arteries. Ischemic heart disease is a deficiency of blood supply to the heart muscle caused by obstruction or constriction of the coronary artery. While atherosclerotic changes are the most common cause of 'coronary artery disease' or 'coronary heart disease,' they are coded to 414.9 and not to 414.0x. Both descriptors, 'coronary artery disease' and 'coronary heart disease,' are not precise enough to assign them to a code other than 414.9. For instance, the term 'coronary heart disease' does not necessarily refer to the presence of clinical manifestations such as acute or chronic myocardial ischemia, stable or unstable angina or coronary insufficiency. The physician using this term may be referring only to the pathological process of atherosclerosis of the coronary artery or to the pathological process plus clinical symptoms or manifestations, such as with stable angina. With variations in classifications and references to coronary heart disease, check with the physician and have him or her clarify the term's meaning and accurate code assignment. The medical staff should be made aware of the ICD-9-CM code classification for diagnoses of 'coronary artery disease' and 'coronary heart disease' and should be encouraged to provide greater specificity in stating the diagnosis. [*Coding Clinic,* J-A, '84, 5]

AHA CC: Assign CAD as the principal diagnosis in cases where the physician has documented the CAD as the underlying cause of the unstable angina (the reason for the admission) even if a diagnostic test has not been performed during the admission for the diagnosis of coronary artery disease. Documentation of previous testing to confirm the presence of CAD would establish the connection between the CAD and unstable angina. Review the medical record carefully because the

414.01   Coronary atherosclerosis of native coronary artery (continued)   DRG 124

physician may document that the angina is due to another condition (i.e., stenosis). In this case, the code for the documented underlying condition is assigned as the principal diagnosis. The angina would be coded secondarily. [*Coding Clinic,* 2Q, '97, 13, effective with discharges May 1, 1997]

AHA CC: Assign code 414.02 when a patient has previously had a CABG but the type of graft material is unknown. [*Coding Clinic,* 2Q, '95, 17, effective with discharges April 15, 1995]

AHA CC: Prior to October 1, 1994, assign code 996.03 for the diagnosis of reocclusion of a graft, both acute and delayed graft closure. With discharges on or after October 1, 1994, new codes provide for the differentiation between a disease process that occurs to a native body part and one affecting a bypass graft for atherosclerosis of the coronary arteries as well as the peripheral arteries. Assign the new codes based on the specific vessel in which the atherosclerosis has been found and is documented. *Do not* assume based on the fact that the patient has atherosclerosis and a history of bypass surgery that they are related. Use code 414.00 to identify atherosclerosis of internal mammary bypass grafts. [*Coding Clinic,* 4Q, '94, 49, effective with discharges October 1, 1994]

AHA CC: When a patient is admitted for unstable angina, CAD may be assigned as the principal diagnosis even when a diagnostic test establishing a diagnosis of CAD is not performed during the patient's stay. The physician must document in the medical record that the CAD is the underlying cause of the unstable angina. The physician may remark in the record that the patient has a known history of CAD. The physician would not need to perform additional testing to re-establish the underlying cause when patients are admitted for treatment of unstable angina. Sequence code 411.1 as the principal diagnosis and code 414.0x as the secondary diagnosis when the physician has not documented the underlying cause of the unstable angina to be CAD. [*Coding Clinic,* 2Q, '94, 15, effective with discharges April 1, 1994]

AHA CC: The following examples illustrate proper sequencing of the diagnoses of angina and coronary heart disease: [*Coding Clinic,* Volume 10, Number 5, '93, 17, effective October 1, 1993. This replaces the advice published in the third quarter 1990 edition of *Coding Clinic.*]

- The reason for admission was progressive episodes of chest pain consistent with crescendo angina. History includes chronic coronary insufficiency and previous myocardial infarctions six years ago. Treatment during the hospitalization included p.o. calcium blockers. At discharge, the patient was pain-free. No complications arose during the hospitalization and no other diagnostic or therapeutic interventions were performed. Assign code 411.1 as the principal diagnosis since this was the condition after study that necessitated admission to the hospital.
- The reason for admission was cardiac catheterization. The patient's diagnosis on admission was unstable angina. The cardiac catheterization showed significant triple-vessel atherosclerotic heart disease. A three-vessel aortocoronary artery bypass was performed. Assign code 414.0x as the principal diagnosis since this was the condition after study that necessitated admission to the hospital. Assign an additional code for the unstable angina as a secondary diagnosis
- The reason for admission was a combined right and left heart cardiac catheterization. The patient's diagnosis on admission was angina. The cardiac catheterization showed significant atherosclerotic heart disease. Triple coronary artery bypass surgery was recommended. No surgery was performed prior to discharge. Later, the patient was readmitted and surgery was performed on the second admission. The patient received his antianginal medication also during this stay. Assign code 414.01 as the principal diagnosis for both admissions since this is the condition that necessitated admission to the hospital. Assign code 413.9 as an additional diagnosis.
- The reason for admission was unstable angina. While in the hospital, the patient was given intravenous nitrate therapy. After stabilization, the patient underwent a diagnostic cardiac catheterization. Results showed atherosclerotic heart disease. Before discharge, the patient was weaned off the nitroglycerin drip and placed on intensified antianginal therapy. The patient was discharged symptom-free without need for further therapeutic interventions. Assign code 414.0x as the principal diagnosis since this condition led to the admission.
- The reason for admission was severe crescendo angina. The physician tried to stabilize the patient by performing an emergency single-vessel PTCA with administration of thrombolytic

414.01   Coronary atherosclerosis of native coronary artery (continued)   DRG 124

agent. However, an acute myocardial infarction of the inferolateral wall occurred. Assign code 410.21 as the principal diagnosis.

- As an outpatient, an asymptomatic patient underwent an exercise stress test and was believed to have ischemic heart disease based on significant ST depression during peak exercise. The reason for admission was cardiac catheterization. Results showed an underlying significant coronary atherosclerosis, thus explaining his abnormal stress test. Treatment included medications. At discharge, the patient was symptom-free and will be followed up as an outpatient. Assign code 414.01 as the principal diagnosis since the patient was admitted without significant anginal symptoms and coronary atherosclerosis is the condition after study that necessitated admission to the hospital.

- As an outpatient, a patient underwent an exercise stress test as part of a routine exercise prescription. The study was abnormal at peak exercise. The reason for the admission was cardiac catheterization. Results were within normal limits. The patient was symptom-free during the hospitalization. Assign code V71.7 as the principal diagnosis as the physician concluded that no cardiac disease was revealed.

- The reason for admission was unstable angina. The patient had been previously hospitalized for an acute myocardial infarction of the anterolateral wall six weeks earlier. During the patient's stay, his angina stabilized and further infarction was avoided. Assign code 411.1 as the principal diagnosis and code 410.02 as a secondary diagnosis.

- The reason for admission was preinfarctional angina. After stabilization, the patient was transferred for further evaluation to a regional hospital specializing in cardiac care. Assign code 411.1 as the principal diagnosis.

- During the patient's stay at the regional hospital, he was maintained on antianginal medications and cardiac catheterization was performed. Results showed coronary atherosclerosis. A CABG was performed. During the stay, the patient had no further anginal episodes. Assign code 414.01 as the principal diagnosis and code 411.1 as a secondary diagnosis.

- Assign code 413.9 as the principal diagnosis for the following scenario: A patient with chest pain visited the physician at his office. After examination, the physician's diagnosis was angina and he decided to admit the patient. Treatment at the hospital consisted of anti-anginal medications. During the stay, the patient had no further anginal episodes.

AHA CC: Included in code 413.9 are stable forms of angina and excluded is preinfarctional angina. For this type of angina, the anginal type of chest pain is at the same level of exertion or stress and is usually relieved in a predictable fashion with rest or nitroglycerin. Treatment of stable angina is on an outpatient basis unless the patient is being admitted for diagnostic studies to determine the extent of coronary artery disease. Assign the underlying cause of the angina, as determined by the diagnostic study, as the principal diagnosis. [*Coding Clinic*, 3Q, '90, 6, effective with discharges July 15, 1990]

AHA CC: Included in code 411.1 are preinfarction angina, crescendo angina, unstable angina or initial onset angina. For this type of angina, the patient experiences pain that lasts longer and/or occurs more frequently. It is also more resistant to an antianginal program and often results in an acute myocardial infarction. Cardiac catheterization or other treatment to interrupt the occlusion process can occur during an inpatient stay. Angina is one symptom of coronary or ischemic heart disease, a disorder resulting from insufficient blood flow secondary to narrowing of the coronary arteries due to atherosclerosis. [*Coding Clinic*, 3Q, '90, 6, effective with discharges July 15, 1990]

AHA CC: Use code 411.81 as the principal diagnosis and codes 411.1 and 414.0x as secondary diagnoses for the following scenario: A patient admitted for coronary occlusion with impending acute myocardial infarction was given tissue plasminogen activator (TPA) to ward off an infarction. Severe coronary arteriosclerosis is also listed as a diagnosis. [*Coding Clinic*, 3Q, '89, 4, effective with discharges October 15, 1989]

DOC: Use code 414.01 when the physician documents coronary (artery) atherosclerosis, arteriosclerosis, arteritis, atheroma, sclerosis or stricture of native coronary artery.

DOC: Use code 414.01 when the physician documents arteriosclerotic heart disease of native coronary artery.

DRG 122 Circulatory Disorders with Acute Myocardial Infarction without Major Complications, Discharged Alive

DRG 125   Circulatory Disorders Except Acute Myocardial Infarction with Cardiac Catheterization without Complex Diagnosis

Issue

The coding of ischemic heart disease is problematic because of the lack of physician documentation on either the known or suspected presence of acute myocardial infarction, determining whether the patient is experiencing an acute episode or has a chronic form of ischemic heart disease, the complexity of ICD-9-CM diagnosis codes and coding guidelines for ischemic heart disease. The following represent the major issues affecting the DRG pairs 122 and 125:

- the known or suspected presence of acute myocardial infarction
- determination of the initial or subsequent episode of care for myocardial infarctions, particularly in transfer cases
- whether the patient is experiencing an acute versus chronic form of ischemic heart disease
- final discharge disposition of the patient
- presence of cardiac catherization during episode of care

Most Common Diagnosis Codes

DRG 122

- 410.11, Acute myocardial infarction of anterolateral wall, initial episode of care
- 410.41, Acute myocardial infarction of other inferior wall
- 410.71, Acute myocardial infarction of other inferior wall
- 410.91, Acute myocardial infarction of unspecified site, initial episode of care

DRG 125

- 414.01, Coronary atherosclerosis of native coronary artery disease
- 786.50, Chest pain, unspecified
- 786.59, Chest pain NEC

Coding and Documentation Guidelines

410.11	Acute myocardial infarction of other anterior wall, initial episode of care	DRG 122

See standards on page 573.

410.41	Acute myocardial infarction of other inferior wall, initial episode of care	DRG 122

See standards on page 573.

410.71	Acute myocardial infarction, subendocardial infarction, initial episode of care	DRG 122

See standards on page 574.

410.91   **Acute myocardial infarction, unspecified site,**   **DRG 122**
            initial episode of care

See standards on page 574.

414.01   **Coronary atherosclerosis of native coronary artery**   **DRG 125**

See standards on page 579.

786.50   **Chest pain, unspecified**   **DRG 125**

AHA CC: Do not use code 786.50 if the physician documents midsternal chest pain. The correct code is 786.51. [*Coding Clinic*, 1Q, '98, 10, effective with discharges January 15, 1998]

AHA CC: Do not use a code describing a symptom when a related definitive diagnosis has been established. [*Coding Clinic*, 2Q, '90, 3, effective with discharges April 1, 1990]

AHA CC: Do not use a code describing a symptom, sign or ill-defined condition from Chapter 16 of ICD-9-CM as the principal diagnosis when a related definitive diagnosis has been established. [*Coding Clinic*, 2Q, '90, 3, effective with discharges April 1, 1990]

AHA CC: Use the code for the symptom as the principal diagnosis if it is followed by contrasting/ comparative diagnoses. The contrasting/comparative diagnoses are coded secondarily. [*Coding Clinic*, 2Q, '90, 3, effective with discharges April 1, 1990]

Doc: Use code 786.50 when the physician documents chest pain.

Doc: Do not use code 786.50 if the physician documents chest discomfort, chest pressure or chest tightness. The correct code is 786.59.

Doc: Do not use code 786.50 if the physician documents anterior chest wall pain. The correct code is 786.52.

786.59   **Chest pain, NEC**   **DRG 125**

AHA CC: Do not use code 786.59 if the physician documents midsternal chest pain. The correct code is 786.51. [*Coding Clinic*, 1Q, '98, 10, effective with discharges January 15, 1998]

AHA CC: Do not use a code describing a symptom when a related definitive diagnosis has been established. [*Coding Clinic*, 2Q, '90, 3, effective with discharges April 1, 1990]

AHA CC: Do not use a code describing a symptom, sign or ill-defined condition from chapter 16 as the principal diagnosis when a related definitive diagnosis has been established. [*Coding Clinic*, 2Q, '90, 3, effective with discharges April 1, 1990]

AHA CC: Use the code for the symptom as the principal diagnosis if it is followed by contrasting/ comparative diagnoses. The contrasting/comparative diagnoses are coded secondarily. [*Coding Clinic*, 2Q, '90, 3, effective with discharges April 1, 1990]

Doc: Use code 786.59 when the physician documents discomfort, pressure, or tightness in the chest.

Doc: Do not use code 786.59 if the physician documents chest pain. The correct code is 786.50.

Doc: Do not use code 786.59 if the physician documents midsternal chest pain. The correct code is 786.51.

Doc: Do not use code 786.59 if the physician documents anterior chest wall pain or pleuritic pain. The correct code is 786.52.

Doc: Do not use code 786.59 if the physician documents breast pain. The correct code is 611.71.

Targeted DRG Listing

DRG 127 Heart Failure and Shock

DRG 140   Angina Pectoris

Issue

The coding of congestive heart failure and angina pectoris is problematic because physician documentation may be unclear as to whether the patient is experiencing an acute episode or has a chronic form of heart disease making it difficult to determine the principal diagnosis, and because of the impact the complexity of the ICD-9-CM diagnosis codes and coding guidelines.

Most Common Diagnosis Codes

DRG 127
- 402.91, Hypertensive heart disease with heart failure
- 428.0, Congestive heart failure, unspecified

DRG 140
- 411.1, Intermediate coronary syndrome
- 411.89, Other acute and subacute forms of ischemic heart disease
- 413.9, Angina pectoris

Coding and Documentation Guidelines

402.91 Hypertensive heart disease with heart failure	DRG 127

CG: Effective October 1, 2002, use an additional code to specify type of heart failure: 428.0, 428.20-428.23, 428.30-428.33, 428.40-428.43 with category 402 codes.

CG: Assign only code 402.91 for a diagnosis of congestive heart failure due to diastolic dysfunction due to hypertension. *Do not* assign an additional code for the diastolic dysfunction.

AHA CC: Use a code for hypertensive heart disease along with the code for congestive heart failure when the physician documents the patient has hypertensive heart disease with congestive heart failure due to hypertension [*Coding Clinic*, 4Q, '02, 50]

AHA CC: Use three codes to accurately report congestive heart failure due to diastolic dysfunction due to hypertension. Assign code 402.91 as the principal diagnosis code and two additional codes to report that the heart failure was diastolic type and congestive. [*Coding Clinic*, 3Q, '02, 22]

AHA CC: If the physician documented only the diastolic dysfunction, assign code 429.9. Diastolic dysfunction can occur as a result of hypertension, coronary artery disease, or cardiomyopathies. There was an index entry change, effective October 1, 1992, regarding the ventricular dysfunction. In addition, this is a revision of the information published in *Coding Clinic*, second quarter 1989. [*Coding Clinic*, 1Q, '93, 19, effective with discharges January 1, 1993]

AHA CC: Assign code 402.91 as the principal diagnosis and code 414.0x as a secondary diagnosis for the following scenario: Principal diagnosis: congestive heart failure. Other diagnoses: arteriosclerotic heart disease; hypertensive cardiovascular disease. [*Coding Clinic*, N-D, '84, 18]

AHA CC: Assign code 402.9x as the principal diagnosis for the diagnostic statement of 'hypertensive cardiomyopathy'when the physician has established hypertension as the cause of the myocardial disease. Assign code 425.8 as an additional diagnosis. [*Coding Clinic*, 2Q, '93, 9, effective with discharges April 1, 1993]

402.91   Hypertensive heart disease with heart failure (continued)   **DRG 127**

AHA CC: Assign the appropriate code from one of categories 401-405 if the physician documents the patient's diagnosis as controlled hypertension. The use of the term 'controlled'indicates an existing state of hypertension under control by therapy. Untreated hypertension or hypertension not responding to current therapeutic regimen may be described by the physician as uncontrolled hypertension. Assign the appropriate code from categories 401-405. The physician should document in the medical record the stage and type of hypertension. [*Coding Clinic*, 3Q, '90, 3, effectve with discharges July 15, 1990]

AHA CC: *Do not* assign a code from category 410 if the physician does not document an established diagnosis of hypertension and the patient's blood pressure is elevated. The correct code assignment is 796.2. This is also the correct code for a statement of elevated blood pressure without further specificity. [*Coding Clinic*, 3Q, '90, 3, effective with discharges July 15, 1990]

AHA CC: When both hypertensive renal disease and hypertensive heart disease are stated in the diagnosis, assign a code from combination category 404. It does not matter whether or not the relationship between the hypertension and the renal disease is stated. [*Coding Clinic*, 3Q, '90, 3, effective with discharges July 15, 1990]

AHA CC: When conditions classified to categories 585-587 are present with hypertension, assign a code from category 403. A cause and effect relationship is presumed. Therefore, renal failure with hypertension is coded as hypertensive renal disease. [*Coding Clinic*, 3Q, '90, 3, effective with discharges July 15, 1990]

AHA CC: When a causal relationship is stated (due to hypertension) or implied (hypertensive) in regard to certain heart conditions (428.0-428.9, 429.0-429.3, 429.8, 429.9), assign only a code from category 402. Code separately these same heart conditions with hypertension but without a stated causal relationship. The principal diagnosis is chosen based on the circumstances of the admission. [*Coding Clinic*, 3Q, '90, 3, effective with discharges July 15, 1990]

AHA CC: Use category 401 when the physician documents arterial, essential or systemic hypertension. A fourth digit is added to this category to indicate that the hypertension is malignant (.0), benign (.1), or unspecified (.9). If the physician does not document in the medical record the stage of hypertension, malignant or benign, the fourth digit of '9' must be used. [*Coding Clinic*, 3Q, '90, 3, effective with discharges July 15, 1990]

AHA CC: Assign codes 428.0 and 401.9 if the physician states that the patient has congestive heart failure and hypertension, but does not indicate that the congestive heart failure is due to hypertension. Before assigning these codes it is best to check with the physician to verify that the patient does not have hypertensive heart disease with congestive heart failure, 401.91, a determination that can be made only by the physician. [*Coding Clinic*, 2Q, '89, 12, effective with discharges July 31, 1989]

AHA CC: Use category 405 for secondary hypertension. Code first the underlying cause, and then the secondary hypertension. [*Coding Clinic*, J-A, '84, 11]

AHA CC: When documentation supports an acute postoperative hypertension, verify with the physician as to whether this is hypertension, as opposed to elevated blood pressure without a diagnosis of hypertension. This type of hypertension is often of nonspecific origin, short-lived and treated with antihypertensive drugs. It may or may not resolve spontaneously as the patient convalesces. Use code 401.1. [*Coding Clinic*, J-A, '84, 11]

AHA CC: Use category 404 for hypertensive heart and renal disease, cardiorenal disease or hypertensive heart disease with nephrosclerosis. When the physician documents the diagnosis of hypertensive cardiovascular and renal disease or hypertensive cardiovascular renal disease, review the medical record for any specific references to the presence of coronary arteriosclerosis, angina pectoris, or chronic coronary insufficiency that would require additional coding. As stated above, cardiovascular hypertension may imply the presence of a coronary artery disease. [*Coding Clinic*, J-A, '84, 11]

402.91   Hypertensive heart disease with heart failure (continued)   DRG 127

AHA CC: Use category 403 for hypertensive renal disease. Hypertension with arteriosclerosis of the kidney, nephrosclerosis, and renal sclerosis refer to structural changes in the arterioles and not in the renal artery. If the physician documented the diagnosis of hypertension and renal failure, ascertain from the physician whether the patient has malignant or accelerated hypertension. Renal failure is not common in hypertensive renal disease until the hypertension has become malignant or accelerated. For example:

- Use code 403.1x when the physician documents hypertensive nephropathy, benign.
- Use code 403.0x when the physician documents hypertensive nephroangiosclerosis.
- Use code 403.01 when the physician documents accelerated hypertension with renal failure. [Coding Clinic, J-A, '84, 11]

AHA CC: Use category 402 for hypertensive heart disease, including that with mention of interstitial, chronic or fibroid myocarditis, with mention of degenerative myocardium and with mention of hyperkinetic heart or cardiomegaly. A fifth-digit subclassification exists to classify casein which congestive heart failure has occurred. If the physician documents the diagnosis of hypertensive cardiovascular disease, use a code from 402.00-402.91. In addition, look for documentation of any mention of coronary arteriosclerosis, angina pectoris, or chronic myocardial ischemia and, if present, code them as well. The use of this clinical diagnosis, hypertensive cardiovascular disease, may include myocardial ischemic conditions that need to be coded separately. For example

- Use code 402.11 when the physician documents hypertensive heart disease, benign, with left ventricular failure.
- Use codes 402.11 and 573.0 when the physician documents hypertensive heart disease, benign, with right and left heart failure and passive congestion of liver.
- Use codes 410.1x, 402.11 and 414.0x when the physician documents acute anterior myocardial infarction with benign hypertensive cardiovascular disease and coronary arteriosclerosis.
- Use code 402.01 when the physician documents congestive heart failure and hypertensive cardiovascular disease with papilledema findings. [Coding Clinic, J-A, '84, 11]

AHA CC: Use category 401 when the physician documents systolic hypertension, i.e., a systolic pressure above 1160 mm Hg but with a diastolic pressure less than 95 mm Hg. This type of hypertension is more common in the elderly, and usually reflects loss of elasticity of the major vessels and atherosclerosis of the central aorta and its branches. A synonymous term is 'arteriosclerotic hypertension'of the elderly. [Coding Clinic, J-A, '84, 11]

AHA CC: Use category 401 for essential hypertension, hypertensive vascular disease and labile hypertension. When hypertension hastens atherosclerosis and both are documented by the physician in the medical record and listed in the final diagnostic statement, code both conditions. [Coding Clinic, J-A, '84, 11]

AHA CC: Use the 401-405 category code series to classify hypertension due to unknown cause (401-404) and hypertension due to an underlying cause (405). Hypertension existing before or arising during pregnancy is classified in the pregnancy chapter of ICD-9-CM. [Coding Clinic, J-A, '84, 11]

AHA CC: The use of the term 'uncontrolled' hypertension does not necessarily indicate malignant hypertension. This descriptor may be used by the physician when there is failure of diuretics to control hypertension and there is a need for the patient to be placed on antihypertensive drugs, such as beta-blockers. Code hypertension described as uncontrolled according to its type and nature. [Coding Clinic, J-A, '84, 11]

AHA CC: Subcategories in ICD-9-CM designated for systemic hypertension indicate the nature of hypertension, i.e., benign, malignant, or unspecified. Attributes of malignant hypertension include rapidly rising blood pressure, usually in excess of 140 mm Hg diastolic, with findings of visual impairment and symptoms or signs of progressive cardiac failure. If the patient does not receive adequate treatment, severe visual loss with hemorrhage, exudates and papilledema may ensue, and death may occur due to uremia, cardiac failure or cerebral hemorrhage. The presence of papilledema

402.91   Hypertensive heart disease with heart failure (continued)   DRG 127

with hypertension by definition is coded to malignant hypertension. Assign the fourth digit '9' when the physician does not document the primary or secondary hypertension as either benign or malignant. Educate the medical staff of the need for stating the hypertension as being either benign or malignant. [Coding Clinic, J-A, '84, 11]

AHA CC: The physician will make a diagnosis of hypertension on a series of blood pressure readings rather than on an isolated reading due to the fact that blood pressures can vary from one occasion of measurement to another. Use code 796.2 to represent an elevated blood pressure reading. A patient may have elevated blood pressure because of emotional factors causing stress, or age. However, if the physician has documented hypertension, the elevated blood pressure may relate to poor toleration of a stressful situation that affects therapy directed at maintaining an acceptable blood pressure level. The term 'transient' hypertension also requires further clarification prior to coding. Check with the physician to determine whether he or she is referring to an established hypertension or to an elevated blood pressure without the diagnosis of hypertension. [Coding Clinic, J-A, '84, 11]

DOC: Use code 402.91 when the physician documents hypertensive cardiomegaly, cardiopathy, cardiovascular disease, heart disease with congestive heart failure.

DOC: Do not assign code 402.91 when the physician does not document a cause and effect relationship between certain heart conditions (428.0-428.9, 429.0-429.3, 429.8, 429.9) and the hypertension. Code these heart conditions and the hypertension separately.

428.0   Congestive heart failure, unspecified   DRG 127

See standards on page 577.

411.1   Intermediate coronary syndrome   DRG 140

AHA CC: Use code 411.1 when the physician documents accelerated angina. [Coding Clinic, 1Q, '03, 50]

AHA CC: When a patient is admitted with severe chest pain resembling an acute MI, but after TPA administration the physician documents that the patient does not demonstrate any myocardial damage or the acute myocardial infarction has been averted use code 411.1. When diagnostic procedures, which may identify coronary artery disease as the underlying cause are not performed, code 411.1 is the correct principal diagnosis in this situation. Code 411.1 includes aborted or impending myocardial infarction and should not be assigned when an infarction has occurred. [Coding Clinic, 2Q, '01, 7]

AHA CC: When a patient is admitted for unstable angina, coronary artery disease (CAD) may be assigned as the principal diagnosis even when a diagnostic test establishing a diagnosis of CAD is not performed during the patient's stay. The physician must document in the medical record that the CAD is the underlying cause of the unstable angina. The physician may remark in the record that the patient has a known history of CAD. The physician would not need to perform additional testing to re-establish the underlying cause when patients are admitted for treatment of unstable angina. Sequence code 411.1 as the principal diagnosis and code 414.0x as the secondary diagnosis when the physician has not documented the underlying cause of the unstable angina to be CAD. [Coding Clinic, 2Q, '94, 15, effective with discharges April 1, 1994, and Coding Clinic, 3Q, '97, 15, effective with discharges September 1, 1998]

AHA CC: In order to code 'postinfarction angina,' the physician must document the type of angina the patient is experiencing. For example, documentation of 'unstable angina' results in the code assignment of 411.1. When 'stable angina' is documented or the type of angina is not further specified, it should be coded to 413.9. [Coding Clinic, 2Q, '95, 19, effective with discharges April 15, 1995]

411.1   Intermediate coronary syndrome (continued)   DRG 140

AHA CC: As described in *Coding Clinic*, angina pectoris is a condition represented by chest pain or discomfort, generally exacerbated by exertion and relieved by medication (nitroglycerin), rest, and/ or treatment of the heart disease. Use code 411.1 when the physician documents pre-infarction, unstable, initial onset or crescendo angina. For this type of angina, the patient's pain is of longer duration and/or happens more often than stable angina. It is difficult to control unstable angina with medication and the angina can develop into an acute myocardial infarction (AMI). An underlying cardiac condition such as coronary arteriosclerosis or aortic stenosis causes the patient to have angina. The physician also may document ischemic heart disease or CAD that can occur because of an insufficient blood flow caused by the narrowing of the coronary arteries due to the formation of atherosclerotic plaque. The patient may undergo additional diagnostic studies such as cardiac catheterization, or treatment to arrest the disease process, such as percutaneous transluminal coronary angioplasty of coronary artery bypass graft (CABG).

Assign code 413.9 for stable forms of angina or angina of effort. This type of angina occurs in patients at certain levels of exertion or stress and is relieved in an expected way with rest or nitroglycerin. Hospitalization is usually not required. When the diagnosis documented is 'angina' without further qualification, the physician should be contacted so that he or she may specify the type of angina. If a patient is hospitalized, it would usually be for preinfarctional or unstable angina. However, without further qualification by the physician, code 'angina' to 413.9.

Code the underlying cause of the angina as the principal diagnosis when a patient is admitted with angina and diagnostic procedure(s) are carried out, showing that the angina was caused by coronary atherosclerosis, aortic stenosis or some other heart disease. Code an AMI as the principal diagnosis when a patient is admitted with symptomatic angina that develops into an AMI. *Do not* assign an additional code for the angina.

Use the appropriate code from category 411 when the physician documents in the medical record a diagnosis of postmyocardial infarction angina or 'postinfarction angina.' Postinfarction angina is not the same as simple angina pectoris or unstable angina. A patient with postinfarction angina is at higher risk and requires more intensive treatment. If the patient's angina leads to myocardial infarction, do not assign a code for the angina. [*Coding Clinic*, 4Q, '94, 55, effective with discharges October 1, 1994]

AHA CC: The following examples illustrate proper sequencing of the diagnoses of angina and coronary heart disease: [*Coding Clinic*, Volume 10, Number 5, '93, 17, effective October 1, 1993. This replaces the advice published in the third quarter 1990 edition of *Coding Clinic*.]

- The patient was admitted due to progressive episodes of chest pain consistent with crescendo angina. History includes chronic coronary insufficiency and previous myocardial infarctions six years ago. Treatment during the hospitalization included p.o. calcium blockers. At discharge, the patient was pain-free. No complications arose during the hospitalization and no other diagnostic or therapeutic interventions were performed. Assign code 411.1 as the principal diagnosis since this was the condition after study that necessitated admission to the hospital.
- The reason for admission was cardiac catheterization. The patient's diagnosis on admission was unstable angina. The cardiac catheterization showed significant triple-vessel atherosclerotic heart disease. A three-vessel aortocoronary artery bypass was performed. Assign code 414.0x as the principal diagnosis since this was the condition after study that necessitated admission to the hospital. Assign an additional code for the unstable angina as a secondary diagnosis.
- The reason for admission was a combined right and left heart cardiac catheterization. The patient's diagnosis on admission was angina. The cardiac catheterization showed significant atherosclerotic heart disease. Triple coronary artery bypass surgery was recommended. No surgery was performed prior to discharge. Later, the patient was readmitted and surgery was performed on the second admission. The patient received his antianginal medication also during this stay. Assign code 414.0x as the principal diagnosis for both admissions since this is the condition that necessitated admission to the hospital. Assign code 413.9 as an additional diagnosis.
- The reason for admission was unstable angina. While in the hospital, the patient was given intravenous nitrate therapy. After stabilization, the patient underwent a diagnostic cardiac

411.1   Intermediate coronary syndrome (continued)   DRG 140

catheterization. Results showed atherosclerotic heart disease. Before discharge, the patient was weaned off the nitroglycerin drip and placed on intensified antianginal therapy. The patient was discharged symptom-free without need for further therapeutic interventions. Assign code 414.0x as the principal diagnosis since this condition led to the admission.

- The reason for admission was severe crescendo angina. The physician tried to stabilize the patient by performing an emergency single-vessel PTCA with administration of thrombolytic agent. However, an acute myocardial infarction of the inferolateral wall occurred. Assign code 410.21 as the principal diagnosis.

- As an outpatient, an asymptomatic patient underwent an exercise stress test and was believed to have ischemic heart disease based on significant ST depression during peak exercise. The reason for admission was cardiac catheterization. Results showed an underlying significant coronary atherosclerosis, thus explaining his abnormal stress test. Treatment included medications. At discharge, the patient was symptom-free and will be followed up as an outpatient. Assign code 414.0x as the principal diagnosis since the patient was admitted without significant anginal symptoms and coronary atherosclerosis is the condition after study that necessitated admission to the hospital.

- As an outpatient, a patient underwent an exercise stress test as part of a routine exercise prescription. The study was abnormal at peak exercise. The patient was admitted for cardiac catheterization. Results were within normal limits. The patient was symptom-free during the hospitalization. Assign code V71.7 as the principal diagnosis as the physician concluded that no cardiac disease was revealed.

- The reason for admission was unstable angina. The patient had been previously hospitalized for an acute myocardial infarction of the anterolateral wall six weeks earlier. During the patient's stay, his angina stabilized and further infarction was avoided. Assign code 411.1 as the principal diagnosis and code 410.02 as a secondary diagnosis.

- The reason for admission was preinfarctional angina. After stabilization, the patient was transferred for further evaluation to a regional hospital specializing in cardiac care. Assign code 411.1 as the principal diagnosis. During the patient's stay at the regional hospital, he was maintained on antianginal medications and cardiac catheterization was performed. Results showed coronary atherosclerosis. A CABG was performed. During the stay, the patient had no further anginal episodes. Assign code 414.0 as the principal diagnosis and code 411.1 as a secondary diagnosis.

- Assign code 413.9 as the principal diagnosis for the following scenario: A patient with chest pain visited the physician at his office. After examination, the physician's diagnosis was angina and he decided to admit the patient. Treatment at the hospital consisted of antianginal medications. During the stay, the patient had no further anginal episodes.

AHA CC: *Do not* assign code 411.1 with code 411.8x. In addition, do not use a code from category 411, except code 411.0, when infarction has occurred. This is different than the example given in the third quarter 1989 issue of *Coding Clinic*, page 5. [*Coding Clinic*, 1Q, '91, 14, effective with discharges January 1, 1991, and *Coding Clinic*, 3Q, '91, 24]

AHA CC: Use code 411.1 when the physician documents the patient's diagnosis as unstable angina, crescendo angina, preinfarction angina, or impending myocardial infarction. The patient's admission and treatment is for unstable angina without documentation of infarction, occlusion, or thrombosis. If the patient's angina leads to myocardial infarction, do not assign a code for the angina. Use the appropriate code from category 410. [*Coding Clinic*, 1Q, '91, 14, effective with discharges January 1, 1991, and *Coding Clinic*, 3Q, '91, 24]

AHA CC: Included in code 411.1 are preinfarction angina, crescendo angina, unstable angina or initial onset angina. For this type of angina, the patient experiences pain that lasts longer and/or occurs more frequently. It is also more resistant to an antianginal program and often results in an acute myocardial infarction. Cardiac catheterization or other treatment to interrupt the occlusion process can occur during an inpatient stay. Angina is one symptom of coronary or ischemic heartdisease, a disorder resulting from insufficient blood flow secondary to narrowing of the coronary arteries due to atherosclerosis. [*Coding Clinic*, 3Q, '90, 6, effective with discharges July 15, 1990]

411.1   Intermediate coronary syndrome (continued)   DRG 140

AHA CC: Use code 411.1 as the principal diagnosis when the physician documentation states that the patient, after undergoing dialysis on an outpatient basis, was admitted to the hospital for heartburn (diagnosed by the cardiologist as unstable angina). *Do not* code the unstable angina as a complication of dialysis unless the cardiologist specifically stated it as such. [*Coding Clinic*, 4Q, '89, 10, effective with discharges January 2, 1989]

AHA CC: Use code 411.81 as the principal diagnosis and codes 411.1 and 414.0x as secondary diagnoses for the following scenario: A patient admitted for coronary occlusion with impending acute myocardial infarction was given TPA to ward off an infarction. Severe coronary arteriosclerosis is also listed as a diagnosis. [*Coding Clinic*, 3Q, '89, 4, effective with discharges October 15, 1989]

AHA CC: Assign CAD as the principal diagnosis in cases where the physician has documented the CAD as the underlying cause of the unstable angina (the reason for the admission) even if a diagnostic test has not been performed during the admission for the diagnosis of coronary artery disease. Documentation of previous testing to confirm the presence of CAD would establish the connection between the CAD and unstable angina. Review the medical record carefully because the physician may document that the angina is due to another condition (i.e., stenosis). In this case, the code for the documented underlying condition is assigned as the principal diagnosis. The angina would be coded secondarily. [*Coding Clinic*, 2Q, '97, 13, effective with discharges May 1, 1997]

AHA CC: Assign code 414.01 as the principal diagnosis when the physician has documented the diagnosis of unstable angina secondary to coronary artery disease of the native vessels. The physician also notes that the CAD is in part due to secondhand tobacco smoke exposure. Additional codes to assign are 411.1 and E869.4. [*Coding Clinic*, 2Q, '96, 10, effective with discharges May 1, 1996 and *Coding Clinic*, 3Q, '97, 15, effective with discharges September 1, 1998]

AHA CC: Assign the appropriate code from category 411, Other acute andsubacute forms of ischemic heart disease, to identify postmyocardial infarction angina. Do not use the codes from categories 410, Acute myocardial infarction unless the angina leads to a myocardial infarction.. [*Coding Clinic*, 4Q, '94, 55, effective with discharges October 1, 1994]

AHA CC: If a patient is admitted with unstable angina and a heart catheterization is done and a definitive diagnosis of CAD is made, assign code 414.0x as the principal diagnosis. Angina is a symptom and should not be coded when a related definitive diagnosis has been established. The known diagnosis rather than a symptom should be coded. However, the physician must state the cause and effect relationship between the angina and underlying coronary atherosclerosis or CAD. Sequence the angina as the principal diagnosis when the cause of the angina is not established or documented. When the physician documents the cause of the angina, list that cause (e.g., CAD) as principal. Since the CAD caused the symptom, angina, the definition of principal diagnosis is met. [*Coding Clinic*, 4Q, '93, 44, effective with discharges September 3, 1993]

AHA CC: Use code 411.81 when the physician's documentation in the medical record indicates clinical evidence of coronary occlusion or thrombosis, or the attending physician includes mention of either of these conditions in the diagnostic statement and the patient does not advance to acute myocardial infarction. Today, treatment with thrombolytic agents may dissolve a developing clot so the infarction does not occur although the patient may sustain occlusion or thrombosis. [*Coding Clinic*, 1Q, '91, 14, effective with discharges January 1, 1991, and *Coding Clinic*, 3Q, '91, 24]

AHA CC: Depending on the circumstances of the admission and the documentation in the medical record, angina may be listed as the principal diagnosis, a secondary diagnosis, or not at all. Documentation of chest pain or discomfort, generally exacerbated by exertion and relieved by medication (nitroglycerin) and/or rest are representative of angina pectoris. If 'angina'is listed in the discharge summary without greater specification, check with the physician and have him or her specify the form of angina. [*Coding Clinic*, 3Q, '90, 6, effective with discharges July 15, 1990]

AHA CC: Included in code 413.9 are stable forms of angina and excluded is preinfarctional angina. For this type of angina, the anginal type of chest pain is at the same level of exertion or stress and is usually relieved in a predictable fashion with rest or nitroglycerin. Treatment of stable angina is on an outpatient basis unless the patient is being admitted for diagnostic studies to determine the

411.1   Intermediate coronary syndrome (continued)   **DRG 140**

extent of coronary artery disease. Assign the underlying cause of the angina, as determined by the diagnostic study, as the principal diagnosis. [*Coding Clinic*, 3Q, '90, 6, effective with discharges July 15, 1990]

AHA CC: When the reason for admission is the symptomatic angina, it is usually assigned as the principal diagnosis. However, if, after study, the patient is found to have an acute myocardial infarction, the AMI is the principal diagnosis and no additional code is assigned for the angina. [*Coding Clinic*, 3Q, '90, 6, effective with discharges July 15, 1990]

AHA CC: Pay careful attention to the reason for hospitalization for those patients who are postmyocardial with a stated duration of 'eight weeks or less.' Admissions or readmissions eight weeks or less from the date of a myocardial infarction do not necessarily constitute a reclassification as acute myocardial infarction. Examples on which code to select for those patients admitted or readmitted eight weeks or less from the time of acute myocardial infarction follow:

- Use the appropriate code from the 410.0-410.8 series if the episode of care is stated to be an extension of the myocardial infarction site, a repeat myocardial infarction, or an infarction of another myocardial site. Code 410.9 should be avoided if possible.
- Use the appropriate code from the 410.0-410.9 series if the diagnosis is stated as an acute ischemia or ischemic attack, postmyocardial infarction.
- In those situations where the patient is admitted six to eight weeks from the time of a myocardial infarction for purposes of diagnostic studies to determine the extent of coronary atherosclerosis or the presence of any sequelae following the myocardial infarction, code the diagnosis as stated by the physician. A physician may admit a patient for diagnostic studies when there are mild or no symptoms of angina, and this may be at six weeks rather than the arbitrary 'eight weeks' stated in the inclusion note under 410 category. For example, a patient admitted for purposes of cardiac catheterization, coronary angiogram, and/or ventriculography may result in a diagnosis of coronary atherosclerosis or arteriosclerosis, vessel disease described as 1, 2, or 3, chronic coronary insufficiency, mitral valve insufficiency with coronary atherosclerosis, ventricular aneurysm, or rupture of papillary muscle. Diagnostic studies after a myocardial infarction are usually carried out to determine how extensive the atherosclerosis is and the need for any operative intervention, such as a coronary bypass. Assign a code from the 410.0-410.9 series if a myocardial infarction occurs during the course of the diagnostic study.
- Use code 411.0 if the postmyocardial diagnosis is pericarditis with friction rub, pericardial effusion, pleurisy, or pleural effusion, and joint pains. [*Coding Clinic*, J-A, '84, 5]

AHA CC: ICD-9-CM directs the coder to use category 410 when the patient's diagnosis is acute ischemia of the coronary artery(ies), heart or myocardium. However, because acute ischemia may not result in a myocardial infarction, the final code assignment depends on the medical record documentation. For example, choose a code from category 411 or 413 when the diagnosis on the medical record is 'acute ischemic (coronary) heart disease' or 'acute myocardial ischemia,' the diagnostic studies show no evidence of a myocardial infarct and the attending physician states or replies that there is no evidence of a myocardial infarction occurring. Ask the physician to clarify the terminology, i.e., which code best represents the patient's condition, 411.1 or 411.8x, or if the reference is to ischemic angina pain classified to category 413. One form of acute myocardial ischemia is unstable angina. Look in the medical record for documentation that the patient received an antithrombolytic agent (streptokinase) during an angiogram or a transluminal (balloon) coronary angioplasty. These procedures may have avoided an infarction. [*Coding Clinic*, J-A, '84, 5]

DOC: Use code 411.1 when the physician documents aborted myocardial infarction

DOC: Use code 411.1 when the physician documents impending infarction

DOC: Use code 411.1 when the physician documents preinfarction angina, preinfarction syndrome, or unstable angina.

DOC: *Do not* use 411.1 when the physician documents angina pectoris. The correct code assignment is 413.9.

411.89 Other acute and subacute forms of ischemic heart disease

AHA CC: Assign the appropriate code from category 411, Other acute and subacute forms of ischemic heart disease, to identify postmyocardial infarction angina. Do not use the codes from categories 410, Acute myocardial infarction unless the angina leads to a myocardial infarction. [*Coding Clinic,* 4Q, '94, 55, effective with discharges October 1, 1994]

AHA CC: Use code 411.81 when the physician's documentation in the medical record indicates clinical evidence of coronary occlusion or thrombosis, or the attending physician includes mention of either of these conditions in the diagnostic statement and the patient does not advance to acute myocardial infarction. Today, treatment with thrombolytic agents may dissolve a developing clot so the infarction does not occur although the patient may sustain occlusion or thrombosis. [*Coding Clinic,* 1Q, '91, 14, effective with discharges January 1, 1991, and *Coding Clinic,* 3Q, '91, 24]

AHA CC: *Do not* assign code 411.1 with code 411.8x. In addition, do not use a code from category 411, except code 411.0, when infarction has occurred. This is different than the example given in the third quarter 1989 issue of *Coding Clinic,* page 5. [*Coding Clinic,* 1Q, '91, 14, effective with discharges January 1, 1991, and *Coding Clinic,* 3Q, '91, 24]

AHA CC: Effective October 1, 1989, category 411 has been revised to include a fifth-digit subclassification to identify coronary embolism or occlusion, without or not resulting in myocardial infarction. [*Coding Clinic,* 3Q, '89, 4, effective with discharges October 15, 1989]

AHA CC: Use code 411.81 as the principal diagnosis and codes 411.1 and 414.0x as secondary diagnoses for the following scenario: A patient admitted for coronary occlusion with impending acute myocardial infarction was given TPA to ward off an infarction. Severe coronary arteriosclerosis is also listed as a diagnosis. [*Coding Clinic,* 3Q, '89, 4, effective with discharges October 15, 1989]

AHA CC: Pay careful attention to the reason for hospitalization for those patients who are postmyocardial with a stated duration of 'eight weeks or less.' Admissions or readmissions eight weeks or less from the date of a myocardial infarction do not necessarily constitute a reclassification as acute myocardial infarction. Examples of which code to select for those patients admitted or readmitted eight weeks or less from the time of acute myocardial infarction follow:

- Use the appropriate code from the 410.0-410.8 series if the episode of care is stated to be an extension of the myocardial infarction site, a repeat myocardial infarction, or an infarction of another myocardial site. Code 410.9x should be avoided if possible.
- Use the appropriate code from the 410.0-410.9 series if the diagnosis is stated as an acute ischemia or ischemic attack, postmyocardial infarction.
- In those situations where the patient is admitted six to eight weeks from the time of a myocardial infarction for purposes of diagnostic studies to determine the extent of coronary atherosclerosis or the presence of any sequelae following the myocardial infarction, code the diagnosis as stated by the physician. A physician may admit a patient for diagnostic studies when there are mild or no symptoms of angina, and this may be at six weeks rather than the arbitrary 'eight weeks' stated in the inclusion note under 410 category. For example, an admission for purposes of cardiac catheterization, coronary angiogram, and/or ventriculography may result in a diagnosis of coronary atherosclerosis or arteriosclerosis, vessel disease described as 1, 2, or 3, chronic coronary insufficiency, mitral valve insufficiency with coronary atherosclerosis, ventricular aneurysm, or rupture of papillary muscle. Diagnostic studies after a myocardial infarction are usually carried out to determine how extensive the atherosclerosis is and the need for any operative intervention, such as a coronary bypass. Assign a code from the 410.0-410.9 series if a myocardial infarction occurs during the course of the diagnostic study.
- Use code 411.0 if the postmyocardial diagnosis is pericarditis with friction rub, pericardial effusion, pleurisy or pleural effusion, and joint pains. [*Coding Clinic,* J-A, '84, 5]
- **AHA CC:** ICD-9-CM directs the coder to use category 410 when the patient's diagnosis is acute ischemia of the coronary artery(ies), heart or myocardium. However, because acute ischemia may not result in a myocardial infarction, the final code assignment depends on the medical record documentation. For example, choose a code from category 411 or 413 when the diagnosis on the medical record is 'acute ischemic (coronary) heart disease' or 'acute myocardial ischemia,' the diagnostic studies show no evidence of a myocardial infarct and the attending physician states or replies that there is no evidence of a myocardialinfarction

411.89   Other acute and subacute forms of ischemic heart disease (continued)

occurring. Ask the physician to clarify the terminology, i.e., which code best represents the patient's condition, 411.1 or 411.8x, or if the reference is to ischemic angina pain classified to category 413. One form of acute myocardial ischemia is unstable angina. Look in the medical record for documentation that the patient received an antithrombolytic agent (streptokinase) during an angiogram or a transluminal (balloon) coronary angioplasty. These procedures may have avoided an infarction. [Coding Clinic, J-A, '84, 5]

DOC: Use code 411.89 when the physician documents (acute) coronary insufficiency or subendocardial ischemia.

DOC: Assign a code from category 410 when the physician documents a diagnosis of acute myocardial ischemia and a myocardial infarction has occurred, and code 411.8x if no infarction is documented. Code 411.81 is used if there is evidence of occlusion or thrombosis; otherwise, assign code 411.89. [Coding Clinic, 3Q, '91, 18, effective with discharges July 1, 1991]

DOC: Use the appropriate code from category 411 when the physician documents in the medical record a diagnosis of postmyocardial infarction angina or 'postinfarction angina.' Postinfarction angina is not the same as simple angina pectoris or unstable angina. A patient with postinfarction angina is at higher risk and requires more intensive treatment. If the patient's angina leads to myocardial infarction, do not assign a code for the angina. [Coding Clinic, 4Q, '94, 55, effective with discharges October 1, 1994]

413.9   Other and unspecified angina pectoris

AHA CC: When the reason for admission is the symptomatic angina, it is usually assigned as the principal diagnosis. However, if, after study, the patient is found to have an acute myocardial infarction, the AMI is the principal diagnosis and no additional code is assigned for the angina. [Coding Clinic, 3Q, '90, 6, effective with discharges July 15, 1990]

The following examples illustrate proper sequencing of the diagnoses of angina and coronary heart disease: [Coding Clinic, volume 10, number 5, '93, 17, effective October 1, 1993. This replaces the advice published in the third quarter 1990 edition of Coding Clinic.]

- The patient was admitted due to progressive episodes of chest pain consistent with crescendo angina. History includes chronic coronary insufficiency and previous myocardial infarctions six years ago. Treatment during the hospitalization included p.o. calcium blockers. At discharge, the patient was pain-free. No complications arose during the hospitalization and no other diagnostic or therapeutic interventions were performed. Assign code 411.1 as the principal diagnosis since this was the condition after study that necessitated admission to the hospital.
- The reason for admission was cardiac catheterization. The patient's diagnosis on admission was unstable angina. The cardiac catheterization showed significant triple-vessel atherosclerotic heart disease. A three-vessel aortocoronary artery bypass was performed. Assign code 414.0x as the principal diagnosis since this was the condition after study that necessitated admission to the hospital. Assign an additional code for the unstable angina as a secondary diagnosis.
- The reason for admission was a combined right and left heart cardiac catheterization. The patient's diagnosis on admission was angina. The cardiac catheterization showed significant atherosclerotic heart disease. Triple coronary artery bypass surgery was recommended. No surgery was performed prior to discharge. Later, the patient was readmitted and surgery was performed on the second admission. The patient received his antianginal medication also during this stay. Assign code 414.0x as the principal diagnosis for both admissions since this is the condition that necessitated admission to the hospital. Assign code 413.9 as an additional diagnosis. patient was discharged symptom-free without need for further therapeutic interventions. Assign code 414.0x as the principal diagnosis since this condition led to the admission.
- The reason for admission was severe crescendo angina. The physician tried to stabilize the patient by performing an emergency single-vessel PTCA with administration of thrombolytic agent. However, an acute myocardial infarction of the inferolateral wall occurred. Assign code

413.9   Other and unspecified angina pectoris (continued)

410.21 as the principal diagnosis.nAs an outpatient, an asymptomatic patient underwent an exercise stress test and was believed to have ischemic heart disease based on significant ST depression during peak exercise. The reason for admission was cardiac catheterization. Results showed an underlying significant coronary atherosclerosis, thus explaining his abnormal stress test. Treatment included medications. At discharge, the patient was symptom-free and will be followed up as an outpatient. Assign code 414.0x as the principal diagnosis since the patient was admitted without significant anginal symptoms and coronary atherosclerosis is the condition after study that necessitated admission to the hospital.

- As an outpatient, a patient underwent an exercise stress test as part of a routine exercise prescription. The study was abnormal at peak exercise. The patient was admitted for cardiac catheterization. Results were within normal limits. The patient was symptom-free during the hospitalization. Assign code V71.7 as the principal diagnosis as the physician concluded that no cardiac disease was revealed.
- The reason for admission was unstable angina. The patient had been previously hospitalized for an acute myocardial infarction of the anterolateral wall six weeks earlier. During the patient's stay, his angina stabilized and further infarction was avoided. Assign code 411.1 as the principal diagnosis and code 410.02 as a secondary diagnosis.
- The reason for admission was preinfarctional angina. After stabilization, the patient was transferred for further evaluation to a regional hospital specializing in cardiac care. Assign code 411.1 as the principal diagnosis. During the patient's stay at the regional hospital, he was maintained on antianginal medications and cardiac catheterization was performed. Results showed coronary atherosclerosis. A CABG was performed. During the stay, the patient had no further anginal episodes. Assign code 414.0 as the principal diagnosis and code 411.1 as a secondary diagnosis.
- Assign code 413.9 as the principal diagnosis for the following scenario: A patient with chest pain visited the physician at his office. After examination, the physician's diagnosis was angina and he decided to admit the patient. Treatment at the hospital consisted of antianginal medications. During the stay, the patient had no further anginal episodes.

AHA CC: Included in code 413.9 are stable forms of angina and excluded is preinfarctional angina. For this type of angina, the anginal type of chest pain is at the same level of exertion or stress and is usually relieved in a predictable fashion with rest or nitroglycerin. Treatment of stable angina is on an outpatient basis unless the patient is being admitted for diagnostic studies to determine the extent of coronary artery disease. Assign the underlying cause of the angina, as determined by the diagnostic study, as the principal diagnosis. [*Coding Clinic*, 3Q, '90, 6, effective with discharges July 15, 1990]

AHA CC: Use code 411.81 as the principal diagnosis if the patient, admitted with severe angina, had a cardiac catheterization that established a diagnosis of coronary artery occlusion, incomplete, and the patient did not suffer an infarction. Assign code 413.9 as an additional diagnosis. [*Coding Clinic*, 3Q, '89, 4, effective with discharges October 15, 1989]

AHA CC: Included in code 411.1 are pre-infarction angina, crescendo angina, unstable angina or initial onset angina. For this type of angina, the patient experiences pain that lasts longer and/or occurs more frequently. It is also more resistant to an antianginal program and often results in an acute myocardial infarction. Cardiac catheterization or other treatment to interrupt the occlusion process can occur during an inpatient stay. Angina is one symptom of coronary or ischemic heart disease, a disorder resulting from insufficient blood flow secondary to narrowing of the coronary arteries due to atherosclerosis. [*Coding Clinic*, 3Q, '90, 6, effective with discharges July 15, 1990]

AHA CC: Depending on the circumstances of the admission and the documentation in the medical record, angina may be listed as the principal diagnosis, a secondary diagnosis, or not at all. Documentation of chest pain or discomfort, generally exacerbated by exertion and relieved by medication (nitroglycerin) and/or rest, is representative of angina pectoris. If 'angina' is listed in the discharge summary without greater specification, check with the physician and have him or her specify the form of angina. [*Coding Clinic*, 3Q, '90, 6, effective with discharges July 15, 1990]

413.9   Other and unspecified angina pectoris (continued)

AHA CC: *Do not* use a code describing a symptom when a related definitive diagnosis has been established. [*Coding Clinic,* 2Q, '90, 3, effective with discharges April 1, 1990]

AHA CC: *Do not* use a code describing a symptom, sign or ill-defined condition from Chapter 16 of ICD-9-CM as the principal diagnosis when a related definitive diagnosis has been established. [*Coding Clinic,* 2Q, '90, 3, effective with discharges April 1, 1990]

AHA CC: Use the code for the symptom as the principal diagnosis if it is followed by contrasting/comparative diagnoses. The contrasting/comparative diagnoses are coded secondarily. [*Coding Clinic,* 2Q, '90, 3, effective with discharges April 1, 1990]

AHA CC: Pay careful attention to the reason for hospitalization for those patients who are postmyocardial with a stated duration of 'eight weeks or less.' Admissions or readmissions eight weeks or less from the date of a myocardial infarction do not necessarily constitute a reclassification as acute myocardial infarction. Examples of which code to select for those patients admitted or readmitted eight weeks or less from the time of acute myocardial infarction follow:

- Use the appropriate code from the 410.0-410.8 series if the episode of care is stated to be an extension of the myocardial infarction site, a repeat myocardial infarction, or an infarction of another myocardial site. Code 410.9 should be avoided if possible.
- Use the appropriate code from the 410.0-410.9 series if the diagnosis is stated as an acute ischemia or ischemic attack, postmyocardial infarction.
- In those situations where the patient is admitted six to eight weeks from the time of a myocardial infarction for purposes of diagnostic studies to determine the extent of coronary atherosclerosis or the presence of any sequelae following the myocardial infarction, code the diagnosis as stated by the physician. A physician may admit a patient for diagnostic studies when there are mild or no symptoms of angina, and this may be at six weeks rather than the arbitrary 'eight weeks' stated in the inclusion note under category 410. For example, an admission for purposes of cardiac catheterization, coronary angiogram, and/or ventriculography may result in a diagnosis of coronary atherosclerosis or arteriosclerosis, vessel disease described as 1, 2, or 3, chronic coronary insufficiency, mitral valve insufficiency with coronary atherosclerosis, ventricular aneurysm, or rupture of papillary muscle. Diagnostic studies after a myocardial infarction are usually carried out to determine how extensive the atherosclerosis is and the need for any operative intervention, such as a coronary bypass. Assign a code from the 410.0-410.9 series if a myocardial infarction occurs during the course of the diagnostic study.
- Use code 411.0 if the postmyocardial diagnosis is pericarditis with friction rub, pericardial effusion, pleurisy or pleural effusion, and joint pains. [*Coding Clinic,* J-A, '84, 5]

AHA CC: ICD-9-CM directs the coder to use category 410 when the patient's diagnosis is acute ischemia of the coronary artery(ies), heart or myocardium. However, because acute ischemia may not result in a myocardial infarction, the final code assignment depends on the medical record documentation. For example, choose a code from category 411 or 413 when the diagnosis on the medical record is 'acute ischemic (coronary) heart disease' or 'acute myocardial ischemia,' the diagnostic studies show no evidence of a myocardial infarct and the attending physician states or replies that there is no evidence of a myocardial infarction occurring. Ask the physician to clarify the terminology, i.e., which code best represents the patient's condition, 411.1 or 411.8x, or if the reference is to ischemic angina pain classified to category 413. One form of acute myocardial ischemia is unstable angina. Look in the medical record for documentation that the patient received an antithrombolytic agent (streptokinase) during an angiogram or a transluminal (balloon) coronary angioplasty. These procedures may have avoided an infarction. [*Coding Clinic,* J-A, '84, 5]

AHA CC: Use code 413.9 and 414.8 to describe a patient with a diagnosis of stable angina and eight or more weeks postmyocardial infarction. [*Coding Clinic,* J-A, '84]

DOC: Use code 413.9 when the physician documents angina pectoris, angina of effort, anginal syndrome, or sternocardia.

DOC: *Do not* use code 413.9 when the physician documents preinfarction angina. The correct code is 411.1.

DRG 130 Peripheral Vascular Disorders with CC
DRG 128 Deep Vein Thrombophlebitis

Issue

The coding of thrombophlebitis and thrombosis is problematic because physician documentation may be unclear as to whether the patient has deep vein thrombosis (DVT) or thrombophlebitis of the deep veins, and because of the complexity of the ICD-9-CM diagnosis codes and coding guidelines.

Most Common Diagnosis Codes

DRG 130
- 453.8, Other venous embolism and thrombosis of other specified sites

DRG 128
- 451.11, Phlebitis and thrombophlebitis of femoral vein
- 451.19, Phlebitis and thrombophlebitis of other deep vessels of lower extremities
- 451.2, Phlebitis and thrombophlebitis of lower extremities

Coding and Documentation Guidelines

453.8 Other venous embolism and thrombosis	DRG 130

AHA CC: When the medical record describes conditions associated with phlebitis (swelling, erythema, pain and induration), but the physician lists only the diagnosis of deep vein thrombosis (DVT), further clarification by the physician is necessary before coding. The acute condition usually has associated inflammation leading to thrombophlebitis. Often DVT is synonymous with thrombophlebitis. A physician statement of only DVT as a diagnosis with documentation of conditions associated with thrombophlebitis requires verification that both conditions are present. If so documented, only a code from category 451, phlebitis and thrombophlebitis, is assigned. An excludes note was added, effective October 1, 1991, under category 453, directing the coder to assign only a code from category 451. However, if the physician states that only deep vein thrombosis is present, assign code 453.8. [*Coding Clinic,* 1Q, '92, 16, effective with discharges January 1, 1992]

AHA CC: Assign only code 451.1x when the diagnostic statement includes both thrombosis and thrombophlebitis of the deep veins of the leg. Thrombophlebitis includes both thrombosis, the formation of a clot in a blood vessel, and phlebitis, the inflammation of the lining of a vein. [*Coding Clinic,* 3Q, '91, 16, effective with discharges July 1, 1991]

DOC: Use code 453.8 when the physician documents thrombosis of a vein other than the cerebral, coronary, intracranial venous sinus, portal, precerebral, mesenteric, pulmonary, hepatic, vena cava or renal vein; femoral thrombosis; jugular (bulb) thrombosis; or leg (deep) (superficial) (vessels) thrombosis.

451.11 Phlebitis and thrombophlebitis of femoral vein	DRG 128

AHA CC: Assign only code 451.1x when the diagnostic statement includes both thrombosis and thrombophlebitis of the deep veins of the leg. Thrombophlebitis includes both thrombosis, the formation of a clot in a blood vessel, and phlebitis, the inflammation of the lining of a vein. [*Coding Clinic,* 3Q, '91, 16, effective with discharges July 1, 1991]

AHA CC: When the medical record describes conditions associated with phlebitis (swelling, erythema, pain and induration), but the physician lists only the diagnosis of deep vein thrombosis (DVT), further clarification by the physician is necessary before coding. The acute condition usually has associated inflammation leading to thrombophlebitis. Often, DVT is synonymous with

451.11   Phlebitis and thrombophlebitis of femoral vein (continued)   DRG 128

thrombophlebitis. A physician statement of only DVT as a diagnosis with documentation of conditions associated with thrombophlebitis requires verification that both conditions are present. If so documented, only a code from category 451, phlebitis and thrombophlebitis, is assigned. An excludes note was added, effective October 1, 1991, under category 453, directing the coder to assign only a code from category 451. However, if the physician states that only deep vein thrombosis is present, assign code 453.8. [*Coding Clinic*, 1Q, '92, 16, effective with discharges January 1, 1992]

DOC: Use code 451.11 when the physician documents thrombophlebitis of the femoral vein, phlebitis of the femoral vein, endophlebitis of the femoral vein, inflammation of the femoral vein, periphlebitis of the femoral vein, or suppurative phlebitis of the femoral vein.

451.19   Phlebitis and thrombophlebitis of deep vessels of lower extremity   DRG 128

AHA CC: When the medical record describes conditions associated with phlebitis (swelling, erythema, pain and induration), but the physician lists only the diagnosis of deep vein thrombosis (DVT), further clarification by the physician is necessary before coding. The acute condition usually has associated inflammation leading to thrombophlebitis. Often DVT is synonymous with thrombophlebitis. A physician statement of only DVT as a diagnosis with documentation of conditions associated with thrombophlebitis requires verification that both conditions are present. If so documented, only a code from category 451, phlebitis and thrombophlebitis, is assigned. An excludes note was added, effective October 1, 1991, under category 453, directing the coder to assign only a code from category 451. However, if the physician states that only deep vein thrombosis is present, assign code 453.8. [*Coding Clinic,* 1Q, '92, 16, effective with discharges January 1, 1992]

AHA CC: Assign only code 451.1x when the diagnostic statement includes both thrombosis and thrombophlebitis of the deep veins of the leg. Thrombophlebitis includes both thrombosis, the formation of a clot in a blood vessel, and phlebitis, the inflammation of the lining of a vein. [*Coding Clinic*, 3Q, '91, 16, effective with discharges July 1, 1991]

DOC: Use code 451.19 when the physician documents thrombophlebitis of the femoropopliteal, popliteal or tibial vein; phlebitis of the femoropopliteal, popliteal or tibial vein; endophlebitis of the femoropopliteal, popliteal or tibial vein; inflammation of the femoropopliteal, popliteal or tibial vein; periphlebitis of the femoropopliteal, popliteal or tibial vein; or suppurative phlebitis of the femoropopliteal, popliteal or tibial vein.

AHA CC: When the medical record describes conditions associated with phlebitis (swelling, erythema, pain and induration), but the physician lists only the diagnosis of deep vein thrombosis (DVT), further clarification by the physician is necessary before coding. The acute condition usually has associated inflammation leading to thrombophlebitis. Often DVT is synonymous with thrombophlebitis. A physician statement of only DVT as a diagnosis with documentation of conditions associated with thrombophlebitis requires verification that both conditions are present. If so documented, only a code from category 451, phlebitis and thrombophlebitis, is assigned. An excludes note was added, effective October 1, 1991, under category 453, directing the coder to assign only a code from category 451. However, if the physician states that only deep vein thrombosis is present, assign code 453.8. [*Coding Clinic,* 1Q, '92, 16, effective with discharges January 1, 1992]

451.2   Phlebitis and thrombophlebitis of lower extremities   DRG 128

AHA CC: Assign only code 451.1x when the diagnostic statement includes both thrombosis and thrombophlebitis of the deep veins of the leg. Thrombophlebitis includes both thrombosis, the formation of a clot in a blood vessel, and phlebitis, the inflammation of the lining of a vein. [*Coding Clinic*, 3Q, '91, 16, effective with discharges July 1, 1991]

DOC: Use code 451.2 when the physician documents thrombophlebitis of the lower extremities, phlebitis of the lower extremities, endophlebitis of the lower extremities, inflammation of the lower extremities, periphlebitis of the lower extremities, or suppurative phlebitis of the lower extremities.

Targeted DRG Listing

DRG 132 Atherosclerosis with CC

DRG 140   Angina Pectoris

Issue

The coding of coronary atherosclerosis and other acute and subacute forms of ischemic heart disease is problematic because physician documentation may be unclear as to whether the patient is experiencing an acute episode or has a chronic form of heart disease making it difficult to determine the principal diagnosis, and because of the complexity of the ICD-9-CM diagnosis codes and coding guidelines.

Most Common Diagnosis Codes

DRG 132
- 414.00, Coronary atherosclerosis of unspecified type of vessel, native or graft
- 414.01, Coronary atherosclerosis of native coronary artery

DRG 140
- 411.1, Intermediate coronary syndrome
- 411.89, Other acute and subacute forms of ischemic heart disease
- 413.9, Angina pectoris

Coding and Documentation Guidelines

414.00   Coronary atherosclerosis of unspecified type of vessel,   DRG 132
native or graft

AHA CC: Assign code 414.00 for the patient with coronary artery disease who had a CABG done years earlier and whose medical record does not specify which vessel is affected by the CAD. *Do not* assign code 414.01 to show the native artery bypassed earlier unless the record supported the current existence of CAD in a native coronary vessel. Use code 414.05 if the physician confirmed that CAD had developed over the previous bypass graft. Also, do not assign CAD of bypass graft based solely on the fact that the patient has atherosclerosis and a history of bypass surgery. [*Coding Clinic*, 3Q, '97, 15, effective with discharges August 1, 1997]

AHA CC: Effective October 1, 1994, fifth digits were added for subcategory code 414.0 to allow for a distinction between a disease process that occurs to a native coronary artery and one affecting a bypass graft. Assign code 414.00 if the physician documents coronary atherosclerosis in the medical record but does not indicate whether this is a native vessel or a graft. Assign code 414.05 if the physician documents in the medical record the diagnosis of coronary atherosclerosis of bypass graft with a patient history of CABG and no further documentation on the bypass graft is available. [*Coding Clinic*, 4Q, '96, 31, effective with discharges October 1, 1996]

AHA CC: Prior to October 1, 1994, assign code 996.03 for the diagnosis of reocclusion of a graft, both acute and delayed graft closure. With discharges on or after October 1, 1994, new codes provide for the differentiation of a disease process that occurs to a native body part and one affecting a bypass graft for atherosclerosis of the coronary arteries as well as the peripheral arteries. Assign the new codes based on the specific vessel in which the atherosclerosis has been found and is documented. *Do not* assume because the patient has atherosclerosis and a history of bypass surgery that they are related. Use code 414.00 to identify atherosclerosis of internal mammary bypass grafts. [*Coding Clinic*, 4Q, '94, 49, effective with discharges October 1, 1994]

414.00 Coronary atherosclerosis of unspecified type of vessel, native or graft (continued)   DRG 132

As described in *Coding Clinic,* angina pectoris is a condition represented by chest pain or discomfort, generally exacerbated by exertion and relieved by medications (nitroglycerin), rest, and/or treatment of the heart disease. Use code 411.1 when the physician documents preinfarction, unstable, initial onset or crescendo angina. For this type of angina, the patient's pain is of longer duration and/or happens more often than stable angina. It is difficult to control unstable angina with medication and the angina can develop into an acute myocardial infarction (AMI). An underlying cardiac condition such as coronary arteriosclerosis or aortic stenosis causes the patient to have angina. The physician also may document ischemic heart disease or CAD that can occur because of an insufficient blood flow caused by the narrowing of the coronary arteries due to the formation of atherosclerotic plaque. The patient may undergo additional diagnostic studies, such as cardiac catheterization, or treatment to arrest the disease process, such as percutaneous transluminal coronary angioplasty of coronary artery bypass graft (CABG).

Assign code 413.9 for stable forms of angina or angina of effort. This type of angina occurs in patients at certain levels of exertion or stress and is relieved in an expected way with rest or nitroglycerin. Hospitalization is usually not required.

When the diagnosis documented is 'angina' without further qualification, the physician should be contacted so that he or she may specify the type of angina. If a patient is hospitalized, it would usually be for preinfarctional or unstable angina. However, without further qualification by the physician, code 'angina' to 413.9.

Code the underlying cause of the angina as the principal diagnosis when a patient is admitted with angina and diagnostic procedure(s) are carried out, showing that the angina was caused by coronary atherosclerosis, aortic stenosis or some other heart disease.

Code an AMI as the principal diagnosis when a patient is admitted with symptomatic angina that develops into an AMI. *Do not* assign an additional code for the angina.

The following examples illustrate proper sequencing of the diagnoses of angina and coronary heart disease: [*Coding Clinic,* Volume 10, Number 5, '93, 17, effective October 1, 1993. This advice replaces the advice published in the third quarter 1990 edition of *Coding Clinic.*]

- The reason for admission was progressive episodes of chest pain consistent with crescendo angina. History includes chronic coronary insufficiency and previous myocardial infarctions six years earlier. Treatment during the hospitalization included p.o. calcium blockers. At discharge, the patient was pain-free. No complications arose during the hospitalization and no other diagnostic or therapeutic interventions were performed. Assign code 411.1 as the principal diagnosis since this was the condition after study that necessitated admission to the hospital.

- The reason for admission was cardiac catheterization. The patient's diagnosis on admission was unstable angina. The cardiac catheterization showed significant triple-vessel atherosclerotic heart disease. A three-vessel aortocoronary artery bypass was performed. Assign code 414.0x as the principal diagnosis since this was the condition after study that necessitated admission to the hospital. Assign an additional code for the unstable angina as a secondary diagnosis.

- The reason for admission was a combined right and left heart cardiac catheterization. The patient's diagnosis on admission was angina. The cardiac catheterization showed significant atherosclerotic heart disease. Triple coronary artery bypass surgery was recommended. No surgery was performed prior to discharge. Later, the patient was readmitted and surgery was performed on the second admission. The patient received his antianginal medication also during this stay. Assign code 414.00 as the principal diagnosis for both admissions since this is the condition that necessitated admission to the hospital. Assign code 413.9 as an additional diagnosis.

414.00 Coronary atherosclerosis of unspecified type of vessel, native or graft (continued)

- The reason for admission was unstable angina. While in the hospital, the patient was given intravenous nitrate therapy. After stabilization, the patient underwent a diagnostic cardiac catheterization. Results showed atherosclerotic heart disease. Before discharge, the patient was weaned off the nitroglycerin drip and placed on intensified antianginal therapy. The patient was discharged symptom-free without need for further therapeutic interventions. Assign code 411.1 as the principal diagnosis since this condition led to the admission. Use code 414.00 as a secondary diagnosis to identify the underlying disease.
- The reason for admission was unstable angina. While in the hospital, the patient was given intravenous nitrate therapy. After stabilization, he underwent a balloon angioplasty. During his stay, antianginal medications were also increased. No myocardial infarction occurred during the hospitalization. Assign code 414.0x as the principal diagnosis since this condition led to the admission.
- The reason for admission was severe crescendo angina. The physician tried to stabilize the patient by performing an emergency single-vessel PTCA with administration of thrombolytic agent. However, an acute myocardial infarction of the inferolateral wall occurred. Assign code 410.21 as the principal diagnosis.
- As an outpatient, an asymptomatic patient underwent an exercise stress test and was believed to have ischemic heart disease based on significant ST depression during peak exercise. The reason for the admission was cardiac catheterization. Results showed an underlying significant coronary atherosclerosis, thus explaining his abnormal stress test. Treatment included medications. At discharge, the patient was symptom-free and will be followed up as an outpatient. Assign code 414.00 as the principal diagnosis since the patient was admitted without significant anginal symptoms and coronary atherosclerosis is the condition after study that necessitated admission to the hospital.
- As an outpatient, a patient underwent an exercise stress test as part of a routine exercise prescription. The study was abnormal at peak exercise. The patient was admitted for cardiac catheterization. Results were within normal limits. The patient was symptom-free during the hospitalization. Assign code V71.7 as the principal diagnosis since the physician concluded that no cardiac disease was revealed.
- The reason for admission was unstable angina. The patient had been previously hospitalized for an acute myocardial infarction of the anterolateral wall six weeks earlier. During the patient's stay, his angina stabilized and further infarction was avoided. Assign code 411.1 as the principal diagnosis and code 410.02 as a secondary diagnosis.
- The reason for admission was preinfarctional angina. After stabilization, the patient was transferred for further evaluation to a regional hospital specializing in cardiac care. Assign code 411.1 as the principal diagnosis. During the patient's stay at the regional hospital, he was maintained on antianginal medications and cardiac catheterization was performed. Results showed coronary atherosclerosis. A CABG was performed. During the stay, the patient had no further anginal episodes. Assign code 414.0x as the principal diagnosis and code 411.1 as a secondary diagnosis.
- Assign code 413.9 as the principal diagnosis for the following scenario: A patient with chest pain visited the physician at his office. After examination, the physician's diagnosis was angina and he decided to admit the patient. Treatment at the hospital consisted of antianginal medications. During the stay, the patient had no further anginal episodes.

AHA CC: *Do not* assign a code from subcategory 414.0 when a patient has a history of CABG and the physician makes no mention of coronary atherosclerosis during this admission. [*Coding Clinic,* 3Q, '97, 15, effective with discharges August 1, 1997]

AHA CC: Assign code 414.01 for the patient with coronary artery disease and no mention of a past history of CABG. Check with the physician if the documentation is unclear regarding the patient's past history of bypass surgery. [*Coding Clinic,* 3Q, '97, 15, effective with discharges August 1, 1997]

414.00   Coronary atherosclerosis of unspecified type of vessel,   DRG 132
native or graft (continued)

AHA CC: Assign the coronary artery disease (CAD) as the principal diagnosis in cases where the physician has documented the CAD as the underlying cause of the unstable angina (the reason for the admission) even if a diagnostic test has not been performed during the admission for the diagnosis of coronary artery disease. Documentation of previous testing to confirm the presence of CAD would establish the connection between the CAD and unstable angina. Review the medical record carefully because the physician may document that the angina is due to another condition (i.e., stenosis). In this case, the code for the documented underlying condition is assigned as the principal diagnosis. The angina would be coded secondarily. [*Coding Clinic*, 2Q, '97, 13, effective with discharges May 1, 1997]

AHA CC: Assign code 414.02 when the physician has indicated a redo of a CABG performed 15 years ago where the arteries have occluded due to atherosclerosis. Use code 414.01 as an additional code if the physician has also documented the presence of atherosclerosis in any remaining native vessels. [*Coding Clinic*, 2Q, '95, 17, effective with discharges April 15, 1995]

AHA CC: Assign code 414.02 for atherosclerosis of the graft vessel and code 414.01 for atherosclerosis of the native vessels when a patient with CAD is admitted with unstable angina. History indicates past CABG. Cardiac catheterization was performed on the current admission, showing occlusion in both the graft vessels and a native vessel. Assign code 411.1 as an additional diagnosis. [*Coding Clinic*, 2Q, '95, 17, effective with discharges April 15, 1995]

AHA CC: Assign code 414.02 for a patient who has previously had a CABG but the type of graft material is unknown. [*Coding Clinic*, 2Q, '95, 17, effective with discharges April 15, 1995]

AHA CC: A patient is admitted with angina and known CAD. Previously, the patient had a PTCA. Cardiac catheterization performed during this admission identifies that the vessels have reoccluded. Assign code 414.01 as the principal diagnosis and code 413.9 and V45.82 as additional diagnoses. [*Coding Clinic*, 2Q, '95, 17, effective with discharges April 15, 1995]

AHA CC: When a patient is admitted with angina, has known CAD and no previous history of any procedures being done, assign code 414.01. Assign code 413.9 as an additional diagnosis. [*Coding Clinic*, 2Q, '95, 17, effective with discharges April 15, 1995]

AHA CC: Assign code 414.01 when the medical record documentation shows no history of prior coronary artery bypass. When the documentation is unclear concerning prior bypass surgery, verify with the physician and have him or her document in the medical record whether previous surgery has occurred. [*Coding Clinic*, 2Q, '95, 17, effective with discharges April 15, 1995]

AHA CC: New codes implemented on October 1, 1994 for subcategory 414.0 have changed previous advice published in *Coding Clinic* November-December 1986 and first quarter 1994 *Coding Clinic*, regarding the use of code 996.03. The October 1, 1994 sequencing advice, published in volume 10, number 5, 1993, and *Coding Clinic* second quarter 1994, page 15, remains unchanged (see above). Assign code 996.03 for conditions such as acute (abrupt) closures and leakage at the anastomosis site. As of October 1, 1994, do not assign code 996.03 when the physician has documented that atherosclerosis has occurred in the bypass graft vessel. Rather, assign a code from subcategory 414.0x since the presence of atherosclerosis in a bypass graft is considered a progression of the disease rather than a mechanical complication. [*Coding Clinic*, 2Q, '95, 17, effective with discharges April 15, 1995]

AHA CC: When a patient is admitted for unstable angina, coronary artery disease (CAD) may be assigned as the principal diagnosis even when a diagnostic test establishing a diagnosis of CAD is not performed during the patient's stay. The physician must document in the medical record that the CAD is the underlying cause of the unstable angina. The physician may remark in the record that the patient has a known history of CAD. The physician would not need to perform additional testing to re-establish the underlying cause when patients are admitted for treatment of unstable angina. Sequence code 411.1 as the principal diagnosis and code 414.0x as the secondary diagnosis when the physician has not documented the underlying cause of the unstable angina to be CAD. [*Coding Clinic*, 2Q, '94, 15, effective with discharges April 1, 1994]

414.00 Coronary atherosclerosis of unspecified type of vessel,   DRG 132
native or graft (continued)

AHA CC: Assign code 414.0x as the principal diagnosis for a patient who is status post heart transplant four years ago and suffers from progressive coronary artery disease (CAD) of the transplanted heart. Code V42.1 may be assigned as an additional diagnosis. [*Coding Clinic*, 2Q, '94, 13, effective with discharges April 1, 1994]

AHA CC: Assign code 414.0x for a postpercutaneous transluminal coronary angioplasty (PTCA) reocclusion of the coronary artery. In a PTCA, the coronary artery is left intact, that is, no 'artificial' grafts are involved and treatment is considered complete. When a PTCA is performed, a balloon is used to apply pressure inside the vessel at the location of the arteriosclerotic plaque. The arteriosclerosis is not removed and remains after PTCA. Therefore, reocclusion of an angioplastied vessel may occur either because of the progression of the arteriosclerotic plaque or the re-expansion of the arteriosclerotic plaque within the vessel. When this happens it is considered to be progression of the atherosclerosis unless the physician specifies this as a complication of the procedure. This situation is different than when a coronary artery bypass graft reoccludes. In this case, the graft itself has the problem and is considered to be a complication. Reasons for the reocclusion include thrombus formation, fibrointimal proliferation or atherosclerotic spread. [*Coding Clinic*, 1Q, '94, 6, effective with discharges January 1, 1994]

AHA CC: If a patient is admitted with unstable angina and a heart catheterization is done, assign code 414.0x as the principal diagnosis. Angina is a symptom and should not be coded when a related definitive diagnosis has been established. The known diagnosis rather than a symptom should be coded. However, the physician must state the cause and effect relationship between the angina and the underlying coronary atherosclerosis or CAD. Sequence the angina as the principal diagnosis when the cause of the angina is not established or documented. When the physician documents the cause of the angina, list that cause (e.g., CAD) as principal. Since the CAD caused the symptom, angina, the definition of principal diagnosis is met. [*Coding Clinic*, 4Q, '93, 44, effective with discharges September 3, 1993]

AHA CC: Included in code 411.1 are pre-infarction angina, crescendo angina, unstable angina or initial onset angina. For this type of angina, the patient experiences pain that lasts longer and/or occurs more frequently. This type of angina is also more resistant to an antianginal program and often results in an acute myocardial infarction. Cardiac catheterization or other treatment to interrupt the occlusion process can occur during an inpatient stay. Angina is one symptom of coronary or ischemic heart disease, a disorder resulting from insufficient blood flow secondary to narrowing of the coronary arteries due to atherosclerosis. [*Coding Clinic*, 3Q, '90, 6, effective with discharges July 15, 1990]

AHA CC: Included in code 413.9 are stable forms of angina and excluded is preinfarctional angina. For this type of angina, the anginal type of chest pain is at the same level of exertion or stress and is usually relieved in a predictable fashion with rest or nitroglycerin. Treatment of stable angina is on an outpatient basis unless the patient is being admitted for diagnostic studies to determine the extent of coronary artery disease. Assign the underlying cause of the angina, as determined by the diagnostic study, as the principal diagnosis. [*Coding Clinic*, 3Q, '90, 6, effective with discharges July 15, 1990]

AHA CC: Use code 411.81 as the principal diagnosis and codes 411.1 and 414.0x as secondary diagnoses for the following scenario: A patient admitted for coronary occlusion with impending acute myocardial infarction was given tissue plasminogen activator (TPA) to ward off an infarction. Severe coronary arteriosclerosis is also listed as a diagnosis. [*Coding Clinic*, 3Q, '89, 4, effective with discharges October 15, 1989]

AHA CC: The physician may use diagnostic study findings such as exercise stress tests and electrocardiographs to determine a diagnosis of asymptomatic or presymptomatic atherosclerotic coronary artery disease. Use code 414.0x for symptomatic or presymptomatic coronary heart or artery disease. If the medical record supports the presence of an old 'silent' myocardial infarct in the findings of asymptomatic coronary heart disease, assign codes 414.0x and 412. [*Coding Clinic*, J-A, '84, 5]

414.00   Coronary atherosclerosis of unspecified type of vessel,   DRG 132
native or graft (continued)

AHA CC: Code 414.0x includes arteriosclerotic coronary artery disease and atherosclerosis of the coronary artery. Arteriosclerosis, a generic term, may be further delineated as to type. For example, atherosclerosis or atheroma is arteriosclerosis of the muscular arteries, including the aortic, coronary, femoral, iliac, internal carotid, and cerebral arteries. Ischemic heart disease is a deficiency of blood supply to the heart muscle caused by obstruction or constriction of the coronary artery. While atherosclerotic changes are the most common cause of 'coronary artery disease' or 'coronary heart disease,' they are coded to 414.9, not to 414.0x. Neither 'coronary artery disease' nor 'coronary heart disease' is a precise enough description to assign a code other than 414.9. For instance, the term 'coronary heart disease' does not necessarily refer to the presence of clinical manifestations such as acute or chronic myocardial ischemia, stable or unstable angina or coronary insufficiency. The physician using this term may be referring only to the pathological process of atherosclerosis of the coronary artery or to the pathological process plus clinical symptoms or manifestations, such as with stable angina. With variations in classifications and references to coronary heart disease, check with the physician and have him or her clarify the term's meaning and accurate code assignment. The medical staff should be made aware of the ICD-9-CM code classification for diagnoses of 'coronary artery disease' and 'coronary heart disease' and should be encouraged to provide greater specificity in stating the diagnosis. [*Coding Clinic,* J-A, '84, 5]

DOC: Use code 414.00 when the physician documents coronary (artery) atherosclerosis, arteriosclerosis, arteritis, atheroma, sclerosis or stricture of an unspecified type of vessel, native or graft.

DOC: Use code 414.00 when the physician documents arteriosclerotic heart disease of an unspecified type of vessel, native or graft.

414.01   Coronary atherosclerosis of native coronary artery   DRG 132

See standards on page 579.

411.1   Intermediate coronary syndrome   DRG 140

See standards on page 589.

411.89   Other acute and subacute forms of ischemic heart disease   DRG 140

See standards on page 594.

413.9   Other and unspecified angina pectoris   DRG 140

See standards on page 595.

DRG 138 Cardiac Arrhythmia and Conduction Disorders with CC

DRG 140   Angina Pectoris

Issue

The coding of cardiac arrhythmias, angina and coronary insufficiency is problematic because physician documentation lacks specificity making it difficult to determine the principal diagnosis, and because of the complexity of the ICD-9-CM diagnosis codes and coding guidelines.

Most Common Diagnosis Codes

DRG 138

- 427.1, Paroxysmal ventricular tachycardia
- 427.31, Atrial fibrillation
- 427.32, Atrial flutter
- 427.89, Other specified cardiac dysrhythmias

DRG 140

- 411.1, Intermediate coronary syndrome
- 411.89, Other acute and subacute forms of ischemic heart disease
- 413.9, Angina pectoris

Coding and Documentation Guidelines

411.1	**Intermediate coronary syndrome**	**DRG 140**

See standards on page 592.

411.89	**Other acute and subacute forms of ischemic heart disease**	**DRG 140**

See standards on page 594.

413.9	**Other and unspecified angina pectoris**	**DRG 140**

See standards on page 595.

427.1	**Paroxysmal ventricular tachycardia**	**DRG 138**

CG: Use code 427.1 when the physician documents ventricular tachycardia.

AHA CC: Assign code 427.1 as the principal diagnosis and code 427.5 as a secondary diagnosis when a patient with ventricular tachycardia resulted in cardiac arrest. [*Coding Clinic,* 3Q, '95, 9, effective with discharges July 15, 1995]

AHA CC: Use code 427.1 when the physician has documented Torsades de pointes, a serious arrhythmia that can lead to ventricular fibrillation, and has listed it in the final diagnostic statement. Torsades de pointes can be an adverse reaction of quinidine sulfate medication. If this is documented by the physician, assign the additional code of E942.0. Torsades de pointes is also known as polymorphous or atypical ventricular tachycardia. [*Coding Clinic,* M-A, '86, 11]

427.31   Atrial fibrillation   DRG 138

CG: Use code 427.31 when the physician documents atrial (established) (paroxysmal) fibrillation.

427.32   Atrial flutter   DRG 138

CG: Use code 427.32 when the physician documents atrial or auricular flutter, atrial heart flutter, or impure flutter.

CG: *Do not* use code 427.32 when the physician documents heart flutter. The correct code is 427.42.

CG: *Do not* use code 427.32 when the physician documents ventricular flutter. The correct code is 427.42.

427.89   Other specified cardiac dysrhythmias   DRG 138

CG: Use code 427.89 when the physician documents sinus bradycardia, coronary sinus rhythm disorder, ectopic rhythm disorder, nodal rhythm disorder, or wandering (atrial) pacemaker.

CG: Do not use code 427.89 when the physician documents carotid sinus syncope. The correct code is 337.0.

CG: Do not use code 427.89 when the physician documents reflex bradycardia. The correct code is 337.0.

CG: Do not use code 427.89 when the physician documents tachycardia. The correct code is 785.0.

AHA CC: Assign code 427.89, Other specified cardiac dysrhythmias, other, for postural orthostatic tachycardia syndrome (POTS).   POTS is excessive tachycardia in the upright position with symptoms such as dizziness, lightheadedness, or syncope. If the patient has orthostatic hypotension, assign an additional code 458.0. [*Coding Clinic,* 3Q, '00, 38, effective with discharges July 15, 2000]

Targeted DRG Listing

DRG 140 Angina Pectoris

DRG 143   Chest Pain

Issue

The coding of cardiac arrhythmias, angina, and coronary insufficiency is problematic because physician documentation lacks detail making it difficult to determine the principal diagnosis, and because of the complexity of ICD-9-CM diagnosis code and coding guidelines.

Most Common Diagnosis Codes

DRG 140

- 411.1, Intermediate coronary syndrome
- 411.89, Other acute and subacute forms of ischemic heart disease
- 413.9, Angina pectoris

DRG 143

- 786.50, Chest pain, unspecified
- 786.59, Chest pain, NEC

Coding and Documentation Guidelines

411.1 Intermediate coronary syndrome	DRG 140
See standards on page 589.	

411.89 Other acute and subacute forms of ischemic heart disease	DRG 140
See standards on page 594.	

413.9 Other and unspecified angina pectoris	DRG 140
See standards on page 595.	

786.50 Chest pain, unspecified	DRG 143
See standards on page 585.	

786.59 Chest pain, NEC	DRG 143
See standards on page 585.	

DRG 174   GI Hemorrhage with CC

DRG 182   Esophagitis, Gastroenteritis and Miscellaneous Digestive Disorders, Age Greater than 17 with CC

Issue

The coding of GI hemorrhage is problematic because of the lack of physician documentation for either the known or suspected location or cause of the bleeding, unclear documentation on the reason for admission, the numerous ICD-9-CM diagnosis codes for the hemorrhage, and the complexity of the ICD-9-CM diagnosis codes and coding guidelines.

Most Common Diagnosis Codes

DRG 174

- 531.40, Chronic or unspecified gastric ulcer with hemorrhage
- 532.40, Chronic or unspecified duodenal ulcer with hemorrhage
- 562.12, Diverticulosis of colon with hemorrhage
- 578.1, Blood in stool
- 578.9, Hemorrhage of gastrointestinal tract

DRG 182

- 008.45, Intestinal infections due to *Clostridium difficile*
- 530.81, Esophageal reflux
- 558.9, Other and unspecified noninfectious gastroenteritis and colitis
- 562.11, Diverticulitis of colon

Coding and Documentation Guidelines

008.45   Intestinal infections due to *Clostridium difficile*   DRG 182

AHA CC: Do not arbitrarily report a diagnosis code on the basis of an abnormal laboratory finding alone. Do not list a diagnosis code on the basis of a single lab value or abnormal diagnostic finding. Many factors influence the value of a lab sample. These include the method used to obtain the sample, the collection device, the method used to transport the sample to the lab, the calibration of the machine that reads the values, and the condition of the patient. Check with the physician and have him or her document the responsible pathogen in the medical record. [*Coding Clinic*, 2Q, '90, 3, effective with discharges April 1, 1990, and *Coding Clinic*, 4Q, '93, 39, effective with discharges August 18, 1993]

AHA CC: *Do not* assign a code for infectious bacteria as the etiology of an infection based solely on gram stains unless the physician has documented the condition in the medical record and has listed it in the final diagnostic statement. [*Coding Clinic*, 4Q, '92, 17, effective with discharges October 1, 1992]

530.81   Esophageal reflux   DRG 182

CG: Use code 530.81 when the physician documents esophageal reflux.

CG: Do not use code 530.81 when the physician documents reflux esophagitis. The correct code is 530.11.

AHA CC: Assign code 530.11 when the physician documents esophageal reflux with reflux esophagitis. Do not use code 530.81 as an additional code. [*Coding Clinic*, 4Q, '95, 82, effective with discharges October 1, 1995]

Targeted DRG Listing

530.81   Esophageal reflux (continued)   DRG 182

AHA CC: Assign code 530.81, Esophageal reflux, and code 723.5, Torticollis, Unspecified for a diagnosis of Sandifer syndrome which is synonymous with gastroesophageal reflux and torticollis. This disorder is usually diagnosed by noting the association of a head tilt (torticollis) in a spitty baby (reflux). Although the etiology is unknown, all of the manifestations seem correlated with the presence of the gastroesophageal reflux. As the child matures and the gastroesophageal reflux improves, the attacks cease and the torticollis disappears. [*Coding Clinic*, 1Q, '95, 7]

558.9   Other and unspecified noninfectious gastroenteritis and colitis   DRG 182

CG: Use code 558.9 when the physician documents allergic, dietetic, noninfectious or not otherwise specified colitis, or enteritis.

CG: Use code 558.9 when the physician documents allergic, dietetic, noninfectious or not otherwise specified gastroenteritis, ileitis, or jejunitis.

CG: Use code 558.9 when the physician documents allergic, dietetic, noninfectious or not otherwise specified sigmoiditis.

CG: Do not use code 558.9 when the physician documents infectious colitis, enteritis, or gastroenteritis. The correct code assignment is chosen from the range 009.0-009.1.

CG: Do not use code 558.9 when the physician documents infectious diarrhea. The correct code assignment is either 009.2 or 009.3.

AHA CC: A patient with a history of status post total proctocolectomy with ileoanal anastomosis, the physician documents a diagnosis of pouchitis.which would be considered a complication of the previous surgery. Assign code 997.4, Digestive system complications, as the principal diagnosis and 558.9, Noninfectious gastroenteritis and colitis, would be assigned as a secondary diagnosis since the pouchitis is inflammation of the intestinal wall. If the condition is documented as an infectious process, assign 009.0, Infectious colitis, enteritis, and gastroenteritis. When there is any question whether or not the gastroenteritis is infectious, query the physician. [*Coding Clinic*, 3Q, '99, 33]

AHA CC: Use code 558.9 when the physician documents gay bowel syndrome unless the physician has documented that the condition is presumed but unproven infectious diarrhea. In that case, assign code 009.3. [*Coding Clinic*, N-D, '87, 7]

AHA CC: Assign code 276.5 as the principal diagnosis and code 558.9 as a secondary diagnosis for the following scenario: The physician documents that the reason for admission was dehydration due to gastroenteritis. IV fluids were administered in order to rehydrate the patient. The physician claims the patient's admission was for treatment of dehydration resulting from gastroenteritis and that he would not have admitted the patient for treatment of the noninfectious gastroenteritis. [*Coding Clinic*, J-A, '84, 19]

562.11   Diverticulitis of colon without mention of hemorrhage   DRG 182

AHA CC: Assign code 562.11 as the principal diagnosis and code 569.5 as an additional diagnosis when the physician documents colon diverticulitis with abscess. Do not assign code 567.2 unless the physician or the medical record documentation indicates that the patient has peritonitis. [*Coding Clinic*, 1Q, '96, 13, effective with discharges February 1, 1996]

AHA CC: Effective October 1, 1991, the issue of choosing between the gastrointestinal condition or its associated hemorrhage as the principal diagnosis has been largely resolved by the addition of fifth digits that indicate whether or not hemorrhage is present. The new codes include the following:

- **Diverticulosis of colon**
  562.10, without mention of hemorrhage
  562.12, with hemorrhage

562.11   Diverticulitis of colon without mention of hemorrhage (continued) **DRG 182**

- Diverticulitis of colon
  562.11, without mention of hemorrhage
  562.13, with hemorrhage
  [*Coding Clinic,* 4Q, '91, 25, effective with discharges October 1, 1991]

AHA CC: Assign codes 562.11 and 560.89 when the physician documents bowel obstruction due to repeated attacks of diverticulitis. [*Coding Clinic,* J-F, '85, 1]

AHA CC: Assign code 562.11 when the physician documents perforation of colonic diverticulum due to diverticulitis. [*Coding Clinic,* J-F, '85, 1]

AHA CC: Assign code 562.10 when the physician documents a false diverticulum of colon or cecum. After the age of 40 the rate of occurrence of diverticula of colon increases. These patients are usually asymptomatic. Documentation of diverticulosis denotes only the presence of diverticula and may be an incidental finding during barium examination of the colon. Review the record for evidence of diverticulitis and, if present, assign code 562.11. Code 562.11 includes any mention of diverticulosis. The physician may elect to perform diagnostic workups for rectal bleeding, including tests to differentiate between diverticulosis and cancer of the large intestine. [*Coding Clinic* J-F, '85, 1]

AHA CC: Assign codes 562.11 and 579.9 when the physician documents diverticulitis of the colon with massive hemorrhage. The hemorrhage is a complication of the diverticulitis. [*Coding Clinic,* J-F, '85, 1]

AHA CC: Prior to October 1, 1991, if the physician documented angiodysplasia of the intestines and stomach, diverticulitis, diverticulosis, gastritis, or duodenitis, and the patient also had an associated gastrointestinal hemorrhage, a code from category 578 was used in addition to a code describing one of the above conditions. Effective October 1, 1991, fifth digits identify the presence or absence of an associated hemorrhage for these conditions, therefore only one code is used to identify the condition as well as the hemorrhage. Assign a code from category 578 when the physician indicates a gastrointestinal bleed but no bleeding site or cause is documented. [*Coding Clinic,* 2Q, '92, 9, effective with discharges April 1, 1992]

AHA CC: The reason for admission was evaluation of intermittent melena, controlled at the time of admission. Patient has diverticulosis of the colon. The physician performed a colonoscopy to determine the cause of the bleeding. Results showed the cause of the bleeding to be angiodysplasia rather than the diverticulosis. Assign code 569.84 as the principal diagnosis since angiodysplasia was determined to be the cause of the melena and no further treatment was given. Assign code 562.10 as a secondary diagnosis. [*Coding Clinic,* 4Q, '90, 20, effective with discharges October 1, 1990]

AHA CC: The reason for admission for the third time in six months was due to bright red blood in the stool. Patient has diverticulosis of the colon. Since previous management had not been effective in controlling the bleeding, the patient received percutaneous embolization. Assign code 578.1 as the principal diagnosis, as the thrust of the treatment was directed at controlling the hemorrhage by percutaneous embolization. Assign code 562.10 as a secondary diagnosis. [*Coding Clinic,* 4Q, '90, 20, effective with discharges October 1, 1990]

AHA CC: Gastrointestinal hemorrhage has different manifestations and various causes. How the patient presents, from that of occult bleeding to acute hemorrhage, can change as well. Manifestations include

- hematemesis, indicating acute upper GI hemorrhage
- melena, indicating upper or lower GI hemorrhage
- occult bleeding seen on laboratory examination only
- hematochezia, usually indicating blood from the rectum

Common causes of upper GI bleeding include gastric or duodenal ulcer and a common cause of lower GI bleeding is diverticulosis. Diverticulosis is one of the most frequent causes of lower GI hemorrhage, although colonoscopy has led to the detection of other causes of bleeding with increasing frequency.

562.11 Diverticulitis of colon without mention of hemorrhage (continued) DRG 182

GI bleeding is not usually seen with diverticulitis. In many cases, diverticular hemorrhage stops spontaneously. Another frequent cause of GI bleeding in the older population is angiodysplasia, often presenting as occult bleeding, but once in a while as an acute hemorrhagic episode.

The initial focus of treatment for a patient with acute hemorrhage manifested by significant hematemesis, melena, and/or hematochezia, is usually assessment and restoration of the individual's blood volume using IV fluids and blood transfusions as needed. Bleeding will usually stop spontaneously with this type of treatment. Endoscopy or arteriography may be performed to determine the site of bleeding, followed by treatment to control the site of hemorrhage. Other treatment, vasopressin infusions, endoscopic coagulation, injection of sclerosing agents, and embolization, may be done when the site of the hemorrhage persists or recurs and the site of hemorrhage has been identified by endoscopy or arteriography. Treatment varies depending on the site and extent of the hemorrhage.

Vomiting of bright red blood denotes upper GI bleeding, which can also be determined by analysis of gastric fluid obtained through a nasogastric tube. Asymptomatic passage of maroon-colored stools or bright red blood may identify lower GI bleeding. Bleeding may occur over several days and be brisk and periodic. [*Coding Clinic*, 4Q, '90, 20, effective with discharges October 1, 1990]

AHA CC: Review the circumstances of admission to determine the principal diagnosis for a patient admitted with GI hemorrhage due to an identified cause. List the GI hemorrhage as the principal diagnosis if the focus of treatment, including diagnostic procedures, is directed toward control of the bleeding. However, if the focal point of treatment is directed toward the underlying cause and the bleeding is minimal and easily controlled, list the underlying condition as the principal diagnosis with an additional code for the bleed. In some instances, a combination code that includes both the identified cause and the hemorrhage is available and should be used. [*Coding Clinic*, 4Q, '90, 20, effective with discharges October 1, 1990]

AHA CC: Assign codes 578.9 and 562.10 when the physician documents massive gastrointestinal bleeding and diverticulosis of colon. No cause and effect relationship has been documented by the physician. [*Coding Clinic*, J-F, '85, 1]

AHA CC: Assign codes 596.1 and 562.10 when the physician documents fistula between colon and bladder due to repeated previous attacks of diverticulitis. [*Coding Clinic*, J-F, '85, 1]

AHA CC: Assign codes 567.2 and 562.10 when the physician documents mesenteric abscess resulting from perforation of colonic diverticulum, and a previous history of repeated attacks diverticulitis. [*Coding Clinic*, J-F, '85, 1]

AHA CC: Assign code 562.10 when the physician documents perforation of one or more diverticula unless the perforation of the diverticulum is accompanied by diverticulitis. In that case, code the diverticulitis first. [*Coding Clinic*, J-F, '85, 1]

AHA CC: A diagnosis of diverticulosis means the presence of a number of diverticula of the   intestine. Use code 562.10 to describe diverticulosis of the large intestine. [*Coding Clinic*, J-F, '85, 1]

DOC: Use code 562.11 when the physician documents diverticulitis (with diverticulosis) of colon.

DOC: Use code 562.11 when the physician documents diverticulitis of (large) intestine.

531.40 Chronic or unspecified gastric ulcer with hemorrhage   DRG 174

AHA CC: Assign code 531.40 as the principal diagnosis when the physician documented a diagnosis of acute onset of upper GI bleeding caused by chronic gastric ulcer and the patient received an endoscopic coagulation with heat probe that achieved hemostasis. [*Coding Clinic*, 4Q, '90, 22, effective with discharges October 1, 1990]

AHA CC: Assign the code for a gastric ulcer with hemorrhage if it has been documented by the physician in the history and/or physical examination even if active bleeding is not demonstrated at the time of endoscopy. Gastric ulcers may bleed at irregular intervals, so it is possible to find a

531.40   Chronic or unspecified gastric ulcer with hemorrhage (continued)   DRG 174

nonbleeding ulcer at the time of endoscopy. Therefore, the fact the ulcer is not bleeding at the time of endoscopy should not preclude the coding of gastric ulcer with hemorrhage. The physician should document in the history and/or physical examination a statement such as "recent history of melena." Gastric ulcer with hemorrhage also should be documented at discharge. [*Coding Clinic*, 1Q, '91, 15, effective with discharges January 1, 1991]

AHA CC: To assign the fifth digit "1," with obstruction, to categories 531.xx-534.xx, look for documentation in the medical record indicating an inability of food or fluid to pass through the outlet of the stomach or the intestinal lumen. Obstruction may be caused by spasm, swelling, edema, and/or scarring when the patient has been diagnosed with ulcer disease. Treatment may include nasogastric suction and other medical management or surgery. [*Coding Clinic*, 4Q, '90, 27, effective with discharges October 1, 1990]

DOC: Use code 531.40 when the physician documents chronic or unspecified prepyloric, pylorus or stomach ulcer.

DOC: Do not use code 531.40 when the physician documents chronic or unspecified peptic ulcer. The correct code is 533 with the appropriate fourth and fifth digits.\

532.40   Chronic or unspecified duodenal ulcer with hemorrhage   DRG 174

AHA CC: To assign the fifth digit "1," with obstruction, to categories 531.xx-534.xx, look for documentation in the medical record indicating an inability of food or fluid to pass through the outlet of the stomach or the intestinal lumen. Obstruction may be caused by spasm, swelling, edema, and/or scarring when the patient has been diagnosed with ulcer disease. Treatment may include nasogastric suction and other medical management or surgery. [*Coding Clinic*, 4Q, '90, 27, effective with discharges October 1, 1990]

DOC: Use code 532.40 when the physician documents chronic or unspecified duodenal or postpyloric ulcer with hemorrhage.

DOC: Use code 532.40 when the physician documents chronic or unspecified erosion of duodenum with hemorrhage.

DOC: Do not use code 532.40 when the physician documents chronic or unspecified peptic ulcer. The category code is 533 with the appropriate fourth and fifth digits.

562.12   Diverticulosis of colon with hemorrhage   DRG 174

AHA CC: Effective October 1, 1991, the issue of choosing between the gastrointestinal condition or its associated hemorrhage as the principal diagnosis has been largely resolved by the addition of fifth digits that indicate whether or not hemorrhage is present. The new codes include the following:

- Diverticulosis of colon
  562.10, without mention of hemorrhage
  562.12, with hemorrhage
- Diverticulitis of colon
  562.11, without mention of hemorrhage
  562.13, with hemorrhage
  [*Coding Clinic*, 4Q, '91, 25, effective with discharges October 1, 1991]

AHA CC: Prior to October 1, 1991, if the physician documented angiodysplasia of the intestines and stomach, diverticulitis, diverticulosis, gastritis or duodenitis and the patient also had an associated gastrointestinal hemorrhage, a code from category 578 was used in addition to a code describing one of the above conditions. Effective October 1, 1991, fifth digits identify the presence or absence of an associated hemorrhage for these conditions, therefore only one code is used to identify the condition as well as the hemorrhage. Assign a code from category 578 when the physician indicates a gastrointestinal bleed but no bleeding site or cause is documented. [*Coding Clinic*, 2Q, '92, 9, effective with discharges April 1, 1992]

562.12 Diverticulosis of colon with hemorrhage (continued) DRG 174

AHA CC: For a patient with a nonbleeding acute gastritis with melena from an unspecified bleeding site, assign code 535.00 as the principal diagnosis and code 578.1 as an additional diagnosis. Two codes, one for the GI condition without bleeding, and code 578.1, are necessary when the medical record documents a GI condition not considered to be the source of bleeding, as well as a GI hemorrhage from an unknown or unspecified site. Be aware that ICD-9-CM assumes that the GI bleeding results from the GI lesion identified (angiodysplasia, ulcers, gastritis, diverticulitis, etc.) and directs you to the combination code. In the event that the physician explicitly states that the bleeding is unrelated to the GI condition, assign both codes (GI condition without hemorrhage, and category code 578, GI hemorrhage). [*Coding Clinic*, 2Q, '92, 8, effective with discharges April 1, 1992]

AHA CC: The reason for admission was evaluation of intermittent melena, controlled at the time of admission. The patient has diverticulosis of the colon. The physician performed a colonoscopy to determine the cause of the bleeding. Results showed the cause of the bleeding to be angiodysplasia rather than the diverticulosis. Assign code 569.84 as the principal diagnosis as angiodysplasia was determined to be the cause of the melena and no further treatment was given. Assign code 562.10 as a secondary diagnosis. [*Coding Clinic*, 4Q, '90, 20, effective with discharges October 1, 1990]

AHA CC: The reason for admission for the third time in six months was bright red blood in the stool. Patient has diverticulosis of the colon. Since previous management had not been effective in controlling the bleeding, the patient received percutaneous embolization. Assign code 578.1 as the principal diagnosis as the thrust of the treatment was directed at controlling the hemorrhage by percutaneous embolization. Assign code 562.10 as a secondary diagnosis. [*Coding Clinic*, 4Q, '90, 20, effective with discharges October 1, 1990]

AHA CC: Gastrointestinal hemorrhage has different manifestations and various causes. How the patient presents, from occult bleeding to acute hemorrhage, can change as well. Manifestations include

- hematemesis, indicating acute upper GI hemorrhage
- melena, indicating upper or lower GI hemorrhage
- occult bleeding seen on laboratory examination only
- hematochezia, usually indicating blood from the rectum

Common causes of upper GI bleeding include gastric or duodenal ulcer, and a common cause of lower GI bleeding is diverticulosis. Diverticulosis is one of the most frequent causes of lower GI hemorrhage, although colonoscopy has led to the detection of other causes of bleeding with increasing frequency. GI bleeding is not usually seen with diverticulitis. In many cases, diverticular hemorrhage stops spontaneously. Another frequent cause of GI bleeding in the older population is angiodysplasia, often presenting as occult bleeding, but once in a while as an acute hemorrhagic episode.

The initial focus of treatment for a patient with acute hemorrhage manifested by significant hematemesis, melena and/or hematochezia is usually assessment and restoration of the individual's blood volume, using IV fluids and blood transfusions as needed. Bleeding will usually stop spontaneously with this type of treatment. Endoscopy or arteriography may be performed to determine the site of bleeding, followed by treatment to control the site of hemorrhage. Other treatment, vasopressin infusions, endoscopic coagulation, injection of sclerosing agents and embolization may be done when the site of the hemorrhage persists or recurs and the site of hemorrhage has been identified by endoscopy or arteriography. Treatment varies depending on the site and extent of the hemorrhage.

Vomiting of bright red blood denotes upper GI bleeding, which can also be determined by analysis of gastric fluid obtained through a nasogastric tube. Asymptomatic passage of maroon-colored stools or bright red blood may identify lower GI bleeding. Bleeding may occur over several days and be brisk and periodic. [*Coding Clinic*, 4Q, '90, 20, effective with discharges October 1, 1990]

562.12   Diverticulosis of colon with hemorrhage (continued)   DRG 174

AHA CC: Review the circumstances of admission to determine the principal diagnosis for a patient admitted with GI hemorrhage due to an identified cause. List the GI hemorrhage as the principal diagnosis if the focus of treatment, including diagnostic procedures, is directed toward control of the bleeding. However, if the focal point of treatment is directed toward the underlying cause and the bleeding is minimal and easily controlled, list the underlying condition as the principal diagnosis, with an additional code for the bleed. In some instances, a combination code that includes both the identified cause and the hemorrhage is available and should be used. [*Coding Clinic,* 4Q, '90, 20, effective with discharges October 1, 1990]

AHA CC: Assign codes 578.9 and 562.10 when the physician documents massive gastrointestinal bleeding and diverticulosis of colon. No cause and effect relationship has been documented by the physician. [*Coding Clinic,* J-F, 85, 1]

AHA CC: Assign codes 596.1 and 562.10 when the physician documents fistula between colon and bladder due to repeated previous attacks of diverticulitis. [*Coding Clinic,* J-F, '85, 1]

AHA CC: Assign codes 567.2 and 562.10 when the physician documents mesenteric abscess resulting from perforation of colonic diverticulum, and a previous history of repeated attacks of diverticulitis. [*Coding Clinic,* J-F, '85, 1]

AHA CC: Assign codes 562.11 and 560.89 when the physician documents bowel obstruction due to repeated attacks of diverticulitis. [*Coding Clinic,* J-F, '85, 1]

AHA CC: Assign code 562.11 when the physician documents perforation of colonic diverticulum due to diverticulitis. [*Coding Clinic,* J-F, '85, 1]

AHA CC: Assign code 562.10 when the physician documents a false diverticulum of colon or cecum. After the age of 40 the rate of occurrence of diverticula of colon increases. These patients are usually asymptomatic. Documentation of diverticulosis denotes only the presence of diverticula and may be an incidental finding during barium examination of the colon. Review the record for evidence of diverticulitis and, if present, assign code 562.11. Code 562.11 includes any mention of diverticulosis. The physician may elect to perform diagnostic workups for rectal bleeding including tests to differentiate between diverticulosis and cancer of the large intestine. [*Coding Clinic,* J-F, '85, 1]

AHA CC: Do not use code 562.10 for congenital diverticulosis of the colon. The correct code, if specified as such, is 751.5. [*Coding Clinic,* J-F, '85, 1]

AHA CC: Assign codes 562.11 and 579.9 when the physician documents diverticulitis of the colon with massive hemorrhage. The hemorrhage is a complication of the diverticulitis. [*Coding Clinic,* J-F, '85, 1]

AHA CC: Assign code 562.10 when the physician documents perforation of one or more diverticula unless the perforation of the diverticulum is accompanied by diverticulitis. In that case, code the diverticulitis first. [*Coding Clinic,* J-F, '85, 1]

AHA CC: Use code 562.10 when the physician documents (acute), (massive), (multiple), (perforated) or (ruptured) diverticulosis, as diverticulosis not specified as to site usually refers to diverticulosis of the colon. [*Coding Clinic,* J-F, '85, 1]

AHA CC: A diagnosis of diverticulosis means the presence of a number of diverticula of the intestine. Use code 562.10 to describe diverticulosis of the large intestine. [*Coding Clinic,* J-F, '85, 1]

DOC: Use code 562.12 when the physician documents diverticulosis of colon without mention of diverticulitis but with hemorrhage.

DOC: Use code 562.12 when the physician documents diverticular disease without mention of diverticulitis but with hemorrhage.

DOC: Do not use code 562.12 when the physician diverticulosis of colon without mention of hemorrhage. The correct category code is 562.10.

578.1   Blood in stool   DRG 174

AHA CC: For a patient with a nonbleeding acute gastritis with melena from an unspecified bleeding site, assign code 535.00 as the principal diagnosis and code 578.1 as an additional diagnosis. Two codes, one for the GI condition without bleeding, and code 578.1, are necessary when the medical record documents a GI condition not considered to be the source of bleeding, as well as a GI hemorrhage from an unknown or unspecified site. Be aware that ICD-9-CM assumes that the GI bleeding results from the GI lesion identified (angiodysplasia, ulcers, gastritis, diverticulitis, etc.) and directs you to the combination code. In the event that the physician explicitly states that the bleeding is unrelated to the GI condition, assign both codes (GI condition without hemorrhage, and category 578, GI hemorrhage). [*Coding Clinic*, 2Q, '92, 8, effective with discharges April 1, 1992]

AHA CC: The reason for admission for the third time in six months was bright red blood in the stool. The patient has diverticulosis of the colon. Since previous management had not been effective in controlling the bleeding, the patient received percutaneous embolization. Assign code 578.1 as the principal diagnosis since the thrust of the treatment was directed at controlling the hemorrhage by percutaneous embolization. Assign code 562.10 as a secondary diagnosis. [*Coding Clinic*, 4Q, '90, 20, effective with discharges October 1, 1990]

AHA CC: A gastrointestinal hemorrhage and occult blood in the stool are not the same. Evidence of a gastrointestinal hemorrhage includes either dark black, tarry, clotted stools, also referred to as melena, or bright red blood in the stool or vomitus. Microscopic exam or a guaiac test is used to identify occult blood in the stool. Laboratory reports will indicate occult blood findings or the physician may note this in his progress notes. The presence of occult blood indicates the occurrence of a small amount of bleeding in the GI tract, but not in sufficient quantity to be categorized as a hemorrhage. Use code 792.1 only when the physician documents a diagnosis of a guaiac positive stool with no additional documentation to identify a more severe GI bleed or the source of the GI bleed. [*Coding Clinic*, 2Q, '92, 9, effective with discharges April 1, 1992]

AHA CC: Prior to October 1, 1991, if the physician documented angiodysplasia of the intestines and stomach, diverticulitis, diverticulosis, gastritis or duodenitis and the patient also had an associated gastrointestinal hemorrhage, a code from category 578 was used in addition to a code describing one of the above conditions. Effective October 1, 1991, fifth digits identify the presence or absence of an associated hemorrhage for these conditions, therefore only one code is used to identify the condition as well as the hemorrhage. Assign a code from category 578 when the physician indicates a gastrointestinal bleed but no bleeding site or cause is documented. [*Coding Clinic*, 2Q, '92, 9, effective with discharges April 1, 1992]

AHA CC: The reason for admission was history of increasingly severe abdominal pain with some melena noted earlier during the day of admission. History showed no previous GI problems but large doses of prescribed aspirin were being consumed by the patient for the relief of pain from arthritis. The physician performed an endoscopy. Results showed an acute erosive gastritis, probably due to the irritant effect of the pain medication. Medications were adjusted and the patient was put on a bland diet. After the second day, no melena was documented. Assign code 535.4 as the principal diagnosis and codes 578.1, E935.3 and 716.90 as secondary diagnoses. [*Coding Clinic*, 4Q, '90, 20, effective with discharges October 1, 1990]

AHA CC: The reason for admission was evaluation of intermittent melena, controlled at the time of admission. The patient has diverticulosis of the colon. The physician performed a colonoscopy to determine the cause of the bleeding. Results showed the cause of the bleeding to be angiodysplasia rather than the diverticulosis. Assign code 569.84 as the principal diagnosis since angiodysplasia was determined to be the cause of the melena and no further treatment was given. Assign code 562.10 as a secondary diagnosis. [*Coding Clinic*, 4Q, '90, 20, effective with discharges October 1, 1990]

Gastrointestinal hemorrhage has different manifestations and various causes. How the patient presents, from occult bleeding to acute hemorrhage, can change as well. Manifestations include

- hematemesis, indicating acute upper GI hemorrhage

578.1   Blood in stool (continued) (continued)   DRG 174

- melena, indicating upper or lower GI hemorrhage
- occult bleeding seen on laboratory examination only
- hematochezia, usually indicating blood from the rectum

Common causes of upper GI bleeding include gastric or duodenal ulcer, and a common cause of lower GI bleeding is diverticulosis. Diverticulosis is one of the most frequent causes of lower GI hemorrhage, although colonoscopy has led to the detection of other causes of bleeding with increasing frequency. GI bleeding is not usually seen with diverticulitis. In many cases, diverticular hemorrhage stops spontaneously. Another frequent cause of GI bleeding in the older population is angiodysplasia, often presenting as occult bleeding, but once in a while as an acute hemorrhagic episode.

The initial focus of treatment for a patient with acute hemorrhage manifested by significant hematemesis, melena and/or hematochezia is usually assessment and restoration of the individual's blood volume using IV fluids and Blood transfusions as needed. Bleeding will usually stop spontaneously with this type of treatment. Endoscopy or arteriography may be performed to determine the site of bleeding, followed by treatment to control the site of hemorrhage. Other treatment, vasopressin infusions, endoscopic coagulation, injection of sclerosing agents and embolization may be done when the site of the hemorrhage persists or recurs and the site of hemorrhage has been identified by endoscopy or arteriography. Treatment varies depending on the site and extent of the hemorrhage.

Vomiting of bright red blood denotes upper GI bleeding, which can also be determined by analysis of gastric fluid obtained through a nasogastric tube. Asymptomatic passage of maroon-colored stools or bright red blood may identify lower GI bleeding. Bleeding may occur over several days and be brisk and periodic. [*Coding Clinic*, 4Q, '90, 20, effective with discharges October 1, 1990]

AHA CC: Review the circumstances of admission to determine the principal diagnosis for a patient admitted with GI hemorrhage due to an identified cause. List the GI hemorrhage as the principal diagnosis if the focus of treatment, including diagnostic procedures, is directed toward control of the bleeding. However, if the focal point of treatment is directed toward the underlying cause and the bleeding is minimal and easily controlled, list the underlying condition as the principal diagnosis with an additional code for the bleed. In some instances, a combination code that includes both the identified cause and the hemorrhage is available and should be used. [*Coding Clinic*, 4Q, '90, 20, effective with discharges October 1, 1990]

DOC: Use code 578.1 when the physician documents melena or blood in stool.

DOC: Do not use code 578.1 when the physician documents occult blood. The correct code is 792.1.

578.9   Hemorrhage of gastrointestinal tract, unspecified   DRG 174

CG: Use code 578.9 when the physician documents hemorrhage of gastrointestinal tract, gastric hemorrhage, or intestinal hemorrhage.

CG: Do not use code 532.40 when the physician documents chronic or unspecified peptic ulcer. The correct code is 533 with the appropriate fourth and fifth digits.

AHA CC: Use code 535.0 as the principal diagnosis and code 578.9 as a secondary diagnosis when the physician documents acute gastritis with hemorrhage or acute hemorrhagic gastritis. [*Coding Clinic*, N-D, '86, 9]

AHA CC: A gastrointestinal hemorrhage and occult blood in the stool are not the same. Evidence of a gastrointestinal hemorrhage includes either dark black, tarry, clotted stools, also referred to as melena, or bright red blood in the stool or vomitus. Microscopic exam or a guaiac test is used to identify occult blood in the stool. Laboratory reports will indicate occult blood findings or the physician may note this in his progress notes. The presence of occult blood indicates the occurrence

578.9   Hemorrhage of gastrointestinal tract, unspecified (continued)   DRG 174

of a small amount of bleeding in the GI tract, but not in sufficient quantity to be categorized as a hemorrhage. Use code 792.1 only when the physician documents a diagnosis of a guaiac positive stool with no additional documentation to identify a more severe GI bleed or the source of the GI bleed. [Coding Clinic, 2Q, '92, 9, effective with discharges April 1, 1992]

AHA CC: Prior to October 1, 1991, if the physician documented angiodysplasia of the intestines and stomach, diverticulitis, diverticulosis, gastritis or duodenitis, and the patient also had an associated gastrointestinal hemorrhage, a code from category 578 was used in addition to a code describing one of the above conditions. Effective October 1, 1991, fifth digits identify the presence or absence of an associated hemorrhage for these conditions, therefore only one code is used to identify the condition as well as the hemorrhage. Assign a code from category 578 when the physician indicates a gastrointestinal bleed but no bleeding site or cause is documented. [Coding Clinic, 2Q, '92, 9, effective with discharges April 1, 1992]

AHA CC: For a patient with a nonbleeding acute gastritis with melena from an unspecified bleeding site, assign code 535.00 as the principal diagnosis and code 578.1 as an additional diagnosis. Two codes, one for the GI condition without bleeding, and code 578.1, are necessary when the medical record documents a GI condition not considered to be the source of bleeding, as well as a GI hemorrhage from an unknown or unspecified site. Be aware that ICD-9-CM assumes that the GI bleeding results from the GI lesion identified (angiodysplasia, ulcers, gastritis, diverticulitis, etc.) and directs you to the combination code. In the event that the physician explicitly states that the bleeding is unrelated to the GI condition, assign both codes (GI condition without hemorrhage, and category 578, GI hemorrhage). [Coding Clinic, 2Q, '92, 8, effective with discharges April 1, 1992]

AHA CC: The reason for admission was history of increasingly severe abdominal pain with some melena noted earlier during the day of admission. History showed no previous GI problems but large doses of prescribed aspirin were being consumed by the patient for the relief of pain from arthritis. The physician performed an endoscopy. Results showed an acute erosive gastritis, probably due to the irritant effect of the pain medication. Medications were adjusted and the patient was put on a bland diet. After the second day, no melena was documented. Assign code 535.4 as the principal diagnosis and codes 578.1, E935.3 and 716.90 as secondary diagnoses. [Coding Clinic, 4Q, '90, 20, effective with discharges October 1, 1990]

AHA CC: The reason for admission was acute onset of vomiting of bright red blood due to acute duodenal ulcer. The physician performed arteriography to determine the site of the bleeding, and transcatheter embolization resulted in hemostasis. Assign code 532.00 as the principal diagnosis since the diagnostic workup was carried out to determine the site of bleeding and the bleeding was treated with transcatheter embolization. ICD-9-CM has a combination code for ulcer with hemorrhage. [Coding Clinic, 4Q, '90, 20, effective with discharges October 1, 1990]

AHA CC: The reason for admission was acute onset of upper GI bleeding caused by a chronic gastric ulcer. The physician performed an endoscopic coagulation with heat probe, resulting in hemostasis. Assign code 531.40 as the principal diagnosis. [Coding Clinic, 4Q, '90, 20, effective with discharges October 1, 1990]

AHA CC: The reason for admission was evaluation of intermittent melena, controlled at the time of admission. The patient has diverticulosis of the colon. The physician performed a colonoscopy to determine the cause of the bleeding. Results showed the cause of the bleeding to be angiodysplasia rather than the diverticulosis. Assign code 569.84 as the principal diagnosis as angiodysplasia was determined to be the cause of the melena and no further treatment was given. Assign code 562.10 as a secondary diagnosis. [Coding Clinic, 4Q, '90, 20, effective with discharges October 1, 1990]

AHA CC: The reason for admission for the third time in six months was bright red blood in the stool. Patient has diverticulosis of the colon. Since previous management had not been effective in controlling the bleeding, the patient received percutaneous embolization. Assign code 578.1 as the principal diagnosis since the thrust of the treatment was directed at controlling the hemorrhage by percutaneous embolization. Assign code 562.10 as a secondary diagnosis. [Coding Clinic, 4Q, '90, 20, effective with discharges October 1, 1990]

578.9 Hemorrhage of gastrointestinal tract, unspecified (continued)   DRG 174

AHA CC: Gastrointestinal hemorrhage has different manifestations and various causes. How the patient presents, from occult bleeding to acute hemorrhage, can change as well. Manifestations include

- hematemesis, indicating acute upper GI hemorrhage
- melena, indicating upper or lower GI hemorrhage
- occult bleeding seen on laboratory examination only
- hematochezia, usually indicating blood from the rectum

Common causes of upper GI bleeding include gastric or duodenal ulcer, and a common cause of lower GI bleeding is diverticulosis. Diverticulosis is one of the most frequent causes of lower GI hemorrhage, although colonoscopy has led to the detection of other causes of bleeding with increasing frequency. GI bleeding is not usually seen with diverticulitis. In many cases, diverticular hemorrhage stops spontaneously. Another frequent cause of GI bleeding in the older population is angiodysplasia, often presenting as occult bleeding, but once in a while as an acute hemorrhagic episode.

The initial focus of treatment for a patient with acute hemorrhage manifested by significant hematemesis, melena and/or hematochezia is usually assessment and restoration of the individual's blood volume using IV fluids and blood transfusions as needed. Bleeding will usually stop spontaneously with this type of treatment. Endoscopy or arteriography may be performed to determine the site of bleeding, followed by treatment to control the site of hemorrhage. Other treatment, vasopressin infusions, endoscopic coagulation, injection of sclerosing agents and embolization may be done when the site of the hemorrhage persists or recurs and the site of hemorrhage has been identified by endoscopy or arteriography. Treatment varies depending on the site and extent of the hemorrhage.

Vomiting of bright red blood denotes upper GI bleeding, which can also be determined by analysis of gastric fluid obtained through a nasogastric tube. Asymptomatic passage of maroon-colored stools or bright red blood may identify lower GI bleeding. Bleeding may occur over several days and be brisk and periodic. [*Coding Clinic*, 4Q, '90, 20, effective with discharges October 1, 1990]

AHA CC: Review the circumstances of admission to determine the principal diagnosis for a patient admitted with GI hemorrhage due to an identified cause. List the GI hemorrhage as the principal diagnosis if the focus of treatment, including diagnostic procedures, is directed toward control of the bleeding. However, if the treatment is directed toward the underlying cause and the bleeding is minimal and easily controlled, list the underlying condition as the principal diagnosis with an additional code for the bleed. In some instances, a combination code that includes both the identified cause and the hemorrhage is available and should be used. [*Coding Clinic*, 4Q, '90, 20, effective with discharges October 1, 1990]

DRG 188 Other Digestive System Diagnoses, Age Greater than 17 with CC

DRG 180   GI Obstruction with CC

Issue

The coding of GI disorders is problematic because of the lack of physician documentation on the known or suspected location or cause of obstruction, unclear documentation on the reason for admission, and the complexity of the ICD-9-CM diagnosis codes and coding guidelines for the obstruction.

Most Common Diagnosis Codes

DRG 188

- 211.3, Benign neoplasm of colon
- 455.2, Internal hemorrhoids with other complication
- 557.0, Acute vascular insufficiency of intestine
- 557.9, Unspecified vascular insufficiency of intestine
- 997.4, Digestive system complications

DRG 180

- 560.1, Paralytic ileus
- 560.39, Other intestinal obstruction without mention of hernia
- 560.81, Intestinal or peritoneal adhesions with obstruction
- 560.89, Other specified intestinal obstruction
- 560.9, Unspecified intestinal obstruction

Coding and Documentation Guidelines

211.3   Benign neoplasm of colon   DRG 188

CG: Use code 211.3 when the physician documents benign neoplasm of the appendix, benign neoplasm of the cecum, benign neoplasm of the ileocecal valve, or benign neoplasm of the large intestine.

CG: Do not use code 211.3 when the physician documents benign neoplasm of rectosigmoid junction. The correct code is 211.4.

455.2   Internal hemorrhoids with other complication   DRG 188

CG: Use code 455.2 when the physician documents bleeding internal hemorrhoids, prolapsed internal hemorrhoids, strangulated internal hemorrhoids, or ulcerated internal hemorrhoids.

CG: Do not use code 455.2 when the physician documents internal thrombosed hemorrhoids. The correct code to use is 455.1.

CG: Do not use code 455.2 when the physician documents internal hemorrhoids without complications. The correct code to use is 455.0.

557.0   Acute vascular insufficiency of intestine   DRG 188

CG: Use code 557.0 when the physician documents acute hemorrhagic enterocolitis, acute ischemic colitis, enteritis or enterocolitis, acute massive necrosis of intestine, bowel infarction, embolism of mesenteric artery, fulminant enterocolitis, hemorrhagic necrosis of intestine, intestinal gangrene, (acute), (agnogenic) (hemorrhagic) (nonocclusive) intestinal infarction, (embolic) (thrombotic) mesenteric infarction, terminal hemorrhagic enteropathy, or thrombosis of mesenteric artery.

CG: Do not use code 557.0 when the physician documents chronic vascular insufficiency of intestines. The correct code is 557.1.

CG: Do not use code 557.0 when the physician documents vascular insufficiency of intestine. The correct code is 557.9.

AHA CC: Assign code 997.71, Vascular complications of mesenteric artery, and code 557.0, Acute vascular insufficiency of intestine for a post-operative mesenteric artery embolism.   [*Coding Clinic*, 4Q, '01, 81]

557.9   Unspecified vascular insufficiency of intestine   DRG 188

CG: Use code 557.9 when the physician documents vascular insufficiency of intestine, alimentary pain due to vascular insufficiency, or ischemic colitis, enteritis or enterocolitis.

CG: Do not use code 557.9 when the physician documents acute vascular insufficiency of intestine. The correct code is 557.0.

CG: Do not use code 557.9 when the physician documents chronic vascular insufficiency of intestine. The correct code is 557.1.

997.4   Digestive system complications   DRG 188

CG: Use code 997.4 when the physician documents complications of intestinal anastomosis and bypass not elsewhere classified except that involving urinary tract.

CG: Use code 997.4 when the physician documents hepatic failure due to a procedure.

CG: Use code 997.4 when the physician documents hepatorenal syndrome.

CG: Use code 997.4 when the physician documents intestinal obstruction due to a procedure.

CG: Do not use code 997.4 when the physician documents blind loop syndrome. The correct code to use is 579.2.

CG: Do not use code 997.4 when the physician documents colostomy or enterostomy complications. The correct code to use is from the 560.60-569.69 series.

CG: Do not use code 997.4 when the physician documents infection of external stoma. The correct code to use is 569.61.

CG: Do not use code 997.4 when the physician documents postcholecystectomy syndrome. The correct code to use is 576.0.

CG: Do not use code 997.4 when the physician documents postgastric surgery syndrome. The correct code to use is 564.2.

AHA CC: Do not use code 997.4 to classify vascular to identify vascular complications of the mesenteric artery (997.71), renal artery (997.72) and other vessels (997.79). complications. Effective October 1, 2001, new codes have been created. [*Coding Clinic*, 4Q, '01, 81]

AHA CC: A patient admitted for treatment of esophageal stricture, reflux and gastric atony, status post Nissen fundoplication should not be coded with 997.4, Digestive system complications. When a patient is experiencing a continuation of the symptoms for which the original surgery was performed, persistent symptoms, which have not been resolved by the procedure, should not be classified as surgical complications. If, however, the physician documents these conditions as

---

Targeted DRG Listing

997.4 Digestive system complications (continued) DRG 188

complications of the Nissen fundoplication surgery, assign code 997.4, Digestive system complications. Codes 530.3, Stricture and stenosis of esophagus, 530.81, Esophageal reflux, and 536.3, Gastroparesis, may be listed to provide further specificity. Query the physician for clarification, if the documentation is unclear, whether these conditions resulted from the Nissen fundoplication surgery. [*Coding Clinic*, 2Q, '01, 42]

AHA CC: A patient with a history of status post total proctocolectomy with ileoanal anastomosis, the physician documents a diagnosis of pouchitis.which would be considered a complication of the previous surgery. Assign code 997.4, Digestive system complications, as the principal diagnosis and 558.9, Noninfectious gastroenteritis and colitis, would be assigned as a secondary diagnosis since the pouchitis is inflammation of the intestinal wall. If the condition is documented as an infectious process, assign 009.0, Infectious colitis, enteritis, and gastroenteritis. When there is any question whether or not the gastroenteritis is infectious, query the physician. [*Coding Clinic*, 3Q, '99, 33]

AHA CC: The correct description of a postoperative biloma in a patient readmitted for this condition is 997.4, Digestive system complications, principal diagnosis. Also assign code 576.8, Other specified disorders of biliary tract. [*Coding Clinic* 2Q,' 99, 14, effective with discharges April 1, 1999]

AHA CC: Do not use code 997.4 when the patient was admitted for cellulitis of the abdominal wall at the gastrostomy site with *Staphylococcus aureus* identified as the organism. Assign code 536.41 for the gastrostomy infection and codes 682.2 and 041.11 for the cellulitis infection. [*Coding Clinic*, 4Q, '98, 42, effective with discharges October 1, 1998]

AHA CC: Do not assign code 997.4 as the principal diagnosis for the following scenario: A patient with a previously placed gastrostomy tube was admitted with bleeding and drainage from the tube. Circumstances were that the G-tube had become stuck in the patient's abdominal wall. The physician removed the tube via an incision and replaced it. Assign code 536.49. [*Coding Clinic*, 4Q, '98, 42, effective with discharges October 1, 1998]

AHA CC: Assign codes 997.4 and 576.1 when the physician documents cholangitis due to percutaneous transhepatic cholangiogram. Since the documented complication, cholangitis, affected the bile duct, a digestive organ, use a code from category 997. [*Coding Clinic*, 2Q, '95, 7, effective with discharges April 15, 1995]

AHA CC: Assign code 997.4 with an additional code of 572.4 when the physician documents a diagnosis of hepatorenal syndrome due to surgery. [*Coding Clinic*, 3Q, '92, 15, effective with discharges July 1, 1992]

AHA CC: Assign code 997.4 when the physician documents subhepatic fluid accumulation following a cholecystectomy. [*Coding Clinic*, 2Q, '89, 15, effective with discharges July 31, 1989]

AHA CC: Assign code 997.4 when the physician documents sump syndrome, a complication of a choledochoenterostomy (either choledochoduodenostomy or choledochojejunostomy). [*Coding Clinic*, 1Q, '88, 14]

AHA CC: Effective October 1, 1998, all gastrostomy complications are to be assigned as follows; gastrostomy complication, unspecified (536.40), infection of gastrostomy (536.41), mechanical complication of gastrostomy (536.42) and other gastrostomy complications (536.49). Gastrostomy complications are no longer to be coded to 997.4. [*Coding Clinic*, 4Q, '98, 42, effective with discharges October 1, 1998]

AHA CC: Since codes in category 997 address a variety of postoperative complications without specifying the nature of the complication, use an additional code whenever possible to describe the specific complication. [*Coding Clinic*, 1Q, '92, 13, effective with discharges January 1, 1992 and *Coding Clinic*, 1Q, '93, 26, effective with discharges January 1, 1993]

AHA CC: Use codes 996.64 and 041.0 when the physician documents that a patient with an indwelling urinary catheter required admission because of streptococcal infection. [*Coding Clinic*, 2Q, '90, 11, effective with discharges April 1, 1990]

997.4   Digestive system complications (continued)   DRG 188

AHA CC: List the complication code as the principal diagnosis when the reason for admission was treatment of a complication resulting from surgery or other medical care. ICD-9-CM states to "use additional code to identify complication" if the complication is classified to the 996-999 series. [*Coding Clinic*, 2Q, '90, 11, effective with discharges April 1, 1990]

560.1   Paralytic ileus   DRG 180

AHA CC: Use code 560.1 when the physician documents spinal anesthesia-induced adynamic ileus of the colon. Use code E938.7 as an additional code for the adverse reaction to tetracaine hydrochloride. [*Coding Clinic*, J-F, '87, 13]

DOC: Use code 560.1 when the physician documents adynamic ileus, ileus of intestine, bowel or colon, or paralysis of intestine or colon.

DOC: Do not use code 560.1 when the physician documents gallstone ileus. The correct code to use is 560.31.

560.39   Other intestinal obstruction without mention of hernia   DRG 180

DOC: Use code 560.39 when the physician documents concretion of intestine, enterolith, or fecal impaction.

560.81   Intestinal or peritoneal adhesions with obstruction   DRG 180

AHA CC: Assign code 560.81 when the physician documents postoperative and postinfective peritoneal adhesions when obstruction is associated with the adhesions. [*Coding Clinic*, 4Q, '95, 55, effective with discharges October 1, 1995]

AHA CC: Assign code 560.81 when the physician documents an intestinal obstruction due to peritoneal adhesions from a pervious surgery. Do not assign a surgical complication code as peritoneal adhesions are ordinarily due to surgery. [*Coding Clinic*, 3Q, 95, 6, effective with discharges July 15, 1995]

AHA CC: Use code 560.81 when the physician documents bowel obstruction with adhesions and a history of multiple abdominal surgeries. Even though the patient may have a history of previous surgery, adhesions are not necessarily due to the surgery. Adhesions may be caused by inflammation, such as acute appendicitis, diverticulitis, avascular degeneration, cholecystitis, pelvic infections, or Crohn's disease, rather than being the result of the surgery performed. [*Coding Clinic*, N-D, '87, 9]

DOC: Use code 560.81 when the physician documents (postoperative) (postinfectional) intestinal or peritoneal adhesion with obstruction.

DOC: Do not use code 560.81 when the physician documents adhesions without obstruction. The correct code to use is 568.0.

560.89   Other specified intestinal obstruction   DRG 180

AHA CC: Assign code 195.2 as the principal diagnosis and code 560.89 as an additional code when the physician documents small bowel obstructions due to abdominal carcinomatosis. The choice of principal diagnosis is not affected by whether the cancer is newly diagnosed or has spread. [*Coding Clinic*, 2Q, '97, 3, effective with discharges May 1, 1997]

AHA CC: Assign code 555.9 as the principal diagnosis and code 560.89 as an additional code when the physician documents admission for non-surgical treatment of bowel obstruction secondary to Crohn's disease. A common complication of Crohn's disease is obstruction; however, not all patients with Crohn's disease develop obstruction. [*Coding Clinic*, 2Q, '97, 3, effective with discharges May 1, 1997]

560.89 Other specified intestinal obstruction (continued) DRG 180

AHA CC: Assign code 560.89 when the physician documents acute pseudo-obstruction of the intestine, also referred to as Ogilvie's syndrome. Assign code 564.8 when the physician documents the condition as chronic or intermittent secondary, idiopathic or primary, and not otherwise specified. Characteristics of acute intestinal pseudo-obstruction, a motility disorder and not a mechanical obstruction of the intestine, include massive dilatation of the colon and occasionally of the small intestine. This condition is usually seen in patients who have undergone major surgery, suffered a myocardial infarction, have a severe infection or septicemia, or are experiencing respiratory failure and are on a respirator. Patients on ventilatory therapy, sedatives or narcotics, and those with metabolic and electrolyte disturbances have also been known to develop acute intestinal pseudo-obstruction. [*Coding Clinic*, 1Q, '88, 6]

DOC: Use code 560.89 when the physician documents mural thickening causing obstruction, or sympathicotonic colon obstruction.

DOC: Do not use code 560.89 when the physician documents obstruction, occlusion, stenosis or stricture of the intestine or colon. The correct code to use is 560.9.

DOC: Do not use code 560.89 when the physician documents ischemic stricture of intestine. The correct code to use is 557.1.

560.9 Unspecified intestinal obstruction DRG 180

AHA CC: Assign code 555.9 as the principal diagnosis and code 560.89 as an additional code when the physician documents admission for non-surgical treatment of bowel obstruction secondary to Crohn's disease. A common complication of Crohn's disease is obstruction; however, not all patients with Crohn's disease develop obstruction. [*Coding Clinic*, 2Q, '97, 3, effective with discharges May 1, 1997]

AHA CC: Assign code 195.2 as the principal diagnosis and code 560.89 as an additional code when the physician documents small bowel obstructions due to abdominal carcinomatosis. The choice of principal diagnosis is not affected by whether the cancer is newly diagnosed or has spread. [*Coding Clinic*, 2Q, '97, 3, effective with discharges May 1, 1997]

AHA CC: Assign code 560.89 when the physician documents acute pseudo-obstruction of the intestine, also referred to as Ogilvie's syndrome. Assign code 564.8 when the physician documents the condition as chronic or intermittent secondary, idiopathic or primary, and not otherwise specified. Characteristics of acute intestinal pseudo-obstruction, a motility disorder and not a mechanical obstruction of the intestine, include massive dilatation of the colon and occasionally of the small intestine. This condition is usually seen in patients who have undergone major surgery, suffered a myocardial infarction, have a severe infection or septicemia, or are experiencing respiratory failure and are on a respirator. Patients on ventilatory therapy, sedatives or narcotics, and those with metabolic and electrolyte disturbances have also been known to develop acute intestinal pseudo-obstruction. [*Coding Clinic*, 1Q, '88, 6]

DOC: Use code 560.9 when the physician documents enterostenosis, obstruction of intestine or colon, occlusion of intestine or colon, stenosis of intestine or colon, or stricture of intestine or colon.

DOC: Do not use code 560.9 when the physician documents congenital stenosis or stricture of the intestine or colon. The correct code to use is either 751.1 or 751.2.

DRG 239 Pathological Fractures and Musculoskeletal and Connective Tissue Malignancy

DRG 243   Medical Back Problems

Issue

The coding of back problems is problematic because of the lack of physician documentation on either the known or suspected location of a fracture/disorder, cause of a fracture/disorder, unclear documentation on the reason for admission, and the complexity of the ICD-9-CM diagnosis codes and coding guidelines for back disorders.

Most Common Diagnosis Codes

DRG 239

- 198.5, Secondary malignant neoplasm of bone and bone marrow
- 733.13, Pathological fracture of vertebra

DRG 243

- 721.3, Lumbosacral spondylosis without myelopathy
- 722.10, Displacement of lumbar intervertebral disc without myelopathy
- 722.52, Degeneration of lumbar or lumbosacral intervertebral disc
- 724.02, Spinal stenosis lumbar region
- 724.2, Spinal stenosis, lumbago
- 805.2, Closed fracture of dorsal vertebra
- 805.4, Closed fracture of lumbar vertebra

Coding and Documentation Guidelines

198.5	Secondary malignant neoplasm of bone and bone marrow	DRG 239

AHA CC: Do not use code 198.5 when the physician documents lymphoma. Code lymphomas regardless of the number of sites involved to the 200–202 series. They are not considered metastatic. For solid tumor (classified to categories 140–199) metastases to the lymphatic system, use a code from category 196, code 197.8 or code 198.5. Never use code 197.8, 198.5 or codes from category 196 for lymphomas. [*Coding Clinic*, 2Q, '92, 3, effective with discharges April 1, 1992]

AHA CC: It is not always appropriate to assign the malignancy as the principal diagnosis when a patient is admitted for a specific condition related to a terminal malignancy and expires. For example, assign code 285.8 as the principal diagnosis and codes 198.5 and V10.3 as secondary diagnoses for the following scenario: Admission was for myelophthisic anemia. The physician stated in her history previously resected carcinoma of the breast and known metastasis to the bone. The patient received a transfusion of packed cells. The patient expired four days into his hospitalization. [*Coding Clinic*, 1Q, '91, 16, effective with discharges January 1, 1991]

AHA CC: Assign only code 203.0 when the physician documents multiple myeloma with bone metastasis. Do not assign two codes, 203.0 and 198.5, for this condition. [*Coding Clinic*, 4Q, '89, 10, effective with discharges January 2, 1990]

AHA CC: When a patient is admitted because of a primary neoplasm with metastasis, and treatment is directed toward the secondary site only, sequence the secondary neoplasm first even though the primary malignancy is still present. [*Coding Clinic*, 2Q, '90, 3, effective with discharges April 1, 1990]

198.5   Secondary malignant neoplasm of bone and bone   DRG 239
         marrow (continued)

AHA CC: In a patient whose pathology report states "metastatic carcinoma of the vertebral body
consistent with prostate primary," but whose reason for admission is a spinal cord injury from a
compression deformity of the same vertebral body, assign 733.13, pathological fracture of vertebra
as principal diagnosis; 336.3, myelopathy in other diseases classified elsewhere 185, malignant
neoplasm of prostate, code 198.5, secondary malignant neoplasm of other specified sites, bone and
bone marrow, are additional diagnoses. [*Coding Clinic* 3Q '99 5, effective with discharges July 1,
1999]

DOC: Use code 198.5 when the physician documents metastasis to the bone or bone marrow.

733.13   Pathologic fracture of vertebrae   DRG 239

AHA CC: In a patient whose pathology report states "metastatic carcinoma of the vertebral body
consistent with prostate primary," but whose reason for admission is a spinal cord injury from a
compression deformity of the same vertebral body, assign 733.13, pathological fracture of vertebra
as principal diagnosis; 336.3, myelopathy in other diseases classified elsewhere 185, malignant
neoplasm of prostate, code 198.5, secondary malignant neoplasm of other specified sites, bone and
bone marrow, are additional diagnoses. [*Coding Clinic* 3Q '99 5, effective with discharges July 1,
1999]

AHA CC: Always verify with the physician when the medical record is unclear as to whether a
fracture was pathological or the result of trauma. Minor trauma can result in a fracture in a patient
with severely diseased bone. The physician is responsible for deciding whether or not the level of
injury is in accordance with the degree of trauma suffered by the patient. The following scenario
represents a situation where the physician must be contacted and further documentation placed in
the medical record prior to coding: Admission to the hospital occurred after a nursing home
patient fell off a sidewalk curb. History shows severe osteoporosis. X-ray revealed advanced
osteoporosis, separation of the acetabulum, and a crumbling fracture of the head of the left femur.
For this case, use a code(s) from the 800-829 series if the physician states that the fracture is due to
trauma. Assign an additional code for the osteoporosis. Use code 733.14 if the physician states
that the fracture is pathological and due to osteoporosis. Assign an additional code for the
osteoporosis. Assign an E code to identify the external cause of injury. [*Coding Clinic*, 4Q, '93, 25,
effective with discharges October 1, 1993]

AHA CC: Do not use subcategory 733.1x with a code from the 800-829 series for traumatic
fractures. To identify the nature of the trauma when pathological fracture follows minor trauma,
assign an external cause of injury code. [*Coding Clinic*, 4Q, '93, 25, effective with discharges
October 1, 1993]

AHA CC: Effective October 1, 1993, fifth digits were added to category 733 to allow
identification of the site of the fracture. [*Coding Clinic*, 4Q, '93, 25, effective with discharges
October 1, 1993]

AHA CC: Use a code from category 733 only if the physician documents a diagnosis of a
pathological fracture. A pathological fracture is a break in a diseased bone due to weakening of the
bone structure by pathologic process (such as osteoporosis or bone tumors) without any
identifiable trauma or following only minor trauma. The physician decides that the fracture is out
of proportion to the degree of trauma, not the coder. The physician may use x-ray indications of
diseased bone to determine a diagnosis of a pathological fracture. [*Coding Clinic*, 4Q, '93, 25,
effective with discharges October 1, 1993]

AHA CC: Use the code for the pathological fracture as the principal diagnosis when the physician
documents that the reason for admission was medical or surgical treatment of a pathological
fracture (that is, due to osteoporosis or metastatic malignant neoplasm). [*Coding Clinic*, N-D, '86,
10]

733.13   Pathologic fracture of vertebrae (continued)   DRG 239

AHA CC: Code a compression fracture as either traumatic (such as those that are work-related or due to sports) or pathological (due to a disease process, such as osteoporosis or cancer) depending on the documentation in the medical record. For example:

- Use a code from the 805.0-805.9 series if the compression fracture of the spine is the result of a blow to the head from diving into shallow water, or from a fall from a height onto the feet, or bounding on a snowmobile.
- Use code 733.1x if the compression fracture of the spine or hip is caused by osteoporosis or malignancy. Assigning codes from the 805.0-805.9 series or 820.8 to identify the fracture sites for a pathological fracture is considered a coding error. [*Coding Clinic*, N-D, '85, 16]

AHA CC: Assign code 733.1x when the physician's written diagnosis is "spontaneous fracture" regardless of whether or not the physician has entered the underlying disease process. [*Coding Clinic*, S-O, '85, 13]

AHA CC: Assign code 733.1x when the physician documents that the patient has a history of osteoporosis but the physician does not designate the fracture as pathological. The spontaneous fracture may or may not be related to osteoporosis. [*Coding Clinic*, S-O, '85, 13]

AHA CC: Assign a code for pathological fracture when the physician documents a spontaneous fracture as it is assumed to have occurred without external injury. A bone weakened by disease can spontaneously fracture with or without minor or slight trauma. Causes of pathological fractures include bone cysts or tumors, hyperparathyroidism, nutritional disturbances, congenital disorders, osteoporosis, Paget's disease, disuse atrophy, and osteomyelitis. [*Coding Clinic*, S-O, '85, 13]

AHA CC: Always verify with the physician when the medical record is unclear as to whether a vertebral fracture is pathological or the result of trauma. A review of the x-ray reports may provide clues about the fracture. In older patients (especially women) with osteoporosis involving the spine, a compression fracture of the vertebral body may occur as a result of the thinning of the cortices or wedging of vertebrae. Other causes of pathological fracture include degeneration of the vertebrae due to osteoarthritis, rarefaction of the bone due to other disorders of the spine or malignant neoplasms. [*Coding Clinic*, N-D, '84, 16]

DOC: Use code 733.13 when the physician documents spontaneous fracture of the vertebrae or collapse of the vertebrae.

DOC: Do not use 733.13 for traumatic fractures. The correct code to use is chosen from the 800-829 series.

721.3   Lumbosacral spondylosis without myelopathy   DRG 243

AHA CC: Neuritis or pain due to spondylosis or degenerative intervertebral disc disorder is included in code 721.3. [*Coding Clinic*, 2Q, '89, 14]

722.10   Displacement of lumbar intervertebral disc without   DRG 243
myelopathy

AHA CC: Use a code from the 722.0-722.2 series when the physician documents lateral disc herniation. [*Coding Clinic*, 1Q, '88, 10]

AHA CC: Do not code symptoms and signs associated with (due to) spondylosis and allied disorders or intervertebral disc disorder (such as slipped disc or arthritic degeneration of intevertebral disc). They are included in the 721-722 code series. For example:

- Use a code from category 722 when the physician documents sciatica due to a slipped or degenerative intervertebral disc. Do not assign code 724.3.
- Use a code from the 721-722 series when the physician documents pain or neuritis due to spondylosis or intervertebral disc disorder. Do not assign a code for the pain or neuritis. [*Coding Clinic*, 2Q, '89, 14, effective with discharges July 31, 1989]

Targeted DRG Listing

722.10   Displacement of lumbar intervertebral disc without myelopathy (continued)   DRG 243

DOC: Use code 722.10 when the physician documents lumbago or sciatica due to displacement of intervertebral disc, neuritis or radiculitis due to displacement or rupture of lumbar intervertebral disc, discogenic syndrome of the lumbar or lubosacral intervertebral disc, herniation of the nucleus pulposus of the lumbar or lubosacral intervertebral disc, extrusion of the lumbar or lubosacral intervertebral disc, prolapse of the lumbar or lubosacral intervertebral disc, protrusion of the lumbar or lubosacral intervertebral disc, rupture of the lumbar or lubosacral intervertebral disc, or neuritis or radiculitis due to displacement to rupture of the lumbar or lumbosacral intervertebral disc.

722.52   Degeneration of lumbar or lumbosacral intervertebral disc   DRG 243

AHA CC: Signs and symptoms due to spondylosis or intervertebral disc disorders are included in code 722.52. [*Coding Clinic*, 2Q, '89, 14]

724.02   Spinal stenosis lumbar region   DRG 243

AHA CC: Use code 724.02 when the physician documents lumbar stenosis is not attributable to a herniated disc. [*Coding Clinic*, 3Q, '94, 14]

724.2   Lumbago   DRG 243

AHA CC: Do not code symptoms and signs associated with (due to) spondylosis and allied disorders or intervertebral disc disorder (such as slipped disc or arthritic degeneration of intevertebral disc). They are included in the 721-722 code series. For example:

- Use a code from category 722 when the physician documents sciatica due to a slipped or degenerative intervertebral disc. Do not assign code 724.3.
- Use a code from the 721–722 series when the physician documents pain or neuritis due to spondylosis or intervertebral disc disorder. Do not assign a code for the pain or neuritis.
- Use a code from category 722 when the physician documents spinal stenosis due to degeneration (arthritic) of the intervertebral disc. If the physician indicates the spinal stenosis is congenital or does not document a cause, it is classified within the 723-724 categories. [*Coding Clinic*, 2Q, '89, 14, effective with discharges July 31, 1989]

AHA CC: Use code 780.9 when the physician documents chronic pain syndrome or, if the site is specified, code to pain by site involved, such as chronic low back pain syndrome (724.2). [*Coding Clinic*, N-D, '85, 12]

DOC: Use code 724.2 when the physician documents low back pain, low back syndrome, or lumbalgia.

DOC: Do not use 724.2 when the physician documents that the low back pain is due to intervertebral disc disorders. The correct code is chosen from the 722.0-722.9 series.

DOC: Do not use 724.2 when the physician documents that the low back pain is due to spondylosis. The correct code is chosen from the 721.0-721.9 series.

805.2   Closed fracture of dorsal (thoracic) vertebra without   DRG 243
mention of spinal cord injury

AHA CC: Always verify with the physician when the medical record is unclear as to whether a fracture was pathological or the result of trauma. Minor trauma can result in a fracture in a patient with severely diseased bone. The physician is responsible for deciding whether or not the level of injury is in accordance with the degree of trauma suffered by the patient. The following scenario represents a situation where the physician must be contacted and further documentation placed in the medical record prior to coding: Admission to the hospital occurred after a nursing home patient fell off a sidewalk curb. History shows severe osteoporosis. X-ray revealed advanced osteoporosis, separation of the acetabulum, and a crumbling fracture of the head of the left femur. For this case, use a code(s) from 800-829 series if the physician states that the fracture is due to trauma. Assign an additional code for the osteoporosis.

Use code 733.14 if the physician states that the fracture is pathological and due toosteoporosis. Assign an additional code for the osteoporosis. Assign an E code to identify the external cause of injury. [*Coding Clinic*, 4Q, '93, 25, effective with discharges October 1, 1993]

AHA CC: *Do not* use subcategory 733.1 with a code from the 800-829 series for traumatic fractures. To identify the nature of the trauma when pathological fracture follows minor trauma, assign an external cause of injury code. [*Coding Clinic*, 4Q, '93, 25, effective with discharges October 1, 1993]

AHA CC: Use a code from category 733 only if the physician documents a diagnosis of a pathological fracture. A pathological fracture is a break in a diseased bone due to weakening of the bone structure by pathologic process (such as osteoporosis or bone tumors) without any identifiable trauma or following only minor trauma. The physician decides that the fracture is out of proportion to the degree of trauma, not the coder. The physician may use x-ray indications of diseased bone to determine a diagnosis of a pathological fracture. [*Coding Clinic*, 4Q, '93, 25, effective with discharges October 1, 1993]

AHA CC: Code a compression fracture as either traumatic (such as those that are work-related or due to sports) or pathological (due to a disease process, such as osteoporosis or cancer) depending on the documentation in the medical record. For example:

- Use a code from the 805.0-805.9 series if the compression fracture of the spine is the result of a blow to the head from diving into shallow water, or from a fall from a height onto the feet, or bounding on a snowmobile.
- Use code 733.1x if the compression fracture of the spine or hip is caused by osteoporosis or malignancy. Assigning codes from the 805.0-805.9 series or 820.8 to identify the fracture sites for a pathological fracture is considered a coding error. [*Coding Clinic*, N-D, '85, 16]

DOC: Use code 805.2 when the physician documents a dorsal (thoracic) fracture of the vertebra without spinal cord injury.

DOC: *Do not use* code 805.2 when the physician documents a dorsal (thoracic) fracture of the vertebra with spinal cord injury. The correct code is 806.2x.

805.4   Closed fracture of lumbar vertebra without mention of spinal cord injury

AHA CC: Always verify with the physician when the medical record is unclear as to whether a fracture was pathological or the result of trauma. Minor trauma can result in a fracture in a patient with severely diseased bone. The physician is responsible for deciding whether or not the level of injury is in accordance with the degree of trauma suffered by the patient. The following scenario represents a situation where the physician must be contacted and further documentation placed in the medical record prior to coding: Admission to the hospital occurred after a nursing home patient fell off a sidewalk curb. History shows severe osteoporosis. X-ray revealed advanced osteoporosis, separation of the acetabulum, and a crumbling fracture of the head of the left femur. For this case, use a code(s) from the 800-829 series if the physician states that the fracture is due to trauma. Assign an additional code for the osteoporosis. Use code 733.14 if the physician states that the fracture is pathological and due to osteoporosis. Assign an additional code for the osteoporosis. Assign an E code to identify the external cause of injury. [*Coding Clinic*, 4Q, '93, 25, effective with discharges October 1, 1993]

AHA CC: Do not use subcategory 733.1 with a code from the 800-829 series for traumatic fractures. To identify the nature of the trauma when pathological fracture follows minor trauma, assign an external cause of injury codes. [*Coding Clinic*, 4Q, '93, 25, effective with discharges October 1, 1993]

AHA CC: Use a code from category 733 only if the physician documents a diagnosis of a pathological fracture. A pathological fracture is a break in a diseased bone due to weakening of the bone structure by pathologic process (such as osteoporosis or bone tumors) without any identifiable trauma or following only minor trauma. The physician decides that the fracture is out of proportion to the degree of trauma, not the coder. The physician may use x-ray indications of diseased bone to determine a diagnosis of a pathological fracture. [*Coding Clinic*, 4Q, '93, 25, effective with discharges October 1, 1993]

AHA CC: Code a compression fracture as either traumatic (such as those that are work-related or due to sports) or pathological (due to a disease process, such as osteoporosis or cancer) depending on the documentation in the medical record. For example:

- Use a code from the 805.0-805.9 series if the compression fracture of the spine is the result of a blow to the head from diving into shallow water, or from a fall from a height onto the feet, or bounding on a snowmobile.
- Use code 733.1x if the compression fracture of the spine or hip is caused by osteoporosis or malignancy. Assigning codes from the 805.0-805.9 series or 820.8 to identify the fracture sites for a pathological fracture is considered a coding error. [*Coding Clinic*, N-D, '85, 16]

DOC: Use code 805.4 when the physician documents a lumbar fracture of the vertebra without spinal cord injury.

DOC: Do not use code 805.4 when the physician documents a lumbar fracture of the vertebra with spinal cord injury. The correct code is 806.4.

DRG 296 Nutritional and Miscellaneous Metabolic Disorders, Age Greater than 17 with CC

DRG 182   Esophagitis, Gastroenteritis and Miscellaneous Digestive Disorders, Age Greater than 17 with CC

Issue

Choosing between dehydration and gastroenteritis as the principal diagnosis is problematic because of the unclear documentation on the reason for admission and the complexity of the ICD-9-CM diagnosis codes and coding guidelines.

Most Common Diagnosis Codes

DRG 296

- 276.1, Hyposmolality and/or hyponatremia
- 276.5, Volume depletion

DRG 182

- 008.45, Intestinal infections due to *Clostridium difficile*
- 530.81, Esophageal reflux
- 558.9, Other and unspecified noninfectious gastroenteritis and colitis
- 562.11, Diverticulitis of colon

Coding and Documentation Guidelines

008.45   Intestinal infections due to *Clostridium difficile*   **DRG 182**

See standards on page 609.

530.81   Esophageal reflux   **DRG 182**

See standards on page 609.

558.9   Other and unspecified noninfectious gastroenteritis and colitis   **DRG 182**

See standards on page 610.

562.11   Diverticulitis of colon without mention of hemorrhage   **DRG 182**

See standards on page 610.

276.1   Hyposmolality and/or hyponatremia   **DRG 296**

AHA CC: Do not arbitrarily report a diagnosis code on the basis of an abnormal laboratory finding alone. Do not list a diagnosis code on the basis of a single lab value or abnormal diagnostic finding. Many factors influence the value of a lab sample. These include the method used to obtain the sample, the collection device, the method used to transport the sample to the lab, the calibration of the machine that reads the values, and the condition of the patient. [*Coding Clinic*, 2Q, '90, 3, effective with discharges April 1, 1990, and *Coding Clinic*, 4Q, '93, 39, effective with discharges August 18, 1993]

DOC: Use code 276.1 when the physician documents sodium [Na] deficiency.

DOC: Do not use code 276.1 when the physician documents hypernatremia. The correct code is 276.0.

276.5   Volume depletion

DRG 296

AHA CC: Assign code 584.9 as the principal diagnosis and code 276.5 when the physician documents that the admission of a patient with acute renal failure was for dehydration. [*Coding Clinic*, 3Q, '02, 22]

AHA CC: Do not arbitrarily report a diagnosis code on the basis of an abnormal laboratory finding alone. Do not list a diagnosis code on the basis of a single lab value or abnormal diagnostic finding. Many factors influence the value of a lab sample. These include the method used to obtain the sample, the collection device, the method used to transport the sample to the lab, the calibration of the machine that reads the values, and the condition of the patient. [*Coding Clinic*, 2Q, '90, 3, effective with discharges April 1, 1990, and *Coding Clinic*, 4Q, '93, 39, effective with discharges August 18, 1993]

AHA CC: Assign code 042 as the principal diagnosis and codes 007.4 and 276.5 when the physician documents that the admission of an AIDS patient was for severe diarrhea and dehydration. The physician documents cryptosporidiosis with dehydration. This advice replaces advice published in *Coding Clinic*, July-August 1987. [*Coding Clinic*, 4Q, '97, 30, effective with discharges October 1, 1997]

AHA CC: A patient with dehydration may present with symptoms and signs of dehydration, such as dryness of mucous membranes, loss of skin turgor, and anorexia. Inadequate fluid intake, vomiting, diarrhea, sweating or polyuria can cause dehydration. The main objective is total replacement of fluid deficit within 48-72 hours. Dehydration can occur in patients with burns, gastrointestinal disease, peritonitis, ascites, diabetic glycosuria, Addison's dis-ease, hypoaldosteronism, renal failure, urinary track infections and other infections. Treatment for dehydration includes oral replenishment of fluids or intravenous administration of fluids. Because dehydration is often the result of another condition as well as a severe management problem in itself, it often is difficult to determine the principal diagnosis. The circumstances of the admission and the judgment of the attending physician govern whether dehydration meets the definition of principal diagnosis. The following are some examples to assist in this determination:

- Dehydration and urinary tract infection are both   present on admission. Treatment consisted of intravenous (IV) fluids for the dehydration and antibiotics for the urinary tract infection. Verify with the physician regarding principal diagnosis, as it is possible that the urinary tract infection could have been treated on an outpatient basis but that the dehydration necessitated the inpatient admission. The reason for admission was nausea, vomiting and diarrhea, complicated by dehydration. The physician documented that the diarrhea was caused by tetracycline given to the patient after recently undergoing a nephrostomy with lithotripsy. History shows the presence of an ileostomy for Crohn's disease. Assign codes 276.5, 564.5, E930.4, 555.9 and V44.2. Verify with the physician regarding the principal diagnosis.
- The reason for admission was diarrhea with dehydration. The physician documents a final diagnosis of diarrhea secondary to infectious gastroenteritis. Treatment included intravenous fluids for the dehydration and Kaopectate for the diarrhea. Assign code 276.5 as the principal diagnosis if review of the medical record shows that the reason for admission was intravenous fluid administration to treat the dehydration, the infectious gastroenteritis having been dealt with (or subsiding) on an outpatient basis. However, assign code 009.0 as the principal diagnosis and 276.5 as a secondary diagnosis if the documentation shows that the patient was admitted for treatment of both the infectious gastroenteritis and the dehydration. The medication prescribed, Kaopectate, is an oral antidiarrheal agent that may be administered on an outpatient basis. Therefore, it is probable that the dehydration necessitating intravenous fluids prompted the admission.
- Assign code 198.7 as the principal diagnosis and codes 276.5 and 162.9 as secondary diagnoses for the following scenario: The reason for admission was syncope, vomiting, diarrhea and dehydration. Patient history states cancer of the lung. The patient received CT scan and the physician documents "bilateral adrenal tumors explaining the patient's dehydration.." Fluids were given but no treatment was given for adrenal metastasis.

276.5   Volume depletion (continued)   DRG 296

- Assign code 276.5 as the principal diagnosis when the physician documents that the reason for admission is dehydration with terminal carcinoma of stomach. History shows carcinoma with generalized metastases. Treatment included rehydration with intravenous fluids. No treatment was provided toward the cancer during the patient's stay. Assign codes 151.9 and 199.0 as secondary diagnoses. [*Coding Clinic*, 2Q, '88, 9]

DOC: Use code 276.5 when the physician documents dehydration, hypovolemia, or depletion of volume of plasma or extracellular fluid.

DOC: Do not use code 276.5 when the physician documents postoperative hypovolemic shock. The correct code is 998.0.

DOC: Do not use code 276.5 when the physician documents traumatic hypovolemic shock. The correct code is 958.4.

DRG 316 Renal Failure

DRG 331   Other Kidney and Urinary Tract Diagnoses, Age Greater than 17 with CC

Issue

The coding of renal disorders is problematic because of the lack of physician documentation on either the known or suspected cause of renal disease, unclear documentation on the reason for admission, and the complexity of the ICD-9-CM diagnosis codes and coding guidelines for the renal disorders.

Most common Diagnosis Codes

DRG 316

- 403.91, Hypertensive renal disease with renal failure
- 584.9, Acute renal failure NOS
- 585, Chronic renal failure

DRG 331

- 250.40, 250.41, Diabetes with renal manifestations, type II and type I, not stated as uncontrolled
- 593.9, Unspecified disorder of kidney and ureter
- 996.64, Infection and inflammatory reaction due to indwelling urinary catheter
- 996.81, Complications of transplanted kidney
- 997.5, Urinary complications

Coding and Documentation Guidelines

250.40	Diabetes with renal manifestations, type II, not stated as uncontrolled	DRG 331

250.41	Diabetes mellitus with renal manifestations, type I, not stated as uncontrolled	

CG: Azotemia is produced by diminished glomerular filtration of nonprotein nitrogenous compounds in the kidney. These compounds are: creatinine, amino acids, uric acids, creatine, and ammonia. Azotemia may be further categorized as prerenal (788.9), postrenal (788.9), or renal azotemia (790.6). The essential meaning conveyed by any of the azotemic states is that the patient suffers from a marked elevation of urea nitrogen and creatine, however, it may be used by a physician as a marker for the presence of either acute or chronic renal failure. The coder should always ask the physician if the patient has either acute or chronic renal failure.

AHA CC: In ICD-9-CM diabetes mellitus is one of several disease categories where one code classifies both the disease and its manifestations. Additional codes may be assigned to more thoroughly describe the manifestations. Diabetic renal failure, diabetic uremia, diabetic intercapillary glomerulosclerosis and chronic renal failure, diabetic nephropathy with chronic renal failure provide a cause and effect relationship that require code 250.4x to be sequenced first. [*Coding Clinic*, 1Q, '03, 20-21]

AHA CC: A patient with type II diabetes, admitted in diabetic coma, is diagnosed with nephrotic syndrome and gangrene of several toes. His case would be coded as follows: Principal diagnosis: 250.30, diabetes with other coma. Other diagnoses: 250.40 diabetes with renal manifestations, 581.81 nephrotic syndrome in diseases classified elsewhere, 250.70 diabetes with peripheral circulatory disorder, 785.4 gangrene. [*Coding Clinic* 3Q '91,12, effective with discharges July 1, 1991]

250.40 Diabetes with renal manifestations, type II, not stated as uncontrolled   **DRG 331**

250.41 Diabetes mellitus with renal manifestations, type I, not stated as uncontrolled (continued)

AHA CC: Use codes 250.4x and 403.91 when the physician documents progressive diabetic nephropathy with hypertension and chronic renal failure. [*Coding Clinic*, 3Q, '91, 3, effective with discharges July 1, 1991]

AHA CC: Use codes 250.4x and 585 when the physician documents diabetes with chronic renal failure. [*Coding Clinic*, 3Q, '91, 3, effective with discharges July 1, 1991]

AHA CC: Use codes 250.4x and 581.81 when the physician documents diabetic nephrotic syndrome. [*Coding Clinic*, 3Q, '91, 3, effective with discharges July 1, 1991]

AHA CC: Use codes 250.4x and 583.81 when the physician documents diabetes with nephritis. [*Coding Clinic*, 3Q, '91, 3, effective with discharges July 1, 1991]

AHA CC: Use codes 250.4x and 791.0 when the physician documents diabetes with mild proteinuria. [*Coding Clinic*, 3Q, '91, 3, effective with discharges July 1, 1991]

AHA CC: Use codes 250.4x and 581.81 when the physician documents diabetic nephrosis or diabetic nephrotic syndrome. [*Coding Clinic*, 3Q, '91, 3, effective with discharges July 1, 1991]

AHA CC: Use codes 250.4x and 583.81 when the physician documents unspecified diabetic nephropathy. [*Coding Clinic*, 3Q, '91, 3, effective with discharges July 1, 1991]

AHA CC: Use as many codes as necessary for category 250 when the physician documents several complications in more than one system. [*Coding Clinic*, 3Q, '91, 3, effective with discharges July 1, 1991]

To further assist the coding of these cases, please read the following:

- Do not assign the codes for prerenal or renal azotemia as the principal diagnosis when the cause of the condition is known. These are symptom codes, and their use should follow the guidelines for coding symptoms.
- Prerenal azotemia is caused by a condition external to the kidney, such as severe dehydration, congestive heart failure or any other edema-forming condition, systemic hypotension, or any condition that causes vascular pooling. These conditions produce inadequate glomerular filtration rates in the kidney.
- Postrenal azotemia occurs with normal renal tubules, but with a diminished glomerular filtration rate due to urinary tract obstruction, such as prostatic enlargement, bladder outlet obstruction, ureteral obstruction. In this form of azotemia, the excretion of urine is functionally impaired.
- Renal azotemia is characterized by damaged renal tubules, in conjunction with diminished glomerular filtration rates. The condition is produced by renal disease and may result in renal failure, either acute (584.9) or chronic (585). The term progressive may be associated with azotemia. Some examples are: acute renal tubular necrosis (584.5), acute renal tubular necrosis due to trauma (958.5), toxic nephropathy (584.5) and analgesic nephropathy inducing papillary necrosis (584.7).
- The coder has the option to use azotemia as an additional code when the cause of the azotemia is known. If the number of codes is tightly restricted, it is better to omit the azotemia code in favor of a more descriptive code. Example: noninsulin dependent nephropathy with azotemia-250.40 and 583.81. [*Coding Clinic*, 4Q '88 1-3, effective with discharges October 1, 1988]
- To code hypertension in end-stage renal disease due to type II diabetes mellitus, one must first ask the physician if the hypertension is due to hypervolemia. If the answer is affirmative, the case is coded as follows: 250.40, 405.99, 276.6, and 585, diabetes with renal failure and hypertension secondary to hypervolemia. However, if the physician's response is that the patient has hypertensive renal disease due to diabetes mellitus, the case would be coded 250.40 and 403.9x. [*Coding Clinic*, S-O '87, 9, effective with discharges September 1, 1987]

250.40   Diabetes with renal manifestations, type II, not stated   **DRG 331**
          as uncontrolled

250.41   Diabetes mellitus with renal manifestations, type I, not stated as
          uncontrolled (continued)

AHA CC: Use code 250.02 when the physician documents uncontrolled diabetes mellitus, adult-onset type, and the patient requires insulin. The determination of the fifth digit is based on whether the patient is a type I or a type II diabetic. When the documentation is not clear as to the patient's type, check with the physician and have him or her state the type in the medical record. The fact that the patient is on insulin has no affect on code assignment. Only the type of diabetes influences code assignment. [*Coding Clinic*, 4Q, '97, 30, effective with discharges October 1, 1997]

AHA CC: Before coding a diagnosis of an adult onset diabetic who is insulin-dependent, check with the physician and have him document in the medical record whether the patient has type I or type II diabetes. The age of the patient at the time of disease onset does not affect the assignment of the appropriate fifth digit for diabetes. The type of diabetes the patient has determines the fifth digit. Type I patients are dependent on insulin to sustain life because the body does not produce insulin. Type II, whose bodies do produce sufficient amounts of insulin, may receive insulin (to correct symptomatic or persistent hyperglycemia) to assist the body in utilizing the insulin that is present in the body, but they are not dependent on the insulin to sustain life. Characteristics of type I diabetics include onset most often prior to age 40 although onset may occur in older adults (particularly in the nonobese) and most frequently in juveniles. Type II characteristics include onset most often in adults, beginning in midlife or beyond, but may have its onset in juvenile. [*Coding Clinic*, 2Q, '97, 14, effective with discharges May 1, 1997]

AHA CC: Effective October 1, 1993, fifth digits have been added and the previous fifth digits modified to indicate uncontrolled diabetes. The term "uncontrolled diabetes" is nonspecific, indicating that the patient's blood sugar level is not kept within acceptable levels by his or her current treatment regimen. Causes of uncontrolled diabetes include noncompliance, insulin resistance, dietary indiscretion, and intercurrent illness. Do not assign a fifth digit indicating uncontrolled diabetes based upon blood glucose levels. Use these fifth digits only when the physician documents a diagnosis of uncontrolled diabetes. [*Coding Clinic*, 4Q, '93, 19, effective with discharges October 1, 1993]

AHA CC: Use the fifth digit "1" when the physician documents an insulin-dependent diabetes regardless of when the diagnosis was made by the attending physician. However, just because the patient received insulin, he or she is not necessarily insulin-dependent. If in doubt as to the patient's type of diabetes, check with the physician and have him clarify this in the medical record. [*Coding Clinic*, 2Q, '92, 5, effective with discharges April 1, 1992]

AHA CC: Use category 250 to classify diabetes mellitus, a disorder of glucose metabolism due to either an absolute decrease in the amount of insulin secreted by the pancreas or to a reduction in the biologic effectiveness of the insulin secreted. Diabetes is broken out into two major groups, type I and type II. Diabetes mellitus can cause two types of complications, the acute metabolic complication and the chronic effect that occurs in another body system due to the diabetes. The latter can affect the kidneys, eyes, peripheral nerves (including the peripheral autonomic nerves) and peripheral blood vessels. The code from the 250.4x-250.8x series for the diabetes mellitus with complicating conditions is coded first, with an additional code to identify the specific complicating condition when the physician qualifies the condition as diabetic or due to diabetes. Assign a code for the condition as a complication only when the physician identifies it as a diabetic complication since a condition listed with a diagnosis of diabetes mellitus or in a diabetic patient is not necessarily a complication of the diabetes. [*Coding Clinic*, 3Q, '91, 3, effective with discharges July 1, 1991]

AHA CC: The assignment of the fifth digit "0" or "1" with a diagnosis of diabetes mellitus is determined by the physician's description of the patient's diabetes. A type II may receive doses of insulin when the patient is having difficulty controlling blood sugar values or when an infection or other illness interferes with control on a temporary basis. Dependence on insulin means the patient must have insulin to avoid a life-threatening situation and implies a true dependence rather

250.40 **Diabetes with renal manifestations, type II, not stated**   **DRG 331**
as uncontrolled

250.41 **Diabetes mellitus with renal manifestations, type I, not stated as**
uncontrolled (continued)

than a matter of simple control on a temporary basis. If a patient is receiving insulin but the physician does not indicate whether the diabetes is insulin-dependent or not, check with the physician and have him or her state in the medical record whether the patient is type I or type II. Do not change the physician's designation of noninsulin dependent, type II diabetes mellitus, to insulin-dependent, type I, without physician agreement. [*Coding Clinic*, 2Q, '90, 22, effective with discharges April 1, 1990]

AHA CC: Use code 250.4 (with the fifth digit) as the primary code when the physician documents a diagnosis of diabetic renal failure, diabetic uremia, diabetic intercapillary glomerulosclerosis and chronic renal failure, diabetic nephropathy with chronic renal failure, or diabetic nephrosis with chronic renal failure. These statements describe a cause and effect relationship. Use 581.81 or 585 as an additional code. In ICD-9-CM, category 250 serves as the primary code to classify both the disease and its major manifestations. An additional code(s) is used as a secondary code to provide more specificity in describing the manifestations. No note exists under code 585 exists under code 585 that excludes that with mention of diabetes mellitusThere is no subterm under "Diabetes mellitus" for chronic renal failure or chronic uremia and diabetes mellitus is not listed as a subterm under "Failure, renal, chronic" or under "Uremia, chronic." Thus, when the physician's diagnosis does not state a cause and effect relationship between the diabetes mellitus and chronic renal failure or chronic uremia, code 585 may be used as the principal diagnosis. [*Coding Clinic*, S-O, '84, 1]

DOC: Use code 250.4x when the physician documents diabetic nephropathy, diabetic nephrosis, intercapillary glomerulosclerosis, or Kimmelstiel-Wilson syndrome.

593.9 **Unspecified disorder of kidney and ureter**   **DRG 331**

AHA CC: Assign code 593.9 when the physician documents early stages of renal impairment as determined by mildly abnormal elevated values of serum creatinine, or BUN, or diminished creatinine clearance. Clinical symptoms or other abnormal laboratory findings may or may not be present and are usually minimal. The treatment of renal insufficiency is dependent to a large extent on the underlying cause. [*Coding Clinic*, 1Q, '93, 17]

DOC: Use code 593.9 when the physician documents renal insufficiency

996.64 **Infection and inflammatory reaction due to indwelling**   **DRG 331**
urinary catheter

AHA CC: Use codes 996.64 and 041.0 when the physician documents that a patient with an indwelling urinary catheter required admission because of streptococcal infection. [*Coding Clinic*, 2Q, '90, 11, effective with discharges April 1, 1990]

AHA CC: List the complication code as the principal diagnosis when the reason for admission was treatment of a complication resulting from surgery or other medical care. ICD-9-CM states to "use additional code to identify complication" if the complication is classified to the 996-999 series. [*Coding Clinic*, 2Q, '90, 11, effective with discharges April 1, 1990]

AHA CC: Use code 996.68 when the physician documents peritoneal infection due to peritoneal dialysis if the infection is due to the presence of the internal device, such as a Tenckhoff catheter. Assign code 041.1 secondarily. [*Coding Clinic*, J-F, '87, 14 and *Coding Clinic*, 4Q, '98, 54, effective with discharges October 1, 1998]

DOC: Use code 996.64 when the physician documents infection due to indwelling urinary catheter.

Targeted DRG Listing

996.64 Infection and inflammatory reaction due to indwelling urinary catheter (continued) DRG 331

DOC: Use code 996.64 when the physician documents inflammation due to indwelling urinary catheter.

DOC: Do not use code 996.64 when the physician documents inflammation or exit site infection due to peritoneal dialysis catheter.

996.81 Complications of transplanted organ, kidney DRG 331

AHA CC: Assign code 996.81,complication of a transplanted organ, kidney, as a secondary diagnosis with a principal diagnosis of 486, pneumonitis when the physician documents the patient was admitted with pneumonitis and in renal failure secondary to transplant rejection. Assign code 586 as an additional diagnosis to identify the renal failure. [*Coding Clinic*, 3Q, '98, 7, effective with discharges September 1, 1998]

AHA CC: Assign code 996.81 as principal diagnosis when the physician documents the patient was admitted in renal failure secondary to transplant rejection. Assign code 586 as a secondary diagnosis to identify the renal failure. [*Coding Clinic*, 3Q, '98, 6, effective with discharges September 1, 1998]

AHA CC: Assign code 996.81 as the principal diagnosis and code 593.3 as an additional diagnosis when the physician documents status post kidney transplant with ureteral stricture of the transplanted ureter. Treatment involved dilation of the ureter, procedure code 59.8. Code assignment is not dependent on the amount of time post organ transplant (e.g., one week, one year, three years). [*Coding Clinic*, 3Q, '94, 8, effective with discharges July 1, 1994]

AHA CC: Assign code 996.81 when the physician documents admission due to acute rejection crisis. Do not use code V42.0 as an additional code. Use the status codes only if there is no current disease. [*Coding Clinic*, 2Q, '94, 9, effective with discharges April 1, 1994]

AHA CC: List the complication code as the principal diagnosis when the reason for admission was treatment of a complication resulting from surgery or other medical care. ICD-9-CM states to "use additional code to identify complication" if the complication is classified to the 996–999 series. [*Coding Clinic*, 2Q, '90, 11, effective with discharges April 1, 1990]

AHA CC: Use code 996.68 when the physician documents peritoneal infection due to peritoneal dialysis if the infection is due to the presence of the internal device, such as a Tenckhoff catheter. Assign code 041.1 secondarily. [*Coding Clinic*, J-F, '87, 14 and *Coding Clinic*, 4Q, '98, 54, effective with discharges October 1, 1998]

DOC: Use code 996.81 when the physician documents transplant failure or rejection of kidney.

997.5 Complications affecting specified body system, not elsewhere classified, urinary complication DRG 331

AHA CC: Do not use code 997.5 to classify vascular to identify vascular complications of the mesenteric artery (997.71), renal artery (997.72) and other vessels (997.79). complications. Effective October 1, 2001, new codes have been created. [*Coding Clinic*, 4Q, '01, 81]

When a patient has failed a voiding trial following surgery and a Foley catheter is inserted, do not code urinary retention unless the physician has documented this condition in themedical record. There may be "clues" in the record, nursing notes, a standing order to straight record. It is possible the physician may not feel it is appropriate to report urinary retention as an additional diagnosis and, if this is the case, do not code it. On the other hand, if the physician states that the urinary retention resulted from a postoperative complication, assign codes 997.5 and 788.20. [*Coding Clinic*, 3Q, '96, 10 and 15, effective August 15, 1996]

AHA CC: Assign code 997.5 as the principal diagnosis when the physician documents urinary incontinence secondary to intrinsic sphincter dysfunction following transurethral resection of prostate or radical prostatectomy. Treatment involved periurethral collagen injections. Use codes 596.59 and 788.30 or 788.32, if specified as stress urinary incontinence, secondarily. [*Coding Clinic*, 4Q, '95, 73, effective with discharges October 1, 1995]

997.5 Complications affecting specified body system, not elsewhere classified, urinary complication (continued) — DRG 331

AHA CC: Assign code 997.5 as the principal diagnosis when the physician documents that the admission was due to a postoperative complication of urinary retention. Outpatient orchiectomy was performed for biopsy-proven adenocarcinoma of the prostate. Use codes 788.2 and 185 secondarily. [*Coding Clinic*, 1Q, '94, 20, effective with discharges January 1, 1994]

AHA CC: Assign two codes, 997.5 and 599.0, when the physician documents postoperative urinary tract infection specified by the physician as a postoperative complication. Codes in category 997 cover a variety of postoperative complications without specifying the nature of the complication. Therefore, assign an additional code to identify the specific complication. [*Coding Clinic*, 1Q, '92, 13, effective with discharges January 1, 1992]

AHA CC: Assign code 997.5 as the principal diagnosis when the physician documents stenosis of the ileal conduit stoma. The presence of chronic inflammation of the skin surrounding the stoma is included in code 997.5 if the inflammation of the skin surrounding the stoma is the result of the stenosis or leakage. If the cause of the inflammation is a covering of the stoma area, such as the adhesive tape, use code 692.4. Do not use code 996.6 for inflammation of the skin around the stoma. [*Coding Clinic*, 2Q, '89, 16, effective with discharges July 31, 1989]

AHA CC: Assign code 595.0 or 599.0 when the physician or the content of the medical record does not state that the "cystitis" or the "urinary tract infection" was a consequence of a surgical or diagnostic procedure (997.5) or due to an internal device, implant or graft (996.31, 996.39, and 996.6). To further specify the effect of complications classified to 996.31, 996.39, 996.6 or 997.5, such as urinary tract infection, urinary retention, oliguria, or acute renal failure, assign additional codes. [*Coding Clinic* S-O, '85, 3]

AHA CC: When the cause of the postoperative cystitis or postoperative urinary tract infection is not documented, the physician must be contacted prior to coding. The physician needs to state in the medical record whether the urinary tract infection or cystitis is related to or resulted from the procedure performed. While these two diagnoses indicate that an infection has occurred postoperatively, there is nothing in the description to assume this occurred as a result of a diagnostic or therapeutic procedure. Some situations that may produce postoperative infection are:

- Placement of a urinary retention catheter to facilitate surgery and to prevent unwanted postoperative urinary conditions, such as urinary retention, may cause postoperative cystitis or urinary tract infection. Use code 996.64.
- Postoperative urinary retention, in particular after pelvic or perineal operations, may lead to urinary tract infection. Use code 997.5 for both conditions.
- A urinary tract procedure, diagnostic or surgical, may be followed by a postprocedure cystitis. Use code 997.5.
- Postoperative oliguria may predispose to urinary tract infection. Use code 997.5 for both conditions.
- Malfunction of urinary retention catheter may cause urinary retention. Use code 996.31.
- A patient may be readmitted with urinary tract infection due to a urinary retention catheter for a chronically distended bladder. Use code 996.64.
- Bacteria may be been present prior to surgery and may surface as acute cystitis or urinary tract infection following surgery. Use either code 595.0 or 599.0. [*Coding Clinic*, S-O, '85, 3]

AHA CC: Assign code 997.4 with an additional code of 572.4 when the physician documents a diagnosis of hepatorenal syndrome due to surgery. [*Coding Clinic*, 3Q, '92, 15, effective with discharges July 1, 1992]

AHA CC: Since the codes in category 997 address a variety of postoperative complications without specifying the nature of the complication, use an additional code whenever possible to describe the specific complication. [*Coding Clinic*, 1Q, '92, 13, effective with discharges January 1, 1992 and *Coding Clinic*, 1Q, '93, 26, effective with discharges January 1, 1993]

AHA CC: Use codes 996.64 and 041.0 when the physician documents that a patient with an indwelling urinary catheter required admission because of streptococcal infection. [*Coding Clinic*, 2Q, '90, 11, effective with discharges April 1, 1990]

997.5   Complications affecting specified body system, not elsewhere   **DRG 331**
classified, urinary complication (continued)

AHA CC: List the complication code as the principal diagnosis when the reason for admission was treatment of a complication resulting from surgery or other medical care. ICD-9-CM states to "use additional code to identify complication" if the complication is classified to the 996-999 series. [*Coding Clinic*, 2Q, '90, 11, effective with discharges April 1, 1990]

DOC: Use code 997.5 when the physician documents complications of external stoma of urinary tract.

DOC: Use code 997.5 when the physician documents complications of internal ansatomosis and bypass of urinary tract, including that involving the intestinal tract.

DOC: Use code 997.5 when the physician documents oliguria or anuria specified as due to a procedure.

DOC: Use code 997.5 when the physician documents renal failure or renal insufficiency specified as due to a procedure.

DOC: Do not use code 997.5 when the physician documents postoperative stricture of the ureter. The correct code to use is 593.3.

DOC: Do not use code 997.5 when the physician documents postoperative stricture of the urethra. The correct code to use is 598.2.

403.91   Hypertensive renal disease, unspecified with renal   **DRG 316**
failure

CG: Effective October 1, 2002, use an additional code to specify type of heart failure: 428.0, 428.200-428.23, 428.30-428.333, 428.40-428.43 with category 402 codes.

AHA CC: Use code 250.40 and code 403.91 to report diabetic nephropathy with chronic renal failure (CRF) and hypertension. Report code 403.91 when physician documentation does not indicate CFR not due to hypertension. [*Coding Clinic*, 1Q, '03, 20-21]

AHA CC: When a note appears at the beginning of the subchapter it applies to all conditions in that subchapter. Therefore, the note, "Excludes hypertensive renal disease (403.0-403.9)" at the beginning of the renal disease subchapter means that if any of the conditions included in the renal disease subchapter are part of hypertensive renal disease, use a code from category 403. Do not interpret this excludes note to mean automatic combination of hypertension with all of the conditions in the subchapter (580-589). The physician must document a specific diagnosis, noting the combination to use a code from 403. For example, documentation of "nephropathy due to hypertension" combines the conditions, therefore the use of category 403 would be correct. In addition, when a condition classified to code range 580-589 is part of hypertensive renal disease, report only one code. For example, when the physician documents chronic renal failure (585) with hypertension (401), use a code only from category 403. [*Coding Clinic*, 4Q, '92, 22, effective with discharges October 1, 1992]

AHA CC: Use category 403 when the physician documents "hypertensive renal failure." However, do not interpret this to mean acute renal failure with hypertension and classify this diganosis to category 403. The index does not direct the coder to this category nor do the tabular notes make this connection. [*Coding Clinic*, 4Q, '92, 22, effective with discharges October 1, 1992]

AHA CC: An excludes note, effective October 1, 1992, was added to category 403 to affirm that acute renal failure and renal disease stated as not due to hypertension are not included in this category. The correct interpretation of the note for category 403 ("any condition classifiable to 585, 586, 587 with any condition classifiable to 401") is that, by the mention of hypertension and chronic renal failure (585), unspecified stage of renal failure (586) or renal sclerosis (587), hypertensive renal disease is assumed to exist. Any other combinations of diseases in the renal and hypertension categories, such as acute renal failure, are not to be presumed for this category. A patient may be diagnosed with acute renal failure separate from hypertensive disease, which may or may not be the result of progressive renal disease. Therefore, the hypertension codes do not

**403.91   Hypertensive renal disease, unspecified with renal   DRG 316
            failure (continued)**

include acute renal failure. It is incorrect to make the assumption that because something is not excluded from an exclusion list that it is included. [*Coding Clinic*, 4Q, '92, 22, effective with discharges October 1, 1992]

AHA CC: Assign a code from category 584 and an additional code from category 401 when the physician documents that the patient was admitted and treated for acute renal failure with essential hypertension. Assign a code from category 584 and an additional code from category 403 when the physician documents that the patient was admitted and treated for acute renal failure with hypertensive renal disease. The hypertension codes do not include acute renal failure. [*Coding Clinic*, 2Q, '92, 5, effective with discharges April 1, 1992]

AHA CC: Assign the appropriate code from categories 401-405 if the physician documents the patient's diagnosis as controlled hypertension. The use of the term "controlled" indicates an existing state of hypertension under control by therapy. Untreated hypertension or hypertension not responding to current therapeutic regimen may be described by the physician as uncontrolled hypertension. Assign the appropriate code from categories 401-405. The physician should document in the medical record the stage and type of hypertension. [*Coding Clinic*, 3Q, '90, 3, effective with discharges July 15, 1990]

AHA CC: When both hypertensive renal disease and hypertensive heart disease are stated in the diagnosis, assign a code from combination category 404. It does not matter whether the relationship between the hypertension and the renal disease is stated. [*Coding Clinic*, 3Q, '90, 3, effective with discharges July 15, 1990]

AHA CC: When conditions classified to categories 585–587 are present with hypertension, assign a code from category 403. A cause and effect relationship is presumed. Therefore, renal failure with hypertension is coded as hypertensive renal disease. [*Coding Clinic*, 3Q, '90, 3, effective with discharges July 15, 1990]

AHA CC: Use category 404 for hypertensive heart and renal disease, cardiorenal disease or hypertensive heart disease with nephrosclerosis. When the physician documents the diagnosis of hypertensive cardiovascular and renal disease or hypertensive cardiovascular renal disease, review the medical record for any specific references to the presence of coronary arteriosclerosis, angina pectoris or chronic coronary insufficiency that would require additional coding. As stated above, cardiovascular hypertension may imply the presence of a coronary artery disease. [*Coding Clinic*, J-A, '84, 11]

AHA CC: Use category 403 for hypertensive renal disease. Hypertension with arteriosclerosis of the kidney, nephrosclerosis, and renal sclerosis refer to structural changes in the arterioles and not in the renal artery. If the physician documented the diagnosis of hypertension and renal failure, verify with the physician whether the patient has malignant or accelerated hypertension, as renal failure is not common in hypertensive renal disease until the hypertension has become malignant or accelerated. For example:

* Use code 403.1 when the physician documents hypertensive nephropathy, benign.
* Use code 403.0 when the physician documents hypertensive nephroangiosclerosis.
* Use code 403.0 when the physician documents accelerated hypertension with renal failure. [*Coding Clinic*, J-A, '84, 11]

AHA CC: Use the 401-405 category code series to classify hypertension due to unknown cause (401-404) and hypertension due to an underlying cause (405). Hypertension existing before or arising during pregnancy is classified in the pregnancy chapter of ICD-9-CM. [*Coding Clinic*, J-A, '84, 11]

AHA CC: The use of the term "uncontrolled hypertension" does not necessarily indicate malignant hypertension. This descriptor may be used by the physician when diuretics have failed to control the hypertension and there is a need for the patient to be placed on antihypertensive drugs, such as beta-blockers. Code hypertension described as uncontrolled according to its type and nature. [*Coding Clinic*, J-A, '84, 11]

Targeted DRG Listing

403.91 Hypertensive renal disease, unspecified with renal failure (continued) **DRG 316**

AHA CC: Subcategories in ICD-9-CM designated for systemic hypertension indicate the nature of the hypertension (i.e., benign, malignant, or unspecified). Attributes of malignant hypertension include rapidly rising blood pressure, usually in excess of 140 mm Hg diastolic, with findings of visual impairment and symptoms or signs of progressive cardiac failure. If the patient does not receive adequate treatment, severe visual loss with hemorrhage, exudates, and papilledema may ensue and death may occur due to uremia, cardiac failure or cerebral hemorrhage. The presence of papilledema with hypertension is, by definition, coded to malignant hypertension. Assign the fourth digit "9" when the physician does not document the primary or secondary hypertension as either benign or malignant. Educate the medical staff of the need for stating the hypertension as being either benign or malignant. [*Coding Clinic*, J-A, '84, 11]

DOC: Use code 403.91 when the physician documents hypertensive renal disease with renal failure.

DOC: Use code 403.91 when the physician documents arteriosclerosis of kidney or renal arterioles with renal failure.

DOC: Use code 403.91 when the physician documents arteriosclerotic nephritis with renal failure.

DOC: Use code 403.91 when the physician documents hypertensive nephropathy with renal failure.

DOC: Use code 403.91 when the physician documents nephrosclerosis with renal failure.

DOC: Use code 403.91 when the physician documents renal sclerosis with hypertension and renal failure.

584.9 Acute renal failure NOS **DRG 316**

AHA CC: Assign code 584.9 as the principal diagnosis and code 276.5 when the physician documents that the admission of a patient with acute renal failure was for dehydration. [*Coding Clinic*, 1Q, '03, 22, 3Q, '02, 22]

AHA CC: Assign code 584.9 as the principal diagnosis and codes 600.00 and 596.0 when the physician documents acute renal failure secondary to benign prostatic hypertrophy (BPH) with obstructive uropathy. [*Coding Clinic*, 3Q, '02, 28]

AHA CC: Assign code 584.9 as the principal diagnosis and code 728.89 when the physician documentation states acute renal failure secondary to rhabdomyolysis. [Coding Clinic, 3Q, '02, 28]

AHA CC: Subaccute renal failure due to urinary obstruction due to benign prostatic hypertrophy should be coded 600.0, Hypertrophy (benign) of prostate, as the principal diagnosis. The urinary obstruction (code 596.0) and acute renal failure (584.9) should be listed as secondary diagnoses. This information is consistent with questions and answers that have been published in previous issues of *Coding Clinic*. See *Coding Clinic* November-December 1984, page 9 and November-December 1986, page 10. [*Coding Clinic* 2Q '01 ,39]

AHA CC: An acute reaction from a blood transfusion that results in acute renal failure should be coded 999.8, Other transfusion reaction, as the principal diagnosis. Code 584.9, Acute renal failure, unspecified and code E934.7, Adverse effect of natural blood and blood products, should be assigned to further describe the exact nature of the complication and the responsible substance. .[*Coding Clinic* 3Q '00 ,38]

AHA CC: Code assignment for the transferring and receiving hospitals in acute renal failure-transferred for renal dialysis is as follows. The original hospital, hospital "A," with no dialysis service, assigns the principal diagnosis as 584.9, Acute renal failure, unspecified. Hospital "B" assigns V56.0, admission for renal dialysis as principal diagnosis, and 584.9, acute renal failure, unspecified, as a secondary diagnosis. [*Coding Clinic* 4Q '93 ,34, effective with discharges October 1, 1993]

585   Chronic renal failure   DRG 316

AHA CC: Assign code 428.0 as the principal diagnosis and codes 585, V15.81, and V45.1 as additional diagnoses for the following scenario: A patient with chronic renal failure goes into fluid overload due to noncompliance with dialysis treatment. [*Coding Clinic*, 2Q, '01, 13]

AHA CC: Two codes should be assigned when Alport's syndrome progresses to end-state renal disease . Assign code 585, Chronic renal failure, as the principal diagnosis. The nephritis does not always advance to chronic renal failure. Therefore, the chronic renal failure is not considered a manifestation of the underlying condition. As the treatment of the chronic renal failure is the reason for the admission, it should be sequenced first, followed by code 759.89, Other specified anomalies, for the Alport's syndrome. [*Coding Clinic*, 1Q, '01, 55]

AHA CC: Assign code 428.0 as the principal diagnosis and codes 584.9, 585, and V15.81 as additional diagnoses for the following scenario: A patient with chronic renal failure is noncompliant with dialysis and diet and goes into volume overload due to salt and fluid levels. As a result, the patient develops congestive heart failure and acute renal failure. Physician documentation indicates that the CHF is due to poor compliance with salt and water restrictions rather than from a primary cardiac dysfunction. [*Coding Clinic*, 3Q, '96, 9, effective with discharges August 15, 1996]

AHA CC: Assign code 403.9 when the physician documents chronic renal failure secondary to nephrosclerosis with uremia. ICD-9-CM presumes nephrosclerosis to be a secondary process and hypertensive renal disease its origin unless otherwise specified. Use code 585 as an additional code. Assign code 274.10 and code 585 when the physician documents chronic renal failure secondary to nephrosclerosis with uremia due to gout. [*Coding Clinic*, N-D, '85, 15]

AHA CC: Code 585 does not exclude secondary hypertension, category 405. When the physician documents that the hypertension is due to renovascular (renal artery) disease or a kidney disease, use code 585. For example:

- Use codes 585, 753.1 and 405.99 when the physician documents chronic renal failure with secondary hypertension due to polycystic kidney disease.
- Use codes 585, 581.1 and 405.99 when the physician documents chronic renal disease with secondary hypertension due to nephrotic syndrome with membranous glomerulonephritis. [*Coding Clinic*, S-O, '84, 1]

AHA CC: Use a code from the range 403.0-403.9 when the physician documents hypertensive renal disease with chronic renal failure (or chronic renal failure due to hypertensive renal disease). The exclusion note under 585 directs the coder to this series for pri mary hypertension with progression to renal involvement. Use code 585 secondarily. [*Coding Clinic*, S-O, '84, 1]

AHA CC: Use code 250.4 (with the appropriate fifth digit) as the primary code when the physician documents a diagnosis of diabetic renal failure, diabetic uremia, diabetic intercapillary glomerulosclerosis and chronic renal failure, diabetic nephropathy with chronic renal failure, ordiabetic nephrosis with chronic renal failure. These statements describe a cause and effect relationship. Use 581.81 and 585 as additional codes. In ICD-9-CM, category 250 serves as the primary code to classify both the disease and its major manifestations. An additional code(s) is used as a secondary code to provide more specificity in describing the manifestations. No note exists under code 585 that excludes that with mention of diabetes mellitus. There is no subterm under "Diabetes mellitus" for chronic renal failure or chronic uremia and diabetes mellitus is not listed as a subterm under "Failure, renal, chronic" or under "Uremia, chronic." Thus, when the physician's diagnosis does not state a cause and effect relationship between the diabetes mellitus and chronic renal failure or chronic uremia, code 585 may be used as the principal diagnosis. [*Coding Clinic*, S-O, '84, 1]

585   **Chronic renal failure (continued)**   **DRG 316**

AHA CC: End-stage renal disease is is a progression of chronic renal failure. Physicians define this condition as the point at which chronic maintenance dialysis or kidney transplantation is required to maintain the patient's life. There are many causes of end-stage renal disease and chronic renal failure, e.g., diabetes mellitus, primary hypertension, glomerulonephritis, renal disease with edema (nephrosis), interstitial nephritis, systemic lupus erythematosis (SLE), obstructive uropathy, polycystic kidney disease, and a number of other congenital disorders. Treatment varies considerably according to the specific disorder. Dialysis may be required once kidney involvement becomes so extensive that kidney function no longer keeps up with the body's needs.

Use code V56.0 as the principal diagnosis when the physician documents that the admission was for renal dialysis in order to manage symptoms arising from renal failure. Use additional code(s) to describe the underlying disease. For example:

- Assign code V56.0 as the principal diagnosis and codes 250.41 and 585 as secondary diagnoses when the physician documents admission for hemodialysis, diabetes mellitus with renal manifestations, insulin dependence and chronic renal failure. The procedures included creation of arteriovenous fistula, 39.27. Code also 39.95 if dialysis was stated during this stay.
- Assign code V56.0 as the principal diagnosis and codes 250.41 and 585 as secondary diagnoses when the physician documents admission for hemodialysis, diabetes mellitus with renal manifestations, insulin dependence and chronic renal failure. The procedures included insertion of Tenckhoff catheter, 54.93, and peritoneal dialysis, 54.98. [*Coding Clinic*, S-O, '84, 1]

AHA CC: Renal failure exists when renal insufficiency progresses to the point where renal function is further impaired and apparent manifestations (see below) have developed.

The treatment of choice for irreversible chronic renal failure is either dialysis or transplantation. However, patients with acute renal fialure may also be placed on dialysis. Review the medical record for the following indications of renal fialure:

- Check the laboratory reports for markedly abnormal elevated values of serum creatinine or BUN, or diminished creatinine clearance.
- Certain manifestations of the degree of renal impairment include anemia, hyerphosphtemia, hypocalcemia, hyperkalemia, acidemia, renal osteodystrophy, uremic symptoms such as nausea, vomiting, itching, hemorrhagic conditions, hypertension, edema, dyspnea, lethargy and coma. [*Coding Clinic*, 1Q, '93, 18, effective with discharges January 1, 1993]

DOC: Use code 585 when the physician documents chronic renal failure.

DOC: Do not use code 585 when the physician documents unspecified renal failure. The correct code is 586.

DRG 320 Kidney and Urinary Tract Infections, Age Greater than 17 with CC

DRG 296 Nutritional and Miscellaneous Metabolic Disorders Greater than 17 with CC

Issue

Choosing between urinary tract infection and dehydration as the principal diagnosis is problematic because of the unclear documentation as to the reason for admission and the complexity of the ICD-9-CM diagnosis codes and coding guidelines.

Most common Diagnosis Codes

DRG 320

- 590.10, Acute pyelonephritis without lesion of renal medullary necrosis
- 599.0, Urinary tract infection, site not specified

DRG 296

- 276.1, Hyposmolality and/or hyponatremia
- 276.5, Volume depletion

Coding and Documentation Guidelines

276.1	**Hyposmolality and/or hyponatremia**	**DRG 296**

See standards on page 631.

276.5	**Volume depletion**	**DRG 296**

See standards on page 632.

590.10	**Acute pyelonephritis without lesion of renal medullary necrosis**	**DRG 320**

DOC: Use code 590.10 when the physician documents acute pyelitis or acute pyonephrosis.

DOC: Do not use code 590.10 when the physician documents acute pyelonephritis with lesion of renal medullary necrosis. The correct code is 590.11.

599.0	**Urinary tract infection, site not specified**	**DRG 320**

CG: If a patient is diagnosed with both UTI and acute cystitis, the code would be assigned based on the site of the infection, if it is known. Usually, it is not possible to determine this solely by clinical means. If the physician states that the bladder is the specific site of the acute infection, use code 595.0, acute cystitis. (Note that any UTI due to sexually transmitted disease is coded elsewhere). Any spread of the UTI to other sites is coded additionally.

AHA CC: When the documentation states urosepsis, the physician should be queried if the use of the term urosepsis was intended to mean generalized sepsis (septicemia) caused by leakage of urine or toxic urine by-products into the general vascular circulation, or if the urine was contaminated by bacteria, bacterial by-products or other toxic material but without other findings (599.0). [*Coding Clinic*, 2Q, '00, 4]

599.0   Urinary tract infection, site not specified (continued)   **DRG 320**

AHA CC: Do not use 599.0 in combination with sites that specifically identify the site(s) if the UTI. Therefore, if a physician documents "acute cystitis" and "urinary tract infection", code only the acute cystitis. Use 599.0 only when the physician is not able to identify the site(s) of the UTI. [*Coding Clinic* 2Q, '99 p15-16, effective with discharges April 1, 1999]

AHA CC: For each individual case, the physician should determine a patient's diagnosis based upon the particulars of the case to avoid inaccurate coding. To ensure accurate coding, check with the physician as to whether a diagnosis documented as urosepsis is intended to mean (1) generalized sepsis (septicemia), code 38.9 or (2) urine contaminated by bacteria, bacterial by-products, or other toxic material but without other findings, code 599.0. The ICD-9-CM system assumes urosepsis to mean urinary tract infection and codes it to 599.0. [*Coding Clinic*, 1Q, '98, 5]

AHA CC: Assign both codes 997.5 and 599.0 when the postoperative urinary tract infection is specified by the physician as a postoperative complication. Category 997 covers a variety of postoperative complications without specifying the nature of the complication. ICD-9-CM instructs coders to assign an additional code to provide this information. [*Coding Clinic*, 1Q, '92, 13, effective with discharges January 1, 1992]

AHA CC: Assign code 427.31 as the principal diagnosis and codes V58.69 and V13.09 as additional diagnoses when the physician documents that the reason for admission is atrial fibrillation. The medical record indicates the patient is on prophylactic Septra for chronic recurrent UTIs. This medication is continued during the current hospitalization. No urinary symptoms or problems are documented by the physician during this hospitalization. Do not assign a code for the UTI as this condition occurs as an acute, episodic condition, which may or may not recur if the prophylactic antibiotic is discontinued. [*Coding Clinic*, 2Q, '96, 7, effective with discharges May 1, 1996]

AHA CC: A patient with dehydration may present with symptoms and signs of dehydration, such as dryness of mucous membranes, loss of skin turgor, and anorexia. Inadequate fluid intake, vomiting, diarrhea, sweating or polyuria can cause dehydration. The main objective is total replacement of fluid deficit within 48-72 hours. Dehydration can occur in patients with burns, gastrointestinal disease, peritonitis, ascites, diabetic glycosuria, Addison's disease, hypoaldosteronism, renal failure, urinary track infections and other infections. Treatment for dehydration includes oral replenishment of fluids or by intravenous administration. Because dehydration is often the result of another condition as well as a severe management problem in itself, it often is difficult to determine the principal diagnosis. The circumstances of the admission and the judgment of the attending physician govern whether dehydration meets the definition of principal diagnosis. The following are some examples to assist in this determination.

- Dehydration and urinary tract infection are both present on admission. Treatment consisted of intravenous (IV) fluids for the dehydration and antibiotics for the urinary tract infection. Verify with the physician regarding the principal diagnosis, as it is possible that the urinary tract infection could have been treated on an outpatient basis but that the dehydration necessitated the inpatient admission. [*Coding Clinic*, 2Q, '88, 9]

DOC: Use code 599.0 when the physician documents a urinary tract infection but does not specify the site.

DOC: Use additional code to identify organism.

DOC: Use code 599.0 when the physician documents a urinary tract infection but does not specify the site.

DOC: Use additional code to identify organism.

DOC: Use code 599.0 if the physician documents urosepsis. The term urosepsis refers to pyuria or bacteria in the urine, not the blood.

DOC: Assign code 599.0 as an additional code when the physician documents urinary tract infection as the underlying cause of autonomic dysreflexia (337.3).

DOC: Do not use code 599.0 when the physician documents candidiasis of the urinary tract. The correct code is 112.2.

DRG 416 Septicemia, Age Greater than 17

DRG 320 Kidney and Urinary Tract Infections, Age Greater than 17 with CC

Issue

Choosing between septicemia and urinary tract infection as the principal diagnosis is problematic because of the unclear documentation on the reason for admission and the complexity of the ICD-9-CM diagnosis codes and coding guidelines.

Most Common Diagnosis Codes

DRG 416

- 038.0, Streptococcal septicemia
- 038.11, Staphylococcal aureus septicemia
- 038.19, Other staphylococcal septicemia
- 038.42, Septicemia due to *Escherichia coli*
- 038.49, Septicemia due to other gram-negative organism
- 038.9, Unspecified septicemia

DRG 320

- 590.10, Acute pyelonephritis without lesion of renal medullary necrosis
- 599.0, Urinary tract infection, site not specified

Coding and Documentation Guidelines

038.0   Streptococcal septicemia   **DRG 416**

CG: Do not arbitrarily assign a code for septicemia based on clinical signs alone. Code assignment should be based strictly on physician documentation. [*Coding Clinic*, 2Q, '00, 3]

AHA CC: Do not arbitrarily report a diagnosis code on the basis of an abnormal laboratory finding alone. Do not list a diagnosis code on the basis of a single lab value or abnormal diagnostic finding. Many factors influence the value of a lab sample. These include the method used to obtain the sample, the collection device, the method used to transport the sample to the lab, the calibration of the machine that reads the values, and the condition of the patient. [*Coding Clinic*, 2Q, '90, 3, effective with discharges April 1, 1990, and *Coding Clinic*, 4Q, '93, 39, effective with discharges August 18, 1993]

AHA CC: As long as there is documentation of clinical evidence of septicemia, negative, or inconclusive blood cultures do not preclude a diagnosis of septicemia in patients with clinical evidence of the condition. [*Coding Clinic*, 2Q, '00, 5]

AHA CC: For each individual case, the physician should determine a patient's diagnosis based upon the particulars of the case to avoid inaccurate coding. To ensure accurate coding, check with the physician as to whether a diagnosis documented as urosepsis is intended to mean: (1) generalized sepsis (septicemia) or (2) urine contaminated by bacteria, bacterial by-products, or other toxic material but without other findings. The ICD-9-CM system assumes urosepsis to mean urinary tract infection and codes it to 599.0. [*Coding Clinic*, 1Q, '98, 5, effective with discharges January 15, 1998]

038.0 Streptococcal septicemia (continued)   DRG 416

AHA CC: Many times, a patient may be suspected of having septicemia and is treated for such even though the blood cultures may not be supportive. The clinical picture of a patient with this condition includes medical record documentation of infection with fever or hypothermia, tachypnea, tachycardia and impaired organ system perfusion, such as altered mental status, oliguria, and relative hypotension. In addition, the patient may have metabolic acidosis secondary to impaired organ perfusion, as evidenced by either an increased lactate level, increased anion gap, or reduced blood pH. As an indication of suspected septicemia or bacteremia, the physician also may treat the patient with intravenous broad-spectrum antibiotics, fluid hydration, and possibly the use of medications to raise the blood pressure. [*Coding Clinic*, 3Q, '88, 12]

AHA CC: If the physician's diagnostic reference is to a site- or organ-specific sepsis, such as urosepsis, further clarification is necessary before coding. To ensure accurate coding, check with the physician as to whether a diagnosis documented as urosepsis is intended to mean: (1) generalized sepsis (septicemia) or (2) urine contaminated by bacteria, bacterial by-products, or other toxic material but without other findings. The ICD-9-CM system assumes urosepsis to mean urinary tract infection and codes it to 599.0. [*Coding Clinic*, 1Q, '88, 1]

AHA CC: Septicemia and shock often occur together. When the physician documents a diagnosis of septicemia with shock, or the diagnosis of general sepsis with septic shock, code and list the septicemia first and report the septic shock code as a secondary condition. If the bacteria is documented, use the specific septicemia code to identify the organism. Use a code from the pregnancy chapter when the sepsis or septic shock is associated with abortion, ectopic pregnancy or molar pregnancy. [*Coding Clinic*, 1Q, '88, 1]

AHA CC: When the documentation states urosepsis, the physician should be queried if the use of the term urosepsis was intended to mean generalized sepsis (septicemia) caused by leakage of urine or toxic urine by-products into the general vascular circulation, or if the urine was contaminated by bacteria, bacterial by-products or other toxic material but without other findings (599.0). [*Coding Clinic*, 2Q, '00, 4]

AHA CC: Blood is often drawn for culturing during the initial workup of a patient with septicemia. The physician will begin treatment (including antibiotics) before the results of the culture are returned. In addition, the patient may show clinical evidence of septicemia while the blood culture may be negative because of the difficulty in culturing fastidious organisms from blood, growth inhibitory factors in the blood, or initiation of specific antibiotic therapy before laboratory test samples are taken. As long as there is documentation of clinical evidence of septicemia, negative or inconclusive blood cultures do not preclude a physician from making a diagnosis of septicemia. [*Coding Clinic*, 1Q, '88, 1]

DOC: Use code 038.0 when the physician documents streptococcal septicemia.

DOC: Do not use code 038.0 when the physician documents septicemia, unspecified or not otherwise specified. The correct code is 038.9.

DOC: Do not assign code 038.0 when the physician documentation states bacteremia. The correct code is 790.7.

038.11 Staphylococcal aureus septicemia   DRG 416

AHA CC: Do not arbitrarily assign a code for septicemia based on clinical signs alone. Code assignment should be based strictly on physician documentation. [*Coding Clinic*, 2Q, '00, 3]

AHA CC: Do not arbitrarily report a diagnosis code on the basis of an abnormal laboratory finding alone. Do not list a diagnosis code on the basis of a single lab value or abnormal diagnostic finding. Many factors influence the value of a lab sample. These include the method used to obtain the sample, the collection device, the method used to transport the sample to the lab, the calibration of the machine that reads the values, and the condition of the patient. [*Coding Clinic*, 2Q, '90, 3, effective with discharges April 1, 1990, and *Coding Clinic*, 4Q, '93, 39, effective with discharges August 18, 1993]

038.11 Staphylococcal aureus septicemia (continued)   DRG 416

AHA CC: The correct coding of staphylococcal aureus septicemia confirmed by attending physician as due to infected tracheostomy site is 519.01, infection of tracheostomy and 038.11, staphylococcal aureus septicemia. [*Coding Clinic*, 4Q, '98 41-42, effective with discharges October 1, 1998]

AHA CC: Prior to October 1, 1997, it was necessary to use two codes to correctly describe Staphylococcal aureus septicemia: 038.1, staphylococcal septicemia and 041.11, Staphylococcal aureus. A new code was introduced after October 1, 1997, to identify staphylococcal aureus septicemia—038.11. Staphylococcal aureus septicemia is probably accurately diagnosed 90 percent of the time, whereas the description of nonaureus staph septicemia cases are probably accurate only 50 percent of the time. [*Coding Clinic*, 4Q, '97, 32, effective with discharges October 1, 1997]

AHA CC: Effective with discharges October 1, 1997, use only one code when the physician documents staphylococcus aureus septicemia. Prior to this date, two codes: 038.1 and 041.11 were used. [*Coding Clinic*, 4Q, '97, 32, effective with discharges October 1, 1997]

AHA CC: As long as there is documentation of clinical evidence of septicemia, negative, or inconclusive blood cultures do not preclude a diagnosis of septicemia in patients with clinical evidence of the condition. [*Coding Clinic*, 2Q, '00, 5]

AHA CC: For each individual case, the physician should determine a patient's diagnosis based upon the particulars of the case to avoid inaccurate coding. To ensure accurate coding, check with the physician as to whether a diagnosis documented as urosepsis is intended to mean (1) generalized sepsis (septicemia) or (2) urine contaminated by bacteria, bacterial by-products, or other toxic material but without other findings. The ICD-9-CM system assumes urosepsis to mean urinary tract infection and codes it to 599.0. [*Coding Clinic*, 1Q, '98, 5, effective with discharges January 15, 1998]

AHA CC: Many times a patient may be suspected of having septicemia and is treated for such even though the blood cultures may not be supportive. The clinical picture of a patient with this condition includes medical record documentation of infection with fever or hypothermia, tachypnea, tachycardia and impaired organ system perfusion, such as altered mental status, oliguria, and relative hypotension. In addition, the patient may have metabolic acidosis secondary to impaired organ perfusion, as evidenced by either an increased lactate level, increased anion gap, or reduced blood pH. As an indication of suspected septicemia or bacteremia, the physician also may treat the patient with intravenous broad-spectrum antibiotics, fluid hydration, and possibly the use of medications to raise the blood pressure. [*Coding Clinic*, 3Q, '88, 12]

AHA CC: If the physician's diagnostic reference is to a site- or organ-specific sepsis, such as urosepsis, further clarification is necessary before coding. To ensure accurate coding, check with the physician as to whether a diagnosis documented as urosepsis is intended to mean: (1) generalized sepsis (septicemia) or (2) urine contaminated by bacteria, bacterial by-products, or other toxic material but without other findings. The ICD-9-CM system assumes urosepsis to mean urinary tract infection and codes it to 599.0. [*Coding Clinic*, 1Q, '88, 1]

AHA CC: Septicemia and shock often occur together. When the physician documents a diagnosis of septicemia with shock, or the diagnosis of general sepsis with septic shock, code and list the septicemia first and report the septic shock code as a secondary condition. If the bacteria is documented, use the specific septicemia code to identify the organism. Use a code from the pregnancy chapter when the sepsis or septic shock is associated with abortion, ectopic pregnancy, or molar pregnancy. [*Coding Clinic*, 1Q, '88, 1]

038.11   Staphylococcal aureus septicemia (continued)   DRG 416

AHA CC: Blood is often drawn for culturing during the initial workup of a patient with septicemia. The physician will begin treatment (including antibiotics) before the results of the culture are returned. In addition, the patient may show clinical evidence of septicemia while the blood culture may be negative because of the difficulty in culturing fastidious organisms from blood, growth inhibitory factors in the blood, or initiation of specific antibiotic therapy before laboratory test samples are taken. As long as there is documentation of clinical evidence of septicemia, negative or inconclusive blood cultures do not preclude a physician from making a diagnosis of septicemia. [*Coding Clinic*, 1Q, '88, 1]

DOC: Use code 038.19 when the physician documents other specified staphylococcal septicemia other than the organism *Staphylococcus aureus*.

DOC: Do not use code 038.19 when the physician documents bacteremia. The correct code is 790.7.

DOC: Do not use code 038.19 when the physician documents staphylococcal aureus septicemia. The correct code is 038.11.

DOC: Do not use code 038.19 when the physician documents unspecified staphylococcal septicemia. The correct code is 038.00.

038.19   Other staphylococcal septicemia   DRG 416

AHA CC: Do not arbitrarily assign a code for septicemia based on clinical signs alone. Code assignment should be based strictly on physician documentation. [*Coding Clinic*, 2Q, '00, 3]

AHA CC: Do not arbitrarily report a diagnosis code on the basis of an abnormal laboratory finding alone. Do not list a diagnosis code on the basis of a single lab value or abnormal diagnostic finding. Many factors influence the value of a lab sample. These include the method used to obtain the sample, the collection device, the method used to transport the sample to the lab, the calibration of the machine that reads the values, and the condition of the patient. [*Coding Clinic*, 2Q, '90, 3, effective with discharges April 1, 1990, and *Coding Clinic*, 4Q, '93, 39, effective with discharges August 18, 1993]

AHA CC: As long as there is documentation of clinical evidence of septicemia, negative, or inconclusive blood cultures do not preclude a diagnosis of septicemia in patients with clinical evidence of the condition. [*Coding Clinic*, 2Q, '00, 5]

AHA CC: For each individual case, the physician should determine a patient's diagnosis based upon the particulars of the case to avoid inaccurate coding. To ensure accurate coding, check with the physician as to whether a diagnosis documented as urosepsis is intended to mean (1) generalized sepsis (septicemia) or (2) urine contaminated by bacteria, bacterial by-products, or other toxic material but without other findings. The ICD-9-CM system assumes urosepsis to mean urinary tract infection and codes it to 599.0. [*Coding Clinic*, 1Q, '98, 5, effective with discharges January 15, 1998]

AHA CC: Many times a patient may be suspected of having septicemia and is treated for such even though the blood cultures may not be supportive. The clinical picture of a patient with this condition includes medical record documentation of infection with fever or hypothermia, tachypnea, tachycardia and impaired organ system perfusion, such as altered mental status, oliguria, and relative hypotension. In addition, the patient may have metabolic acidosis secondary to impaired organ perfusion, as evidenced by either an increased lactate level, increased anion gap, or reduced blood pH. As an indication of suspected septicemia or bacteremia, the physician also may treat the patient with intravenous broad-spectrum antibiotics, fluid hydration, and possibly the use of medications to raise the blood pressure. [*Coding Clinic*, 3Q, '88, 12]

038.19 Other staphylococcal septicemia (continued)   DRG 416

AHA CC: If the physician's diagnostic reference is to a site- or organ-specific sepsis, such as urosepsis, further clarification is necessary before coding. To ensure accurate coding, check with the physician as to whether a diagnosis documented as urosepsis is intended to mean (1) generalized sepsis (septicemia) or (2) urine contaminated by bacteria, bacterial by-products, or other toxic material but without other findings. The ICD-9-CM system assumes urosepsis to mean urinary tract infection and codes it to 599.0. [*Coding Clinic*, 1Q, '88, 1]

AHA CC: Septicemia and shock often occur together. When the physician documents a diagnosis of septicemia with shock, or the diagnosis of general sepsis with septic shock, code and list the septicemia first and report the septic shock code as a secondary condition. If the bacteria is documented, use the specific septicemia code to identify the organism. Use a code from the pregnancy chapter when the sepsis or septic shock is associated with abortion, ectopic pregnancy, or molar pregnancy. [*Coding Clinic*, 1Q, '88, 1]

AHA CC: Blood is often drawn for culturing during the initial workup of a patient with septicemia. The physician will begin treatment (including antibiotics) before the results of the culture are returned. In addition, the patient may show clinical evidence of septicemia while the blood culture may be negative because of the difficulty in culturing fastidious organisms from blood, growth inhibitory factors in the blood, or initiation of specific antibiotic therapy before laboratory test samples are taken. As long as there is documentation of clinical evidence of septicemia, negative or inconclusive blood cultures do not preclude a physician from making a diagnosis of septicemia. [*Coding Clinic*, 1Q, '88, 1]

DOC: Use code 038.19 when the physician documents other specified staphylococcal septicemia other than the organism *Staphylococcus aureus*.

DOC: Do not use code 038.19 when the physician documents bacteremia. The correct code is 790.7.

DOC: Do not use code 038.19 when the physician documents staphylococcal aureus septicemia. The correct code is 038.11.

DOC: Do not use code 038.19 when the physician documents unspecified staphylococcal septicemia. The correct code is 038.00.

038.42 Septicemia due to *Escherichia coli*   DRG 416

AHA CC: Do not arbitrarily assign a code for septicemia based on clinical signs alone. Code assignment should be based strictly on physician documentation. [*Coding Clinic*, 2Q, '00, 3]

AHA CC: Do not arbitrarily report a diagnosis code on the basis of an abnormal laboratory finding alone. Do not list a diagnosis code on the basis of a single lab value or abnormal diagnostic finding. Many factors influence the value of a lab sample. These include the method used to obtain the sample, the collection device, the method used to transport the sample to the lab, the calibration of the machine that reads the values, and the condition of the patient. [*Coding Clinic*, 2Q, '90, 3, effective with discharges April 1, 1990, and *Coding Clinic*, 4Q, '93, 39, effective with discharges August 18, 1993]

AHA CC: As long as there is documentation of clinical evidence of septicemia, negative, or inconclusive blood cultures do not preclude a diagnosis of septicemia in patients with clinical evidence of the condition. [*Coding Clinic*, 2Q, '00, 5]

AHA CC: For each individual case, the physician should determine a patient's diagnosis based upon the particulars of the case to avoid inaccurate coding. To ensure accurate coding, check with the physician as to whether a diagnosis documented as urosepsis is intended to mean (1) generalized sepsis (septicemia) or (2) urine contaminated by bacteria, bacterial by-products, or other toxic material but without other findings. The ICD-9-CM system assumes urosepsis to mean urinary tract infection and codes it to 599.0. [*Coding Clinic*, 1Q, '98, 5, effective with discharges January 15, 1998]

038.42   Septicemia due to *Escherichia coli* (continued)   DRG 416

AHA CC: Many times a patient may be suspected of having septicemia and is treated for such even though the blood cultures may not be supportive. The clinical picture of a patient with this condition includes medical record documentation of infection with fever or hypothermia, tachypnea, tachycardia and impaired organ system perfusion, such as altered mental status, oliguria, and relative hypotension. In addition, the patient may have metabolic acidosis secondary to impaired organ perfusion, as evidenced by either an increased lactate level, increased anion gap, or reduced blood pH. As an indication of suspected septicemia or bacteremia, the physician also may treat the patient with intravenous broad-spectrum antibiotics, fluid hydration, and possibly the use of medications to raise the blood pressure. [*Coding Clinic*, 3Q, '88, 12]

AHA CC: If the physician's diagnostic reference is to a site- or organ-specific sepsis, such as urosepsis, further clarification is necessary before coding. To ensure accurate coding, check with the physician as to whether a diagnosis documented as urosepsis is intended to mean (1) generalized sepsis (septicemia) or (2) urine contaminated by bacteria, bacterial by-products, or other toxic material but without other findings. The ICD-9-CM system assumes urosepsis to mean urinary tract infection and codes it to 599.0. [*Coding Clinic*, 1Q, '88, 1]

AHA CC: Septicemia and shock often occur together. When the physician documents a diagnosis of septicemia with shock, or the diagnosis of general sepsis with septic shock, code and list the septicemia first and report the septic shock code as a secondary condition. If the bacteria is documented, use the specific septicemia code to identify the organism. Use a code from the pregnancy chapter when the sepsis or septic shock is associated with abortion, ectopic pregnancy, or molar pregnancy. [*Coding Clinic*, 1Q, '88, 1]

AHA CC: Blood is often drawn for culturing during the initial workup of a patient with septicemia. The physician will begin treatment (including antibiotics) before the results of the culture are returned. In addition, the patient may show clinical evidence of septicemia while the blood culture may be negative because of the difficulty in culturing fastidious organisms from blood, growth inhibitory factors in the blood, or initiation of specific antibiotic therapy before laboratory test samples are taken. As long as there is documentation of clinical evidence of septicemia, negative or inconclusive blood cultures do not preclude a physician from making a diagnosis of septicemia. [*Coding Clinic*, 1Q, '88, 1]

DOC: Use code 038.42 when the physician documents septicemia due to *Escherichia coli*.

DOC: Do not use code 038.42 when the physician documents bacteremia. The correct code is 790.7.

038.49   Septicemia due to other gram-negative organism   DRG 416

AHA CC: Do not arbitrarily assign a code for septicemia based on clinical signs alone. Code assignment should be based strictly on physician documentation. [*Coding Clinic*, 2Q, '00, 3]

AHA CC: Do not arbitrarily report a diagnosis code on the basis of an abnormal laboratory finding alone. Do not list a diagnosis code on the basis of a single lab value or abnormal diagnostic finding. Many factors influence the value of a lab sample. These include the method used to obtain the sample, the collection device, the method used to transport the sample to the lab, the calibration of the machine that reads the values, and the condition of the patient. [*Coding Clinic*, 2Q, '90, 3, effective with discharges April 1, 1990, and *Coding Clinic*, 4Q, '93, 39, effective with discharges August 18, 1993]

AHA CC: As long as there is documentation of clinical evidence of septicemia, negative, or inconclusive blood cultures do not preclude a diagnosis of septicemia in patients with clinical evidence of the condition. [*Coding Clinic*, 2Q, '00, 5]

038.49   Septicemia due to other gram-negative organism (continued)   DRG 416

AHA CC: For each individual case, the physician should determine a patient's diagnosis based upon the particulars of the case to avoid inaccurate coding. To ensure accurate coding, check with the physician as to whether a diagnosis documented as urosepsis is intended to mean (1) generalized sepsis (septicemia) or (2) urine contaminated by bacteria, bacterial by-products, or other toxic material but without other findings. The ICD-9-CM system assumes urosepsis to mean urinary tract infection and codes it to 599.0. [*Coding Clinic*, 1Q, '98, 5, effective with discharges January 15, 1998]

AHA CC: Many times a patient may be suspected of having septicemia and is treated for such even though the blood cultures may not be supportive. The clinical picture of a patient with this condition includes medical record documentation of infection with fever or hypothermia, tachypnea, tachycardia and impaired organ system perfusion, such as altered mental status, oliguria, and relative hypotension. In addition, the patient may have metabolic acidosis secondary to impaired organ perfusion, as evidenced by either an increased lactate level, increased anion gap, or reduced blood pH. As an indication of suspected septicemia or bacteremia, the physician also may treat the patient with intravenous broad-spectrum antibiotics, fluid hydration, and possibly the use of medications to raise the blood pressure. [*Coding Clinic*, 3Q, '88, 12]

AHA CC: If the physician's diagnostic reference is to a site- or organ-specific sepsis, such as urosepsis, further clarification is necessary before coding. To ensure accurate coding, check with the physician as to whether a diagnosis documented as urosepsis is intended to mean (1) generalized sepsis (septicemia) or (2) urine contaminated by bacteria, bacterial by-products, or other toxic material but without other findings. The ICD-9-CM system assumes urosepsis to mean urinary tract infection and codes it to 599.0. [*Coding Clinic*, 1Q, '88, 1]

AHA CC: Septicemia and shock often occur together. When the physician documents a diagnosis of septicemia with shock, or the diagnosis of general sepsis with septic shock, code and list the septicemia first and report the septic shock code as a secondary condition. If the bacteria is documented, use the specific septicemia code to identify the organism. Use a code from the pregnancy chapter when the sepsis or septic shock is associated with abortion, ectopic pregnancy, or molar pregnancy. [*Coding Clinic*, 1Q, '88, 1]

AHA CC: Blood is often drawn for culturing during the initial workup of a patient with septicemia. The physician will begin treatment (including antibiotics) before the results of the culture are returned. In addition, the patient may show clinical evidence of septicemia while the blood culture may be negative because of the difficulty in culturing fastidious organisms from blood, growth inhibitory factors in the blood, or initiation of specific antibiotic therapy before laboratory test samples are taken. As long as there is documentation of clinical evidence of septicemia, negative or inconclusive blood cultures do not preclude a physician from making a diagnosis of septicemia. [*Coding Clinic*, 1Q, '88, 1]

DOC: Use code 038.49 when the physician documents septicemia due to *Aerobacter aerogenes*, septicemia due to *Enterobacter aerogenes*, septicemia due to Friedländer's bacillus, septicemia due to *Proteus vulgaris*, or septicemia due to *Yersinia enterocolitica*.

DOC: Do not use code 038.49 when the physician documents anaerobic gram-negative organism. The correct code is 038.3.

038.9 Unspecified septicemia DRG 416

AHA CC: Assign code 038.9 first when the diagnosis of septicemia with shock or the diagnosis of general sepsis with septic shock is documented and report 785.59 as a secondary condition. [*Coding Clinic*, 2Q, '00, 4 and *Coding Clinic*, 1Q, '98, 1]

AHA CC: Assign code 038.9 as the principal diagnosis and code 288.0 as an additional diagnosis when the physician documents admission for septicemia and a final diagnosis of neutropenic sepsis. Neutropenia, a reduction in the blood neutrophil (granulocyte) count, can result in an increased susceptibility to bacterial and fungal infections. [*Coding Clinic*, 2Q, '96, 6, effective with discharges May 1, 1996]

AHA CC: Assign code 038.43 for the following scenario: The reason for admission was a chief complaint of nausea, fever and lethargy. The physician ordered blood and urine cultures. Results showed the presence of an organism, in this case pseudomonas. The physician documented a diagnosis of "Sepsis secondary to urinary tract infection (pseudomonas)." Assign code 599.0 as an additional diagnoses. Do not assign code 041.7 as the organism is already captured in the code for the septicemia. [*Coding Clinic*, 4Q, '88, 10, effective with discharges July 1, 1989]

AHA CC: As long as there is documentation of clinical evidence of septicemia, negative, or inconclusive blood cultures do not preclude a diagnosis of septicemia in patients with clinical evidence of the condition. [*Coding Clinic*, 2Q, '00, 5]

AHA CC: For each individual case, the physician should determine a patient's diagnosis based upon the particulars of the case to avoid inaccurate coding. To ensure accurate coding, check with the physician as to whether a diagnosis documented as urosepsis is intended to mean (1) generalized sepsis (septicemia) or (2) urine contaminated by bacteria, bacterial by-products, or other toxic material but without other findings. The ICD-9-CM system assumes urosepsis to mean urinary tract infection and codes it to 599.0. [*Coding Clinic*, 1Q, '98, 5, effective with discharges January 15, 1998]

AHA CC: Assign code 038.9 when the physician documents a diagnosis of nadir sepsis. In this type of sepsis the temperature and the white cell count are at a low point. In addition, bacteria are present. Do not assign only a code for the neutropenia as this is only one manifestation of the condition. This would not represent a complete picture of a patient with the final diagnostic statement of nadir sepsis. Assign code 288.0 as a secondary diagnosis. [*Coding Clinic*, 3Q, '96, 16, effective with discharges August 15, 1996]

AHA CC: Many times, a patient may be suspected of having septicemia and is treated for such even though the blood cultures may not be supportive. The clinical picture of a patient with this condition includes medical record documentation of infection with fever or hypothermia, tachypnea, tachycardia, and impaired organ system perfusion, such as altered mental status, oliguria, and relative hypotension. In addition, the patient may have metabolic acidosis secondary to impaired organ perfusion, as evidenced by either an increased lactate level, increased anion gap, or reduced blood pH. As an indication of suspected septicemia or bacteremia, the physician also may treat the patient with intravenous broad-spectrum antibiotics, fluid hydration, and possibly the use of medications to raise the blood pressure. [*Coding Clinic*, 3Q, '88, 12]

AHA CC: If the physician's diagnostic reference is to a site- or organ-specific sepsis, such as urosepsis, further clarification is necessary before coding. To ensure accurate coding, check with the physician as to whether a diagnosis documented as urosepsis is intended to mean (1) generalized sepsis (septicemia) or (2) urine contaminated by bacteria, bacterial by-products, or other toxic material but without other findings. The ICD-9-CM system assumes urosepsis to mean urinary tract infection and codes it to 599.0. [*Coding Clinic*, 1Q, '88, 1]

AHA CC: Septicemia and shock often occur together. When the physician documents a diagnosis of septicemia with shock, or the diagnosis of general sepsis with septic shock, code and list the septicemia first and report the septic shock code as a secondary condition. If the bacteria is documented, use the specific septicemia code to identify the organism. Use a code from the pregnancy chapter when the sepsis or septic shock is associated with abortion, ectopic pregnancy, or molar pregnancy. [*Coding Clinic*, 1Q, '88, 1]

038.9   Unspecified septicemia (continued)   DRG 416

AHA CC: Blood is often drawn for culturing during the initial workup of a patient with septicemia. The physician will begin treatment (including antibiotics) before the results of the culture are returned. In addition, the patient may show clinical evidence of septicemia while the blood culture may be negative because of the difficulty in culturing fastidious organisms from blood, growth inhibitory factors in the blood, or initiation of specific antibiotic therapy before laboratory test samples are taken. As long as there is documentation of clinical evidence of septicemia, negative or inconclusive blood cultures do not preclude a physician from making a diagnosis of septicemia. [*Coding Clinic*, 1Q, '88, 1]

DOC: Use code 038.9 when the physician documents unspecified septicemia.

DOC: Do not use code 038.9 when the physician documents bacteremia. The correct code is 790.7.

590.10   Acute pyelonephritis without lesion of renal medullary necrosis   DRG 320

See standards on page 645.

599.0   Urinary tract infection, site not specified   DRG 320

See standards on page 645.

DRG Desk Reference

DRG 430 Psychoses

DRG 425 Acute Adjustment Reactions and Disturbances of Psychosocial Dysfunction

Issue

The coding of psychotic and neurotic disorders is problematic because of the lack of physician documentation on the type of disorder, the overlap of mental health disorders with other acute nonmental health disorders, and the complexity of the ICD-9-CM diagnosis codes and coding guidelines.

Most Common Diagnosis Codes

DRG 430

- 295.34, Schizophrenic disorders, paranoid type with acute exacerbation
- 295.70, Schizophrenic disorders, schizoaffective type
- 296.20, Major depressive disorder, single episode
- 296.30, 296.33, 296.34, Major depressive disorder, recurrent episode
- 298.9, Nonorganic psychoses, unspecified

DRG 425

- 293.0, Acute delirium
- 300.00, Anxiety state, unspecified
- 300.01, Panic disorder
- 300.11, Conversion disorder

Coding and Documentation Guidelines

293.0	Acute delirium	DRG 425

AHA CC: The physician may document a diagnosis of metabolic encephalopathy, referring to an altered state of consciousness, usually denoting delirium. Physicians also use the term "acute confusional state" to represent metabolic encephalopathy. Use code 293.0 for both acute delirium and acute confusional state. Review the medical record for the associated condition or cause of the metabolic encephalopathy (delirium), such as brain tumors, malignant metastasis to brain, cerebral infarction or hemorrhage, subdural or epidural hematoma, hypoxia, cerebral ischemia, uremia, nutritional deficiency, poisoning, cumulative effect of a prescribed drug, effect of drugs in various combinations, systemic infection, meningitis, postoperative or post-traumatic states, postictal state, hypoglycemia, severe burns, and drug or alcohol withdrawal. Verify with the physician the meaning behind "metabolic encephalopathy," as this term can refers to any number of the conditions and code assignment. For example:

- Use code 293.0 if the physician documents acute delirium.
- Use code 291.0 if the physician documents acute alcohol withdrawal with delirium tremens.
- Use code 291.0 if the physician documents alcoholic delirium.
- Use code 292.81 if the physician documents drug-induced delirium (prescribed drug) (non-prescribed drug) (cumulative effect of drug) (various combination of drugs).
- Use code 293.0 if the physician documents acute brain syndrome with transient delirium.
- Use code 290.11 if the physician documents Alzheimer's disease with delirium.
- Use code 293.0 if the physician documents postictal state with delirium (confusional state in twilight epilepsy). [Coding Clinic, 1Q, '88, 3]

293.0   Acute delirium (continued)   **DRG 425**

AHA CC: Assign metabolic encephalopathy (delirium) as the principal diagnosis if it meets the definition. In addition, an instructional note under category 293 states "Code first the associated physical or neurological condition." Otherwise, it is listed as an associated condition. [*Coding Clinic*, 1Q, '88, 3]

DOC: Use code 293.0 when the physician documents acute confusional state, acute infective psychosis, acute organic reaction, acute post-traumatic organic psychosis, acute psycho-organic syndrome, acute psychosis associated with endocrine, metabolic, or cerebrovascular disorder, epileptic confusional state, or epileptic twilight state.

DOC: Do not use code 293.0 when the physician documents confusional state or delirium superimposed on senile dementia. The correct code is 290.3.

DOC: Do not use code 293.0 when the physician documents dementia due to alcohol. The correct code is chosen from the 291.0-291.9 series.

DOC: Do not use code 293.0 when the physician documents dementia due to arteriosclerosis. The correct code is chosen from the series 290.40-290.43.

DOC: Do not use code 293.0 when the physician documents dementia due to drugs The correct code is 292.82.

DOC: Do not use code 293.0 when the physician documents dementia due to senility. The correct code is 290.0.

300.00   Anxiety state, unspecified   **DRG 425**

AHA CC: A patient presenting with non-cardiac chest pain with severe anxiety is coded is 786.59, Chest pain, Other, and 300.00, Anxiety state, unspecified. The chest pain is not integral to a diagnosis of anxiety. [*Coding Clinic*, 1Q, '02, 37]

DOC: Use code 300.00 when the physician documents anxiety neurosis, anxiety reaction, anxiety state (neurotic), or atypical anxiety disorder.

DOC: Do not use code 300.00 when the physician documents anxiety in acute stress reaction. The correct code is 308.0.

DOC: Do not use code 300.00 when the physician documents anxiety in transient adjustment reaction. The correct code is 309.24.

DOC: Do not use code 300.00 when the physician documents separation anxiety. The correct code is 309.21.

DOC: Do not use code 300.00 when the physician documents neurasthenia. The correct code is 300.5.

DOC: Do not use code 300.00 when the physician documents psychophysiological disorders. The correct code is chosen from the 306.0-306.9 series.

300.01   Panic disorder   **DRG 425**

DOC: Use code 300.01 when the physician documents panic attack or panic state.

DOC: Do not use code 300.01 when the physician documents anxiety in acute stress reaction. The correct code is 308.0.

DOC: Do not use code 300.01 when the physician documents anxiety in transient adjustment reaction. The correct code is 309.24.

DOC: Do not use code 300.01 when the physician documents separation anxiety. The correct code is 309.21.

DOC: Do not use code 300.01 when the physician documents neurasthenia. The correct code is 300.5.

DOC: Do not use code 300.01 when the physician documents psychophysiological disorders. The correct code is chosen from the 306.0-306.9 series.

300.11   Conversion disorder   DRG 425

DOC: Use code 300.11 when the physician documents hysterical astasia-abasia, conversion hysteria or reaction, hysterical blindness, hysterical deafness, or hysterical paralysis.

DOC: Do not use code 300.11 when the physician documents an adjustment reaction. The correct code is chosen from the 309.0-309.9 series.

DOC: Do not use code 300.11 when the physician documents anorexia nervosa. The correct code is 307.1.

DOC: Do not use code 300.11 when the physician documents gross stress reaction. The correct code is chosen from the 308.0-308.9 series.

DOC: Do not use code 300.11 when the physician documents a hysterical personality. The correct code is chosen from the 301.50-301.59 series.

DOC: Do not use code 300.11 when the physician documents psychophysiologic disorders. The correct code is chosen from the 306.0-306.9 series.

DOC: Assign code 300.11 when the physician documents pseudoseizure. This is another term for hysterical seizure.

295.70   Schizophrenic disorders, schizoaffective type, unspecified   DRG 430

DOC: Use code 295.7x when the physician documents cyclic schizophrenia, mixed schizophrenic and affective psychosis, schizoaffective psychosis, or schizophreniform psychosis, affective type.

296.20   Major depressive disorder, single episode, unspecified   DRG 430

AHA CC: Check with the physician before assigning a code for "major affective disorder." Under the main term "disorder" and the subterm "affective," code 296.90 is referenced. However, it may be appropriate to use a code to indicate major depression, a subentry under category 296. When a diagnosis is unclear or questionable, the physician needs to clarify the condition in the medical record prior to coding. It also may be beneficial to review the subentries under category 296 and the fifth-digit code assignments with the physician. [*Coding Clinic*, M-A, '85, 14]

DOC: Use code 296.2x when the physician documents depressive psychosis, endogenous depression, involutional melancholia, manic-depressive psychosis or reaction, depressed type, monopolar depression, or psychotic depression.

DOC: Do not use code 296.2x when the physician documents depression. The correct code is 311.

DOC: Do not use code 296.2x when the physician documents reactive depression. The correct code is 300.4.

DOC: Do not use code 296.2x when the physician documents psychotic reactive depression. The correct code is 298.0.

DOC: Do not use code 296.2x when the physician documents manic-depressive psychosis, circular type, if previous type was manic. The correct code is 296.5x.

296.30 **Major depressive disorder, recurrent episode, unspecified** **DRG 430**

296.33 **Major depressive disorder, recurrent episode, severe, without mention of psychotic behavior**

296.34 **Major depressive disorder, recurrent episode, severe, specified as with psychotic behavior**

AHA CC: Check with the physician before assigning a code for "major affective disorder." Under the main term "disorder" and the subterm "affective," code 296.90 is referenced. However, it may be appropriate to use a code to indicate major depression, a subentry under category 296. When a diagnosis is unclear or questionable, the physician needs to clarify the condition in the medical record prior to coding. It also may be beneficial to review the subentries under category 296 and the fifth-digit code assignments with the physician. [*Coding Clinic*, M-A, '85, 14]

DOC: Use code 296.3x when the physician documents recurrent depressive psychosis, recurrent endogenous depression, recurrent involutional melancholia, recurrent manic-depressive psychosis or reaction, depressed type, recurrent monopolar depression, or recurrent psychotic depression.

DOC: Do not use code 296.3x when the physician documents depression. The correct code is 311.

DOC: Do not use code 296.3x when the physician documents reactive depression. The correct code is 300.4.

DOC: Do not use code 296.3x when the physician documents psychotic reactive depression. The correct code is 298.0.

DOC: Do not use code 296.3x when the physician documents manic-depressive psychosis, circular type, if previous type was manic. The correct code is 296.5x.

298.9 **Nonorganic psychoses, unspecified** **DRG 430**

DOC: Do not use 298.9 when the physician documents altered mental status. The correct code is 780.9.

DRG 475 Respiratory System Diagnosis with Ventilator Support

DRG 121 Circulatory Disorders with Acute Myocardial Infarction and Major Complications, Discharged Alive

Issue

The coding of hospital stays for patients who have received continuous mechanical ventilation support is problematic because of the numerous diagnoses relating to the respiratory system. Physician documentation may be unclear as to the condition established after study to be chiefly responsible for admission of the patient to the hospital. Although respiratory complications may arise during a patient stay that justify assigning additional ICD-9-CM diagnosis codes for the respiratory condition and continuous mechanical ventilation support, the first partitioning in DRG assignment is made according to the principal diagnosis, not the secondary diagnosis of respiratory disease with continuous mechanical ventilation support. Assignment of DRG 475 is appropriate only when the medical record documentation supports both the principal diagnosis of respiratory disease and that mechanical ventilation support was provided.

Most Common Diagnosis Codes

DRG 475
- 486, Pneumonia, organism unspecified
- 491.21, Obstructive chronic bronchitis with acute exacerbation
- 507.0, Pneumonitis due to inhalation of food or vomitus
- 518.81, Acute respiratory failure

DRG 121
- 410.11, Acute myocardial infarction of anterolateral wall
- 410.41, Acute myocardial infarction of other inferior wall
- 410.71, Acute subendocardial infarction
- 410.91, Acute myocardial infarction of unspecified site
- 428.0, Congestive heart failure

Coding and Documentation Guidelines

410.11	Acute myocardial infarction of other anterior wall, initial episode of care	DRG 121

See standards on page 573.

410.41	Acute myocardial infarction of other inferior wall, initial episode of care	DRG 121

See standards on page 573.

410.71	Acute myocardial infarction, subendocardialinfarction, initial episode of care	DRG 121

See standards on page 574

410.91   Acute myocardial infarction, unspecified site,   **DRG 121**
initial episode of care

See standards on page 574.

428.0   Congestive heart failure   **DRG 121**

See standards on page 578.

486   Pneumonia, organism unspecified   **DRG 475**

See standards on page 554.

491.21   Obstructive chronic bronchitis with acute exacerbation   **DRG 475**

See standards on page 566.

507.0   Pneumonitis due to inhalation of food or vomitus   **DRG 475**

See standards on page 554.

518.81   Acute respiratory failure   **DRG 475**

See standards on page 558.

Targeted DRG Listing

DRG 475 Respiratory System Diagnosis with Ventilator Support

DRG 127 Heart Failure and Shock

Issue

The coding of hospital stays of patients who have received continuous mechanical ventilation support is problematic because of the numerous diagnoses relating to the respiratory system. Physician documentation may be unclear as to the condition established after study to be chiefly responsible for admission of the patient to the hospital. Although respiratory complications may arise during a patient stay that justify assigning additional ICD-9-CM diagnosis codes for the respiratory condition and continuous mechanical ventilation support, the first partitioning in DRG assignment is made according to the principal diagnosis, not the secondary diagnosis of respiratory disease with continuous mechanical ventilation support. Assignment of DRG 475 is appropriate only when the medical record documentation supports both the principal diagnosis of respiratory disease and that mechanical ventilation support was provided.

Most Common Diagnosis Codes

DRG 475

- 486, Pneumonia, organism unspecified
- 491.21, Obstructive chronic bronchitis with acute exacerbation
- 507.0, Pneumonitis due to inhalation of food or vomitus
- 518.81, Acute respiratory failure

DRG 127

- 402.91, Hypertensive heart disease with heart failure
- 428.0, Congestive heart failure

Coding and Documentation Guidelines

402.91 Hypertensive heart disease with congestive heart failure	DRG 127

See standards on page 564.

428.0 Congestive heart failure	DRG 127

See standards on page 555.

486 Pneumonia, organism unspecified	DRG 475

See standards on page 532.

491.21 Obstructive chronic bronchitis with acute exacerbation	DRG 475

See standards on page 539.

507.0 Pneumonitis due to inhalation of food or vomitus	DRG 475

See standards on page 532.

518.81 Acute respiratory failure	DRG 475

See standards on page 536.

New Medical Services and Technologies Under IPPS

On December 21, 2000, Congress passed the Medicare, Medicaid, and SCHIP (State Children's Health Insurance Program) Benefits Improvement and Protection Act (BIPA) of 2000. Section 533 of the Public Law 106-554 requires the establishment of a mechanism to recognize costs of new services and technologies under the hospital inpatient prospective payment system by October 1, 2001. The proposed rule was issued with the Medicare Program Notice of Proposed Rule Making (NPRM) annual inpatient prospective payment system (IPPS) proposed changes on May 4, 2001, and the final rule published on September 7, 2001, *Federal Register* "Medicare Program; Payments for New Medical Services and New Technologies Under the Acute Care Hospital Inpatient Prospective Payment System." The provisions of the final rule address the following policy changes required to accommodate new technology payments:

- Due to rapid innovations in technology, the identification of ICD-9-CM codes require a more expeditious process than currently in place, prior length of time does not accommodate technologic advances. The annual process for code identification and approval has been reduced from 11 months to six months beginning FY 2002.
- ICD-9-CM provides a limited expansion of codes for assigning new technology categories. A new code category has been identified as a short-term solution. A new chapter in volume 3, ICD-9-CM procedures numbered 00 and titled "Procedures and interventions, Not Elsewhere Classified," will be used to identify future new technology codes. Other new services and technologies fall within their respective chapters, for example, 84.52, Insertion of recombinant bone morphogenetic protein.
- Even though the tracking of new codes will be accommodated on an annual basis, newly assigned codes for technologies will not result in any changes in payment, diagnosis-related group (DRG) construction, or reweighting until October of the following year. Therefore, the interim payment would initially be the same as the predecessor technologies.
- The new technology add-on payment policy will provide for additional payment for cases with high costs that include eligible new technologies. The payment methodology is based on the cost to the hospitals of the new technology. Medicare will pay a marginal cost factor of 50 percent for the costs of the new technology in excess to the DRG payment. If the actual costs of a new technology case exceed the DRG payment by more than the estimated costs of the new technology, Medicare payment will be limited to the DRG payment plus 50 percent of the estimated costs of the new technology.
- To qualify for payment, charges for the new technology must exceed one standard deviation from the mean charge in all cases for an individual DRG. This threshold was established to maintain budget neutrality. Since only a few applications for new tecnology add-on payments are received each year, FY 2005 and subsequent years, the threshold will be reduced to 75 percent of one standard deviation beyond the geometric mean standard for all cases in te DRG to which the new technology is assigned.

Criteria for Identifying New Medical Services and Technology

A medical service or technology will be considered new and appropriate and eligible for additional payment if it represents an advance in medical technology that substantially improves, relative to technologies previously available, the diagnosis or treatment of Medicare beneficiaries. A panel of federal clinical and outside experts will provide oversight to adequately review the services. At least one or more of the following criteria will be required as evidence for recognition as a new medical service or technology under IPPS:

- The device offers a treatment option for a patient population unresponsive to, or ineligible for, currently available treatments.
- The device offers the ability to diagnose a medical condition in a patient population where that medical condition is currently undetectable or offers the ability to diagnose a medical condition earlier in a patient population than allowed by currently available methods.
- There must be clear evidence that use of the device to make a diagnosis affects the management of the patient.
- Use of the device significantly improves clinical outcomes for a patient population as compared to currently available treatments. Some examples of outcomes that are frequently evaluated in studies of medical devices are the following:
  — reduced mortality rate with use of the device
  — reduced rate of device-related complications
  — decreased rate of subsequent diagnostic or therapeutic interventions (e.g., due to reduced rate of recurrence of the disease process)
  — decreased number of future hospitalizations or physician visits
  — more rapid beneficial resolution of the disease process treatment because of the use of the device
  — decreased pain, bleeding, ore other quantifiable symptom
  — reduced recovery time

High-dose Infusion Interleukin-2 (IL-2)

The ICD-9-CM Coordination and Maintenance Committee approved the creation of a new ICD-9-CM code for high-dose infusion of interleukin-2 (IL-2) effective for discharges on or after October 1, 2003.

High-dose infusion interleukin-2 (IL-2) regimen is administered by oncology professionals in an inpatient setting for the treatment of advanced renal cell carcinoma and advanced melanoma. Interleukin-2 activated the immune system and stimulates the growth and activity of cancer-killing cells rather than acting as a cytotoxin that attack cancer cells directly.

High-dose interleukin-2 therapy is administered during two separate inpatient admissions. The first cycle is administered every eight hours over the course of five days. The patient returns after several days to undergo the second cycle of the same regimen and dosing as the first cycle. This two-cycle regimen may be repeated at eight- to twelve-week intervals. The average number of courses of treatment is five.

The prevalence in the United States of cases of advanced renal cell carcinoma and advanced melanoma is estimated between 15,000 and 20,000. Only 20 percent are considered appropriate candidates for this particular treatment. Due to high-costs associated with interleukin-2 therapy many of the eligible cases do not receive therapy.

Patients who receive this therapy for treatment of advanced renal cell carcinoma and advanced melanoma have been assigned to DRGs according to the principal diagnosis. The average charges for the interleukin-2 therapy is approximately $54,000, which is significantly more that the average DRG payment for the DRG to which the patients are assigned based upon principal diagnosis.

With the approval of the new code 00.15 High-dose infusion interleukin-2 (IL-2), effective for discharges on or after October 1, 2003, the mechanism for identifying patients receiving this therapy has been established. After cost data analysis, CMS determined that patients undergoing high-dosed interleukin therapy are more clinically similar to cases assigned to DRG 492 Chemotherapy With Acute Leukemia as a Secondary Diagnosis. Therefore, for FY 2004 the title of DRG 492 has been revised to Chemotherapy With Acute Leukemia or With Use of High-Dose Chemotherapy Agent. ICD-9-CM code 00.15 has been assigned to DRG 492.

While high-dose interleukin therapy is considered new technology and assigned a code in the 00 chapter, Procedures and Interventions NEC, CMS had sufficient data to assign the procedure to a DRG that provided appropriate reimbursement to cover the costs associated with the case management. Therefore, high-dose interleukin-2 infusion therapy was not eligible to be considered under the Add-on Payments New Service and Technology Provision.

Add-on Payment for New Services and Technologies

The Centers for Medicare and Medicaid Services (CMS) established that an additional payment would be appropriate for a new technology that substantially improves the diagnosis and treatment. Besides the above mentioned clinical and cost criteria, a new technology must meet the definition of "new." To be considered new and eligible for add-on payments, costs for the new technology must be in a DRG weight recalibration cycle no less than two years and no more than three.

Bone Morphogenic Proteins (BMPs) for Spinal Fusion

An application for consideration of eligibility was submitted for InFUSE Bone Graft/LT-Cage Lumbar Tapered Fusion Device. A similar application was submitted for FY 2003 and denied based on lack of sufficient data to make a determination as to whether the technology met the criteria for add-on payments.

BMPs have been recognized for the capacity to induced new bone formation in a variety of clinical applications. Using recombinant techniques, some BMPs (referred to as rhBMPs) can be produced in large quantities for clinical use. In 2002 the FDA approved BMP for spinal fusion procedures in skeletally mature patients with degenerative disc disease at one level from L4-S1. Multilevel use was not approved. The product is applied through the use of an absorbable collagen sponge or an interbody fusion device, which is then implanted at the fusion site. This procedure replaces the more traditional use of autogenous iliac crest bone graft.

Because the average charges for the use of the technology for single level spinal fusion did not exceed the threshold to qualify for additional payment, the application was denied in FY 2003. A new ICD-9-CM code, 84.52, was established, effective October 1, 2002, to capture the insertion of recombinant bone morphogenic protein (rhBMP).

Single level spinal fusions are assigned to DRGs 497 and 498 Spinal Fusion Except Cervical, With and Without CC, respectively. The DRGs do not differentiate cases on the basis of the number of levels of the spine fused. Through analysis of MedPAR data for DRG 497 and 498,

CMS determined that single level fusions represented about 78 percent of the average charges across all spinal fusion including multi-level fusions. CMS estimated that since the FDA approval of InFUSET™ was recent and that over the course of a year, the final estimated percent of the average charge for single-level spinal fusion using InFUSE™ might be as much as 90 percent, this would bring the average charge for spinal fusion using InFUSE™ above the threshold amount. Therefore, this technology met the cost threshold for add-on payment.

Also CMS evaluated whether this technology met the substantial improvement criteria. Evidence indicated InFUSE™ reduces operative time, blood loss and hospitalization, obviates iliac crest bone graft donor site morbidity, results in greater fusion success, enables faster return to work, and lowers the Oswestry Low Back Pain and Disability score. Therefore, InFUSE™ was approved for add-on payment under the Add-on Payments for New Services Technologies provision.

GLIADEL® Wafer

GLIADEL® Wafer (prolifeprostan 20 with carmustine implant) was approved by the FDA in 1996 for use as an adjunct therapy to surgery to prolong survival in patients with recurrent glioblastoma multiforme (GBM) for whom surgical resection was indicated. The GLIADEL® Wafer is an implantable drug that delivers chemotherapy directly to the site of the removed tumor. Effective with discharges on or after October 1, 2002, the implantation of brain wafter chemotherapy is reported using ICD-9-CM code 00.10 Implantation of chemotherapeutic agent.

Cases involving the use of GLIADEL® Wafter are assigned to DRG 1 and 2 (Craniotomy, Age Greater than 17, With and Without CC, respectively). MedPAR data analysis indicates that the average cost associated with the implantation of GLIADEL® Wafer does not meer the threshold criteria for add-on payment.

Infusion of Drotrecogin Alfa (Activated)- Xigris™

Drotrecogin alfa (activated) is a biotechnology agent used to treat severe sepsis. Naturally occurring activated protein C (APC) is needed to ensure the control of infammation and clotting in the blood vessels. In patients with severe sepsis, protein C cannot be converted in sufficient quantities to the activated form. It appears that drotrecogin alfa (activated), which is a recombinant version of APC, has the ability to bring inflammation and clotting into balance and restore blood flow to organs. The FDA approved the use of Xigris™ in November 2001.

A new code (00.11) was created to report the infusion of drotrecogin alfa (activated) effective October 1, 2002 and drotrecogin alfa (Xigris™) was approved for add-on payments FY 2003. Under the statutory requirements the technology is considered new within the two or three years after the data becomes available. Since Xigris™ did not qualify for add-on payments until October 1, 2002, Xigris™ will continue to be eligible for add-on payments in FY 2004 under the new technology provision.

Application of Coding for New Technology and Medical Services ICD-9-CM Codes

Only new technologies that represent significant advances are to be considered under the add-on payment provision for new services and technologies. The determination of whether a new technology meets the criteria for add-on payments is published in the annual proposed and final rules for the inpatient prospective payment system.

ICD-10-PCS: A Possible Long-term Solution

The ICD-10-PCS proposed draft is being considered as a long-term approach in assigning codes for new technology. The system provides a great flexibility and capacity to accommodate temporary coding categories. In addition, the transition from ICD-9-CM to ICD-10-PCS would drastically increase the number of procedural codes available for reporting. ICD-9-CM currently is limited to a maximum of 10,000 codes and the current draft of ICD-10-PCS contains 197,769 codes and the code set could be expanded.

ICD-10-CM Coding System

ICD-10-CM is a revision of the International Classification of Diseases (ICD). In April 2003, Medicare reform legislation was introduced in the U.S. House requesting the HHS Secretary take action on the proposed adoption of ICD-10-CM and ICD-10-PCS code set standards if the National Committee on Vital and Health Statistics (NCVHS) did not make a recommendation. NCVHS is slated to present a final recommendation to the HHS secretary in the fall of 2003. The American Hospital Association (AHA) and AHIMA are testing ICD-10-CM in order to provide information for both NCVHS and HHS. The ICD-9-CM coding system has been the standard coding system for the United States since 1979. The evolution of ICD-10-CM began in 1994 in cooperation with the World Health Organization, National Center for Health Statistics and CMS. The intent of the revision is to address the limitations of the current ICD-9-CM system and enhance the classifications of mortality and morbidity data.

ICD-10-CM (clinical modification) was drafted to encompass the classification of diseases and related health problems as classified in the current ICD-9-CM, volumes 1 and 2. ICD-10-PCS (procedural coding system) was drafted for reporting of procedures as currently used in ICD-9-CM, volume 3.

The pre-release draft of ICD-10-CM was released in August 2002. Under the Health Insurance Portability and Accountability Act (HIPAA) of 1996 the adoption of final approved code sets and implementation schedules is part of an effort to set standards for electronic transactions and other administrative simplification issues for all health plans, health care clearinghouses, and health care providers. The federal regulation will provide for standard code sets to be used and applied by all entities when providing health information electronically. All three volumes of ICD-9-CM are included as the standard coding system under current HIPAA final rules. If ICD-10-CM is adopted the HIPAA regulation will need to be modified to include this as an approved transaction code set standard.

DRG List

DRG	Title	MDC	Med/Surg	RW	AMLOS	GMLOS
1	Craniotomy, Age Greater than 17 with CC	1	S	3.6186	10.90	8.00
2	Craniotomy, Age Greater than 17 without CC	1	S	2.0850	5.30	4.10
3	Craniotomy, Age 0-17	1	S	1.9753	12.70	12.70
6	Carpal Tunnel Release	1	S	0.0000	0.00	0.00
7	Peripheral and Cranial Nerve and Other Nervous System Procedures with CC	1	S	0.0000	0.00	0.00
8	Peripheral and Cranial Nerve and Other Nervous System Procedures without CC	1	S	0.8092	3.10	2.20
9	Spinal Disorders and Injuries	1	M	2.6519	9.80	6.60
10	Nervous System Neoplasms with CC	1	M	1.5453	2.80	1.90
11	Nervous System Neoplasms without CC	1	M	1.4214	6.90	4.70
12	Degenerative Nervous System Disorders	1	M	1.2448	6.50	4.80
13	Multiple Sclerosis and Cerebellar Ataxia	1	M	0.8571	4.10	3.00
14	Intracranial Hemorrhage and Stoke with Infarction	1	M	0.9259	5.90	4.50
15	Nonspecific Cerebrovascular and Precerebral Occlusion without Infarction	1	M	0.8176	5.00	4.00
16	Nonspecific Cerebrovascular Disorders with CC	1	M	1.2682	6.10	4.70
17	Nonspecific Cerebrovascular Disorders without CC	1	M	0.9677	4.90	3.90
18	Cranial and Peripheral Nerve Disorders with CC	1	M	1.2618	6.40	4.80
19	Cranial and Peripheral Nerve Disorders without CC	1	M	0.6991	3.20	2.50
20	Nervous System Infection Except Viral Meningitis	1	M	1.0026	5.50	4.20
21	Viral Meningitis	1	M	0.7041	3.50	2.80
22	Hypertensive Encephalopathy	1	M	2.7394	10.50	8.00
23	Nontraumatic Stupor and Coma	1	M	1.5138	6.60	5.00
24	Seizure and Headache, Age Greater than 17 with CC	1	M	1.0737	5.10	3.90
25	Seizure and Headache, Age Greater than 17 without CC	1	M	0.8239	4.30	3.20
26	Seizure and Headache, Age 0-17	1	M	1.0121	5.00	3.70
27	Traumatic Stupor and Coma, Coma Greater than One Hour	1	M	0.6109	3.20	2.50
28	Traumatic Stupor and Coma, Coma Less than One Hour, Age Greater than 17 with CC	1	M	1.3730	4.10	2.20

DRG	Title	MDC	Med/Surg	RW	AMLOS	GMLOS
29	Traumatic Stupor and Coma, Coma Less than One Hour, Age Greater than 17 without CC	1	M	0.7087	3.50	2.70
30	Traumatic Stupor and Coma, Coma Less than One Hour, Age 0-17	1	M	0.3341	2.00	2.00
31	Concussion, Age Greater than 17 with CC	1	M	0.9117	4.10	3.10
32	Concussion, Age Greater than 17 without CC	1	M	0.5684	2.50	2.00
33	Concussion, Age 0-17	1	M	0.2098	1.60	1.60
34	Other Disorders of Nervous System with CC	1	M	0.9931	5.00	3.70
35	Other Disorders of Nervous System without CC	1	M	0.6355	3.10	2.50
36	Retinal Procedures	2	S	0.6298	1.50	1.20
37	Orbital Procedures	2	S	1.0575	3.80	2.50
38	Primary Iris Procedures	2	S	0.4669	2.80	1.90
39	Lens Procedures with or without Vitrectomy	2	S	0.6285	2.10	1.50
40	Extraocular Procedures Except Orbit, Age Greater than 17	2	S	0.8937	3.80	2.70
41	Extraocular Procedures Except Orbit, Age 0-17	2	S	0.3401	1.60	1.60
42	Intraocular Procedures Except Retina, Iris and Lens	2	S	0.7064	2.70	1.90
43	Hyphema	2	M	0.5382	3.40	2.40
44	Acute Major Eye Infections	2	M	0.6597	5.00	4.00
45	Neurological Eye Disorders	2	M	0.7250	3.10	2.50
46	Other Disorders of the Eye, Age Greater than 17 with CC	2	M	0.7936	4.50	3.40
47	Other Disorders of the Eye, Age Greater than 17 without CC	2	M	0.5317	3.10	2.40
48	Other Disorders of the Eye, Age 0-17	2	M	0.2996	2.90	2.90
49	Major Head and Neck Procedures	3	S	1.7277	4.50	3.20
50	Sialoadenectomy	3	S	0.8317	1.90	1.50
51	Salivary Gland Procedures Except Sialoadenectomy	3	S	0.8410	2.80	1.90
52	Cleft Lip and Palate Repair	3	S	0.8018	1.80	1.40
53	Sinus and Mastoid Procedures, Age Greater than 17	3	S	1.2520	3.60	2.20
54	Sinus and Mastoid Procedures, Age 0-17	3	S	0.4856	3.20	3.20
55	Miscellaneous Ear, Nose, Mouth and Throat Procedures	3	S	0.9247	3.00	2.00
56	Rhinoplasty	3	S	0.9233	2.90	1.90
57	Tonsillectomy and Adenoidectomy Procedures Except Tonsillectomy and/or Adenoidectomy Only, Age Greater than 17	3	S	1.1029	3.70	2.40

DRG	Title	MDC	Med/Surg	RW	AMLOS	GMLOS
58	Tonsillectomy and Adenoidectomy Procedures Except Tonsillectomy and/or Adenoidectomy Only, Age 0-17	3	S	0.2757	1.50	1.50
59	Tonsillectomy and/or Adenoidectomy Only, Age Greater than 17	3	S	0.9557	2.70	1.90
60	Tonsillectomy and/or Adenoidectomy Only, Age 0-17	3	S	0.2099	1.50	1.50
61	Myringotomy with Tube Insertion, Age Greater than 17	3	S	1.2334	5.20	3.10
62	Myringotomy with Tube Insertion, Age 0-17	3	S	0.2973	1.30	1.30
63	Other Ear, Nose, Mouth and Throat OR Procedures	3	S	1.3759	4.40	3.00
64	Ear, Nose, Mouth and Throat Malignancy	3	M	1.3089	6.50	4.30
65	Dysequilibrium	3	M	0.5748	2.80	2.30
66	Epistaxis	3	M	0.5811	3.10	2.40
67	Epiglottitis	3	M	0.7780	3.70	2.90
68	Otitis Media and URI, Age Greater than 17 with CC	3	M	0.6531	3.90	3.10
69	Otitis Media and URI, Age Greater than 17 without CC	3	M	0.4987	3.00	2.50
70	Otitis Media and URI, Age 0-17	3	M	0.3188	2.40	2.00
71	Laryngotracheitis	3	M	0.7065	3.40	2.50
72	Nasal Trauma and Deformity	3	M	0.6954	3.40	2.60
73	Other Ear, Nose, Mouth and Throat Diagnoses, Age Greater than 17	3	M	0.8184	4.50	3.30
74	Other Ear, Nose, Mouth and Throat Diagnoses, Age 0-17	3	M	0.3380	2.10	2.10
75	Major Chest Procedures	4	S	3.0437	10.00	7.70
76	Other Respiratory System O.R. Procedures with CC	4	S	2.8184	11.10	8.40
77	Other Respiratory System O.R. Procedures without CC	4	S	1.2378	4.80	3.50
78	Pulmonary Embolism	4	M	1.2731	6.60	5.60
79	Respiratory Infections and Inflammations, Age Greater than 17 with CC	4	M	1.5974	8.50	6.70
80	Respiratory Infections and Inflammations, Age Greater than 17 without CC	4	M	0.8400	5.40	4.30
81	Respiratory Infections and Inflammations, Age 0-17	4	M	1.5300	6.10	6.10
82	Respiratory Neoplasms	4	M	1.3724	6.90	5.10
83	Major Chest Trauma with CC	4	M	0.9620	5.40	4.30
84	Major Chest Trauma without CC	4	M	0.5371	3.30	2.60
85	Pleural Effusion with CC	4	M	1.1927	6.30	4.80

DRG	Title	MDC	Med/Surg	RW	AMLOS	GMLOS
86	Pleural Effusion without CC	4	M	0.6864	3.60	2.80
87	Pulmonary Edema and Respiratory Failure	4	M	1.3430	6.40	4.80
88	Chronic Obstructive Pulmonary Disease	4	M	0.9031	5.10	4.10
89	Simple Pneumonia and Pleurisy, Age Greater than 17 with CC	4	M	1.0463	5.90	4.90
90	Simple Pneumonia and Pleurisy, Age Greater than 17 without CC	4	M	0.6147	4.00	3.40
91	Simple Pneumonia and Pleurisy, Age 0-17	4	M	0.7408	5.10	3.10
92	Interstitial Lung Disease with CC	4	M	1.2024	6.30	5.00
93	Interstitial Lung Disease without CC	4	M	0.7176	4.00	3.30
94	Pneumothorax with CC	4	M	1.1340	6.30	4.70
95	Pneumothorax without CC	4	M	0.6166	3.80	3.00
96	Bronchitis and Asthma, Age Greater than 17 with CC	4	M	0.7464	4.60	3.70
97	Bronchitis and Asthma, Age Greater than 17 without CC	4	M	0.5505	3.50	2.90
98	Bronchitis and Asthma, Age 0-17	4	M	0.9662	3.70	3.70
99	Respiratory Signs and Symptoms with CC	4	M	0.7032	3.20	2.40
100	Respiratory Signs and Symptoms without CC	4	M	0.5222	2.10	1.80
101	Other Respiratory System Diagnoses with CC	4	M	0.8654	4.40	3.30
102	Other Respiratory System Diagnoses without CC	4	M	0.5437	2.60	2.10
103	Heart Transplant	PRE	S	18.6081	42.40	26.10
104	Cardiac Valve Procedures and Other Major Cardiothoracic Procedures with Cardiac Catheterization	5	S	7.9351	14.40	12.20
105	Cardiac Valve Procedures and Other Major Cardiothoracic Procedures without Cardiac Catheterization	5	S	5.7088	9.90	8.20
106	Coronary Bypass with PTCA	5	S	7.2936	11.40	9.60
107	Coronary Bypass with Cardiac Catheterization	5	S	5.3751	10.40	9.20
108	Other Cardiothoracic Procedures	5	S	5.3656	9.80	7.30
109	Coronary Bypass without Cardiac Catheterizaton	5	S	3.9401	7.70	6.70
110	Major Cardiovascular Procedures with CC	5	S	4.0492	8.90	6.20
111	Major Cardiovascular Procedures without CC	5	S	2.4797	4.10	3.20
112	No Longer Valid	5		0.0000	0.00	0.00
113	Amputation for Circulatory System Disorders Except Upper Limb and Toe	5	S	3.0106	13.30	10.40
114	Upper Limb and Toe Amputation for Circulatory System Disorders	5	S	1.6436	8.70	6.30

DRG	Title	MDC	Med/Surg	RW	AMLOS	GMLOS
115	Permanent Cardiac Pacemaker Implant with Acute Myocardial Infarction, Heart Failure or Shock or AICD Lead or Generator Procedure	5	S	3.5465	7.40	5.00
116	Other Cardiac Pacemaker Implantation	5	S	2.3590	4.40	3.10
117	Cardiac Pacemaker Revision Except Device Replacement	5	S	1.3951	4.30	2.60
118	Cardiac Pacemaker Device Replacement	5	S	1.6089	2.90	2.00
119	Vein Ligation and Stripping	5	S	1.3739	5.30	3.20
120	Other Circulatory System OR Procedures	5	S	2.3164	9.00	5.60
121	Circulatory Disorders with Acute Myocardial Infarction and Major Complications, Discharged Alive	5	M	1.6169	6.60	5.30
122	Circulatory Disorders with Acute Myocardial Infarction without Major Complications, Discharged Alive	5	M	1.0297	3.70	2.90
123	Circulatory Disorders with Acute Myocardial Infarction, Expired	5	M	1.5645	4.80	2.90
124	Circulatory Disorders Except Acute Myocardial Infarction with Cardiac Catheterization and Complex Diagnosis	5	M	1.4367	4.40	3.30
125	Circulatory Disorders Except Acute Myocardial Infarction with Cardiac Catheterization without Complex Diagnosis	5	M	1.0947	2.80	2.20
126	Acute and Subacute Endocarditis	5	M	2.5418	11.80	9.20
127	Heart Failure and Shock	5	M	1.0265	5.30	4.20
128	Deep Vein Thrombophlebitis	5	M	0.7285	5.50	4.60
129	Cardiac Arrest, Unexplained	5	M	1.0229	2.60	1.70
130	Peripheral Vascular Disorders with CC	5	M	0.9505	5.70	4.50
131	Peripheral Vascular Disorders without CC	5	M	0.5676	4.10	3.30
132	Atherosclerosis with CC	5	M	0.6422	2.90	2.30
133	Atherosclerosis without CC	5	M	0.5559	2.30	1.80
134	Hypertension	5	M	0.5954	3.20	2.50
135	Cardiac Congenital and Valvular Disorders, Age Greater than 17 with CC	5	M	0.9282	4.50	3.40
136	Cardiac Congenital and Valvular Disorders, Age Greater than 17 without CC	5	M	0.5740	2.70	2.20
137	Cardiac Congenital and Valvular Disorders, Age 0-17	5	M	0.8243	3.30	3.30
138	Cardiac Arrhythmia and Conduction Disorders with CC	5	M	0.8355	4.00	3.10
139	Cardiac Arrhythmia and Conduction Disorders without CC	5	M	0.5160	2.50	2.00
140	Angina Pectoris	5	M	0.5305	2.50	2.00

DRG	Title	MDC	Med/Surg	RW	AMLOS	GMLOS
141	Syncope and Collapse with CC	5	M	0.7473	3.60	2.80
142	Syncope and Collapse without CC	5	M	0.5761	2.60	2.10
143	Chest Pain	5	M	0.5480	2.10	1.70
144	Other Circulatory System Diagnoses with CC	5	M	1.2260	5.60	3.90
145	Other Circulatory System Diagnoses without CC	5	M	0.5787	2.60	2.00
146	Rectal Resection with CC	6	S	2.7376	10.20	8.80
147	Rectal Resection without CC	6	S	1.5375	6.20	5.60
148	Major Small and Large Bowel Procedures with CC	6	S	3.4025	12.30	10.10
149	Major Small and Large Bowel Procedures without CC	6	S	1.4590	6.30	5.80
150	Peritoneal Adhesiolysis with CC	6	S	2.8711	11.30	9.20
151	Peritoneal Adhesiolysis without CC	6	S	1.3061	5.60	4.40
152	Minor Small and Large Bowel Procedures with CC	6	S	1.9134	8.40	6.90
153	Minor Small and Large Bowel Procedures without CC	6	S	1.1310	5.30	4.70
154	Stomach, Esophageal and Duodenal Procedures, Age Greater than 17 with CC	6	S	4.0212	13.30	9.90
155	Stomach, Esophageal and Duodenal Procedures, Age Greater than 17 without CC	6	S	1.3043	4.10	3.00
156	Stomach, Esophageal and Duodenal Procedures, Age 0-17	6	S	0.8489	6.00	6.00
157	Anal and Stomal Procedures with CC	6	S	1.3152	5.80	4.00
158	Anal and Stomal Procedures without CC	6	S	0.6517	2.60	2.00
159	Hernia Procedures Except Inguinal and Femoral, Age Greater than 17 with CC	6	S	1.3744	5.10	3.80
160	Hernia Procedures Except Inguinal and Femoral, Age Greater than 17 without CC	6	S	0.8219	2.70	2.20
161	Inguinal and Femoral Hernia Procedures, Age Greater than 17 with CC	6	S	1.1676	4.30	3.00
162	Inguinal and Femoral Hernia Procedures, Age Greater than 17 without CC	6	S	0.6446	1.90	1.60
163	Hernia Procedures, Age 0-17	6	S	0.6965	2.10	2.10
164	Appendectomy with Complicated Principal Diagnosis with CC	6	S	2.3306	8.40	7.00
165	Appendectomy with Complicated Principal Diagnosis without CC	6	S	1.2302	4.50	3.90
166	Appendectomy without Complicated Principal Diagnosis with CC	6	S	1.4317	4.70	3.60

DRG	Title	MDC	Med/Surg	RW	AMLOS	GMLOS
167	Appendectomy without Complicated Principal Diagnosis without CC	6	S	0.8889	2.40	2.00
168	Mouth Procedures with CC	3	S	1.3158	4.90	3.30
169	Mouth Procedures without CC	3	S	0.7525	2.40	1.80
170	Other Digestive System OR Procedures with CC	6	S	2.8245	10.90	7.50
171	Other Digestive System OR Procedures without CC	6	S	1.1912	4.30	3.30
172	Digestive Malignancy with CC	6	M	1.3670	7.00	5.20
173	Digestive Malignancy without CC	6	M	0.7528	3.80	2.80
174	GI Hemorrhage with CC	6	M	1.0025	4.80	3.90
175	GI Hemorrhage without CC	6	M	0.5587	2.90	2.50
176	Complicated Peptic Ulcer	6	M	1.0998	5.20	4.10
177	Uncomplicated Peptic Ulcer with CC	6	M	0.9259	4.60	3.70
178	Uncomplicated Peptic Ulcer without CC	6	M	0.6940	3.10	2.60
179	Inflammatory Bowel Disease	6	M	1.0885	6.00	4.60
180	GI Obstruction with CC	6	M	0.9642	5.50	4.20
181	GI Obstruction without CC	6	M	0.5376	3.40	2.80
182	Esophagitis, Gastroenteritis and Miscellaneous Digestive Disorders, Age Greater than 17 with CC	6	M	0.8223	4.40	3.40
183	Esophagitis, Gastroenteritis and Miscellaneous Digestive Disorders, Age Greater than 17 without CC	6	M	0.5759	2.90	2.30
184	Esophagitis, Gastroenteritis and Miscellaneous Digestive Disorders, Age 0-17	6	M	0.4813	3.30	2.40
185	Dental and Oral Diseases Except Extractions and Restorations, Age Greater than 17	3	M	0.8685	4.70	3.30
186	Dental and Oral Diseases Except Extractions and Restorations, Age 0-17	3	M	0.3236	2.90	2.90
187	Dental Extractions and Restorations	3	M	0.7778	4.00	3.00
188	Other Digestive System Diagnoses, Age Greater than 17 with CC	6	M	1.1088	5.60	4.10
189	Other Digestive System Diagnoses, Age Greater than 17 without CC	6	M	0.5987	3.10	2.40
190	Other Digestive System Diagnoses, Age 0-17	6	M	0.8104	5.20	3.70
191	Pancreas, Liver and Shunt Procedures with CC	7	S	4.2787	13.80	9.80
192	Pancreas, Liver and Shunt Procedures without CC	7	S	1.8025	6.20	4.70
193	Biliary Tract Procedures Except Only Cholecystectomy with or without Common Duct Exploration with CC	7	S	3.4211	12.80	10.40

DRG	Title	MDC	Med/Surg	RW	AMLOS	GMLOS
194	Biliary Tract Procedures Except Only Cholecystectomy with or without Common Duct Exploration without CC	7	S	1.6030	6.70	5.70
195	Cholecystectomy with Common Duct Exploration with CC	7	S	3.0613	10.60	8.70
196	Cholecystectomy with Common Duct Exploration without CC	7	S	1.6117	5.60	4.80
197	Cholecystectomy Except by Laparoscope without Common Duct Exploration with CC	7	S	2.5547	9.20	7.50
198	Cholecystectomy Except by Laparoscope without Common Duct Exploration without CC	7	S	1.1831	4.40	3.80
199	Hepatobiliary Diagnostic Procedure for Malignancy	7	S	2.3953	9.80	7.00
200	Hepatobiliary Diagnostic Procedure for Nonmalignancy	7	S	3.0415	10.50	6.70
201	Other Hepatobiliary or Pancreas OR Procedures	7	S	3.6841	14.20	10.20
202	Cirrhosis and Alcoholic Hepatitis	7	M	1.3120	6.40	4.80
203	Malignancy of Hepatobiliary System or Pancreas	7	M	1.3482	6.70	5.00
204	Disorders of Pancreas Except Malignancy	7	M	1.1675	5.80	4.40
205	Disorders of Liver Except Malignancy, Cirrhosis and Alcoholic Hepatitis with CC	7	M	1.2095	6.20	4.60
206	Disorders of Liver Except Malignancy, Cirrhosis and Alcoholic Hepatitis without CC	7	M	0.7071	3.80	2.90
207	Disorders of the Biliary Tract with CC	7	M	1.1539	5.30	4.00
208	Disorders of the Biliary Tract without CC	7	M	0.6601	2.90	2.30
209	Major Joint and Limb Reattachment Procedures of Lower Extremity	8	S	2.0327	4.90	4.40
210	Hip and Femur Procedures Except Major Joint Procedures, Age Greater than 17 with CC	8	S	1.8477	7.00	6.10
211	Hip and Femur Procedures Except Major Joint Procedures, Age Greater than 17 without CC	8	S	1.2544	4.90	4.50
212	Hip and Femur Procedures Except Major Joint Procedures, Age 0-17	8	S	1.4152	6.40	3.20
213	Amputation for Musculoskeletal System and Connective Tissue Disorders	8	S	1.8904	9.20	6.70
214	No Longer Valid	8		0.0000	0.00	0.00
215	No Longer Valid	8		0.0000	0.00	0.00
216	Biopsies of Musculoskeletal System and Connective Tissue	8	S	2.1107	8.00	5.00

DRG	Title	MDC	Med/Surg	RW	AMLOS	GMLOS
217	Wound Debridement and Skin Graft Except Hand for Musculoskeletal and Connective Tissue Disorders	8	S	3.0020	13.40	9.00
218	Lower Extremity and Humerus Procedures Except Hip, Foot and Femur, Age Greater than 17 with CC	8	S	1.5750	5.50	4.30
219	Lower Extremity and Humerus Procedures Except Hip, Foot and Femur, Age Greater than 17 without CC	8	S	1.0258	3.20	2.70
220	Lower Extremity and Humerus Procedures Except Hip, Foot and Femur, Age 0-17	8	S	0.5881	5.30	5.30
221	No Longer Valid	8		0.0000	0.00	0.00
222	No Longer Valid	8		0.0000	0.00	0.00
223	Major Shoulder/Elbow Procedures or Other Upper Extremity Procedures with CC	8	S	1.0573	3.00	2.20
224	Shoulder, Elbow or Forearm Procedures Except Major Joint Procedures without CC	8	S	0.7898	1.90	1.60
225	Foot Procedures	8	S	1.1704	5.30	3.60
226	Soft Tissue Procedures with CC	8	S	1.5529	6.60	4.50
227	Soft Tissue Procedures without CC	8	S	0.8190	2.60	2.10
228	Major Thumb or Joint Procedures or Other Hand or Wrist Procedures with CC	8	S	1.1639	4.20	2.70
229	Hand or Wrist Procedures Except Major Joint Procedures without CC	8	S	0.7064	2.30	1.80
230	Local Excision and Removal of Internal Fixation Devices of Hip and Femur	8	S	1.3147	5.60	3.60
232	Arthroscopy	8	S	0.0000	0.00	0.00
233	Other Musculoskeletal System and Connective Tissue O.R. Procedures with CC	8	S	0.9674	2.70	1.80
234	Other Musculoskeletal System and Connective Tissue O.R. Procedures without CC	8	S	2.0024	7.40	5.00
235	Fractures of Femur	8	M	1.1977	3.10	2.20
236	Fractures of Hip and Pelvis	8	M	0.7580	4.90	3.80
237	Sprains, Strains and Dislocations of Hip, Pelvis and Thigh	8	M	0.7358	4.80	3.90
238	Osteomyelitis	8	M	0.5983	3.70	2.90
239	Pathological Fractures and Musculoskeletal and Connective Tissue Malignancy	8	M	1.3564	8.70	6.50
240	Connective Tissue Disorders with CC	8	M	1.0614	6.40	5.10
241	Connective Tissue Disorders without CC	8	M	1.3153	6.70	4.90
242	Septic Arthritis	8	M	0.6358	3.80	3.00

DRG	Title	MDC	Med/Surg	RW	AMLOS	GMLOS
243	Medical Back Problems	8	M	0.7525	4.70	3.70
244	Bone Diseases and Specific Arthropathies with CC	8	M	0.7155	4.70	3.70
245	Bone Diseases and Specific Arthropathies without CC	8	M	0.4786	3.30	2.60
246	Nonspecific Arthropathies	8	M	0.6063	3.80	3.00
247	Signs and Symptoms of Musculoskeletal System and Connective Tissue	8	M	0.5724	3.30	2.60
248	Tendonitis, Myositis and Bursitis	8	M	0.8585	4.90	3.80
249	Aftercare, Musculoskeletal System and Connective Tissue	8	M	0.6744	3.60	2.50
250	Fractures, Sprains, Strains and Dislocations of Forearm, Hand and Foot, Age Greater than 17 with CC	8	M	0.7091	4.10	3.20
251	Fractures, Sprains, Strains and Dislocations of Forearm, Hand and Foot, Age Greater than 17 without CC	8	M	0.4578	2.80	2.30
252	Fractures, Sprains, Strains and Dislocations of Forearm, Hand and Foot, Age 0-17	8	M	0.2553	1.80	1.80
253	Fractures, Sprains, Strains and Dislocations of Upper Arm and Lower Leg Except Foot, Age Greater than 17 with CC	8	M	0.7581	4.70	3.70
254	Fractures, Sprains, Strains and Dislocations of Upper Arm and Lower Leg Except Foot, Age Greater than 17 without CC	8	M	0.4464	3.20	2.60
255	Fractures, Sprains, Strains and Dislocations of Upper Arm and Lower Leg Except Foot, Age 0-17	8	M	0.2974	2.90	2.90
256	Other Musculoskeletal System and Connective Tissue Diagnoses	8	M	0.8190	5.10	3.80
257	Total Mastectomy for Malignancy with CC	9	S	0.8913	2.60	2.10
258	Total Mastectomy for Malignancy without CC	9	S	0.7018	1.80	1.60
259	Subtotal Mastectomy for Malignancy with CC	9	S	0.9420	2.70	1.80
260	Subtotal Mastectomy for Malignancy without CC	9	S	0.6854	1.40	1.20
261	Breast Procedure for Nonmalignancy Except Biopsy and Local Excision	9	S	0.8944	2.10	1.60
262	Breast Biopsy and Local Excision for Nonmalignancy	9	S	0.9533	4.30	2.90
263	Skin Graft and/or Debridement for Skin Ulcer or Cellulitis with CC	9	S	2.0556	11.50	8.30
264	Skin Graft and/or Debridement for Skin Ulcer or Cellulitis without CC	9	S	1.0605	6.60	5.00

DRG	Title	MDC	Med/Surg	RW	AMLOS	GMLOS
265	Skin Graft and/or Debridement Except for Skin Ulcer or Cellulitis with CC	9	S	1.5984	6.60	4.20
266	Skin Graft and/or Debridement Except for Skin Ulcer or Cellulitis without CC	9	S	0.8791	3.20	2.30
267	Perianal and Pilonidal Procedures	9	S	0.9574	4.50	2.90
268	Skin, Subcutaneous Tissue and Breast Plastic Procedures	9	S	1.1513	3.80	2.40
269	Other Skin, Subcutaneous Tissue and Breast Procedures with CC	9	S	1.7747	8.50	6.00
270	Other Skin, Subcutaneous Tissue and Breast Procedures without CC	9	S	0.8129	3.60	2.50
271	Skin Ulcers	9	M	1.0280	7.20	5.60
272	Major Skin Disorders with CC	9	M	1.0185	6.00	4.60
273	Major Skin Disorders without CC	9	M	0.6192	3.90	3.00
274	Malignant Breast Disorders with CC	9	M	1.1574	6.50	4.70
275	Malignant Breast Disorders without CC	9	M	0.5729	3.40	2.40
276	Nonmalignant Breast Disorders	9	M	0.6471	4.50	3.50
277	Cellulitis, Age Greater than 17 with CC	9	M	0.8805	5.80	4.70
278	Cellulitis, Age Greater than 17 without CC	9	M	0.5432	4.20	3.50
279	Cellulitis, Age 0-17	9	M	0.7779	5.30	4.00
280	Trauma to Skin, Subcutaneous Tissue and Breast, Age Greater than 17 with CC	9	M	0.7109	4.10	3.20
281	Trauma to Skin, Subcutaneous Tissue and Breast, Age Greater than 17 without CC	9	M	0.4866	2.90	2.30
282	Trauma to Skin, Subcutaneous Tissue and Breast, Age 0-17	9	M	0.2586	2.20	2.20
283	Minor Skin Disorders with CC	9	M	0.7322	4.70	3.50
284	Minor Skin Disorders without CC	9	M	0.4215	2.90	2.30
285	Amputation of Lower Limb for Endocrine, Nutritional and Metabolic Disorders	10	S	2.0825	10.60	7.90
286	Adrenal and Pituitary Procedures	10	S	2.0342	5.90	4.40
287	Skin Grafts and Wound Debridement for Endocrine, Nutritional and Metabolic Disorders	10	S	1.8899	10.30	7.70
288	O.R. Procedures for Obesity	10	S	2.1498	5.00	3.90
289	Parathyroid Procedures	10	S	0.9441	2.70	1.80
290	Thyroid Procedures	10	S	0.8938	2.20	1.70
291	Thyroglossal Procedures	10	S	0.6468	1.60	1.40
292	Other Endocrine, Nutritional and Metabolic O.R. Procedures with CC	10	S	2.7336	10.60	7.30
293	Other Endocrine, Nutritional and Metabolic O.R. Procedures without CC	10	S	1.3896	4.70	3.20
294	Diabetes, Age Greater than 35	10	M	0.7800	4.60	3.50
295	Diabetes, Age 0-35	10	M	0.7975	4.00	3.00

DRG	Title	MDC	Med/Surg	RW	AMLOS	GMLOS
296	Nutritional and Miscellaneous Metabolic Disorders, Age Greater than 17 with CC	10	M	0.8639	5.10	4.00
297	Nutritional and Miscellaneous Metabolic Disorders, Age Greater than 17 without CC	10	M	0.5085	3.30	2.70
298	Nutritional and Miscellaneous Metabolic Disorders, Age 0-17	10	M	0.4537	3.10	2.40
299	Inborn Errors of Metabolism	10	M	0.9466	5.50	3.80
300	Endocrine Disorders with CC	10	M	1.1001	6.20	4.70
301	Endocrine Disorders without CC	10	M	0.6158	3.60	2.80
302	Kidney Transplant	11	S	3.2343	8.50	7.20
303	Kidney, Ureter and Major Bladder Procedures for Neoplasm	11	S	2.3659	8.00	6.40
304	Kidney, Ureter and Major Bladder Procedures for Non-neoplasms with CC	11	S	2.3856	8.90	6.20
305	Kidney, Ureter and Major Bladder Procedures for Non-neoplasms without CC	11	S	1.1854	3.60	2.80
306	Prostatectomy with CC	11	S	1.2257	5.40	3.50
307	Prostatectomy without CC	11	S	0.6145	2.10	1.70
308	Minor Bladder Procedures with CC	11	S	1.5993	6.20	4.00
309	Minor Bladder Procedures without CC	11	S	0.8991	2.10	1.70
310	Transurethral Procedures with CC	11	S	1.1502	4.40	2.90
311	Transurethral Procedures without CC	11	S	0.6258	1.80	1.50
312	Urethral Procedures, Age Greater than 17 with CC	11	S	1.0841	4.50	3.00
313	Urethral Procedures, Age Greater than 17 without CC	11	S	0.6814	2.20	1.70
314	Urethral Procedures, Age 0-17	11	S	0.4984	2.30	2.30
315	Other Kidney and Urinary Tract OR Procedures	11	S	2.0796	7.00	3.70
316	Renal Failure	11	M	1.2987	6.60	4.90
317	Admission for Renal Dialysis	11	M	0.8503	3.60	2.40
318	Kidney and Urinary Tract Neoplasms with CC	11	M	1.1871	6.10	4.40
319	Kidney and Urinary Tract Neoplasms without CC	11	M	0.6771	2.90	2.20
320	Kidney and Urinary Tract Infections, Age Greater than 17 with CC	11	M	0.8853	5.40	4.30
321	Kidney and Urinary Tract Infections, Age Greater than 17 without CC	11	M	0.5685	3.70	3.10
322	Kidney and Urinary Tract Infections, Age 0-17	11	M	0.4625	3.30	2.80
323	Urinary Stones with CC and/or ESW Lithotripsy	11	M	0.8088	3.20	2.40
324	Urinary Stones without CC	11	M	0.4797	1.90	1.60

DRG	Title	MDC	Med/Surg	RW	AMLOS	GMLOS
325	Kidney and Urinary Tract Signs and Symptoms, Age Greater than 17 with CC	11	M	0.6553	3.80	2.90
326	Kidney and Urinary Tract Signs and Symptoms, Age Greater than 17 without CC	11	M	0.4206	2.60	2.10
327	Kidney and Urinary Tract Signs and Symptoms, Age 0-17	11	M	0.3727	3.10	3.10
328	Urethral Stricture, Age Greater than 17 with CC	11	M	0.7613	3.80	2.70
329	Urethral Stricture, Age Greater than 17 without CC	11	M	0.5296	2.10	1.70
330	Urethral Stricture, Age 0-17	11	M	0.3210	1.60	1.60
331	Other Kidney and Urinary Tract Diagnoses, Age Greater than 17 with CC	11	M	1.0618	5.60	4.20
332	Other Kidney and Urinary Tract Diagnoses, Age Greater than 17 without CC	11	M	0.5982	3.20	2.40
333	Other Kidney and Urinary Tract Diagnoses, Age 0-17	11	M	0.9483	5.70	3.70
334	Major Male Pelvic Procedures with CC	12	S	1.4810	4.60	3.90
335	Major Male Pelvic Procedures without CC	12	S	1.0835	3.00	2.80
336	Transurethral Prostatectomy with CC	12	S	0.8595	3.40	2.60
337	Transurethral Prostatectomy without CC	12	S	0.5869	2.00	1.80
338	Testes Procedures for Malignancy	12	S	1.2316	5.50	3.50
339	Testes Procedures for Nonmalignancy, Age Greater than 17	12	S	1.1345	4.80	2.90
340	Testes Procedures for Nonmalignancy, Age 0-17	12	S	0.2853	2.40	2.40
341	Penis Procedures	12	S	1.2739	3.20	1.90
342	Circumcision, Age Greater than 17	12	S	0.7800	3.20	2.40
343	Circumcision, Age 0-17	12	S	0.1551	1.70	1.70
344	Other Male Reproductive System O.R. Procedures for Malignancy	12	S	1.3306	2.50	1.60
345	Other Male Reproductive System O.R. Procedures Except for Malignancy	12	S	1.1671	4.90	3.00
346	Malignancy of Male Reproductive System with CC	12	M	1.0213	5.90	4.50
347	Malignancy of Male Reproductive System without CC	12	M	0.5417	3.00	2.20
348	Benign Prostatic Hypertrophy with CC	12	M	0.7472	4.40	3.30
349	Benign Prostatic Hypertrophy without CC	12	M	0.4608	2.50	2.00
350	Inflammation of the Male Reproductive System	12	M	0.7370	4.50	3.60

DRG	Title	MDC	Med/Surg	RW	AMLOS	GMLOS
351	Sterilization, Male	12	M	0.2379	1.30	1.30
352	Other Male Reproductive System Diagnoses	12	M	0.7097	4.00	2.90
353	Pelvic Evisceration, Radical Hysterectomy and Radical Vulvectomy	13	S	1.8390	6.50	4.90
354	Uterine and Adnexa Procedures for Nonovarian/Adnexal Malignancy with CC	13	S	1.4808	5.70	4.70
355	Uterine and Adnexa Procedures for Nonovarian/Adnexal Malignancy without CC	13	S	0.8912	3.20	3.00
356	Female Reproductive System Reconstructive Procedures	13	S	0.7556	2.10	1.80
357	Uterine and Adnexa Procedures for Ovarian or Adnexal Malignancy	13	S	2.2737	8.40	6.70
358	Uterine and Adnexa Procedures for Nonmalignancy with CC	13	S	1.1807	4.20	3.40
359	Uterine and Adnexa Procedures for Nonmalignancy without CC	13	S	0.8099	2.60	2.30
360	Vagina, Cervix and Vulva Procedures	13	S	0.8661	2.80	2.20
361	Laparoscopy and Incisional Tubal Interruption	13	S	1.0793	3.20	2.20
362	Endoscopic Tubal Interruption	13	S	0.3041	1.40	1.40
363	D and C, Conization and Radio-Implant for Malignancy	13	S	0.9374	3.60	2.60
364	D and C, Conization Except for Malignancy	13	S	0.9098	4.10	2.90
365	Other Female Reproductive System OR Procedures	13	S	2.1284	8.20	5.30
366	Malignancy of Female Reproductive System with CC	13	M	1.2826	6.80	4.80
367	Malignancy of Female Reproductive System without CC	13	M	0.5588	3.10	2.30
368	Infections of Female Reproductive System	13	M	1.1657	6.70	5.10
369	Menstrual and Other Female Reproductive System Disorders	13	M	0.6065	3.30	2.40
370	Cesarean Section with CC	14	S	1.0119	5.70	4.20
371	Cesarean Section without CC	14	S	0.6317	3.50	3.20
372	Vaginal Delivery with Complicating Diagnoses	14	M	0.5520	3.50	2.70
373	Vaginal Delivery without Complicating Diagnoses	14	M	0.3856	2.30	2.00
374	Vaginal Delivery with Sterilization and/or D and C	14	S	0.7402	3.00	2.50
375	Vaginal Delivery with OR Procedure Except Sterilization and/or D and C	14	S	0.5806	4.40	4.40
376	Postpartum and Postabortion Diagnoses without OR Procedure	14	M	0.5693	3.40	2.50

DRG	Title	MDC	Med/Surg	RW	AMLOS	GMLOS
377	Postpartum and Postabortion Diagnoses with O.R. Procedure	14	S	1.0321	4.10	3.10
378	Ectopic Pregnancy	14	M	0.7950	2.60	2.00
379	Threatened Abortion	14	M	0.3626	3.00	2.00
380	Abortion without D and C	14	M	0.4323	2.00	1.60
381	Abortion with D and C, Aspiration Curettage or Hysterotomy	14	S	0.5257	1.90	1.50
382	False Labor	14	M	0.2190	1.70	1.30
383	Other Antepartum Diagnoses with Medical Complications	14	M	0.5123	3.80	2.70
384	Other Antepartum Diagnoses without Medical Complications	14	M	0.3485	2.60	1.90
385	Neonates, Died or Transferred to Another Acute Care Facility	15	M	1.3855	1.80	1.80
386	Extreme Immaturity or Respiratory Distress Syndrome of Neonate	15	M	4.5687	17.90	17.90
387	Prematurity with Major Problems	15	M	3.1203	13.30	13.30
388	Prematurity without Major Problems	15	M	1.8827	8.60	8.60
389	Full Term Neonate with Major Problems	15	M	3.2052	4.70	4.70
390	Neonate with Other Significant Problems	15	M	1.1344	3.40	3.40
391	Normal Newborn	15	M	0.1536	3.10	3.10
392	Splenectomy, Age Greater than 17	16	S	3.3164	9.70	7.10
393	Splenectomy, Age 0-17	16	S	1.3571	9.10	9.10
394	Other O.R. Procedures of the Blood and Blood-Forming Organs	16	S	1.9338	7.60	4.70
395	Red Blood Cell Disorders, Age Greater than 17	16	M	0.8307	4.40	3.20
396	Red Blood Cell Disorders, Age 0-17	16	M	0.6986	4.20	2.90
397	Coagulation Disorders	16	M	1.2648	5.20	3.70
398	Reticuloendothelial and Immunity Disorders with CC	16	M	1.2360	5.90	4.50
399	Reticuloendothelial and Immunity Disorders without CC	16	M	0.6651	3.50	2.70
401	Lymphoma and Nonacute Leukemia with Other O.R. Procedure with CC	17	S	0.0000	0.00	0.00
402	Lymphoma and Nonacute Leukemia with Other O.R. Procedure without CC	17	S	2.8946	11.60	8.10
403	Lymphoma and Nonacute Leukemia with CC	17	M	1.1430	4.00	2.70
404	Lymphoma and Nonacute Leukemia without CC	17	M	1.8197	8.20	5.80
405	Acute Leukemia without Major O.R. Procedure, Age 0-17	17	M	0.8658	4.10	3.00
406	Myeloproliferative Disorders or Poorly Differentiated Neoplasms with Major O.R. Procedures with CC	17	S	1.9241	4.90	4.90

DRG	Title	MDC	Med/Surg	RW	AMLOS	GMLOS
407	Myeloproliferative Disorders or Poorly Differentiated Neoplasms with Major O.R. Procedures without CC	17	S	1.2410	4.10	3.20
408	Myeloproliferative Disorders or Poorly Differentiated Neoplasms with Other O.R. Procedures	17	S	2.1984	8.20	4.80
409	Radiotherapy	17	M	1.2439	6.10	4.60
410	Chemotherapy without Acute Leukemia as Secondary Diagnosis	17	M	1.0833	4.10	3.20
411	History of Malignancy without Endoscopy	17	M	0.3948	4.70	4.70
412	History of Malignancy with Endoscopy	17	M	0.5679	3.60	2.50
413	Other Myeloproliferative Disorders or Poorly Differentiated Neoplasm Diagnoses with CC	17	M	1.3224	7.10	5.20
414	Other Myeloproliferative Disorders or Poorly Differentiated Neoplasm Diagnoses without CC	17	M	0.7370	4.20	3.20
415	O.R. Procedure for Infectious and Parasitic Diseases	18	S	3.6276	14.40	10.40
416	Septicemia, Age Greater than 17	18	M	1.5918	7.50	5.60
417	Septicemia, Age 0-17	18	M	0.9612	5.70	4.40
418	Postoperative and Posttraumatic Infections	18	M	1.0672	6.30	4.80
419	Fever of Unknown Origin, Age Greater than 17 with CC	18	M	0.8476	4.60	3.60
420	Fever of Unknown Origin, Age Greater than 17 without CC	18	M	0.6107	3.40	2.80
421	Viral Illness, Age Greater than 17	18	M	0.7464	4.10	3.10
422	Viral Illness and Fever of Unknown Origin, Age 0-17	18	M	0.7248	3.70	2.50
423	Other Infectious and Parasitic Diseases Diagnoses	18	M	1.8155	8.40	5.90
424	O.R. Procedure with Principal Diagnosis of Mental Illness	19	S	2.4074	13.10	8.00
425	Acute Adjustment Reactions and Psychosocial Dysfunction	19	M	0.6781	3.80	2.80
426	Depressive Neuroses	19	M	0.5087	4.50	3.20
427	Neuroses Except Depressive	19	M	0.5012	4.40	3.10
428	Disorders of Personality and Impulse Control	19	M	0.7291	7.10	4.50
429	Organic Disturbances and Mental Retardation	19	M	0.8291	6.10	4.50
430	Psychoses	19	M	0.6801	7.90	5.60
431	Childhood Mental Disorders	19	M	0.6620	6.90	4.40
432	Other Mental Disorder Diagnoses	19	M	0.6513	4.00	2.90
433	Alcohol/Drug Abuse or Dependence, Left Against Medical Advice	20	M	0.2904	3.10	2.20

DRG	Title	MDC	Med/Surg	RW	AMLOS	GMLOS
434	No Longer Valid	20		0.0000	0.00	0.00
435	No Longer Valid	20		0.0000	0.00	0.00
436	No Longer Valid	20		0.0000	0.00	0.00
437	No Longer Valid	20		0.0000	0.00	0.00
438	No Longer Valid	20		0.0000	0.00	0.00
439	Skin Grafts for Injuries	21	S	1.7547	8.20	5.20
440	Wound Debridements for Injuries	21	S	1.8878	9.10	5.80
441	Hand Procedures for Injuries	21	S	0.9662	3.10	2.10
442	Other O.R. Procedures for Injuries with CC	21	S	2.4200	8.60	5.60
443	Other O.R. Procedures for Injuries without CC	21	S	0.9787	3.40	2.50
444	Traumatic Injury, Age Greater than 17 with CC	21	M	0.7475	4.20	3.20
445	Traumatic Injury, Age Greater than 17 without CC	21	M	0.5015	2.90	2.30
446	Traumatic Injury, Age 0-17	21	M	0.2983	2.40	2.40
447	Allergic Reactions, Age Greater than 17	21	M	0.5238	2.50	1.90
448	Allergic Reactions, Age 0-17	21	M	0.0981	2.90	2.90
449	Poisoning and Toxic Effects of Drugs, Age Greater than 17 with CC	21	M	0.8352	3.70	2.60
450	Poisoning and Toxic Effects of Drugs, Age Greater than 17 without CC	21	M	0.4246	2.00	1.60
451	Poisoning and Toxic Effects of Drugs, Age 0-17	21	M	0.2648	2.10	2.10
452	Complications of Treatment with CC	21	M	1.0455	4.90	3.50
453	Complications of Treatment without CC	21	M	0.5113	2.80	2.10
454	Other Injury, Poisoning and Toxic Effect Diagnoses with CC	21	M	0.8153	4.20	3.00
455	Other Injury, Poisoning and Toxic Effect Diagnoses without CC	21	M	0.4773	2.40	1.80
456	No Longer Valid	22		0.0000	0.00	0.00
457	No Longer Valid	22		0.0000	0.00	0.00
458	No Longer Valid	22		0.0000	0.00	0.00
459	No Longer Valid	22		0.0000	0.00	0.00
460	No Longer Valid	22		0.0000	0.00	0.00
461	OR Procedure with Diagnosis of Other Contact with Health Services	23	S	1.1692	3.60	2.20
462	Rehabilitation	23	M	0.9747	11.00	9.00
463	Signs and Symptoms with CC	23	M	0.6856	4.10	3.10
464	Signs and Symptoms without CC	23	M	0.4982	3.00	2.40
465	Aftercare with History of Malignancy as Secondary Diagnosis	23	M	0.8881	3.90	2.00
466	Aftercare without History of Malignancy as Secondary Diagnosis	23	M	0.8088	3.90	2.20
467	Other Factors Influencing Health Status	23	M	0.5274	3.70	1.90

DRG	Title	MDC	Med/Surg	RW	AMLOS	GMLOS
468	Extensive O.R. Procedure Unrelated to Principal Diagnosis	ALL	S	3.8454	13.10	9.40
469	Principal Diagnosis Invalid as Discharge Diagnosis	14	M	0.0000	0.00	0.00
470	Ungroupable	15	M	0.0000	0.00	0.00
471	Bilateral or Multiple Major Joint Procedures of Lower Extremity	8	S	3.0576	5.40	4.70
472	No Longer Valid	22		0.0000	0.00	0.00
473	Acute Leukemia without Major OR Procedure, Age Greater than 17	17	M	3.4885	12.70	7.40
474	No Longer Valid	4		0.0000	0.00	0.00
475	Respiratory System Diagnosis with Ventilator Support	4	M	3.6000	11.30	8.00
476	Prostatic O.R. Procedure Unrelated to Principal Diagnosis	ALL	S	2.2477	11.10	8.00
477	Nonextensive O.R. Procedure Unrelated to Principal Diagnosis	ALL	S	1.8873	8.30	5.40
478	Other Vascular Procedures with CC	5	S	2.3743	7.30	4.90
479	Other Vascular Procedures without CC	5	S	1.4300	3.20	2.40
480	Liver Transplant	PRE	S	9.7823	21.10	14.00
481	Bone Marrow Transplant	PRE	S	6.1074	21.80	19.20
482	Tracheostomy for Face, Mouth and Neck Diagnoses	PRE	S	3.4803	12.50	9.60
483	Tracheostomy with Mechanical Ventilation 96+ Hours or Principal Diagnosis Except Face, Mouth, and Neck	PRE	S	16.7762	41.60	34.20
484	Craniotomy for Multiple Significant Trauma	24	S	5.4179	14.50	9.70
485	Limb Reattachment, Hip and Femur Procedures for Multiple Significant Trauma	24	S	3.2121	10.00	7.90
486	Other O.R. Procedures for Multiple Significant Trauma	24	S	4.8793	12.90	8.70
487	Other Multiple Significant Trauma	24	M	2.0057	7.30	5.30
488	HIV with Extensive O.R. Procedure	25	S	4.8118	17.00	11.70
489	HIV with Major Related Condition	25	M	1.8603	8.60	6.00
490	HIV with or without Other Related Condition	25	M	1.0512	5.50	3.90
491	Major Joint and Limb Reattachment Procedures of Upper Extremity	8	S	1.7139	3.40	2.80
492	Chemotherapy With Acute Leukemia or With Use of a High-Dose Chemotherapy agent	17	M	3.8371	14.90	9.30
493	Laparoscopic Cholecystectomy without Common Duct Exploration with CC	7	S	1.8302	6.00	4.40
494	Laparoscopic Cholecystectomy without Common Duct Exploration without CC	7	S	1.0034	2.50	2.00

DRG	Title	MDC	Med/Surg	RW	AMLOS	GMLOS
495	Lung Transplant	PRE	S	8.5551	16.20	13.40
496	Combined Anterior/Posterior Spinal Fusion	8	S	5.6839	8.90	6.80
497	Spinal Fusion Except Cervical with CC	8	S	3.4056	6.30	5.20
498	Spinal Fusion Except Cervical without CC	8	S	2.5319	4.00	3.60
499	Back and Neck Procedures Except Spinal Fusion with CC	8	S	1.4244	4.50	3.30
500	Back and Neck Procedures Except Spinal Fusion without CC	8	S	0.9369	2.40	2.00
501	Knee Procedures with Principal Diagnosis of Infection with CC	8	S	2.6393	10.70	8.30
502	Knee Procedures with Principal Diagnosis of Infection without CC	8	S	1.4192	6.20	5.10
503	Knee Procedures without Principal Diagnosis of Infection	8	S	1.2233	3.90	3.00
504	Extensive Third Degree Burn with Skin Graft	22	S	11.6215	28.00	20.30
505	Extensive Third Degree Burn without Skin Graft	22	M	2.0006	5.60	2.30
506	Full Thickness Burn with Skin Graft or Inhalation Injury with CC or Significant Trauma	22	S	4.1070	16.90	12.10
507	Full Thickness Burn with Skin Graft or Inhalation Injury without CC or Significant Trauma	22	S	1.8154	9.20	6.50
508	Full Thickness Burn without Skin Graft or Inhalation Injury with CC or Significant Trauma	22	M	1.3775	8.00	5.60
509	Full Thickness Burn without Skin Graft or Inhalation Injury without CC or Significant Trauma	22	M	0.6426	4.40	3.10
510	Nonextensive Burns with CC or Significant Trauma	22	M	1.1812	6.80	4.60
511	Nonextensive Burns without CC or Significant Trauma	22	M	0.6753	4.70	3.20
512	Simultaneous Pancreas/Kidney Transplant	PRE	S	5.3405	13.20	11.10
513	Pancreas Transplant	PRE	S	6.1594	10.00	8.70
515	Cardiac Defibrillator Implant without Cardiac Catheterization	5	S	0.0000	0.00	0.00
516	Percutaneous Cardiovascular Procedures with Acute Myocardial Infarction	5	S	5.3366	5.20	3.00
517	Percutaneous Cardiovascular Procedures without Acute Myocardial Infarction, with Coronary Artery Stent Implant	5	S	2.6911	4.80	3.80

DRG	Title	MDC	Med/Surg	RW	AMLOS	GMLOS
518	Percutaneous Cardiovascular Procedures without Acute Myocardial Infarction without Coronary Artery Stent Implant	5	S	1.7494	3.40	2.30
519	Cervical Spinal Fusion with CC	8	S	2.4266	5.10	3.20
520	Cervical Spinal Fusion without CC	8	S	1.5780	2.10	1.70
521	Alcohol/Drug Abuse or Dependence with CC	20	M	0.7115	5.80	4.30
522	Alcohol/Drug Abuse or Dependence with Rehabilitation Therapy without CC	20	M	0.5226	9.70	7.70
523	Alcohol/Drug Abuse or Dependence without Rehabilitation Therapy without CC	20	M	0.3956	4.10	3.30
524	Transient Ischemia	1	M	0.7320	3.40	2.70
525	Heart Assist System Implant	5	S	11.4372	17.00	8.90
526	Percutaneous Cardiovascular Procedure with Drug-eluting Stent with AMI	5	S	2.9891	4.50	3.60
527	Percutaneous Cardiovascular Procedure with Drug-eluting Stent without AMI	5	S	2.4483	2.50	1.80
528	Intracranial Vascular Procedure with a Principal Diagnosis of Hemorrhage	1	S	7.2205	17.50	14.20
529	Ventricular Shunt Procedures with CC	1	S	2.2529	8.20	5.30
530	Ventricular Shunt Procedures without CC	1	S	1.2017	3.60	2.80
531	Spinal Procedures with CC	1	S	3.0552	9.90	6.80
532	Spinal Procedures without CC	1	S	1.4482	4.00	2.90
533	Extracranial Procedures with CC	1	S	1.6678	4.10	2.70
534	Extracranial Procedures without CC	1	S	1.0748	2.00	1.60
535	Cardiac Defibrillator Implant with Cardiac Catheterization with Acute Myocardial Infarction, Heart Failure, or Shock	5	S	8.1560	11.00	8.10
536	Cardiac Defibrillator Implant with Cardiac Catheterization without Acute Myocardial Infarction, Heart Failure, or Shock	5	S	6.2775	5.80	3.90
537	Local Excision and Removal of Internal Fixation Devices Except Hip and Femur with CC	8	S	1.8185	7.00	4.70
538	Local Excision and Removal of Internal Fixation Devices Except Hip and Femur without CC	8	S	0.9919	2.90	2.10
539	Lymphoma and Leukemia with Major O.R. Procedure with CC	17	S	3.3846	11.20	7.40
540	Lymphoma and Leukemia with Major O.R. Procedure without CC	17	S	1.2891	4.00	2.90

Glossary

against medical advice. The discharge status of patients who leave the hospital after signing a form that releases the hospital from responsibility, or who leave the hospital premises without notifying hospital personnel.

arithmetic mean length of stay (AMLOS). The average number of days patients within a given DRG stay in the hospital, also referred to as the average length of stay. The AMLOS is used to determine payment for outlier cases.

audit. An examination or review that establishes the extent to which performance or a process conforms to predetermined standards or criteria.

average resources. Refers to the relative volume and types of diagnostic, therapeutic, and bed services used in the management of a particular illness.

base rate. A number assigned to a hospital used to calculate DRG reimbursement. Base rates vary from hospital to hospital. The base rate adjusts reimbursement to allow for such individual characteristics of the hospital as geographic location, status (urban/rural, teaching), and local labor costs.

case mix index (CMI). The sum of all DRG relative weights, divided by the number of Medicare cases. A low CMI may denote DRG assignments that do not adequately reflect the resources used to treat Medicare patients.

CC. Complication or comorbid condition.

charges. The dollar amount of hospital bills.

comorbidity. Pre-existing condition that, because of its presence with a specific diagnosis, causes an increase in length of stay by at least one day in approximately 75 percent of the cases.

complication. A condition that arises during the hospital stay that prolongs the length of stay by at least one day in approximately 75 percent of the cases.

diagnosis-related group (DRG). One of the 527 (510 valid) classifications of diagnoses in which patients demonstrate similar resource consumption and length-of-stay patterns.

discharge. A situation in which the patient leaves an acute care (prospective payment) hospital after receiving complete acute care treatment.

discharge status. Disposition of the patient at discharge (for example: left against medical advice, discharged home, transferred to an acute care hospital, expired).

coding specificity. Refers to assigning codes to the highest level of specificity by assigning a three-digit disease code only when there are no four-digit codes within that category, assigning a four-digit code only when there is no fifth-digit subclassification within that category, or assigning a fifth-digit for any category for which a fifth-digit subclassification is provided.

complex diagnoses. Specific diagnoses that affect DRG 124, Circulatory Disorders (except acute myocardial infarction) with Cardiac Catheterization.

durable medical equipment (DME). Medical equipment that can withstand repeated use, is not disposable, is used to serve a medical purpose, is generally not useful to a person in the absence of a sickness or injury, and is appropriate for use in the home. Examples of durable medical equipment include hospital beds, wheelchairs, and oxygen equipment.

False Claims Act. Governs civil actions for filing false claims. Liability under this act pertains to any person who knowingly presents or causes to be presented a false or fraudulent claim to the government for payment or approval.

geometric mean length of stay (GMLOS). Used to compute reimbursement, the GMLOS is a statistically adjusted value for all cases for a given DRG, allowing for the outliers, transfer cases, and negative outlier cases that would normally skew the data. The GMLOS is used to determine payment only for transfer cases (i.e., the per diem rate).

grouper. The software program that assigns DRGs.

homogeneous. Adjective describing patients consuming similar types and amounts of hospital resources.

major diagnostic category (MDC). Broad classification of diagnoses typically grouped by body system.

medical necessity. Generally, the evaluation of health care services to determine if they are medically appropriate and necessary to meet basic health needs; consistent with the diagnosis or condition and rendered in a cost-effective manner; and consistent with national medical practice guidelines regarding type, frequency, and duration of treatment.

noninvasive diagnostic test. Denotes a procedure that does not require insertion of an instrument or device through the skin or body orifice for diagnosis.

nonoperating room procedure. A procedure that does not normally require the use of the operating room and that can affect DRG assignment.

operating room (OR) procedure. A procedure that falls into a defined group of procedures that normally requires the use of an operating room.

Office of Inspector General (OIG). The OIG is an agency within the Department of Health and Human Services that is ultimately responsible for investigating instances of fraud and abuse in the Medicare and Medicaid programs.

other diagnosis (*see also* comorbidity and complication). All conditions (secondary) that exist at the time of admission or that develop subsequently that affect the treatment received and/or the length of stay. Diagnoses that relate to an earlier episode and that have no bearing on the current hospital stay are not to be reported.

outliers. There are two types of outliers: day outliers and cost outliers. Payment for day outliers was eliminated with discharges occurring on or after October 1, 1997. A cost outlier is a case in which the costs for treating the patient are extraordinarily high in relation to the costs for other patients in the DRG. An increase in cost outlier payments will compensate for the elimination of day outlier payments. For cost outliers, CMS allows a fixed loss threshold equal to the DRG payment plus $31,000 (FY 2004) with a marginal cost factor at 80 percent. The cost outlier must be requested either at the time bills are submitted for payment or within 60 days of receipt of the intermediary's initial determination.

per diem rate. Payment made to the hospital from which a patient is transferred for each day of stay. Per diem rate is determined by dividing the full DRG payment by the GMLOS for the DRG. The payment rate for the first day of stay is twice the per diem rate, and subsequent days are paid at the per diem rate up to the full DRG amount.

PMDC (Pre-MDC). There are eight DRGs to which cases are directly assigned based upon procedure codes. Cases are assigned to these DRGs before classification to an MDC. The PMDC includes DRGs for heart, liver, bone marrow, simultaneous pancreas/kidney transplant, pancreas transplant, lung transplant, and two DRGs for tracheostomies. These DRGs are listed in the section of this manual entitled "DRGs Associated with All MDCs and Pre-MDC."

principal diagnosis. The condition established after study to be chiefly responsible for occasioning the admission of the patient to the hospital for care.

principal procedure. A procedure performed for definitive treatment rather than diagnostic or exploratory purposes, or that was necessary to treat a complication. The principal procedure usually is related to the principal diagnosis.

relative weight (RW). An assigned weight that is intended to reflect the relative resource consumption associated with each DRG. The higher the relative weight, the greater the payment to the hospital. The relative weights are calculated by CMS and published in the final prospective payment system rule.

severity of illness. Refers to the relative levels of loss of function and mortality that may be experienced by patients with a particular disease.

surgical hierarchy. Surgical hierarchy is defined as an ordering of surgical cases from most to least resource intensive. Application of this decision rule is necessary in those cases when patient stays involve multiple surgical procedures, each of which, occurring by itself, could result in the assignment to a different DRG. All patients must be assigned to only one DRG per admission.

therapeutic treatment. The medical or surgical management of a patient.

transfer. A situation in which the patient is transferred to another acute care hospital for related care.

uniform hospital discharge data set (UHDDS). A minimum data set that acute-care, short-term hospitals are required to complete and report for Medicare and Medicaid discharges.

utilization review (UR). A formal assessment of the medical necessity, efficiency, and/or appropriateness of health care services and treatment plans on a prospective, concurrent, or retrospective basis.

volume. The total number of patients assigned each DRG.